Clinical Surgery in General
RCS Course Manual

JIM MAHON LIBRARY

For Churchill Livingstone

Commissioning Editor: Laurence Hunter
Project Editor: Janice Urquhart
Project Controller: Nancy Arnott
Design direction: Erik Bigland
Page Layout: Gerard Heyburn

Clinical Surgery in General

RCS Course Manual

Edited by

R. M. Kirk MS FRCS
Honorary Consulting Surgeon, Royal Free Hospital, London, UK

Averil O. Mansfield ChM FRCS
Professor of Surgery, St Mary's Hospital, Imperial College of Science, Technology and Medicine, London, UK

John P. S. Cochrane MS FRCS
Consultant Surgeon, Whittington Hospital, London, UK

THIRD EDITION

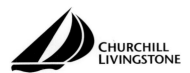
CHURCHILL
LIVINGSTONE

EDINBURGH LONDON NEW YORK PHILADELPHIA ST LOUIS SYDNEY TORONTO 1999

CHURCHILL LIVINGSTONE
An imprint of Harcourt Publishers Limited

© Royal College of Surgeons of England

 is a registered trade mark of Harcourt Publishers Limited

First edition 1993
Second edition 1996
Third edition 1999

ISBN 0 443 06219 6

British Library Cataloguing in Publication Data
A catalogue record for this book is available from the British
Library.

Library of Congress Cataloging in Publication Data
A catalog record for this book is available from the Library of
Congress.

Medical knowledge is constantly changing. As new information
becomes available, changes in treatment, procedures,
equipment and the use of drugs become necessary.
The editors, contributors and the publishers have, as far as it
is possible, taken care to ensure that the information given in
this text is accurate and up to date. However, readers are
strongly advised to confirm that the information, especially
with regard to drug usage, complies with current legislation
and standards of practice.

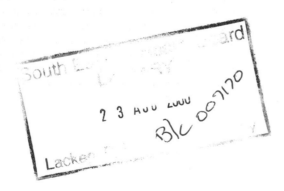

The
publisher's
policy is to use
**paper manufactured
from sustainable forests**

Printed in China
NPCC/01

Preface

A good surgeon knows how to operate
A better surgeon knows when to operate
The best surgeon knows when not to operate

Now that the new MRCS/AFRCS examinations have been fully introduced that assess trainees at the end of Basic Surgical Training, it is time to revise this book to cover the new curricula. Furthermore, those who are taking the specialist FRCS at the end of Higher Surgical Training, and who have not covered the curriculum of the modern basic assessment, will find that this book covers many topics that are relevant to the final examination.

Emergency management has been given pride of place, with concentration on the principles, rather than attempting to deal with the whole variety of problems encountered.

Although taking a history and examining a patient may seem rather elementary, failure to carry these out competently, are probably the commonest cause of misdiagnosis and examination failure. The overuse and misuse of investigations has stimulated the inclusion of chapters offering guidance on their use, followed by consideration of general assessment and preparation of patients who will require operation.

How do we attain 'best surgeon,' in the aphorism at the top of the page? The general public cannot understand why different surgeons offer varying treatments for a single condition. They see surgical problems in terms of black and white. We know that most surgical problems are various shades of grey – and that the particular shade of grey cannot always be universally agreed upon. In the chapters on 'Evidence based practice' and 'Decision making', are discussed the means that can be applied in some areas to make sensible, defensible choices. In the last section of the book are chapters offering guidance on the logic of gathering and interpreting evidence applied to surgery.

No longer do we accept that operation is the individual domain and responsibility of the surgeon. The section on 'Preparation for surgery' covers many of the aspects that are often overlooked. Although individual operations are not described in Section 4, relevant aspects of important general principles are discussed.

Malignant disease is encountered in most branches of surgery. As management becomes more interdisciplinary, we need to understand the principles underlying the developments of newer and more effective treatments.

Good operative surgery must be followed by good aftercare and effective management of complications. Some important aspects are covered in Sections 6 and 7.

The final section of the book deals with a number of topics that were often ignored in the past. How valuable is it to screen for certain diseases, identify genetic aspects and study cost/benefits? How important is it for us to keep records of our results, discuss them with our colleagues and jointly learn from our cumulative experience? Do some of our problems stem from our failure to communicate well with our patients and our colleagues? Finally, because our ability to practice surgery depends on gaining the approval of our teachers, two outstanding surgeons, teachers and examiners offer advice on gaining success in the examinations.

1999

R.M.K.
A.O.M.
J.P.S.C.

Acknowledgements

All the contributions have been written without any fee. The authors have generously given a great deal of effort and expertise in order that the royalties should go to the Royal College of Surgeons of England, earmarked for the Audiovisual Department.

I would like to thank the team at Churchill Livingstone for their cooperation and support.

Contributors

P. L. Amlot MB BS FRCP
Senior Lecturer, Department of Immunology, Royal
Free and University College Medical School, London

W. Aveling MA MB BChir FRCA
Consultant Anaesthetist, University College London
Hospitals, London, UK

Daryll Baker PhD FRCS(Gen)
Consultant Vascular Surgeon, Royal Free Hospital,
London, UK

Tom Bates MBBS FRCS
Consultant Surgeon, The Breast Unit, William Harvey
Hospital, Ashford, Kent, UK

T. J. Beale FRCS(Eng) FRCR
Consultant Radiologist, Central Middlesex Hospital,
London, UK

S. Bhattacharya MS FRCS(Gen Surg)
Lecturer in Surgery, University Department of
Surgery, Royal Free Hospital, London, UK

Laura J. Buist MD FRCS
Consultant Transplant Surgeon, Queen Elizabeth
Hospital, Birmingham, UK

N. J. W. Cheshire MD FRCS
Consultant Vascular Surgeon, Regional Vascular Unit,
St Mary's Hospital, London; Vascular Tutor,
The Royal College of Surgeons of England and The
Vascular Society of Great Britain and Ireland

John P. S. Cochrane MS FRCS
Consultant Surgeon, Whittington Hospital, London,
UK

Carmel A. E. Coulter FRCP FRCR
Consultant in Clinical Oncology, St Mary's Hospital,
London, UK

M. K. H. Crumplin FRCS
Consultant General Surgeon, Wrexham Maelor
Hospital, Wrexham, Wales, UK

Brian Davidson MB ChB MD FRCS
Professor of Surgery, Royal Free and University
College School of Medicine, London, UK

A. P. Davies MA MRCP
Specialist Registrar, Department of Medical Microbiology,
Royal Free Hospital and Medical School, London, UK

Dai Davies FRCS
Consultant Plastic Surgeon, Charing Cross Hospital,
Hammersmith Hospitals Trust and The Stomford
Institute of Cosmetic Reconstruction Plastic Surgery,
Stomford Hospital, London, UK

A. Darzi MD FRCSI FRCS
Professor of Surgery, Imperial College of Science,
Technology and Medicine, St Mary's Hospital,
London, UK

J. L. Dawson CVO FKC MS FRCS
Former Consultant Surgeon, King's College Hospital,
London, UK

Amar P. Dhillon MD FRCP FRCPath
Senior Lecturer and Honorary Consultant,
Department of Histopathology, Royal Free Hospital,
London, UK

Len Doyal BA MSc
Reader in Medical Ethics, Department of Human
Science and Medical Ethics, London Hospital Medical
College, London, UK

P. A. Driscoll BSc MD FRCS FFAEM
Consultant in Emergency Medicine, Hope Hospital,
Salford, UK

Karen Eagle MRCP
Macmillan Consultant in Medical Oncology,
Peterborough District Hospital, Peterborough, UK

Brian W. Ellis MB FRCS
Consultant Urological Surgeon, Ashford Hospital,
Middlesex; Honorary Senior Clinical Research Fellow,
St Mary's Hospital, London, UK

Roshan Fernando FRCA
Consultant Anaesthetist, Department of Anaesthesia,
Royal Free Hospital, London, UK

Jane Fothergill FRCP FRCSEd FFAEM
Consultant in Accident and Emergency Medicine,
St Mary's Hospital, London, UK

Stuart W. T. Gould BSc MB BS FRCS
Surgical Specialist Registrar, Minimal Access Unit,
St Mary's Hospital, London

C. S. Gricks BSc
PhD Student, Department of Immunology, Royal Free
and University College Medical School, London

P. J. Guillou BSc(Hons) MD FRCS FRCPSGlasg(Hon) FAMS
Professor of Surgery at the University of Leeds (Based
at St James's University Hospital); Dean, School of
Medicine, University of Leeds, Leeds, UK

Colin Hamilton-Davies MBBS MD FRCA
Consultant Anaesthetist, University College Hospital,
London, UK

Michael Hobsley MChir PhD DSc FRCS
Emeritus Professor, Department of Surgery, Royal
Free and University College Medical School, London,
UK

Daniel Hochhauser MRCP DPhil
Senior Lecturer in Medical Oncology, Royal Free and
University College Medical School, London, UK

R. W. Hoile MS(Lond) FRCS(Eng)
Consultant General Surgeon, Medway NHS Trust and
Principal Surgical Coordinator of National
Confidential Enquiry into Perioperative Deaths, UK

Robert A. Huddart MA MBBS MRCP FRCR
Senior Lecturer and Honorary Consultant, Institute of
Cancer Research and Royal Marsden Hospital, Surrey,
UK

Katharine D. Hunt MBBS
Specialist Registrar, Department of Anaesthetics,
Royal Free Hospital, London, UK

Lucian L.E. Ion FRCS
Specialist Registrar in Plastic Surgery, Charing Cross
Hospital, London, UK

Donald J. Jeffries BSc MB BS FRCPath
Professor and Head of Department of Medical
Microbiology,St Bartholomew's and the Royal London
School of Medicine and Dentistry, London, UK

Jennifer Jones BSc FRCP FFARCS
Consultant Anaesthetist, St Mary's Hospital, London,
UK

R. M. Jones MD FRCA
Professor of Anaesthetics, St Mary's Hospital,
London, UK

Christopher C. Kibbler MA FRCP FRCPath
Consultant in Medical Microbiology, Department of
Medical Microbiology, Royal Free Hospital, London

R. M. Kirk MS FRCS
Honorary Consulting Surgeon, Royal Free Hospital,
London, UK

Anna Kurowska BSc BA FRCP
Consultant in Palliative Medicine, Whittington
Hospital, London; Consultant and Deputy Medical
Director, Edenhall Marie Curie Centre, London, UK

Sunil R. Lakhani BSc MBBS MD MRCPath
Senior Lecturer and Consultant in Histopathology,
University College London Medical School, London, UK

David John Leaper MD ChM FRCS FRCSEd FRCPS Glasg
(Hon) FACS
Professor of Surgery, North Tees Hospital, Stockton-
on-Tees, UK

Margaret Lloyd MD FRCP FRCGP
Reader in General Practice, Royal Free and University
College Medical School, London, UK

John W. McClenahan MA MS PhD FOR
Fellow in Leadership Development, King's Fund,
London, UK

Kay D. MacDermot MPhil FRCP
Consultant and Senior Lecturer in Clinical Genetics,
Royal Free and University College Medical School,
University of London, London, UK

C. Geraldine McMahon BScAnat FRCSEd(A & E)
Consultant, Accident and Emergency Department,
St James's Hospital, Dublin

Paul McMaster MA MB ChM FRCS FICS
Professor of Liver and Hepatobiliary Surgery, Clinical
Director, Liver Unit, Queen Elizabeth Hospital,
Birmingham, UK

Averil O. Mansfield ChM FRCS
Professor of Surgery, St Mary's Hospital, Imperial
College of Science, Technology and Medicine,
London, UK

Caroline Marshall MBBS MRCP FRCA
Consultant Anaesthetist, Southampton General
Hospital, Southampton, UK

Atul B. Mehta MA MD FRCP FRCPath
Consultant Haematologist/Senior Lecturer, Royal Free
and University College, London, UK

Jason Payne-James LLM FRCS(Eng & Edin) FLLA
Honorary Senior Research Fellow, Gastroenterology
and Nutrition, Central Middlesex Hospital, London,
UK

A. L. G. Peel MA MChir FRCS
Consultant Surgeon, North Tees Hospital, Stockton-
on-Tees, UK

R. M. Pemberton MA MS FRCS
Senior Clinical Fellow, St Mary's Hospital, London,
UK

Michael Pietroni MB BS FRCS
Consultant Surgeon, Whipps Cross Hospital,
Associate Dean of Postgraduate Medicine,
University of London, UK

M. W. Platt MB BS FRCA
Consultant and Honorary Senior Lecturer,
Department of Anaesthesia, St Mary's Hospital,
London, UK

R. C. G. Russell MS FRCS
Consultant Surgeon, The Middlesex Hospital,
London, UK

Gordon J. S. Rustin MD MSc FRCP
Director of Medical Oncology, Mount Vernon
Hospital, Middlesex, UK

Michael Schachter BSc MB BS MRCP
Senior Lecturer and Honorary Consultant Physician,
Imperial College School of Medicine, St Mary's
Hospital, London, UK

John E. Scoble MA MD FRCP
Clinical Director, Renal Services, Guy's and St
Thomas' Trust, London, UK

Jean Simpson BSc MSc
Public Health Specialist, Ealing Hammersmith and
Hounslow Health Authority, Middlesex, UK

J. A. R. Smith MB ChB PhD FRCS(Eng) FRCSEd
Consultant Surgeon, The Northern General NHS
Trust, Sheffield, UK

Jeremy J. T. Tate MS FRCS
Consultant, Gastrointestinal Surgery, Royal United
Hospital, Bath, UK

Adrian Tookman MRCP
Medical Director, Edenhall Marie Curie Centre,
London; Consultant in Palliative Medicine, Royal Free
Hospital Trust, London, UK

Robin Touquet MD FRCS FFAEM DCH
Consultant in Accident and Emergency Medicine,
St Mary's Hospital, London, UK

Naomi Vaughan MBBS FRCS
Research Fellow, Minimal Access Surgical Unit,
St Mary's Hospital, London, UK

Marc Winslet MS FRCS
Professor of Surgery, University Department of
Surgery, Royal Free Hospital, London, UK

Neville Woolf MB ChB Mmed (Path) PhD FRCPath
Vice Dean, Faculty of Clinical Sciences, University
College, London, UK

Contents

Emergency

1

Resuscitation

R. Touquet, J. Fothergill, M. W. Platt

'Scientia vincit timorem'

Objectives

- **Recognize the wide variety of patient presentations to an accident and emergency (A&E) department; these are often multidisciplinary and complex, being neither solely medical nor solely surgical.**
- **Understand the rationale for prioritization of the resuscitation sequences and recognize that decisions are based on the responses of the patient to interventions.**
- **Use protocols to prevent sins of omission.**
- **Understand how to read a set of arterial blood gases, both in terms of acid–base balance and gas exchange.**
- **Understand the difference between oxygen tension (Po_2, partial pressure) and oxygen saturation.**
- **Respect that the doctor in A&E may be the last generalist to manage the patient before admission under a more specialist team.**

The cause of the collapse or coma (a symptom of a broad spectrum of life-threatening conditions that depress or injure the central nervous system) precipitating a patient's arrival in the resuscitation room is often unknown. Furthermore, there may be more than one pathology, for example the patient with hypoglycaemia who has fallen, striking his head.

When a patient is brought into an accident and emergency (A&E) department with an altered level of consciousness, the resuscitation sequence described in the American College of Surgeons' Advanced Trauma Life Support Course is appropriate, whether the cause is a medical or a surgical emergency. The initial sequence is known as the primary survey (ABCDE, see below). This is a systematic form of assessment that is carried out at the same time that any resuscitative procedures are undertaken. There is ongoing monitoring of the vital signs and, in particular, monitoring of the vital signs in response to any procedure undertaken, such as the immediate infusion of 2 litres of crystalloid for the adult in hypovolaemic shock.

The standard sequence of the initial primary survey is as follows:

Airway, with cervical spine control
Breathing
Circulation
Disability – a brief neurological assessment
Exposure – undress the patient completely temperature control.

Due notice must be taken of the history from the ambulance crew. The ambulance transfer form must be signed by a member of the A&E staff. It is prudent to involve the ambulance crew in the initial resuscitation and to have that crew immediately available to give any further details about the history.

When the patient has stabilized, with clinically acceptable vital signs, the patient is examined from head to toe in order to prevent any pathology being missed. It is not infrequent that the A&E doctor is the last doctor to examine the patient in their totality. This systematic methodical examination is known as the secondary survey. However, if the patient has to be taken to theatre urgently then this secondary survey will have to be carried out later, on the ward, by the responsible admitting team.

PART 1: PRIMARY SURVEY WITH INITIAL RESUSCITATION

Greet the conscious patient from the ambulance by talking to him and reassuring him that he is in the right place and that you know what to do. Do not treat the patient as an inanimate object.

Airway

In all trauma victims apply an appropriately sized head cervical collar. Steady the head – in-line cervical spine immobilization – to prevent those with unsuspected neck injury from sustaining an iatrogenic injury to the cervical spinal cord during manoeuvres on the airway. The neck is at particular risk during orotracheal intubation, when extreme vigilance is mandatory in those in whom a cervical spine injury has not been ruled out.

Assessment

Assess the patency of the airway by talking to the patient, looking for signs of confusion or agitation which may indicate cerebral hypoxia. Listen for stridor or gurgling sounds from a compromised airway. Feel for warm air against your hand in a patient who is breathing. Following smoke inhalation there may be carbon deposits in the mouth or nostrils, raising the possibility of upper airway burns and associated carbon monoxide poisoning. In this situation call an anaesthetist, as early tracheal intubation will be required.

Look to see whether chest movements are adequate.

Management

Keep the airway open and clear it. Remove any foreign bodies such as sweets, or vomit which must be sucked out. Lift the chin forwards to bring the tongue off the back of the nasopharynx, and if the gag reflex is diminished insert an oral (Guedel) airway. If a Guedel airway is not tolerated, but obstruction is still present, consider gently inserting a well-lubricated nasopharyngeal airway, ensuring that this is done automatically. Once the airway is secured deliver 10–15 1 min^{-1} of oxygen via a face mask with a reservoir device, providing 95% oxygen.

None of these basic airway manoeuvres protects the lungs from aspiration of gastric contents or blood. In those unable to protect their own airway (absent gag reflex) a cuffed tracheal tube must be inserted via the oral or nasal route, both to facilitate efficient ventilation and to protect the lungs.

If the airway cannot be secured by any of the above methods, urgently carry out a needle cricothyroidotomy followed, if necessary, by a surgical cricothyroidotomy.

Breathing

Assessment

Note any degree of cyanosis. Assess the neck veins and if they are engorged consider the possibility of a tension pneumothorax, cardiac tamponade, air embolus, pulmonary embolus or myocardial contusion. Feel for the position of the trachea, and if it is deviated to one side decide whether it has been pushed over by a tension pneumothorax on the other side. Count the respiratory rate (normally 12–20 per minute) and expose, inspect and palpate the anterior chest wall. Assess air entry or the lack of it by auscultation. A severe asthmatic may present with collapse and have a silent chest because with extreme airway narrowing no air can move in or out of the lungs. In a flail chest there are three or more consecutive ribs, each fractured in two or more places, with a segment of paradoxical chest wall motion, the underlying pulmonary contusion may cause acute respiratory failure. If there is any doubt about the adequacy of a patient's airway or breathing, urgently obtain expert help from physicians and anaesthetists.

Management: control of ventilation

Preventing hypoventilation, hypercarbia, cerebral vasodilatation and a resultant increase in intracerebral pressure is vital in trauma patients, especially if they have suffered a head injury. Both adults and children have a normal tidal volume of 7 ml kg^{-1}. If the patient is obviously unable to sustain a normal tidal volume (with obvious shallow respirations, often associated with tachypnoea, signs of fatigue and distress), there is a high risk of hypercarbia and resultant increased cerebral perfusion and oedema, necessitating assisted respiration, initially by bag–valve–mask positive pressure ventilation. An arterial blood sample will demonstrate a high arterial carbon dioxide tension ($P_a CO_2$) level if the patient is breathing inadequately. Ventilate and oxygenate the hypoxic or apnoeic patient if possible for at least 3 minutes prior to attempted intubation, and do not prolong any attempt for more than 60 seconds before returning to bag–valve–mask ventilation. Any patient who is apnoeic obviously needs ventilation urgently.

The aim of assisted ventilation is to keep the arterial blood oxygen above 10 kPa (80 mmHg) and the carbon dioxide below 5.5 kPa (40 mmHg), but above 30 mmHg to prevent brain ischaemia. A reduction of the $P_a CO_2$ to just above 4 kPa (30 mmHg) will reduce cerebral oedema and intracerebral acidosis in a patient with a head injury and a decreased level of consciousness.

In those who are breathing spontaneously, assume that agitation, aggression or depressed level of consciousness is due to hypoxia, demonstrating how all collapsed patients who are not likely to recover immediately must have arterial blood samples taken urgently for measurement of oxygen, carbon dioxide and acid–base balance. (Also consider, where appropriate, a full bladder or tight plaster of Paris as causes of restlessness.) Aspirate arterial blood into a heparinized syringe (a 2-ml syringe whose dead space has been filled with heparin 1000 unit ml^{-1}) from the radial artery or, failing this, the femoral artery.

The arterial oxygen tension (P_aO_2) should be maintained above 10 kPa (80 mmHg), with added inspired oxygen, for tissue viability. The exception is the patient with chronic obstructive airways disease (COAD), who depends on hypoxic drive rather than P_aCO_2 to breathe and will tend to hypoventilate when given added oxygen of more than 35%. The only way to diagnose this problem is by the arterial blood gas, which will show a high P_aCO_2 with a normal pH. All collapsed patients should initially be given 95% oxygen, as the problem of the patient whose respiration is dependent on hypoxic drive is uncommonly encountered in A&E.

Oxygen administration may also be necessary to produce a higher than normal P_aO_2. This is indicated to correct a pathological state the treatment of which is with an elevated P_aO_2; some examples are carbon monoxide poisoning, elevated pulmonary vascular resistance, sickle cell crisis and anaerobic infections.

Circulation

This is the third priority after **A**irway with cervical spine control, and **B**reathing.

Assessment

Assessment of the patient for shock requires skill. Remember that the earliest signs of shock are anxiety, a tachycardia of 100–120 beats per minute, tachypnoea of 20–30 breaths per minute, skin mottling and a prolonged capillary refill time of more than 2 seconds, and postural hypotension. If there is postural hypotension with a fall of systolic blood pressure of 20 mmHg, a fall of diastolic blood pressure of 10 mmHg and a rise of pulse of 20 beats per minute (20 : 10 : 20 rule), diagnose hypovolaemia due to an occult bleeding until proved otherwise. Supine systolic blood pressure does not drop until an adult has lost around 1500–2000 ml of blood, or 30–40% of the blood volume of 70 ml kg^{-1} body weight; by this time the patient is ashen in colour because of blood-drained extremities.

The level of consciousness is also decreased because of inadequate cerebral circulation, particularly if blood loss was rapid. As a guide, a palpable carotid pulse indicates a systemic blood pressure of at least 60 mmHg. If the carotid pulse is absent, initiate immediate basic cardiopulmonary resuscitation (CPR, see below).

Management

Control haemorrhage from any external bleeding points by direct pressure, with limb elevation where appropriate.

Intravenous access. Poiseuille's law states that the rate of flow of fluid through a pipe is proportional to the fourth power of the radius, and inversely proportional to the length. In a severely traumatized or hypovolaemic patient, never fail to insert two short widebore cannulae of 14 gauge or larger, sited in peripheral veins, whether introduced percutaneously or by surgical cutdown.

Preferred sites for cutdown are the long saphenous vein anterior to the medial malleolus, or the basilic vein in the elbow crease. Cutdown is a safe, simple and quick procedure in which every surgical trainee should be skilled.

Technique for venous cutdown. Make a transverse 2 cm incision anterior to the medial malleolus or to the medial epicondyle of the humerus. By blunt dissection delineate the long saphenous vein or basilic vein. Ligate the vein distally with 2/0 black silk. Control the vein proximally with a similar loose ligature. Make a transverse incision for one-third of the circumference of the vein, such that it is possible to insert a 14- to 12-gauge cannula into the vein. Secure the cannula in place by tightening the proximal suture. This technique is applicable for collapsed infants.

Intraosseous infusion. An even simpler technique for children under 7 is to use an intraosseous trocar and cannula: these are specially designed to be inserted through the cortex of bone into the bone marrow. The site for introduction of the needle is two fingers distal to the tibial tuberosity on the anteromedial surface of the tibia. Clean the area thoroughly as osteomyelitis is a possible complication of the technique. Crystalloid and colloid may slowly be injected into the marrow (20 ml kg^{-1} initially for the collapsed child) together with drugs used in resuscitation, with the exception of sodium bicarbonate and bretylium. The circulation time from here to the heart is only 20 seconds.

Central venous cannulation may be dangerous, even in experienced hands, for the trauma patient, who is often restless. Such patients may not survive an iatrogenic pneumothorax or cervical spinal cord injury caused by the turning of an unsuspected neck injury, and as the above routes of access avoid the possibility of these complications they are to be preferred. Central venous pressure monitoring is useful in the stabilized patient, but these lines are not for resuscitation other than in patients with cardiac arrest, when drugs should be administered centrally.

Correct hypovolaemia with the rapid intravenous infusion of warmed crystalloid or colloid solution followed by blood. Rapid loss of greater than 40% of a patient's blood volume produces electromechanical dissociation leading to circulatory standstill unless immediate resuscitation is carried out. It is not possible to measure the blood volume of a patient in the resuscitation room. Therefore you must monitor the vital signs (delineated in Part 2), especially in response to treatment such as fluid replacement, and tailor your treatment accordingly.

If the carotid pulse is impalpable, the heart has become an ineffective pump, and irreversible brain damage results unless immediate action is taken to correct the specific causes of electromechanical dissociation such as massive blood loss, tension pneumothorax or cardiac tamponade. If there is no improvement or these conditions are not present, commence cardiac massage for cardiac arrest (Fig. 1.1). Check the heart's electrical rhythm on the monitor. Place the leads in the correct positions as quickly as possible. If no rhythm shows, ensure that the gain knob is turned up on the monitor and check for a rhythm in two different ECG leads; alternatively, monitor through the paddles of a defibrillator, one placed just to the left of the expected position of the apex beat and one inferior to the right clavicle.

External chest compression. When the carotid pulse is not palpable after you have controlled ventilation, place one hand over the other on the sternum, the lower border of the hands being two fingers above the xiphisternal–sternal junction. If the hands are lower there is risk of damage to the liver. Keep the arms straight, with the shoulders in a direct line over the hands in order that you do not tire. Depress the sternum smoothly for 4–5 cm, at a rate of 100 per minute, with a ratio of one ventilation to about five compressions, both actions being carried out synchronously. Keep the compression rate regular so that the ventilation between compression five and the next compression runs from the fifth compression into the next compression. In this way the pressure is increased generally in the chest both during part of compression five and compression one by that ventilation. In addition, the expanding lungs drive the diaphragm down, leading to compression of the vena cava. This further facilitates blood being forced up the carotid arteries (the thoracic pump effect); feel for the carotid or femoral pulse every 2 minutes.

The correct cardiac rhythm must be diagnosed quickly. In a non-traumatic cardiac arrest patient the rhythm is ventricular fibrillation in 70% of cases, and the chances of a successful resuscitation are directly proportional to the speed of applying DC shock in the correct manner and sequence (see Fig. 1.1). Therefore there must be no delays from the time of arrest, and this is why ambulance crews are now being trained to use, and are issued with, defibrillators.

Internal cardiac massage. External chest compression does not effectively resuscitate an empty heart in cardiac arrest due to hypovolaemic shock. However this is indicated, in the Accident and Emergency Department, only for direct penetrating trauma, *not* for blunt trauma, when the patient, at the very least, just has a palpable pulse on arrival. When there is not an appropriate response to prompt rapid transfusion, you should consider internal cardiac massage for penetrating trauma. This is the only indication for an emergency thoracotomy for internal cardiac massage in the A&E department by trained personnel. Internal cardiac massage is, in the hands of those with appropriate training, both safe and haemodynamically superior to external cardiac massage, although the latter can be initiated without delay and performed by non-surgeons. Openchest cardiopulmonary resuscitation (CPR) enables direct palpation and observation of the heart and direct electric defibrillation.

The technique for internal cardiac massage (by trained personnel) is as follows: make a left-sided thoracotomy through the fourth or fifth intercostal space once the patient is receiving intermittent positive pressure ventilation through a tracheal tube. Immediately compress the heart using the left hand, without at first opening the pericardial sac, by placing the thumb over the left ventricle posteriorly and the fingers anteriorly in front of the heart. The heart is compressed at the rate of 100 per minute, adjusting the compression force and rate to the filling of the heart. Open the pericardium, avoiding the phrenic and vagus nerves. Adrenaline, atropine and lignocaine, but not sodium bicarbonate, may be injected directly into the left ventricle, avoiding the coronary arteries. For internal defibrillation use internal 6 cm paddle electrodes with saline-soaked gauze pads and insulated handles. Place one paddle posteriorly over the left ventricle and one over the anterior surface of the heart (10–20 J).

Drugs. In a patient with cardiac arrest, drugs such as adrenaline should, if possible, be given centrally, and for this reason you must be proficient in at least one method of central venous cannulation. You should use the approach with which you are most familiar; however, the infraclavicular approach is often the most convenient and practicable means of access for the surgeon.

Technique for central vein cannulation

1. *Preparation:* clean the area with surgical antiseptic solution.

2. *Position:* use a 20° head-down tilt (in patients without head injury) to fill the vein and to reduce the risk of air embolus. The easiest route for an anaesthetist

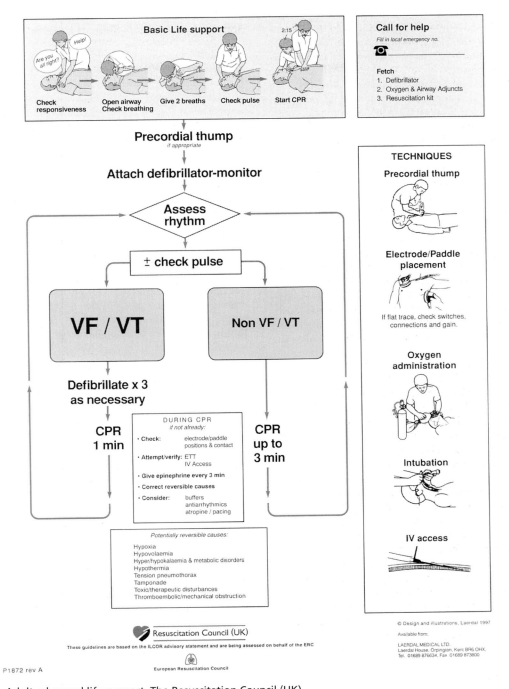

Fig 1.1 Adult advanced life support. The Resuscitation Council (UK).

is via the right internal jugular vein, which gives the most direct access to the right atrium. This can be palpated, with the head facing contralaterally, as the softest part of the neck usually lateral to the carotid artery in a line from the mastoid process to the supratracheal notch. For access to the right subclavian vein, which may be the easiest route for the A&E clinician or surgeon, pull the right arm caudally, to place the vein in the most convenient position to the clavicle for cannulation. If the shoulder is obstructing access, place a sandbag below the upper thoracic spine so that the shoulders lie more posteriorly, unless there is any possibility of spinal injury.

3. *Access*: for jugular vein cannulation, introduce the needle into the skin approximately at the mid-point of a line running from the mastoid process to the supratracheal notch, aiming laterally at 30° to the skin, towards the right big toe or right nipple, or towards the previously palpated jugular vein. For subclavian vein access, introduce the needle through the skin 2 cm inferior to the junction of the lateral and middle thirds of the clavicle. Advance the needle, aspirating continuously and snugging the inferior bony surface of the clavicle, aiming at the superior aspect of the right sternoclavicular joint for not more than 6 cm.

4. *Technique*: aspirate until blood freely appears, ensure the bevel of the needle is now directed caudally, remove the syringe and immediately insert the Seldinger wire, flexible end first, through the needle. Remove the needle, railroad the plastic cannula over the Seldinger wire, then remove the wire. Check that the cannula is in the central vein by briefly allowing retrograde blood flow into the attached intravenous giving set.

5. *Aftercare*: secure the line with a black silk suture through the skin and dress with sterile dressing. Return the patient to the horizontal position and obtain a chest X-ray to check the position of the central venous cannula and to exclude a pneumothorax. Note that the absence of a pneumothorax on this film does not exclude the possibility of one developing subsequently, possibly under tension. If there is trauma to only one side of the chest, then use this side for cannulation because there is already a risk of pneumothorax there. Jugular vein cannulation carries less risk of pneumothorax, but is more difficult to perform if cervical spine immobilization is required.

If this direct venous access is not obtained during CPR for immediate drug therapy to the heart muscle, then drugs should be given via a peripheral venous line, with an infusion of 5% dextrose solution running after each drug to flush it into the central circulation. Certain drugs such as adrenaline, atropine, lignocaine and naloxone may be given via the tracheal tube route, in double the intravenous dosage diluted to 10 ml.

Disability

This term is used to signify a brief neurological assessment which must be carried out at this stage of the initial examination. The mnemonic used in the Advanced Trauma Life Support Course is useful:

A = **A**lert
V = responds to **V**erbal stimuli
P = responds to **P**ainful stimuli
U = **U**nresponsive

In addition, now assess the presence or absence of orientation in time (knows day and month), space (knows where he is) and person (knows who he is). These perceptions are usually lost in this sequence with lessening of consciousness. Alternatively use the Glasgow Coma Scale at the outset.

Record the pupil size and response to light (Table 1.1). Bilateral small pupils denote opiate poisoning unless disproved by failure of naloxone to reverse the constriction. If necessary, up to 2 mg of naloxone (i.e. five vials of 0.4 mg) are given.

If there is a response, more may have to be given because it has a short half-life; it may be given via an endotracheal tube if you do not have intravenous access. The other common cause of bilateral small pupils is a pontine haemorrhage, for which there is no specific treatment.

Exposure

In a severely traumatized patient always carry out a complete examination of all the skin. This necessitates the removal of every scrap of clothing, being careful to protect the spine. Full examination includes log-rolling with a minimum of four trained personnel to examine the back. Perform this earlier if there is a specific indication (e.g. trauma to the posterior chest wall) or at the latest at the end of the secondary survey. Protect the child from hypothermia.

Consider inserting a nasogastric tube or, if there is a suspicion of a cribriform plate fracture, an orogastric tube. Insert a urinary catheter after inspecting the perineum for bruising and blood, and carrying out a rectal examination in an injured patient (see Ch. 2).

PART 2: MONITORING

Throughout this initial assessment, resuscitation proceeds with constant ongoing monitoring of vital signs and simple clinical measurements. You must constantly tailor your resuscitation according to the results of your monitoring and keep an open mind to possible diagnoses and, therefore, appropriate treatment.

Table 1.1 Pupil size and response to light in comatose patients

	One pupil	Both pupils

Dilated	Atropine in eye
	3rd nerve lesion normal consensual light reflex, e.g. posterior communicating artery aneurysm
	Enlarging mass lesion above the tentorium, causing a pressure cone
	
	Optic nerve lesion:
	Old: pale disc and afferent pupil
	New: afferent pupil with normal disc, loss of direct light reflex, loss of consensual reflex in other eye – both constrict with light in other eye
		Cerebral anoxia
		Very poor outlook if increasing supratentorial pressure – if dilated pupils preceded by unilateral dilation or if due to diffuse cerebral damage
		
		Overdose: e.g. amphetamines
		               carbon monoxide
		               phenothiazines
		               cocaine
		               glutethimide
		               antidepressants
		Hypothermia

Constricted	Pilocarpine in eye Horner's, e.g. brachial plexus lesion Acute stroke uncommonly (brain stem occlusion or carotid artery ischaemia: small pupil opposite side to weakness)	Pilocarpine in both eyes (glaucoma treatment) Opiates, organophosphate insecticides and trichloroethanol (chloral) Pontine haemorrhage or ischaemia (brisk tendon reflexes, and temperature increased: poor prognostic sign) Alcohol poisoning (dilatation shaking (Macewan's pupil'))
	If pupils normal in size, and reacting to light, consider metabolic, systemic non-cerebral causes (N.B. Normal pupils do not exclude an overdose)	

Pulse

Remember that in an elderly or even middle-aged person a rate of more than 140 per minute is very unlikely to be sinus tachycardia as this is too fast for someone of that age. Atrial flutter runs at around 300 beats per minute, and therefore if there is 2–1 atrioventricular block the ventricular rate is 150 per minute. The rate of supraventricular tachycardia is usually 160–220 beats per minute.

Respiratory rate

The importance of this is all too easily forgotten. The normal range is 12–20 breaths per minute. It rises early with blood loss or hypoxia, and as well as being a very useful indication of the patient's clinical state it is one of the physiological parameters that is mandatory for the calculation of the Revised Trauma Score.

Blood pressure

With hypovolaemia this drops when the blood loss is greater than 1500–2000 ml. Fit young adults, and especially children, maintain their blood pressure resiliently, but then it falls precipitously when compensatory mechanisms are overwhelmed.

Pulse pressure

This is the difference between systolic pressure and diastolic pressure. Initially, with haemorrhage the diastolic pressure rises due to vasoconstriction from circulating catecholamines, while the systolic stays constant. Therefore the pulse pressure decreases. This is followed by a greater decrease in the pulse pressure as the systolic blood pressure falls once 30% of the patient's blood volume has been lost.

Capillary refill time

This is the time it takes for blood to return to a compressed nail bed on release of pressure – the time can be longer because of hypothermia, peripheral microvascular disease and collagen diseases as well as in hypovolaemia. The normal value is 2 seconds, but this time increases early in shock, following a 15% loss of blood volume.

Temperature

Quite apart from primary hypothermia, in a hypovolaemic patient a decreased temperature is an indication of the degree of blood loss. Blood volume must be restored adequately because if the hypovolaemic patient is simply warmed the blood pressure falls further by virtue of the resulting vasodilation. The patient with primary hypothermia is usually hypovolaemic as well, which is why rapid rewarming results in a drop in blood pressure unless blood volume is replaced. Every resuscitation room should have a warming cabinet so that intravenous fluid at 37°C can be immediately infused to the hypovolaemic or hypothermic patient or better still, a rapid transfuser which warms fluids to 37–38°C.

Urinary output

The minimal normal obligatory output is 30 ml h^{-1}. In a child it is easily remembered as 1 ml kg^{-1} h^{-1}. Consider renal pathology if greater than +protein on stick testing.

Central venous pressure (CVP)

This is measured in centimetres of water by positioning the manometer on a stand such that the zero point is level with the patient's right atrium. The normal pressure is around 5 cmH$_2$O from the angle of Louis, with the patient at 45° to the horizontal.

The CVP is a measure of the filling pressure (preload) to the right atrium. It reflects the volume of blood in the central veins relative to the venous tone. It is not a measure of left heart function, until right ventricular function is compromised as a result of poor left heart function.

The CVP may be low if the patient is hypovolaemic, and rises to normal with correction. If the CVP rises slowly with a fluid challenge, this is usually indicative of hypovolaemia. Particularly in the young, peripheral vasoconstriction to conserve central blood volume occurs when hypovolaemic shock is present, resulting in preservation of central venous pressure to a limited degree. The CVP is raised if the circulating volume is too large, as might happen with renal failure or with overtransfusion. Overtransfusion not only precipitates heart failure, due to dilatation of the heart, but in a patient with a head injury the resultant rise in intracranial pressure may cause irreversible damage to the already bruised brain. Monitoring the CVP in these circumstances is therefore crucial.

The CVP also rises if the right side of the heart is malfunctioning. The CVP cannot then be used as an indication of the filling of the systemic circulation, except as a measure of changing cardiac function. It may be raised for mechanical reasons such as a tension pneumothorax or cardiac tamponade. It is raised in the presence of pulmonary embolism, or when the heart is failing for lack of muscular power due to contusion or infarction.

Arterial blood gases

1. pH (normal range 7.35–7.45)

Does the patient have an acidosis, alkalosis or neither (Table 1.2)?

pH is the negative logarithm to base 10 of the hydrogen ion concentration. It is measured in the blood gas machine using an electrode that produces an electrical current in direct linear proportion to this value. It also so happens that the body's hydrogen ion levels tend to change in logarithmic fashion, making this a very useful measure indeed. Some gas machines do give an absolute concentration of hydrogen ions, in nanomoles per litre, but this is derived from the logarithm.

Table 1.2 Reading of arterial blood gases for acid–base balance	
Acidosis or alkalosis?	pH 7.35–7.45
Respiratory component?	If P_{CO_2} < 4.5 kPa, suggests respiratory alkalosis (pH > 7.45), or attempted compensation of a metabolic acidosis (pH < 7.35 and BE < –3) If PCO_2 > 5.5 kPa, suggests respiratory acidosis (pH < 7.35), or attempted compensation of a metabolic alkalosis (pH > 7.45 and BE > +3)
Metabolic component?	Base excess (BE) is always affected by metabolic acid–base changes: Metabolic acidosis causes BE < –3 Metabolic alkalosis causes BE > +3

The lower the pH, the more acid is the blood sample, the opposite being the case for alkalosis. Acid (as hydrogen ions) is produced continually from metabolizing cells, mostly as carbon dioxide. More is produced from lactic acid production during conditions of hypoxia, for example in shock, or in cardiac or respiratory arrest. Inadequate tissue perfusion results in acid build-up. Most acid–base abnormalities are the result of an imbalance between production and removal of H^+ ions (Table 1.3).

Hydrogen is adsorbed by buffers, the largest being proteins, both intra- and extracellularly. In the extracellular fluid, the largest buffer is haemoglobin. However, bicarbonate is a highly dynamic buffer, enabling an exchange to occur between hydrogen and carbon dioxide. This enables hydrogen to be excreted via the lungs rapidly as carbon dioxide:

$$H^+ + HCO_3^- \Leftrightarrow H_2CO_3 \Leftrightarrow CO_2 + H_2O$$

Hydrogen ions are also excreted via the kidneys, but over hours or days, leaving the respiratory compensation to be the most rapid method the body has for correction.

The complex proteins of the body are optimally conformed at ideal pH. When the pH of tissues changes, conformational changes occur in proteins affecting their function, especially enzymes and cell membrane channels. This is why the maintenance of normal pH is crucial. Carbon dioxide is the largest generator of H^+ ions, ten times more than the production of lactic or other metabolic acids (Table 1.3).

2. P_aCO_2 (normal range 35–45 mmHg, 4.5–5.5 kPa)

PCO_2 is high: suggests a respiratory acidosis (if pH is low); or a compensated metabolic alkalosis (see below).

PCO_2 is low: suggests a respiratory alkalosis (if pH is high); or a compensated metabolic acidosis (see below).

The partial pressure of carbon dioxide is related to degree of lung ventilation. Hyperventilation produces a reduction in PCO_2 and vice-versa. If the patient is not breathing adequately, CO_2 is not adequately excreted

Table 1.3 Production and elimination of hydrogen ions

Class		Daily production (mol)	Source	Excreted in breath	Metabolic removal possible	Normal organ of elimination
I	CO_2	15	Tissue respiration	+	–	Lungs
II	*Organic acids and urea synthesis*					
	Lactic	1.2	Muscle, brain erythrocytes, skin, etc.	–	+	Liver (50%), kidneys, heart Many tissues (not liver)
	Hydroxybutyric and acetoacetic	0.6*	Liver	–	+	
	Fatty free acids (FFA)	0.7	Adipose tissue	–	+	Most tissues
	H^+ generated during urea synthesis	1.1†	Liver	–	+	Most tissues (see text), small fraction in urine
III	*'Fixed acids'* Sulphuric Phosphoric	0.1	Dietary sulphur-containing amino acids Organic phosphate metabolism	–	–	Urinary excretion (partly)

The daily production rates for the organic acids are calculated from results obtained in resting 70 kg man after an overnight fast, and are proportioned up to 24-hour values.
*Because of ingestion of food during daytime and consequent suppression of FFA and ketone body production, the values for these acids may be considerable overestimates.
†On 100 g protein diet.

and hydrogen ions build up, leading to an acidosis caused by inadequate ventilation, that is, a respiratory acidosis. pH will fall, indicating an acidosis.

Anxious patients and those in early hypovolaemic shock have a tachypnoea, resulting in over-excretion of CO_2, resulting in loss of hydrogen and a resulting respiratory alkalosis.

When the patient is being mechanically or manually ventilated, the use of an end-tidal CO_2 measuring device will give a good correlation of arterial CO_2 (unless there is significant lung disease). End-tidal CO_2 partial pressure reflects that in the pulmonary artery, and indicates correct siting of the tracheal tube.

3. Base excess (or deficit) (normal range – 3 to + 3)

High negative value: (e.g. – 10) always means metabolic acidosis. pH will try to normalize as there is normally an attempt to compensate by hyperventilation to reduce P_aCO_2, producing a compensatory 'respiratory alkalosis'.

High positive value: (e.g. +10) always means metabolic alkalosis. Similarly, hypoventilation to increase P_aCO_2 will compensate somewhat to try to normalize the pH.

A metabolic acidosis indicates an inability of the kidneys to shift an increased hydrogen load, as occurs in shock, diabetes or renal failure.

Chronic respiratory acidosis, with normal pH. Chronic lung disease associated with chronic hypercarbia, results in the kidneys retaining bicarbonate ion, causing an increase in plasma bicarbonate concentration and a normalizing of blood pH, despite the hypercarbia (metabolic compensation). These changes take several days to occur, but will identify those patients who normally run high P_aCO_2 levels, and not those with just acute changes. Whenever there is an attempted compensation, the pH never quite reaches completely normal values, which is how we can tell if there has been compensation.

Treatment with sodium bicarbonate has in the past been overenthusiastic and there are definite hazards in its uses (see Table 1.4). It is now recognized that bicarbonate should not be given during the first 15 minutes of a cardiac arrest in a previously healthy patient. The principal method of controlling acid–base status during a cardiorespiratory arrest is adequate ventilation to ensure CO_2 excretion. If the pH is < 7.1 at 15 minutes with a normal or low PCO_2, give either 50 ml of 8.4% sodium bicarbonate (1 ml = 1 mmol) or calculate the amount of bicarbonate needed to correct the metabolic acidosis from the blood gas result. Multiply the base deficit by the estimated extracellular volume (i.e. divide the product of the patient's weight in kilograms and their base deficit by 3). Base deficit is defined as the millimoles of alkali required to restore the pH of 1 litre of the patient's blood to normal at PCO_2 = 5.33 kPa. In practice, the initial amount to be given should seldom exceed 1 mmol kg^{-1}. In the traumatized patient, what is of paramount importance, in addition to ventilation, is restoration of blood volume and reperfusion of the tissues.

A lowered pH is desirable provided that it does not fall below 7.1. Below this, further acidosis lowers the threshold of the heart to ventricular fibrillation and inhibits normal cell metabolism, and should therefore be corrected.

4. P_aO_2 and oxygen saturation

The partial pressure of oxygen in the arterial blood (also called the *oxygen tension*) is that pressure which oxygen gas would produce if it was in a gaseous phase (e.g. if the blood was in a glass vessel with a gaseous phase immediately above it). Gases move down pressure gradients, and so oxygen in the body will always move from an area of higher partial pressure to an area of lower pressure (e.g. from lung alveoli to mixed venous blood in the pulmonary artery). The P_aO_2 gives some idea of the amount of oxygen reaching the arterial blood from the lungs, or if there is some dilution with venous blood (shunting).

Oxygen saturation is that amount of the haemoglobin concentration which is bound to oxygen, expressed as a percentage. Oxygen carriage is dependent on haemoglobin and it is the haemoglobin-bound oxygen that is

Table 1.4	Hazards of bicarbonate therapy

1. Inactivates simultaneously administered catecholamines
2. Shifts the oxyhaemoglobin dissociation curve to the left, inhibiting the release of oxygen to the tissues
3. Exacerbates central venous acidosis and may, by production of carbon dioxide, produce a paradoxical acidosis
4. Induces hypernatraemia, hyperosmolarity and an extracellular alkalosis; the latter causes an acute intracellular shift of potassium and a decreased plasma ionized calcium

the main supply for the tissues. The amount of oxygen in solution in the blood is tiny, only becoming significant at ambient pressures which are multiples of atmospheric pressure. This is demonstrated in the oxygen flux equation, which gives the amount of oxygen flowing to the tissues per minute:

$$O_2 \text{ Flux} = CO \left[(S_aO_2 \times Hb \times 1.34) + F \right]$$

where CO is the cardiac output, S_aO_2 is the arterial oxygen saturation, 1.34 is Hoeffner's constant (the amount of oxygen that is capable of combining to Hb) and F is the small amount of oxygen dissolved in the blood. The values are converted to give ml/minute: normal oxygen flux is 1000 ml min^{-1}; the minimum flux compatible with life is 400 ml min^{-1}.

Oxygen saturation is now routinely measured non-invasively by shining several infra-red wavelengths of light across a finger or nose or other piece of skin. A sensor detects those waves not absorbed by haemoglobin. Oxyhaemoglobin and deoxyhaemoglobin have different infra-red absorption spectra, and so the machine can calculate the mean oxygen saturation of blood reaching the part with each pulse, compensating for tissue absorption by an algorithm.

The relationship between Po_2 and So_2 is shown in the oxygen dissociation curve (Fig. 1.2). Note how the curve becomes steep below 90% saturation – the situation that many patients with lung disease are in.

This curve is calculated for HbA, with normal characteristics. Other haemoglobins produce curves in different positions (e.g. sickle cell anaemia shows a marked shift to the right, and fetal haemoglobin is shifted to the left).

Acidosis increases ease of unloading oxygen from the blood into tissues ('Bohr effect' of pH on the oxygen dissociation curve (see Fig. 1.2)). Increasing temperature and increasing partial pressure of carbon dioxide have the same effect, the latter not just because of an associated acidosis but also because carbon dioxide combines directly with haemoglobin to form carbamino compounds. Anaemia, heat, raised CO_2, acidosis and increased 2,3-DPG cause a rightward shift to the oxygen dissociation curve, the opposite effects producing a leftward shift.

Blood sugar

Order an immediate blood glucose estimation using a reagent strip on every patient who has an altered level of consciousness, otherwise hypoglycaemia will be missed. This is followed by a laboratory estimation. When giving glucose in A&E, be aware of the possibility of precipitating Wernicke's encephalopathy and give B vitamins (Pabrinex®) intravenously at the same time if there is any evidence of alcohol misuse.

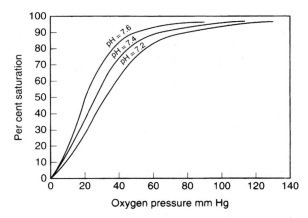

Fig 1.2 Effect of pH on the oxyhaemoglobin dissociation curve of human blood at 38°C.

PART 3: THE SECONDARY SURVEY: DETERMINING THE CAUSE OF THE PATIENT'S COLLAPSE

After carrying out the initial assessment (primary survey) and resuscitation of a collapsed patient presenting to the A&E department with no history, a deceptively incomplete history or, worse, an incorrect history, you must now go on to make a full head-to-toe examination. This is the secondary survey, during which you aim to gain a clearer picture of the cause of the patient's collapse. Ensure that there is no occult injury. Examine all the skin, including the mouth and throat, the external auditory meati and the perineum. Always remember the possibility of non-accidental injury in children, and in the elderly. Consider all the forensic possibilities, noting needle marks, pressure blisters and the presence of any visible soft tissue injuries. Remember that bruising may appear at a distance from the site of injury.

You must:

1. Keep an open mind to all diagnostic possibilities while both collecting the clinical evidence and monitoring the response of the vital signs to treatment.

2. Actively consider the common causes of collapse. This is especially important when there is a problem of communication, perhaps because of language, or when obvious initial clinical signs deflect you from finding the hidden life-threatening pathology. An example is a patient found by the police smelling of alcohol but developing an acute intracranial haematoma after a relatively trivial head injury. *Beware!* Involve your anaesthetist early with preparation for the CT scan of brain and possibly cervical spine. Patients with a head injury who misuse alcohol may have a larger subdural space and prolonged clotting times.

It is wise to leave on the cervical collar in all trauma patients while they are in the resuscitation room. This is mandatory for all patients who have evidence of trauma above the level of the clavicle and have any decrease in their level of consciousness, whether it be from the trauma itself or from drugs, especially alcohol.

A synopsis of the main causes of collapse is best considered under systems in order that sins of omission are not committed in the frenetic atmosphere of the resuscitation room of the A&E department (Table 1.5). The synopsis is not comprehensive, but does include the common causes, together with less common causes

Table 1.5 Synopsis of causes of collapse to be considered during secondary survey

System	Diagnosis	Notes
Respiratory	Upper airway obstruction	Inhaled foreign body (try Heimlich manoeuvre) Infection such as epiglottitis (occurs in adults although commoner in children) Call help urgently Trauma including respiratory burns
	Ventilatory failure	Asthma Chest trauma such as sucking open wound Paralysis such as in Guillain–Barré syndrome
	Failure of alveolar gas exchange	Pneumonia Pulmonary contusions Cardiogenic pulmonary oedema Adult respiratory distress syndrome
	Tension pneumothorax	From trauma (including iatrogenic) ruptured emphysematous bulla
Cardiac	Ventricular fibrillation Asystole	Follow Resuscitation Council (UK) guidelines for treatment of cardiac arrest
	Electromechanical dissociation	Look for treatable cause: tension pneumothorax, cardiac tamponade, hypoxia or hypovolaemia, drug overdose
	Cardiogenic shock or failure	Acute myocardial infarct Arrhythmia Pulmonary embolism Cardiac contusions after blunt chest trauma Valve rupture
Vascular	Hypovolaemic shock	Revealed or concealed haemorrhage Diarrhoea and vomiting Fistulae Heat exhaustion
	Anaphylactic shock	From stings and bites, drugs or iodine-containing contrast used for radiological investigation
	Dissecting thoracic aorta	Usually in previously hypertensive patients, pain radiates to back
	Leaking abdominal aortic aneurysm	Always check femoral pulses so that you consider aortic pathology (although pulses may not be lost)
	Septic shock	Initially massive peripheral vasodilation: 'warm shock'. Temperature may be normal
	Neurogenic shock	From loss of sympathetic vascular tone in cervical or high thoracic spinal cord injury
Gastrointestinal	Haemorrhage Perforated peptic ulcer Pancreatitis Mesenteric embolism	Always check serum amylase Abdominal signs may be absent initially

Table 1.5 (contd.)

System	Diagnosis	Notes
Gynaecological	Ruptured ectopic pregnancy	Usually at 4–6 weeks' gestation. Always think of diagnosis in collapsed young woman
Obstetric	Supine hypotension	The gravid uterus obstructs venous return from the vena cava unless the pregnant woman is turned onto her left side
	Eclampsia	
	Pulmonary embolism	
	Amniotic fluid embolism	
Neurological	Head injury	Isolated head injuries do not cause shock in adults. Look for sites of blood loss elsewhere
	Infection	Meningitis in children (often meningococcal in UK), tetanus, botulism, poliomyelitis, rabies
	Cerebrovascular	Intracranial embolism or haemorrhage. Subarachnoid haemorrhage may present solely as a severe headache
	Epilepsy	Including the postictal state
	Poisoning	See Table 1.6
	Alcohol	
Haematological	Sickle cell crisis	May lead to respiratory failure
	Malaria	Cerebral malaria causes coma
	Coagulopathy	Thrombocytopenia may present with bleeding
Metabolic	Hypoglycaemia	Check blood glucose in *every* patient
	Hyperglycaemia	Coma may be first presentation of diabetes mellitus
	Hyponatraemia	May be Addisonian crisis
	Hypocalcaemia	May present with fits
	Hepatic failure	Precipitated by paracetamol overdose in previously fit people, and by intestinal haemorrhage, drugs, or high-protein diet in those with chronic liver disease
	Renal failure	Pre-renal from dehydration. Renal, e.g. from crush syndrome and myoglobinuria. Post-renal from ureteric obstruction (dangerous hyperkalaemia causes tall tented T waves and widening of the QRS complexes)
	Hypothermia	Resuscitation may include passive or active core rewarming. Sepsis and hypovolaemia often coexist
Endocrine	Addisonian crisis	Give 200 mg hydrocortisone i.v. (hypotension, low serum sodium, raised serum potassium)
	Myxoedema	Always consider in hypothermic patients

that are easily missed, with dire consequences for the patient (Table 1.6).

If the gag reflex is depressed the patient cannot protect his own airway. Provided he is breathing spontaneously, place the patient in the recovery position on his side (ensure first there is no evidence whatever of a spinal injury). Otherwise intubate the trachea in order to protect the lungs. This applies if the patient is to receive gastric lavage and cannot protect his own airway with complete certainty. If gastric contents are aspirated into the lungs they must be promptly sucked out because they produce a chemical pneumonitis and bacterial pneumonia. The clinical picture may well develop into adult respiratory distress syndrome (ARDS).

Rhabdomyolysis and myoglobinuria may develop in any comatose patient after prolonged tissue pressure and muscle ischaemia, which is then relieved. Local swelling of muscles may be evident and compartment

Table 1.6 Common drugs and poisons

Drug	Symptoms and signs	Treatment
Paracetamol	Liver and renal failure, hypoglycaemia May be asymptomatic initially	Charcoal Acetylcysteine
Salicylates	Tinnitus, abdominal pain Vomiting, hypoglycaemia, hyperthermia, sweating Acid–base disturbances	Lavage and charcoal Rehydration Urinary alkalization haemodialysis
Tricyclic antidepressants	Arrhythmias and hypotension Dilated pupils, convulsions Coma	Lavage and charcoal Cardiopulmonary support Sodium bicarbonate
Benzodiazepines	Respiratory depression	(Flumazenil)
Opiates	Pinpoint pupils Loss of consciousness Respiratory depression Needle marks	Respiratory agent Naloxone
Phenothiazines	Dyskinesia, torticollis	Procyclidine
Lignocaine	Tingling tongue Perioral paraesthesia Convulsions Ventricular fibrillation	Cardiopulmonary support Diazepam for convulsions
Carbon monoxide	33% of fatal poisoning in UK insidious from inefficient gas fires Nausea and vomiting Headache, drowsiness Hallucinations, convulsions	100% or hyperbaric oxygen
Cyanide	Headache, vomiting, weakness Tachypnoea, convulsions Coma	Amyl nitrate inhalation Dicobalt edetate i.v.
Iron	Hypotension, vasodilatation Gastric haemorrhage	Lavage Desferrioxamine
Organophosphates (pesticides, nerve gases)	Nausea, vomiting, diarrhoea Salivation, pulmonary oedema Pinpoint pupils, convulsions, coma	Lavage Atropine Pyridostigmine

syndromes can develop because of positional obstruction of the circulation. Muscle death starts after 4 hours of complete ischaemia.

Look for the early symptoms and signs of pain and paraesthesiae in a pallid, cool, weak limb. Passively extend the fingers or flex the foot to test for a developing compartment syndrome (anterior tibial compartment syndrome is the commonest). Losses of distal pulses, numbness, paralysis and development of a flexion contracture are all late signs.

With myoglobinuria ensure that the urinary output is maintained at over 100 ml h^{-1} in an adult, or $2 \text{ ml kg}^{-1} \text{ h}^{-1}$ in a child. Alkalinization of the urine increases the excretion of myoglobin, and will help prevent renal failure.

Summary

1. Patients are often brought into the resuscitation room in a physical condition which is very alarming to the inexperienced trainee. Unless the patient is rapidly transported to the operating theatre, adhere to the methodical sequence of Primary Survey with Initial Resuscitation (see Part 1, above), Monitoring (see Part 2, above), Secondary Survey (see Part 3, above) while the patient is in the resuscitation room of the A&E department. By having a known sequence of procedures to go through you and the nurse will gain confidence as the resuscitation continues, and you will not miss pathology. The patient then has the best chance of survival and also the least chance of morbidity.

2. Keep an open mind as to the cause of the clinical signs. Monitor the vital signs and level of consciousness, and do not jump to preconceived conclusions – this is all too easy to do under pressure. If there is any clinical deterioration return to the basic initial sequence of the primary survey and recheck AIRWAY, BREATHING, CIRCULATION yet again.

3. Do not allow the patient to leave the A&E department without stable vital signs, appropriate intravenous lines in place, and having been thoroughly examined, unless there is an acceptable reason. A patient may all too easily deteriorate clinically in the X-ray room or, even more dangerously by reasons of secluded space, in the computed tomography (CT) scanner.

4. Patients with a diminished level of consciousness must be seen by an anaesthetist, at the very latest before they leave the A&E department. Patients must be in the best possible clinically supported condition for transportation, whether their journey is to the CT scanner, to a ward or to another hospital. If necessary the patient must be ventilated, depending on the length of journey and the vehicle employed, and must be accompanied by appropriate attendants such as an anaesthetist.

5. Strictly adhere to standard guidelines for protection of medical and nursing staff from contamination with body fluids: wear gloves, waterproof gowns and masks with visors. Staff must be immunized against hepatitis B virus.

6. Keep clear, precise medical records of any resuscitation sequence, remembering that since 1 November 1991 patients or their relatives have had the legal right to see medical records. This record keeping is the responsibility of the senior doctor present. Take appropriate care with forensic evidence, especially from terrorist incidents – anything removed from victims must be removed by a named person and must also be handed to a named person who personally seals the item in a labelled bag.

7. There must be at the very least a doctor of registrar grade in command of the resuscitation team. For an A&E department to receive patients who need immediate resuscitation from a 'blue-light' ambulance, the hospital must have a minimum of an anaesthetic registrar, a medical registrar and a surgical registrar 'living in' on-site 24 hours a day. Even if the patient does not survive you will be able to tell the relatives truthfully that everything possible was done.

   Both medical audit and medicolegal considerations dictate the above minimal adequate standards of care. All doctors who are expected to resuscitate the collapsed patient as part of their work practice are expected to be trained in the above. This is your responsibility, but more especially of the supervising consultant and above all of the employing authority.

Further reading

Advanced Life Support Course Sub-Committee. 1998 Advanced Life Support Course Provider Manual. 3rd edn. Resuscitation Council UK

Advanced Life Support Group. 1997 Advanced Paediatric Life Support. 2nd edn. BMJ Publishing Group

Advanced Trauma Life Support Course Manual 1998. American College of Surgeons

Driscoll P, Brown T, Gwinnutt C, Wardle T 1997 A simple guide to blood gas analysis. BMJ Publishing Group

Driscoll P, Gwinnutt C, Jimmerson CL, Goodall O 1993 Trauma resuscitation. MacMillan

Evans T R 1995 ABC of resuscitation. British Medical Association, London

Henry JA 1997 Poisoning. In: Skinner D, Swain A, Peyton R, Robertson C (eds) Cambridge textbook of accident and emergency. Cambridge University Press, Cambridge

Jones R M 1989 Drug therapy in cardiopulmonary resuscitation. In: Baskett P J F (ed) Cardiopulmonary resuscitation. Elsevier, Amsterdam p 99–101

Royal College of Physicians of London 1991 Some aspects of the medical management of casualties of the Gulf War. February

Skinner D, Driscoll P, Earlam R. 1996 ABC of major trauma. British Medical Journal, London

Touquet R, Fothergill J, Henry JA, Harris NH (in press) Accident and emergency medicine. In: Powers MJ, Harris NH (eds) Medical negligence 3rd edn. Butterworths, London

APPENDIX: CHEMICAL WEAPONS

In the 1990–91 Gulf War it was considered possible that the chemical weapons of nerve gases and mustard gas would be used.

Nerve gases (e.g. Tabun)

These agents are organophosphorus compounds which act by inhibiting the enzyme acetylcholinesterase and therefore preventing the breakdown of acetylcholine at motor endplates. The symptoms and signs are the same as for organophosphorus insecticide poisoning (i.e. overactivity of the parasympathetic system and paralysis of the muscles of respiration). Early treatment involves the reversal of the effects of acetylcholine at muscurinic receptors by atropine, 2 mg being given intravenously every 10–15 minutes in severe poisoning. Management also involves the support of respiration, the reactivation of inhibited acetylcholinesterase by oximes (pralidoxime mesylate) and the suppression of convulsions by diazepam. Pretreatment with pyridostigmine (reversible inhibitor of acetylcholinesterase) protects a proportion of the total quantity of enzyme present against a subsequent attack by nerve gas.

Mustard gas (sulphur mustard)

Exposure to the liquid or vapour produces blistering of the skin and damage to the cornea and conjunctiva. Classically there is an asymptomatic latent period of up to 6 hours, before reddening of the skin, leading to blistering. Burns are initially superficial, and blister fluid does not contain free sulphur mustard.

Eye damage usually resolves over a number of weeks, but treat with saline irrigations, mydriatics, vaseline to prevent sticking of the eyelids, dark glasses and antibiotic drops.

Inhalation produces damage to the upper respiratory tract, with sloughing of the epithelium of the airways and nasal passages. The most severely affected patients need assisted ventilation with oxygen. Absorption leads to depression of the bone marrow and a fall in the white count, with a maximum effect at about 2 weeks post-exposure.

In the First World War the death rate from mustard gas was 2% of those exposed, resulting from burns, respiratory damage and bone marrow depression.

We are grateful to Professor J. A. Henry for his advice on toxicology.

2

Trauma

P. A. Driscoll, C. G McMahon

Objectives

- **Describe the biomechanics of injury commonly seen in clinical practice.**
- **Revise those aspects of human anatomy important in trauma care.**
- **Discuss the normal and pathophysiological response to trauma.**
- **Quantify trauma severity by using the anatomical and physiological assessments.**

INTRODUCTION

As a result of a number of primary, secondary and tertiary initiatives there has been a gradual fall in the number of UK deaths and serious injuries following trauma. A good example of this is seen in the case of road traffic accidents (RTA) (Table 2.1). Between 1974 and 1993 the number of fatalities has fallen by 45% to 3814 and the number of seriously injured by 52% to 45 009. In contrast, the number of minor injuries has risen by around 9% to 257 000.

Even with these improvements, trauma remains a major cause of death in this country, only being surpassed by ischaemic heart disease and carcinoma. Irrespective of gender, it is the leading cause of death in people aged 1–35 years and accounts for 8.3% of all potential years of life lost under age 75. In England and Wales, approximately 11 500 people die each year; over a half of these deaths are as a result of road traffic accidents, and just over a third occur at home. In addition to these fatalities, trauma also gives rise to a much larger group of people who remain permanently disabled. It is estimated that for every trauma death there are approximately 2–3 victims who are disabled, a proportion of whom will require continuing health-care facilities for life.

Clearly this has financial implications. Recent estimates indicate that trauma care could account for up to 7% of all hospital care and be responsible for 7% of all NHS expenditure.

Trimodal distribution of death following trauma

Over a decade ago, Trunkey, an American pioneer in studying trauma, showed that trauma deaths in San Francisco followed a trimodal distribution over time.

Table 2.1 Initiatives in reducing RTA trauma

Initiative	Definition	Examples
Primary	Prevents the RTA occurring	Better roads, speed restrictions, better car brakes, drink driving legislation
Secondary	Reduces the effect of the collision	Seat belts, air bags, pedestrian-'friendly' cars
Tertiary	Improvements in medical care	Speedy and effective resuscitation, integrated trauma care, early rehabilitation

The first peak occurred at, or shortly after, the time of injury. These patients died of major neurological or vascular injury and most were unsalvageable with current technology. However, it is estimated that up to 40% of these injuries could be avoided by various prevention programmes.

The second peak occurred several hours after the injury. These patients commonly died from airway, breathing or circulatory problems and many were potentially treatable. This period became known as the 'golden hour', to emphasize the time following injury when optimum resuscitation and stabilization are critical.

The final peak occurred days or weeks after the injury. These victims died from multi-system organ failure (MSOF), sepsis syndrome or septic shock. It is now known that sub-optimal resuscitation in the immediate or early post-injury phase leads to an increased incidence of mortality and morbidity during this phase.

> Recent work indicates that the relative sizes of these peaks varies between countries. In Scotland the first peak accounts for 76% of all the trauma deaths, the second 7% and the third 17%. This contrasts with San Francisco's figures of 50%, 30% and 20% respectively.

BIOMECHANICS OF INJURY

Trauma can be divided into categories depending upon its causative mechanism:

- Blunt
- Penetrating
- Burns
- Blast.

BLUNT TRAUMA

> Over 90% of trauma in the UK is a result of a blunt mechanism.

This mechanism of injury dissipates its force over a wide area, minimizing the energy transfer at any one spot and so reducing tissue damage. In low-energy impacts, the clinical consequences are dependent on the organs involved. In contrast, when high energies are involved, considerable tissue disruption can be produced, irrespective of the underlying organs.

Blunt trauma gives rise to three types of force:

1. *Shearing* results from two forces acting in opposite directions. Skin lacerations and abrasions following this tend to be irregular and have a higher risk of infection. They are also associated with more damage to the surrounding tissue and more excessive scarring than low energy penetrating trauma.

With regard to the abdominal viscera, shearing forces have a maximal effect at the points where the organs are tethered down. Common examples include the peritoneal attachments at the duodenojejunal flexure, the spleen and the ileocaecal junction, as well as the vascular attachments of the liver.

2. *Tension* occurs when a force hits a tissue surface at an angle of less than 90°. It gives rise to avulsions and flap formation. Both are associated with more tissue damage and necrosis than that found after a shearing force.

3. *Compression* follows a force hitting a tissue surface at 90° and can result in significant damage and necrosis of the underlying structures. The site of the impact can usually be identified by the presence of contusion, haematoma (if a significant number of blood vessels are damaged), and possibly a breach in the surface tissue. In addition to this direct damage, compression forces may produce a sufficient rise in internal pressure to rupture the outer layer of closed gas or fluid-filled organs such as the bowel.

A combination of these forces frequently contributes to the pattern of injury seen in victims of blunt trauma. Typically multiple injuries occur, with usually one system being severely affected and one to two other areas damaged to a lesser degree. Overall, the UK incidence of life-threatening injuries in different systems is: head 50.2%, chest 21.8%, abdomen 23.9% and spine 8.55%. In excess of 69% of trauma victims also have orthopaedic injuries, but these are not usually life threatening.

Determining how these various forces result in patient injury is complicated. However, an important clue can be gained from members of the emergency services who have had the opportunity to inspect the scene. For example, a frontal impact with a 'bulls-eye' pattern on the windscreen, a collapsed steering column and indentations on the dashboard indicate that the driver of this vehicle may have sustained the following injuries:

- Facial fractures
- Obstructed airway
- Cervical injury
- Cardiac contusion

- Pneumothorax
- Flail chest/fractured ribs
- Liver and/or splenic injury
- Posterior dislocation of the hip
- Acetabular fracture
- Fractured femur
- Patella fracture
- Carpometacarpal injuries
- Tarsometatarsal injuries.

Following a frontal impact, the patient is at risk of sustaining a flexion–distraction type injury to the lumbar vertebrae if only a lap seat belt has been worn. This can produce a Chance fracture in addition to some or all of the injuries listed above. Motorcyclists, pedestrians and victims ejected from a car have a significant risk of multiple injuries, including head, spinal, wrist and lower limb damage.

A completely different pattern of injuries is produced in the patient who has sustained a rapid deceleration injury following a fall from a height onto a solid surface. If the victim lands on his feet, the following injuries could be expected:

- Tarsometatarsal injuries
- Calcaneal compression fractures
- Ankle fracture
- Tibial plateau fractures
- Pelvic vertical shear fracture
- Vertebral wedge fracture
- Cervical injury
- Rupture of the thoracic aorta
- Tracheo-bronchial disruption
- Liver avulsion.

It follows that with knowledge of the mechanism of injury, the clinician will be in a position to consider the presence of potentially life-threatening secondary injuries which may not be immediately apparent (see Ch. 1). It can also give a clue as to the degree of energy transfer and, consequently, the level of tissue damage. Mechanisms that indicate a high energy transfer are:

- Road traffic accident
- Falls from a height
- Crushing.

> Knowing the mechanism of injury, the clinician can estimate the degree of energy transfer as well as suspect particular patterns of injuries.

PENETRATING TRAUMA

> Around 7% of the annual trauma deaths in the UK are a result of a penetrating mechanism.

The clinical consequences of penetrating trauma are dependent on both energy transfer and anatomical factors.

Energy transfer

Several factors affect the degree of energy transferred to tissues surrounding the track of the weapon or missile:

- The kinetic energy of the weapon or missile
- The mean presenting area of the weapon or missile
- The weapon or missile's tendency to deform and fragment
- Density of the tissues
- Mechanical characteristics of the tissues.

It follows that if the missile has a high velocity (e.g. a rifle bullet), then it will carry a considerable amount of kinetic energy, even though its mass may be small. It is important to realize that the crucial speed is the impact velocity (i.e. the speed of the missile when it hits the patient), not its initial velocity (i.e. the speed of the projectile when it leaves the barrel of the gun). Unlike the bullet, a knife has a much lower kinetic energy, because it is travelling at a much slower speed.

The neighbouring tissues may be injured when the kinetic energy of the missile is transferred to the surrounding structures. If the missile impacts in the tissue and fails to exit, all the kinetic energy will be transferred, and the maximum amount of damage will have been achieved for that particular missile. The chances of this occurring increase considerably if the missile tumbles or fragments once it enters the tissues.

With high energy transfer, neighbouring tissues are pushed away from the missile track and a temporary cavity is created. Although this lasts only a few milliseconds it can reach 30–40 times the diameter of the missile, depending on the amount of energy transferred to these tissues and their elastic properties. As the energy waves dissipate, the tissues rapidly retract to a permanent cavity formed by the immediate destruction of tissue in the direct path of the missile.

This has three consequences. Firstly, there is functional and mechanical disruption of the neighbouring tissues. The extent is related to energy transfer and the tissue characteristics. Solid organs, such as the liver and spleen, sustain more damage than the lungs and other low-density organs such as muscle, skin and blood vessels. These tissues have greater elastic properties, which minimizes the amount of damage they sustain.

Secondly, a core of any clothing that was originally over the skin surface is carried in front of the missile deep into the wound. The higher the velocity of the projectile, the finer the shearing of material and the wider it is spread. Further contamination can be caused by material being sucked into the wound from the negative pressure at the missile's exit site. These grossly contaminated wounds have a high chance of becoming infected.

Thirdly, as a general rule, if a missile traverses a narrow part of the body, then the exit wound is usually larger than the entry one. This is due to the temporary cavitation effect extending along the wound track. Conversely, the temporary cavitation effect would have finished if the missile had given up enough kinetic energy to behave as a low-energy missile before it left the body. Nevertheless, there are no absolute certainties, and variations in the relative sizes of exit and entry wounds are well recognized.

Anatomical factors

An incision produced by low-energy penetrating trauma (e.g. a stab wound) results in a wound with little oedema and inflammation which heals quickly and with minimum scarring (see Ch. 30). However, low-energy transfer injuries can still be fatal, for example a stab wound to the heart. Consequently, the significance of a penetrating wound is also dependent upon the type and extent of the organs involved.

BURNS

> Fire and flames account for 5% of the annual trauma deaths in the UK.

Thermal

These are the most common type of burns and are caused by heat from flames, scalds and contact with hot surfaces or flashes. Children and the elderly are the most frequent victims, but scalds are also the most prevalent type of industrial burn.

Electrical

There are several factors that affect the severity of the injury:

- Type of current (AC or DC)
- The voltage of the shock
- Duration of the contact
- Resistance of the tissues
- The pathway in which the current travels.

Although the entrance and exit wounds are treated as thermal wounds, they do not give an accurate indication of the extent of the burn. This is because the electric current will have travelled through the body along the path of least resistance. For example, skin is highly resistant and consequently the current travels preferentially along arteries, veins, nerves, bones and tendons. It follows that the true extent of the tissue damage cannot be measured on superficial inspection.

BLAST INJURIES

Following the detonation of a bomb, there is a sudden release of considerable energy. Initially, there is an almost instantaneous rise in pressure in the surrounding air known as the *shock front* (or blast wave). This moves through the surrounding air in all directions, faster than the speed of sound. As it spreads out it gets weaker as the distance from the edge of the band to the epicentre of the explosion increases.

Behind the shock front comes the *blast wind*, which is movement of the air itself. As the blast wind rapidly spreads out from the epicentre, it carries fragments, either from the bomb or from surrounding debris. In view of the velocity at which they are travelling, many of these fragments can produce 'high energy transfer' wounds.

Bomb blasts can therefore injure people in a variety of ways:

Primary effect

This is a result of the shock front and mainly affects air-containing organs such as the lung. bowel and ears. Once the band of pressure hits the surface of the body it causes distortion, the magnitude and rate of onset of which has a direct effect on the extent of the tissue damage. In particular, the higher the rate, the bigger the pressure wave traversing the body. It is these waves which produce most of the damage associated with 'blast' lung, gut and tympanic membrane, with most of the pathology occurring at the air–tissue boundary. Pathological features of 'blast' lung, gut and tympanic membrane are:

- Haemorrhage into alveolar spaces
- Damage to alveolar septae
- Stripping of bronchial epithelium
- Emphysematous blebs produced on the pleural surface

- Contusion of the gut wall
- Leakage of blood into the gut lumen
- Perforation
- Rupture or congestion of the tympanic membrane.

If these pulmonary changes are extensive, a ventilation–perfusion (V/Q) mismatch will develop and hypoxia will result. High blast pressures may also lead to air emboli and, if they obstruct the cerebral or coronary arteries, sudden death can occur.

Secondary effects

These are the result of the direct impact of fragments carried in the blast wind. In most explosions, the lethal area for these fragments is much greater than that of the shock front. Furthermore, at distances outside this area, they can still produce considerable damage. The patient usually presents with multiple, extensive wounds of varying depth, which are grossly contaminated. As the distance from the epicentre increases, the wounds become more superficial.

Tertiary effects

These are a result of the dynamic force of the wind itself, which can be so great as to carry all or part of the patient along with it. This results in impact (deceleration) injuries and, in extreme cases, amputations.

In addition to these effects, the patient may also sustain injuries from falling masonry, as well as fires, toxic chemicals and flash burns. Acute and chronic psychological disturbances resulting from explosions are also well recognized.

> In addition to the primary effects, blasts can give rise to penetrating, blunt and burn trauma.

RELEVANT ANATOMY

In addition to being aware of the biomechanics, the clinician should understand how the anatomical relationship of the body can have a profound effect on the type of injuries the patient sustains. Listed below are the more relevant aspects of each body system with regard to trauma. These are dealt with in the order in which they tend to be managed clinically:

- Airway
- Thorax
- Circulation
- Skull

- Face
- Abdomen and genitourinary system
- Bony pelvis
- Limbs
- Spinal column
- Skin.

AIRWAY

The important structures and surface landmarks of the upper airway are shown in Figure 2.1.

THORAX

Chest wall

The upper two ribs are extensively protected by the scapula and overlying muscle. Consequently, the patient has to be subjected to a considerable force for these structures to be broken. Therefore, when breaks do occur, there is a high chance of coexisting damage to vital structures such as the thoracic aorta, the main bronchi, the lungs and the spinal cord. It follows that the clinician must closely assess these vital structures if

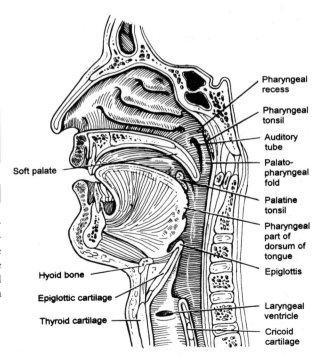

Labels:
Pharyngeal recess
Pharyngeal tonsil
Auditory tube
Palato-pharyngeal fold
Palatine tonsil
Pharyngeal part of dorsum of tongue
Epiglottis
Laryngeal ventricle
Cricoid cartilage
Soft palate
Hyoid bone
Epiglottic cartilage
Thyroid cartilage

Fig 2.1 Line diagram of the upper airway.

fractures to the first two ribs are discovered during the resuscitation.

It is also important to remember that the top is mobile and the pleural cavity and apex of the lung can project above the clavicle. Consequently, a pneumothorax or lung injury may occur following penetrating injuries to the lower neck. Similarly the lower six ribs overlie the abdominal cavity when the diaphragm is elevated during expiration. Therefore trauma in this area may cause injury to both the lung and the upper abdominal viscera.

The incidence of abdominal visceral involvement following penetrating injury to the lower chest is dependent upon the weapon used. With stabbings it is 15% but with shootings it rises to 46%.

> Trauma to the 'midzone' of the trunk may be associated with both abdominal and chest injuries.

A flail segment is when two or more ribs are fractured in two or more places. It also applies to the situation when the clavicle and first rib are similarly affected. In this case paradoxical movement of the chest may be visible on inspection. Nevertheless, in the early stages, the spasm of the chest wall musculature will splint these fractures, and so eliminate this sign. Later, however, the muscles fatigue and paradoxical movement becomes apparent. A flail segment can be a life-threatening condition, particularly if there is an underlying pulmonary contusion which adds to the hypoxia already produced as a result of the impaired ventilation.

As the neurovascular bundle lies underneath the ribs in the subcostal groove, these structures can be torn when ribs are fractured. When there are several fractures and/or significant disruption this can give rise to a massive haemothorax. Other sources include the internal mammary artery and large lacerations of the lung surface which do not stop bleeding once the lung has been re-expanded following the insertion of a chest drain.

Trauma can lead to a one-way valve developing on the lung surface, allowing air into the pleural cavity during inspiration but blocking its escape during expiration. This will give rise to a tension pneumothorax unless the intrapleural pressure is relieved.

Mediastinum

The trachea, oesophagus and major blood vessels lie in close proximity to one another in the mediastinum. Consequently, penetrating injuries in this area may damage one or more of these structures. The surface landmarks of the mediastinum are medial to the nipple line anteriorly, or medial to the medial edges of the scapulae posteriorly.

CIRCULATION

The heart is covered with the tough, inelastic fibrous pericardium. In the healthy state, even a small collection of blood within the pericardium could create a pericardial tamponade, compromising ventricular filling and hence cardiac output. This condition usually follows penetrating trauma of the heart.

Blunt trauma to the heart can give rise to cardiac contusion which, due to its anatomical location, may be associated with an overlying sternal fracture. This condition can lead to coronary artery occlusion due to a combination of vascular spasm, neighbouring tissue oedema and intimal tearing. As a result of the myocardial ischaemia, the patient may develop dysrhythmias, infarction and impaired cardiac performance (see below). Significant blunt trauma can also rupture the chordae tendinae and, therefore, produce mitral or tricuspid incompetence.

The distal part of the arch of the aorta is anchored just inferior to the left subclavian artery. Patients who sustain deceleration injury have a significant risk of aortic disruption due to the mobile aortic arch shearing off the fixed descending aorta. Examples of this mechanism of injury include crashes over 30 m.p.h. or falls over 30 feet. In 10% of cases a thoracic aortic disruption results but the escaping blood is contained by the outer (adventitial) layer of the aorta. With time, however, this outer layer is also breached, and the patient will rapidly exsanguinate without surgical intervention.

SKULL

The scalp is made up of five layers:

- Skin
- Subcutaneous layer
- Aponeurosis
- Loose (areolar) layer
- Periosteum.

(A useful mnemonic to help remember these layers is SCALP.) The subcutaneous layer is very vascular and is divided into loculi by fibrous bands. The areolar layer is much looser and therefore has a greater capacity for expansion. This is the layer where scalp haematomas usually collect. Scalp wounds tend to pout open if the aponeurosis is breached.

The inside of the neurocranium is divided into two levels by a fibrous structure called the tentorium cerebelli ('tent'). The midbrain passes through the opening in the anterior aspect of this layer and is partially covered on its anterolateral aspects by the corticospinal tract. The oculomotor nerve leaves the anterior aspect of the midbrain and runs forward lying between the free and attached edges of the tent. In the intact state, there is free communication above and below the tentorium as well as between the intracranial and spinal subarachnoid spaces.

Following head trauma, the development of a mass lesion above the tent (e.g. from a haematoma or cerebral oedema) can cause a pressure gradient to develop. If this is unrelieved it can result in one or both medial surfaces of the temporal lobes herniating through the opening in the tent. In so doing, this brain tissue presses on, and damages, structures in this region, namely the oculomotor nerve and motor fibres in the corticospinal tract. This is called *tentorial herniation* and results in an ipsilateral fixed dilated pupil and contralateral weakness in the limbs. If the pressure increases further, the medulla and cerebellum are forced downwards into the foramen magnum – a process known as *coning*. This is a preterminal condition resulting in compression of the vital centres, and disturbance of cardiovascular and respiratory function.

The base of the neurocranium is irregular, with the sphenoid wings and the petrous processes projecting from its surface. Following acceleration and deceleration forces, the brain moves over the base of the skull. Consequently, its inferior surface can be damaged by colliding with these two large projections.

The internal surface of the neurocranium is lined with a thick, hard, fibrous cover called the *dura mater* (Fig. 2.2). Its blood supply is closely adherent to the bone surface and even grooves it in places. Consequently these vessels can be torn when forces are applied to the overlying bone. The resulting haematoma collects between the bone and dura and is known as an *extradural haematoma*; 90% of these are associated with a fractured skull. The middle meningeal artery is the vessel most prone to this type of injury and the thin temporoparietal area is the commonest site.

The arachnoid mater is connected to the pia mater, across the cerebrospinal fluid (CSF)-filled subarachnoid space, by thin fibrous strands. Running between these strands are bridging veins which carry blood from the brain to the venous sinuses. With age, the brain atrophies and the subarachnoid and subdural spaces increase. This stretches the bridging veins and makes them more likely to tear following a head injury. The bleeding which results collects in the subdural and subarachnoid spaces.

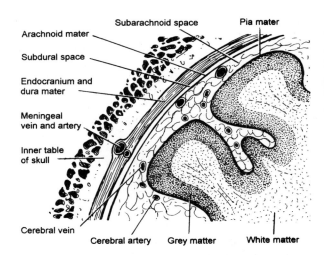

Fig 2.2 Line diagram of the meninges and their blood supply.

MAXILLOFACIAL SKELETON

> The major acute problem associated with significant facial fractures is the potential for associated airway obstruction secondary to haemorrhage and structural damage.

This consists of a complex series of mainly aerated bones which provide a firm but light foundation to the face (Fig. 2.3). The nasal, frontal and zygomatic–maxillary buttresses provide vertical support, with lateral stability coming from the zygomatic–temporal buttresses. Several of these bones, especially those making up the bony orbits, are closely associated with nerves and blood vessels which can consequently be damaged when these bones are broken or crushed following trauma. In addition, the associated bleeding and deformity can lead to obstruction of the patient's airway.

Nasoethmoidal–orbital fractures

These occur with trauma to the bridge of the nose or medial orbital wall. In view of their location they are associated with lacrimal injury, dural tears and traumatic telecanthus.

Blow-out fractures

When a blunt object hits the globe it can cause the intraorbital pressure to rise such that the thin orbital

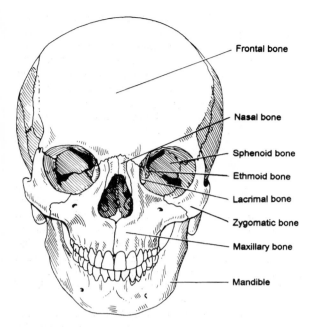

Fig 2.3 Line diagram of the facial skeleton (individual bones labelled).

floor breaks. It is commonly associated with a fracture of the medial orbital wall. The infraorbital nerve is usually damaged in the process, giving rise to anaesthesia of the cheek, upper lip and upper gum. Diplopia, especially to upward gaze, is also common and results from a combination of muscle haematoma, third nerve damage, entrapment of periorbital fat and, in a minority of cases, true entrapment of extraocular muscles. Subcutaneous emphysema occurs if the fracture extends into a sinus or nasal antrum.

Zygomatic complex fractures

Blunt trauma can produce two types of zygomatic fracture. Zygomatic arch fractures are produced by a direct blow and can give rise to an open bite due to the fracture impinging on the temporomandibular joint. The more serious 'tripod' type of fracture involves the displacement of the whole zygoma. This bone can be compared to a four-legged stool with the 'legs' being the floor and lateral wall of the orbit, the zygomatic arch and the lateral wall of the antrum. The 'seat' of the stool cannot be moved without displacement of at least two of the 'legs'. This is associated with lateral subconjunctival haemorrhage and infraorbital anaesthesia. In addition, the displacement leads to a downward angulation of the lateral canthus and either trismus or an open bite.

Fractures of the middle third of the facial skeleton

It takes approximately 100 times the force of gravity to break the middle third of the face. Consequently, patients with this condition have significant multisystem trauma in addition to the malocclusion, facial anaesthesia and visual symptoms described above.

Traditionally, the fractures are classified using the Le Fort system (Fig. 2.4). It should be remembered, however, that the grade of fracture is often asymmetrical (i.e. different on the right and left sides). The Le Fort I fracture runs in a transverse plane above the alveolar ridge to the pterygoid region. Le Fort II extends from the nasal bones into the medial orbital wall and crosses the infraorbital rim. Le Fort III detaches the middle third of the facial skeleton from the cranial base; it is therefore commonly associated with fractures of the base of the skull and bloody CSF rhinorrhoea and otorrhoea. A characteristic 'dish face' may be evident due to retropositioning of the midface along the base of the skull.

Mandibular fractures

These are the second most common facial fractures after nasal fractures. As with the pelvis, the mandible is a ring structure and is therefore rarely fractured in isola-

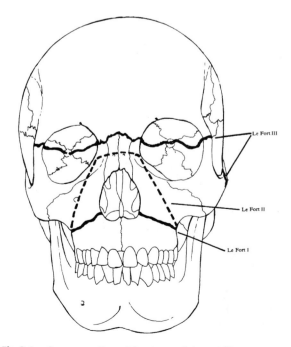

Fig 2.4 Common sites of fracture of the midface.

tion. Usually there are multiple fractures or an injury to the temporomandibular joint. Common fracture sites are the condylar process, through the posterior alveolar margin, and through the alveolar margin anterior to the premolar teeth. In both of the latter cases the fracture extends to the lower border of the mandible (Fig. 2.5). Numbness of the lower lip on the affected side and mal-occlusion are common findings.

ABDOMEN AND GENITOURINARY SYSTEM

The contents of the abdomen occupy the following regions:

- Peritoneal cavity
- Retroperitoneum
- Pelvis.

Peritoneal cavity

This can be subdivided further into intrathoracic and abdominal regions. It is important to remember, however, that on expiration, the diaphragm rises to the level of the fourth intercostal space. As a result, several of the 'peritoneal' organs, such as the liver, spleen and stomach, actually lie within the bony thorax and are therefore at risk of injury if the patient suffers trauma to the lower chest.

Diaphragm

Injury to this structure is uncommon, but may result from both blunt and penetrating trauma. The former

tends to occur with greater force than the latter. It also commonly leads to larger tears in the diaphragm through which abdominal contents may enter the thorax. Injuries to the diaphragm may be so slight that the patient is asymptomatic and the damage not discovered until weeks, months or even years later. In contrast, when the tear in the diaphragm is large, the abdominal contents may herniate into the thoracic cavity, compromising the patient's respiration.

Liver and biliary tree

This is covered over a large part of its surface by the rib cage, which affords it some protection from injury. Although numerically less common than splenic injury, liver injuries account for more deaths as a result of unsuspected intra-abdominal haemorrhage. A high index of suspicion is essential when assessing trauma victims. Therefore, any injury to the right lower chest or upper abdomen should alert you to the possibility of underlying liver damage.

Due to their location, the gallbladder and extrahepatic biliary tract are usually damaged in association with other viscera. Liver trauma is the most common coexisting pathology (50% of cases), but there is a significant chance of the pancreas also being injured (17% of cases). As a consequence of this, the clinical presentation of trauma to the gallbladder and biliary tree is usually masked by symptoms resulting from damage to the surrounding viscera. This condition has an overall mortality of 16% due to coexisting organ injuries. Blunt trauma is the usual cause of gallbladder damage, and rupture is more likely when the gallbladder is distended, such as between meals.

Spleen

As the spleen is the most commonly injured solid organ in the abdomen following blunt trauma, it is a frequent cause of shock in patients with abdominal injury. Any trauma to the left lower chest or upper abdomen may lead to splenic damage ranging from small tears to complete shattering of the organ.

Bowel

Injury to the stomach following blunt trauma is rare. However, the stomach is sometimes damaged as a result of penetrating trauma, and usually presents as peritonitis. Damage to the small bowel may result from both blunt and penetrating trauma, as well as blast injuries.

Blunt trauma and blasts commonly cause bowel injury in one of three ways. Firstly, the force may squeeze the viscus between the anterior abdominal wall

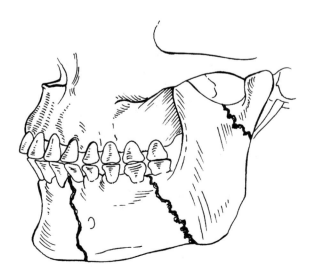

Fig 2.5   Common sites of fracture of the mandible.

and the vertebral column. Secondly, the bowel may rupture as a result of a sudden increase in pressure within the lumen, such as may occur when the abdomen is compressed (the closed-loop phenomenon). Finally, the bowel may become ischaemic because of damage to the mesentery and its arteries. This usually arises when the abdomen is subjected to deceleration or shearing forces, and is particularly common at points where the bowel crosses the interface between the intra- and retroperitoneum. Examples of the latter include the duodenojejunal flexure and the ileocaecal junction. Blast injuries can also lead to multiple intestinal perforations and areas of infarction.

Penetrating injury to the bowel usually results in small tears in the bowel wall. Occasionally, the bowel may become completely transected.

Unlike injuries to the liver and spleen, trauma to the bowel is rarely immediately life-threatening. As with the stomach, the major problem is peritonitis, which develops over several hours as a result of leakage of bowel contents into the peritoneum.

Retroperitoneum

Injury to organs in this region are much more difficult to diagnose compared with those in the peritoneal cavity. The main reasons for this are that the viscera contained within this region are less accessible to physical examination and investigation.

Pancreas and duodenum

These may be injured as a result of both blunt and penetrating trauma, with the commonest mechanism being that of the unrestrained car driver impacting with the steering wheel.

Bowel

All of the caecum and ascending colon, as well as one-to two-thirds of the circumference of the descending colon lie within the retroperitoneal space. The remainder of the colon is located within the peritoneal cavity. Blunt or penetrating trauma can damage any part of the colon and cause leakage of the bowel contents. However, in cases of retroperitoneal perforation, the symptoms are usually ill-defined and slow to develop. This often leads to delays in diagnosis and increases the chances of abscess formation.

Vascular

The abdominal aorta is susceptible to damage as a result of penetrating injury. Severe trauma is almost invariably lethal, but lesser degrees of injury will manifest as hypotension and/or symptoms of ischaemia. If the haemorrhage is contained within the retroperitoneum then the hypotension may be mild and respond to fluid resuscitation. Later, a retroperitoneal haematoma may be visible as bruising in the flank or back (Grey Turner's sign).

The inferior vena cava (IVC) is susceptible to the same types of injury as the aorta. It can result in significant blood loss but this is usually less than from an equivalent injury to the aorta. This is because of the lower pressure within the vessel, and the relatively high pressure in the surrounding tissues. However, if this pressure is lost, as occurs in the presence of a large wound, haemorrhage from the IVC is severe and may be life-threatening.

Renal system

The kidneys are well protected by soft tissue in front and bone and muscle behind. As a result, isolated injury to the kidneys is uncommon barring sporting incidents. However, following major penetrating or blunt trauma, significant renal damage is associated with multiple organ injuries. Trauma to the ureters, as a result of either blunt or penetrating injury, is uncommon.

Pelvis

Injuries to the bladder and the posterior urethra are the most frequent types of urological trauma seen.

Urinary system

The bladder lies within the pelvis, but remember that, when full, it may extend as high as the umbilicus. This means that it is susceptible to injury following trauma to the lower abdomen. Injury to the bladder may follow compression of the abdomen, thus increasing intravesical pressure. More commonly, it is damaged as a result of penetrating injury from fragments of bone produced when the pelvis is fractured.

When the bladder is ruptured, the urine leaks into either the peritoneal cavity, causing peritonitis, or the perineum and surrounding structures. The latter usually produces a less dramatic picture than intraperitoneal leakage, but it is important to diagnose this condition early, as necrosis of the tissues will follow if it is missed.

The urethra is rarely injured in women, due to its short length. In men, injuries are divided into those above the urogenital diaphragm (posterior) and those below (anterior). This level is indicated by the sphincter urethrae. Posterior urethral injury usually arises as a result of pelvic fracture, and is therefore often associated with injuries to other body regions. Anterior urethral injury occurs as a result of blunt trauma to the perineum (e.g. falling astride a beam) and therefore is usually an isolated injury. If the rupture is complete, the patient will be unable to pass urine. In contrast, a lesser injury, such as a submucosal haematoma, will make micturition slow and painful, but possible.

Bowel and reproductive system

The pelvis also contains the rectum and the female reproductive organs. In addition to perforation from bony pelvic fragments following trauma, injuries to the rectum are similar to those described for the colon and bowel above. Injuries to the uterus are uncommon but can result from both blunt and penetrating trauma. Due to the increase in size, the chances of damage from either mechanism is increased during pregnancy.

Abdominal wall

In the fit, athletic individual this forms a firm muscular layer which can offer considerable protection from blunt trauma. The level of protection is much less in children and those with poor muscle development. Rupture of anterior abdominal muscles can occur spontaneously, for example following vigorous exercise or coughing. More commonly, however, these muscles are torn by compression from a seat belt in a deceleration injury. When this force is sufficient to produce an imprint of the overlying clothes and seat belt on the skin, there is a high probability of significant intra-abdominal injury.

Though penetrating trauma can breach the anterior abdominal wall, it may not necessarily cause intra-abdominal injury. The degree of damage sustained is dependent on the nature of the weapon used:

- Stab wound
- Gunshot wound.

Perineum

The penis can be subjected to both blunt and penetrating trauma. Fracture of the penis is rare but does occur following forceful bending of the erect organ. It leads to rupture of one or both corpora cavernosa, resulting in a large subcutaneous haematoma and detumescence.

The testes can be damaged by blunt or, rarely, penetrating trauma. Rupture of the testis following the former is uncommon because of the scrotal position, cremasteric retraction and the frictionless surface of the

tunica vaginalis. All these features allow the testis to evade the direct effects of blunt trauma.

BONY PELVIS

The bony pelvis is usually injured as a result of road traffic accidents (60%) or falls from a height (30%). These mechanisms give rise to anteroposterior compression, lateral compression or vertical shear acting on the pelvis either singularly or in combination. They are all capable of producing pelvic instability and haemorrhage because of the vascular and bony damage. Due to the nature of this high energy transfer, 98% of patients with major pelvic trauma have other injuries (Table 2.2). The mortality rate is therefore high at 15–25% but rises even further to 50% when the fracture is open. In the latter case, reports indicate that the rate can approach 100% if the open fracture is missed.

The bones of the pelvis can only be separated if the ligaments joining them together are torn. When this occurs, structures which run close to the ligaments (i.e. vessels and nerves) can be damaged. The bleeding which results is usually venous, extraperitoneal and can be life–threatening. However, some tamponading effect can be achieved if fractures occur whilst the ligaments remain intact. In these cases the degree of haemorrhage is less severe, and the mortality rate is reduced.

LIMBS

Bone

The size, shape and consistency of bone varies with age. Old bones require less force to break them than young ones because they are more brittle and often osteoporotic. In children, fractures may involve the growth plate (physis), which if not accurately reduced can subsequently lead to deformity.

Bone is a living tissue with a generous blood supply and can bleed profusely after injury. Furthermore,

Table 2.2 Associations with pelvic fractures	
Major haemorrhage	over 70%
Musculoskeletal injury	over 80%
Intra-abdominal injury	18–35%
Urological injury	12–20%
Lumbosacral plexus injury	8–30%

blood loss from adjacent vessels and oedema in the surrounding tissues can be severe enough to cause hypovolaemic shock. The approximate blood loss with some closed fractures is:

- Pelvis   1.0–5.0 litres
- Femur   1.0–2.5 litres
- Tibia   0.5–1.5 litres
- Humerus   0.5–1.5 litres.

These volumes can be much higher if there is an open fracture (see below).

Nerves

In the limbs, nerves tend to lie close to the long bones in neurovascular fascial bundles. This close proximity is particularly noticeable around joints and makes them prone to nerve damage following fractures and dislocations.

Structure and function of a peripheral nerve

The neurons making up a nerve trunk are grouped into fascicles. In the more proximal segments there is considerable crossing over and rearrangement between fascicles, but more distally (below the elbow, for example) the fascicular arrangement is constant and predictable, and corresponds to the eventual motor and cutaneous branches. Some nerves, such as the ulnar nerve, have small numbers of well-defined fascicles; others, such as the median nerve, have large numbers of smaller ones.

Understanding the connective-tissue framework of the nerve is essential for thinking about nerve repair. The outermost layer is the epineurium, the chief characteristic of which is mechanical strength. It is usually in a state of longitudinal tension, which is why the ends of a cut nerve spring apart. Each fascicle is surrounded by perineurium; this functions as a blood–nerve barrier and determines the biochemical environment of the nerve tissue. The individual axons are invested in endoneurium, which forms conduits guiding each axon to the appropriate end organ.

The nerve is nourished by an internal longitudinal plexus of vessels, fed at intervals by perforators from the adventitia. This plexus becomes occluded if the nerve is subjected to undue tension, otherwise it can support the nerve trunk even when it has been lifted from its bed over quite a distance. The cell body and axonal parts of the neuron communicate with each other chemically by means of a highly efficient, two-way axoplasmic transport system. This carries transmitter substances centrifugally under normal conditions and structural proteins during regeneration after injury. It also carries, to the cell body, signalling molecules from the end organs or from axons which are damaged. In this way they can influence the nucleus in its control of the cell.

Vessels

Following trauma, the intimal layer may be the only part of a limb artery damaged. This can be very difficult to detect clinically, initially because distal pulses and capillary refill are maintained. Subsequently, the intimal tear can become a focus for intravascular thrombosis formation and can also give rise to distal embolization.

More overt acute signs are only seen if a significant area of the lumen is occluded. When all the layers of the artery are transected transversely, the vessel will go into spasm, due to constriction of the muscle fibres in the media, limiting the degree of blood loss. Conversely, if there is a partial or longitudinal laceration, the muscle spasm tends to keep the hole in the artery open, and blood loss continues.

Veins have little muscle fibre in their walls and therefore cannot contract when they are damaged. Consequently, blood continues to leak from the lumen until direct pressure is applied.

Limb compartments

These are regions in the limbs where skeletal muscle is enclosed by relatively non-compliant fascia. Running through these areas are blood vessels and nerves, the function of which can be affected if intracompartmental pressure rises above capillary pressure. This is most commonly seen in the four compartments around the tibia and fibula. Nevertheless, compartments also occur in the shoulder, forearm, hand, buttocks and thigh, and therefore these can also give rise to the compartment syndrome (see below).

SPINAL COLUMN

The stability of the vertebral column depends mainly on the integrity of a series of ligaments, including the intervertebral discs. Schematically, these can be divided into three vertical complexes. The anterior one consists of the anterior longitudinal ligaments and the anterior half of the intervertebral discs. The middle complex is made up of the posterior longitudinal ligaments and the posterior half of the intervertebral discs. The posterior complex is made up of the remaining intervertebral ligaments and joints, and is structurally the most important. If any two of these complexes are torn the vertebral column becomes unstable.

The spinal cord runs down the spinal canal to the level of the second (adult) or third (baby) lumbar vertebrae. The size of the space around the cord in the canal varies depending on the relative diameters of the spinal cord and spinal canal. In the region of the thorax it is very small because the spinal cord is relatively wide. In contrast, there is a large potential space at the level of C2. Consequently, injuries in this area are not automatically fatal because there is a potential space behind the dens. This has been described in *Steel's rule of three*:

> One-third of the spinal canal area of C1 is occupied by the odontoid, one-third by the intervening space and one-third by the spinal canal.

The space in the spinal canal may be reduced in some patients due to spinal stenosis, or the presence of posterior osteophytes. An awareness of this space is therefore important because it controls the body's ability to adapt to injuries which further reduce the size of the spinal canal.

The incidents which commonly lead to spinal injury are:

- Road traffic accident   48%
- Falls   21%
- Violent acts   14%
- Sport   14%
- Other   3%

Road traffic accidents account for approximately 50% of the spinal injuries in the UK and can result from side, rear or front collision. Ejection from a car increases the chance of a spinal injury to approximately 1 in 13. Rear-end collisions can produce hyperextension of the neck followed by hyperflexion (the 'whiplash phenomenon'). Unprotected victims, such as pedestrians hit by cars or motorcyclists, have a higher chance of sustaining a spinal injury compared to those who remain in the vehicle.

The sporting activities which are infamous for producing spinal trauma are rugby (especially after a collapse of the scrum), gymnastics, trampolining, horse-riding, skiing, bungee jumping and hang-gliding. Diving is a common cause of neck injuries during the spring and summer months, particularly in young males who have recently drunk alcohol. The victim usually misjudges the depth of the water or dives from too steep an angle, hitting his head on a solid surface.

Due to the mechanism of injury, 50% of patients with spinal trauma have injuries elsewhere. In particular, 7–20% have head injuries, 15–20% have chest injuries and about 2.5% have abdominal injuries.

The common feature of all the mechanisms leading to spinal injury is that the vertebral column is subjected to a series of forces. These can act either singly or in combination to produce flexion, extension, rotation, lateral flexion, compression and distraction. The vertebral column is usually injured at C5/C6/C7 and T12/L1. At these sites flexibility is reduced because the direction of the curve of the spine changes.

SKIN

The principal soft tissue in the body is the skin. With increasing age, there is a decrease in the amount of collagen in the skin and subcutaneous tissues as well as a weakening of the elastic fibres. These changes reduce the tensile strength of skin and thus allow extensive lacerations to develop with minor trauma. Similar effects are seen following long-term steroid use.

PATHOPHYSIOLOGICAL RESPONSE

Injury initiates many well-developed physiological responses. Consequently, clinicians dealing with trauma victims are presented with a combination of physiological changes, some of which are a direct result of the injury and others the body's response to the initial insult. The more important physiological changes are listed and described below:

- The metabolic response to injury
- Shock and cardiovascular pathophysiology
- Coagulopathy
- Multi-system organ failure (MSOF)
- Neuropathophysiology
- Spinal injuries
- Fractures
- Peripheral nerve injury
- Compartment syndrome
- Crush syndrome
- Fat emboli
- Wound healing
- Burns.

THE METABOLIC RESPONSE TO INJURY

The response to injury can be usefully divided into three phases: the early, acute *ebb* phase, which is followed by either the *flow* phase if resuscitation and homeostasis are able to overcome the initial insult, or by *necrobiosis* if treatment fails and death ensues (Fig. 2.6).

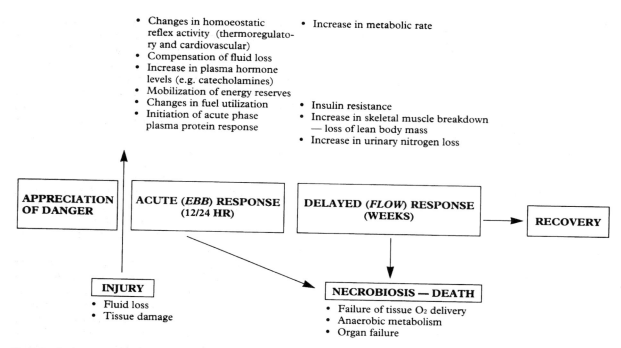

- Changes in homoeostatic reflex activity (thermoregulatory and cardiovascular)
- Compensation of fluid loss
- Increase in plasma hormone levels (e.g. catecholamines)
- Mobilization of energy reserves
- Changes in fuel utilization
- Initiation of acute phase plasma protein response

- Increase in metabolic rate

- Insulin resistance
- Increase in skeletal muscle breakdown — loss of lean body mass
- Increase in urinary nitrogen loss

| APPRECIATION OF DANGER | ACUTE (*EBB*) RESPONSE (12/24 HR) | DELAYED (*FLOW*) RESPONSE (WEEKS) | RECOVERY |

INJURY
- Fluid loss
- Tissue damage

NECROBIOSIS — DEATH
- Failure of tissue O_2 delivery
- Anaerobic metabolism
- Organ failure

Fig 2.6 Defence reaction.

After very severe injuries the ebb phase may be short and necrobiosis may have already started by the time the patient reaches the accident and emergency (A&E) department.

The ebb phase

This phase includes the pattern of physiological and metabolic changes associated with the preparation for fight or flight (the defence reaction). On this are superimposed the responses elicited by the hypoxia, tissue damage, nociceptive (Latin: *noceo* = to injure) afferent activity and fluid loss from the circulation associated with the injury. Broadly speaking, these changes are related to the severity of the injury.

The ebb phase is characterized by mobilization of energy reserves and changes in cardiovascular reflex activity. The latter corresponds to the clinical state commonly referred to as 'shock' (see below). A link between these factors is the increased activity of the sympathetic nervous system. This is initiated by the appreciation of danger, and is sustained by afferent neural impulses arising from the site of injury and cardiovascular reflexes triggered by reductions in blood pressure and volume. The increase in sympathetic activity is reflected by rises in plasma catecholamine concentrations which are directly related to the severity

of injury. In addition, in the ebb phase there is a rapid secretion of hormones from the posterior and anterior pituitary as well as from the adrenal medulla.

Increased sympathetic activity stimulates the breakdown of liver and muscle glycogen, leading, either directly or indirectly, to increases in plasma glucose levels. This hyperglycaemia is potentiated by the reduction in glucose utilization by skeletal muscle due to an inhibition (by the raised adrenaline levels) of insulin secretion and the development of relative intracellular insulin resistance. The mechanism of insulin resistance is unclear, although glucocorticoids may be involved.

The changes in carbohydrate metabolism in the ebb phase can be interpreted as defensive. In addition to providing a fuel for fight or flight, the hyperglycaemia may also play a role in the compensation for post-traumatic fluid loss, both through the mobilization of water associated with glycogen and through its osmotic effects. The decrease in glucose clearance associated with the development of insulin resistance can be considered as a mechanism for preventing the wasteful use of the mobilized carbohydrate, which is an essential fuel for the brain and the wound, at a time when the supply of nutrients may be limited.

The increases in sympathetic activity also cause mobilization of fat (triacylglycerol) in adipose tissue. Plasma concentrations of non-esterified fatty acids

(NEFAs) and glycerol are raised after accidental injury in man, although the relationship with injury severity is complex. For example, plasma NEFA is lower after severe injuries than after moderate ones; this may be related to metabolic (e.g. stimulation of re-esterification within adipose tissue by the raised plasma lactate levels associated with severe injury) or circulatory (poor perfusion of adipose tissue) factors.

An increase in plasma cortisol, mediated by adrenocorticotrophic hormone (ACTH), occurs rapidly after all forms of injury, although the relationship with severity is, once again, complex. Unexpectedly low cortisol concentrations have been found after severe injuries which cannot be related to a failure of the ACTH response. It has been suggested that an impairment of adrenocortical blood flow in the severely injured is responsible.

The original description of the ebb phase characterized it as a period of depressed metabolism, and there is good evidence for this from experimental studies. The fall in metabolic rate following haemorrhage which is due to a reduction in tissue oxygen delivery can be reversed by transfusion; however, if hypovolaemia is accompanied by tissue damage, transfusion is less effective. It seems that neural impulses, associated with tissue injury ascending to the brain via the spinal cord, cause the release of noradrenaline in the hypothalamus which, in turn, leads to an inhibition of thermoregulatory heat production and, at ambient temperatures below thermoneutral, a fall in oxygen consumption and body temperature.

The evidence for such an inhibition of thermoregulatory heat production shortly after injury in man is, however, not nearly so clear. Indeed, what evidence there is suggests that oxygen consumption is maintained at or, more commonly, above normal levels shortly after injury in man. There is, however, clinical evidence for changes in the control of thermoregulation at this time; for example, severely injured patients do not shiver, despite having body temperatures below the normal threshold for its onset, and the selection of the ambient temperature for thermal comfort is modified.

In addition to modifying thermoregulation, nociceptive stimulation also modifies the cardiovascular response to fluid loss. For example, the heart rate response to simple haemorrhage is an initial tachycardia (mediated by the baroreflex) followed, as the severity of haemorrhage increases, by a bradycardia (mediated by the stimulation of neural afferents arising from the heart). This vagally induced bradycardia can be markedly attenuated, and blood pressure better maintained, if the blood loss is superimposed on a background of nociceptive stimulation. The sensitivity of the baroreflex is itself reduced by injury, although an increase is seen after haemorrhage. This impairment of the baroreflex, which can persist for several weeks after even quite modest injuries (e.g. fracture dislocation of the ankle), means that vasopressors such as vasopressin (ADH) released acutely after injury will be more effective in helping maintain blood pressure than normally, when the baroreflex buffers their pressor effects. This complex interaction between the cardiovascular responses to haemorrhage and injury may not be beneficial, as it has been demonstrated that the ability to tolerate haemorrhage is reduced by concomitant tissue damage. Thus it seems that the better maintenance of blood pressure after haemorrhage and injury is achieved at the expense of intense vasoconstriction in peripheral vascular beds. This may lead to further tissue damage and increase the likelihood of the development of multiple organ failure.

If the magnitude of tissue damage and fluid loss from the circulation is so severe that endogenous homoeostatic mechanisms are overwhelmed and resuscitation is inadequate, the phase of necrobiosis is initiated. This is characterized by a progressive imbalance between oxygen demand and supply in the tissues, leading to a downward spiral of anaerobic metabolism. As a result, irreversible tissue damage is initiated, leading to death. However, if treatment is successful and tissue oxygen delivery maintained, the ebb phase is followed by the flow phase.

The flow phase

The main features of the flow phase are increases in metabolic rate and in urinary nitrogen excretion. These are associated with weight loss and muscle wasting, which reach a maximum at 7–10 days after injury in uncomplicated cases. If sepsis and/or multiple organ failure supervene, this pattern of response may be prolonged for many weeks.

The increase in metabolic rate, which is directly related to the severity of injury, is due to a number of factors, probably the most important of which is an increased sympathetic drive secondary to an upward central resetting of metabolic activity. The wound, whether it is a fracture site or a burned surface, can be considered as an extra organ which is metabolically active and has a circulation which is not under neural control. The wound consumes large amounts of glucose which is converted to lactate; this in turn is carried to the liver, where it is reconverted to glucose. This is an energy-consuming process, which is reflected by an increase in hepatic oxygen consumption. Other factors that might contribute to the hypermetabolism are: increases in cardiac output (needed to sustain a hyperdynamic circulation); the energy cost of the latent heat of evaporation of water from, for example, the surface of the burn; and the energy costs of substrate cycling (metabolic processes which involve the expenditure of energy without any change in the amount of either substrate or product) and increased protein turnover.

Metabolic rates measured in the flow phase seldom exceed 3000–4000 kcal per day (twice normal resting metabolic expenditure), with the highest values noted after major burns. The levels of energy expenditure are often lower than expected and may be close to or even lower than values predicted from standard tables. The explanation for this is that the hypermetabolic stimulus of injury or sepsis is superimposed on a background of inadequate calorie intake, immobility and loss of muscle mass, all of which tend to reduce metabolic rate.

The hypermetabolism of the flow phase is fuelled by increases in the rates of turnover of both fat and glucose. Turnover of NEFAs is raised in relation to their plasma concentration, and the normal suppression of fat oxidation following the administration of exogenous glucose is not seen in these hypermetabolic patients. Both these changes have been attributed to increased sympathetic activity, although plasma catecholamine concentrations are not always increased at this time. The rate of hepatic gluconeogenesis is increased from a number of precursors (e.g. lactate and pyruvate from the wound and muscle, amino acids from muscle protein breakdown, and glycerol from fat mobilization). This increase in hepatic glucose production is not suppressed by the infusion of large quantities of glucose in patients with burns or sepsis. This apparent resistance to the effects of insulin is mirrored by the failure of peripheral glucose utilization to rise to the extent predicted from the raised plasma glucose and insulin concentrations. This insulin resistance in, for example, uninjured skeletal muscle seems to be an intracellular (post-receptor) change.

The balance between whole-body protein synthesis and breakdown is obviously disturbed in the flow phase. It seems that the changes observed represent the interaction between the degree of injury and the nutritional state: increasing severity of injury causes increasing rates of both synthesis and breakdown, while undernutrition tends to depress synthesis. Thus, increasing nutritional intake ought to move a patient towards nitrogen balance; however, it seems that, despite advances in techniques for administering nutrients and modifications to the type and composition of feeding regimens, no amount of nitrogen is sufficient to produce a positive balance after severe injuries. Nevertheless, the use of anabolic agents, such as growth hormone, and manipulations of ambient temperature may be of advantage as the patient moves from the catabolic flow phase into the anabolic convalescent phase.

A major site of net protein loss is skeletal muscle, both in the injured area as well as distant from it. For example, after moderate injury the patient can lose 2 kg of lean body mass. The loss can be sufficient to compromise mobility, especially in the elderly, whose reserves of muscle mass and strength are already reduced. Although the changes in skeletal muscle are very obvious, the liver is another tissue in which changes in protein synthesis are of particular interest after injury. The liver is the source of the acute-phase reactants (e.g. C-reactive protein, fibrinogen and α_1-antitrypsin) the concentrations of which rise in response to infection, inflammation and trauma.

These metabolic changes, which cannot be attributed to starvation or immobility, can be mimicked to some extent by the infusion of the counterregulatory hormones glucagon, adrenaline and cortisol. However, the plasma concentrations required to elicit relatively modest increases in nitrogen excretion and metabolic rate and induce peripheral insulin resistance are much higher than those found in the flow phase, although they are similar to those noted in the ebb phase. It has been suggested that other factors must be involved, and the cytokines, most probably interleukin-6, released by activated macrophages may play an important role.

SHOCK AND CARDIOVASCULAR PATHOPHYSIOLOGY

Shock can be defined as inadequate organ perfusion and tissue oxygenation. It is therefore dependent upon pulmonary function (see above), oxygen delivery and release to the tissues and tissue oxygen consumption.

Oxygen delivery

This is governed by level of saturation of haemoglobin with oxygen, the haemoglobin concentration, the cardiac output, systemic vascular resistance and individual organ autoregulation.

The vast majority of oxygen carried in the blood is taken up by the haem molecule, with only a small amount dissolving in the plasma. The relationship between the P_{O_2} and oxygen uptake by haemoglobin is not linear, because each O_2 molecule added facilitates the uptake of the next O_2 molecule. This is known as the quaternary function of haemoglobin and it gives rise to a sigmoid oxygen association curve (Fig. 2.7). Furthermore, because haemoglobin is virtually fully saturated at a P_{O_2} of 100 mmHg (i.e. the level found in the normal healthy state), increasing the P_{O_2} further has little effect on oxygen transport.

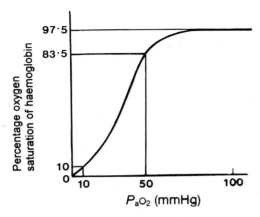

Fig 2.7 Line diagram of the oxygen dissociation curve. (With permission from Driscoll, P, Gwinnutt, C, Jimmerson, C, Goodall, O, from Trauma Resuscitation: The Team Approach, Macmillan Press Ltd)

The affinity of haemoglobin for oxygen at a particular Po_2 (commonly known as the O_2–Hb association) is also affected by other factors. It is increased (i.e. shifting the curve to the left) by an alkali environment, low Pco_2, low concentrations of 2,3-diphosphoglycerate (2,3–DPG) in the red cells, carbon monoxide (CO) and a fall in temperature.

At first sight, it would seem logical that a greater haemoglobin concentration would allow more oxygen to be carried. However, increasing this leads to an increase in blood viscosity, which impedes blood flow, and so offsets this advantage. This normal haemoglobin concentration (as measured by haematocrit) is usually just above the point at which the oxygen transportation is optimal. Consequently, a slight fall in haemoglobin concentration actually increases oxygen transportation.

Oxygen release to tissue

At the tissue level, the capillary P_aO_2 is approximately 20 mmHg and the cellular Po_2 only 2–3 mmHg. This facilitates the release of oxygen by the haemoglobin molecule to the surrounding tissues. Local factors, such as an increase in P_aCO_2, temperature, acidosis and an increase in 2,3-DPG have a similar effect.

Tissue oxygen consumption

In the normal subject, the total consumption of oxygen per minute (Vo_2) is constant throughout a wide range of oxygen delivery (Do_2). The normal Vo_2 for a resting male is 100–160 ml min^{-1} m^{-2} and the normal value of Do_2 in the same person is 500–720 ml min^{-1} m^{-2}.

Therefore, tissues are taking up only 20–25% of the oxygen brought to them. This is known as the oxygen extraction ratio (OER) and demonstrates that normally there is great potential for the tissues of the body to extract more oxygen from the circulating blood.

Following trauma, both oxygen delivery and consumption can be affected. Tissue damage results in an early increase in consumption, despite the fact that the delivery of oxygen falls because of the reduced blood volume. The increase in consumption is achieved by increasing the extraction of oxygen from the blood. This compensatory response only works if the delivery of oxygen is greater than 300 ml min^{-1} m^{-2}. At levels below this the tissues cannot increase oxygen extraction any further. Oxygen consumption therefore progressively falls because it is now directly dependent on the rate of delivery to the tissues.

Compensatory mechanisms

When a sufficient cell mass has been damaged, the shocked state becomes irreversible and death of the patient is inevitable. Fortunately, the body has several compensatory mechanisms which attempt to maintain adequate oxygen delivery to the essential organs of the body and help prevent this stage being reached.

Circulatory control

Pressure receptors in the heart and baroreceptors in the carotid sinus and aortic arch trigger a reflex sympathetic response via control centres in the brain stem in response to hypovolaemia. The sympathetic discharge stimulates many tissues in the body, including the adrenal medulla, which leads to an increased release of systemic catecholamines, enhancing the effects of direct sympathetic discharge, particularly on the heart. This has the effect of preventing or limiting the fall in cardiac output by positive inotropic and chronotropic effects on the heart and by increasing venous return as a result of venoconstriction. Furthermore, selective arteriolar and precapillary sphincter constriction of non-essential organs (e.g. skin and gut) maintains perfusion of vital organs (e.g. brain and heart). Selective perfusion also leads to a lowering of the hydrostatic pressure in those capillaries serving non-essential organs. This also reduces the diffusion of fluid across the capillary membrane into the interstitial space, thereby decreasing any further loss of intravascular volume. Any reduction in renal blood flow is detected by the juxtaglomerular apparatus in the kidney, which releases renin. This leads to the formation of angiotensin II and aldosterone which, together with antidiuretic hormone released from the pituitary, increase the reabsorption of sodium and water by the kidney (reducing urine volume), which helps maintain the circulating volume. Renin, angiotensin II and ADH can also produce generalized vasoconstriction and so help increase the venous return. In addition, the body attempts to enhance the circulating volume by releasing osmotically active substances from the liver. These increase plasma osmotic pressure, and so cause interstitial fluid to be drawn into the intravascular space.

Oxygen delivery

Although sympathetically induced tachypnoea occurs, it does not produce any increase in oxygen uptake because the haemoglobin in blood passing ventilated alveoli is already fully saturated.

Causes of shock

Reduced venous return

The most common cause of shock in the trauma patient is haemorrhage. This may be occult, as the thorax, abdomen and pelvis have large potential spaces in which blood may collect. Significant haematomas can also develop in potential spaces in the body (e.g. the intrapleural and retroperitoneal spaces), as well as in muscles and tissues around the long-bone fractures. In addition, intravascular volume may be reduced by fractures as a result of leakage of plasma into the interstitial spaces. This can account for up to 25% of the volume of tissue swelling following blunt trauma.

The rate of blood returning to the heart is dependent on the pressure gradient created by the high hydrostatic pressure in the peripheral veins and low hydrostatic pressure in the right atrium of the heart. Any reduction in this gradient (e.g. tension pneumothorax or cardiac tamponade increasing right atrial pressure) will lead to a fall in the venous return to the heart. External compression on the thorax or abdomen can have a similar action in obstructing the venous return.

Cardiogenic

Both ischaemic heart disease and cardiac contusions have negative inotropic effects. Nevertheless, cardiogenic shock does not occur unless more than 40% of the left ventricular myocardium has died or has been severely damaged. In cardiogenic shock the compensatory sympathetic and catecholamine responses only serve to increase the myocardial oxygen demand and further increase the degree of ischaemia.

Certain dysrhythmias on their own significantly reduce cardiac performance. They are usually a result of pre-existing myocardial ischaemia, but can result de novo following cardiac contusion. It is also important to be aware that all antiarrhythmic agents may have a significant negative inotropic effect and can therefore impede the patient's physiological response to the injury. Cardiac tamponade, in addition to its effect on venous return, also restricts ventricular filling.

Reduction of arterial tone

A spinal injury above T6 will impair the sympathetic nervous system outflow from the spinal cord below this level. As a consequence, both the reflex tachycardia and vasoconstriction responses to hypovolaemia are restricted to a degree proportional to the level of sympathetic block. With high level spinal injuries, generalized vasodilation, bradycardia and loss of temperature control can occur. This is known as *neurogenic shock*; it leads to a reduction in blood supply to the spinal column and so additional nervous tissue damage ensues. Any associated haemorrhage from the injury will aggravate this situation, further reducing spinal blood flow. In addition, these patients are very sensitive to any vagal stimulation. For example, pharyngeal suction can aggravate the bradycardia and lead to cardiac arrest.

In *septic shock*, circulating endotoxins, commonly from Gram-negative organisms, produce vasodilation and impair energy utilization at a cellular level. In this type of shock tissue hypoxia can occur even with normal or high oxygen delivery rates because the tissue oxygen demand is extremely high and there is direct impairment of oxygen uptake by the cells. In addition, the capillary walls at the site of infection become leaky due to the endotoxin. Later on this becomes more generalized, allowing sodium and water to move from the interstitial to the intracellular space. With time, this leads to hypovolaemia, and the condition becomes indistinguishable from hypovolaemic shock.

Further cellular damage by endotoxins causes the release of proteolytic enzymes. These paralyse precapillary sphincters, enhance capillary leakage and increase hypovolaemia. The situation is aggravated by the endotoxin acting as a negative inotrope on the myocardium. It follows that in the late stage of sepsis there are several causes of the shock state.

COAGULOPATHY

This is defined as inappropriate intravascular activation of the coagulation and fibrinolytic systems, causing depletion of platelets, coagulation and fibrinolytic factors. It is associated with the formation of platelet-fibrin thrombi in the microvasculature and raised fibrin degradation products in the plasma.

Massive blood transfusion, with resulting dilution of platelets and coagulation factors, and hypothermia are the usual causes of coagulopathy in trauma victims. However, injury and damage to the microvascular endothelium are also common initiating factors. This can be in the presence of either low tissue blood flow (e.g. hypoxia, thromboxanes and leukotrienes) or high tissue blood flow (e.g. endotoxins, cytokines such as tumour necrosis factor, interleukins and free radicals).

By vascular occlusion, coagulopathy can give rise to end-organ ischaemia, infarction and failure. At the same time it can lead to haemorrhage and uncontrolled bleeding at many sites, such as surgical wounds, the pulmonary system, the gastrointestinal tract, and retroperitoneal and intracranial spaces.

MULTI-SYSTEM ORGAN FAILURE (MSOF)

> Multi-system organ failure is a deadly condition with a mortality rate of about 60%.

This is defined as the presence of altered organ function in an acutely ill patient such that intervention is required to maintain homeostasis. It represents the final common pathway of many disease processes which give rise to a condition known as the systemic inflammatory response syndrome (SIRS). With regard to trauma it usually results from prolonged hypoperfusion. Conditions that lead to MSOF are:

- Prolonged inadequate perfusion
- Persistent infection
- Persistent inflammatory source (e.g. pancreatitis and dead tissue).

Despite intensive research there is still no encompassing theory accounting for the link between trauma and MSOF. The two most commonly discussed are the 'gut hypothesis' and the 'two hit model'. The former states that trauma victims developing MSOF do so because of translocation of bacteria and endotoxins from the gut into the portal circulation. The latter hypothesis states that the initial injury primes the inflammatory machinery to a subclinical level. This only gives rise to the exaggerated response seen in MSOF if the patient is subjected to a 'second hit' such as hypoxia, infection or further trauma.

Irrespective of the actual cause, it is suspected that following a stimulus (e.g. trauma or infection) there are a number of mediators released from macrophages,

monocytes and endothelial cells. These include tumour necrosis factor, interleukin-6 and -8 as well as platelet activating factor. Within the first few hours after trauma there is also a fall in the circulating level of interleukin-1. These changes cause further white cell activation in addition to adhesion of leukocytes to endothelial cells lining blood vessels. This occurs in virtually all organs of the body, but particularly the lungs, liver and intestine. The process leads to the migration of white cells into the interstitial space and the release of proteases, oxygen radicals and the activation of arachidonic acid. These changes add to the existing capillary damage, thus causing widespread leakage of fluid into the interstitial space. In addition, the activation of arachidonic acid gives rise to prostacyclin, thromboxane A_2 and leukotrienes. At the same time, tissue damage is also resulting from vasoconstriction and intravascular thrombosis in the microvascular circulation. In the lungs, this can give rise to right heart failure due to the increases in the pulmonary vascular resistance and pulmonary artery pressure.

In managing these patients it is important to realize that the normal relationship between oxygen delivery to tissue (DO_2) and oxygen consumption (VO_2) is altered. In MSOF, partly due to the marked increase in VO_2, tissues become flow dependent (i.e. reliant upon DO_2). Consequently, any hypovolaemia, pulmonary disease or myocardial dysfunction will jeopardize the delivery of oxygen even further, and so increase the degree of tissue hypoxia and organ dysfunction.

Adult respiratory distress syndrome (ARDS)

> ARDS represents the extreme form of acute lung injury (ALI). Though only approximately 2% of trauma patients go on to develop ARDS, they have a mortality rate of 50–60%.

ARDS is often an early manifestation of SIRS (see above) and is therefore frequently allied with the later development of MSOF. Less often it results from a direct lung insult which does not give rise to the multiple organ dysfunction associated with MSOF.

The main functions of the lungs are oxygen (O_2) uptake and carbon dioxide (CO_2) elimination. To do this air has to get to the alveoli (*ventilation*, V), blood has to reach the pulmonary capillaries (*perfusion*, Q), and O_2 and CO_2 have to cross the gas–blood interface (*diffusion*). Finally, the balance between ventilation and perfusion (V/Q ratio) has to be correct. ARDS represents an example of a combined ventilatory, perfusion and diffusional pathology.

Aetiology

ARDS may be caused by, or is associated with, the following conditions:

• Direct lung injury due to lung trauma i.e. blunt injury to the chest, resulting in pulmonary contusion, aspiration of gastric contents, near drowning, inhalation of toxic fumes and thermal injury to the respiratory tract, and bacterial, viral or drug-induced (e.g. bleomycin) pneumonia, radiation injury and oxygen toxicity.

• Indirect causes (i.e. the primary insult is remote from the lungs) include sepsis, massive haemorrhage, multiple transfusions, shock from any cause, disseminated intravascular coagulation, massive burns, major and multiple trauma, pre-eclampsia, amniotic fluid embolism, pancreatitis, head injuries and cardiopulmonary bypass.

The above list is not exhaustive and it has been suggested that any critical illness which leads to inadequate cellular oxygenation can precipitate the syndrome. The chances of developing ARDS increases with the number of risk factors: 25% for one risk factor; 42% for two and 85% for three.

Despite diverse causative factors, the structural changes in the lungs follow a common pattern (Fig. 2.8). Due to the capillary leak there is oedema of the lung tissue and movement of neutrophils and erythrocytes into the lung parenchyma. The lung lymph flow is increased and there is thickening of the alveolar capillary membrane. This results in impaired oxygen diffusion and reduced lung compliance as the alveolus is surrounded by fluid. In addition some of the fluid in the pulmonary parenchyma may leak into the alveoli, giving the characteristic appearance of a hyaline membrane. In the later stages of the disease, fibrosis may be seen.

Clinical presentation

Not all patients presenting with sepsis and multiple trauma develop ARDS. However, they invariably have suffered from hypoxia and/or hypotension at some stage. The diagnosis is based upon finding:

• A cause
• Refractory hypoxaemia (i.e. $P_aO_2 < 8$ kPa with an $FiO_2 > 0.4$ or $P_aO_2/FiO_2 < 20$ kPa)
• Radiological evidence of bilateral diffuse pulmonary infiltrates
• A total compliance less than 30 ml/cmH$_2$O
• A POAP <15–18 mmHg with normal oncotic pressures

Acute lung injury passes through four progressively worsening phases. ARDS is used to define the worst state:

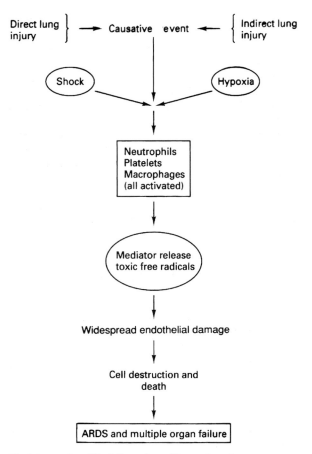

Fig 2.8 A simplified flow chart illustrating the development of ARDS.

Phase I. This may start 16–24 hours after the onset of the presenting clinical condition. Apart from tachypnoea and tachycardia, no other abnormalities may be present. Chest X-ray at this stage is normal.

Phase II. This phase develops up to 48 hours after the initial insult and 12–24 hours after phase I. The patient appears clinically stable but shows increasing dyspnoea with cyanosis. The skin may appear moist. The effort of breathing is greatly increased and hypoxaemia is present despite oxygen therapy. Clinically, only minor chest signs (such as inspiratory ronchi) may be present.

Phase III. This follows phase II and there is now marked tachypnoea and dyspnoea, with increasing involvement of the accessory muscles of respiration. Auscultation of the lung fields reveals high-pitched ronchi. Chest X-ray shows bilateral diffuse pulmonary infiltration. These are often most visible initially in the upper and middle lobes.

Phase IV. This is the terminal phase of ARDS if effective treatment has not been started. The patient shows increasing lethargy and restlessness and may lapse into a coma. There is respiratory and metabolic acidosis with severe hypoxaemia and hypotension. Urine output is usually low (<0.5 ml kg^{-1} h^{-1}). The prognosis at this stage is poor, even if effective treatment is started, as multiple organ failure has already set in.

Therapeutic intervention may alter many of these signs and phases, depending on when the treatment is started. Experience has shown that patients in phases I and II have a better prognosis because the lungs show only mild to moderate injury. Therefore it must be emphasized that the syndrome should be recognized and treatment started, preferably early in the disease process.

NEUROLOGICAL PATHOPHYSIOLOGY

> The number of deaths from falls resulting in head injuries has remained reasonably constant for the last 40 years. This implies that there is little evidence either of prevention of this condition or of its successful management.

Head injuries are common. Over 10 million people per year present to A&E departments in the USA after sustaining a head injury. In the UK the figure is approximately 1.4 million, or 11% of all A&E attendances. Of all trauma deaths, 50–70% are associated with this type of injury, with 4000 children dying each year in the USA alone, due to the resulting brain damage. The combination of head injury and peripheral injury is a particularly dangerous one, as the presence of hypoxia and hypotension is associated with a 75% increase in mortality from severe head injury. The mechanism of this is due in part to the impaired autoregulatory capacity of the injured brain, resulting in the development of secondary brain injury.

Intracranial pressure (ICP)

As the neurocranium is a rigid box in the adult, the pressure generated inside it (the ICP) is dependent on the relationship between its volume and its contents. In the normal state the latter consists of the brain, CSF, blood and blood vessels. Together, these produce an ICP of 5.8–13 mmHg in the horizontal position.

If the ICP is to be kept at normal levels, any increase in the volume of one component must be accompanied by a decrease in either or both of the other components.

CSF can be displaced into the spinal system and its absorption increased. The volume of cerebral venous blood within the dural sinuses can also decrease. Furthermore, the brain is a compliant organ, so it can mould to accommodate changes. Once the limit of these compensatory mechanisms is reached, the ICP rises.

Head trauma results not only in mass lesions but also in an increase in the permeability of the intracerebral microvasculature. This leads to interstitial oedema and cerebral swelling, making the brain relatively 'stiff'. Consequently, the brain has less ability to adapt to changes in the intracranial contents. This situation is worsened if ventilation is impaired, as hypoxia produces additional cerebral swelling. Hypercarbia results in vasodilatation of the blood vessels in the uninjured parts of the brain (see below), thereby increasing intracranial pressure.

Alterations in the intracranial contents, including haematoma, not only produce an elevation in the ICP, but also make the brain, CSF and blood less adaptable to any further additions. In this situation, even a small rise in volume of the intracranial contents causes a steep rise in the ICP. Eventually, tentorial herniation occurs, causing pupillary dilatation (III N compression) and motor weakness (corticospinal tract compression). With a further rise in ICP, coning occurs and the vital centres are compressed. *Cushing's response* includes:

- Decrease in the respiratory rate
- Decrease in the heart rate
- Increase in the systolic blood pressure
- Increase in the pulse pressure.

Without treatment, pontine compression gives rise to a further deterioration in motor function and bilateral pupillary constriction. In the preterminal situation, pupillary dilatation returns, the heart rate increases, the respiratory rate becomes very slow and irregular and the blood pressure falls. Finally, there is a respiratory arrest from haemorrhage or infarction of the brain stem.

Cerebral perfusion

To supply the brain with oxygenated blood there needs to be adequate ventilation and cerebral perfusion. The ability to carry out the latter is dependent on the mean arterial pressure (MAP), the resistance to blood flow due to the ICP and, to a lesser extent, the central venous pressure (CVP).

In the multiply injured patient, not only is the ICP rising due to the head injury, but also the MAP may be falling because of blood loss from an extracranial trauma. In these situations, therefore, the cerebral perfusion pressure (CPP) is markedly reduced. If the CPP is 50 mmHg or less, cerebral ischaemia will develop. As described above, this leads to additional brain swelling and further rises in ICP as the cycle perpetuates itself. A CPP less than 30 mmHg causes death.

Consciousness

This is dependent on two features: a network of neurons in the midbrain and brain stem, known as the reticular activating system; and both cerebral cortices. If either or both of these features are damaged, then consciousness is lost. Hypercapnia, from any cause, can lead to a reduction in the level of consciousness. Mild hypoxia tends to make the patient restless, and only when it is profound does a fall in consciousness result.

Other important causes of an alteration in the conscious level can be remembered from the mnemonic 'TIPPS on the vowels':

Trauma	**A**lcohol
Infection	**E**pilepsy
Poisons	**I**ncrease in ICP
Psychiatric	**O**piates
Shock	**U**raemia/metabolic

Clinically, the level of consciousness is measured from the best eye opening, verbal and motor responses using the Glasgow Coma Scale (Greek *koma* = a deep sleep) (Table 2.3). The scale is an objective measure of the condition and can be used to monitor the patient's progress. The three scores are added; the minimum score is 3 and any score below 8 carries a poor prognosis.

Fractures

Skull fractures usually result from direct trauma and are classified as being linear, depressed or open. The term 'open' is used when there is a direct communication between the brain surface and either the scalp or mucous membrane laceration.

Primary and secondary brain injury

Primary brain injury is the neurological damage produced by the causative event, e.g. the blow to the head. It is now also suspected that progressive primary brain damage may occur subsequently due to endogenous neurochemical changes leading to further cellular injury. Secondary brain injury is the neurological damage produced by subsequent insults such as hypoxia, ischaemia, hypovolaemia, metabolic imbalance, infection and elevations in the ICP.

A purely focal injury can follow a contact force. However, there is usually sufficient associated diffuse brain injury to produce an altered level of consciousness from a temporary disruption of the reticular formation. Furthermore, a space-occupying lesion is often accompanied by a swollen brain due to primary and secondary brain damage. This accelerates the rise in intracranial pressure and the development of additional brain damage. Consequently, the trauma patient invariably has diffuse and specific neurological injuries.

The presenting signs and symptoms from a focal injury depend on the site injured, as different parts of the brain carry out different functions. A focal lesion above the tentorium can produce ipsilateral unilateral herniation of the medial part of the temporal lobes (diffuse brain injuries tend to be bilateral). This produces an ipsilateral fixed dilated pupil in 90% of cases, and contralateral hemiplegia. With further rises in the ICP the brain stem begins to be compressed and the patient develops the signs described previously.

Selective herniation of the cerebellum through the foramen magnum can be produced by an expanding posterior fossa intracranial haematoma. This can lead to a whole collection of presenting signs, the most common being pupil dilatation, respiratory abnormalities, bradycardia, head tilt and cranial nerve palsies. Most alarming is the sudden respiratory arrest due to distal brain stem compression. This is the only cerebral haematoma to do this without a preceding deterioration in conscious level. It is a rare condition but must be

Table 2.3	The Glasgow Coma Scale					

Eye opening	Score	Verbal response	Score	Motor response	Score
Spontaneous	4	Orientated	5	Obeys commands	6
To speech	3	Confused	4	Localizes to pain	5
To pain	2	Inappropriate words	3	Withdraws	4
None	1	Inappropriate sounds	2	Flexion to pain	3
		None	1	Extension to pain	2

considered early on, especially in patients who are found to have an occipital fracture.

Concussion

Concussion occurs when the head has been subjected to minor inertial forces. The patient is always amnesic of the event and there may also be post- and antegrade amnesia. A transient loss of consciousness (usually less than 5 minutes) may occur. On examination, these patients do not have any localizing signs, but there can be nausea, vomiting and headache. Originally it was thought that no organic brain damage occurred in this condition. This has been found not to be the case – microscopic changes occur and, while the net effect of one episode is minor, the effect of more than one episode can be cumulative.

Diffuse axonal injury (DAI)

This is a result of widespread, mainly microscopic, disruption of the brain consisting of axonal damage, microscopic haemorrhages, tears in the brain tissue and interstitial oedema. As a consequence, it can cause prolonged periods of coma (days or weeks) and has an overall mortality rate of 33–50%. Autonomic dysfunction giving rise to high fever, hypertension and sweating are also common in this condition.

The brain, lying under the impact point of a contact force, is subjected to a series of strains resulting from the inward deformation of bone and the shock waves spreading out from the site of impact. Strain can also occur as the base of the brain impinges on projections on the base of the skull. These strains produce gross neurological damage, with haemorrhages, neuronal death and brain swelling. The patient therefore invariably loses consciousness at the time of the incident and has usually developed neurological signs by the time he is examined by a doctor. The most common signs are an altered consciousness level, hemiparesis, ataxia and seizures.

The brain is not fixed inside the neurocranium but floats in a bath of CSF, tethered by the arachnoid fibres and blood vessels. If the head moves due to an accelerating or decelerating force, the skull, and then the brain, will move in the direction of the force. As a consequence, strains develop in the brain tissue and small blood vessels opposite the impact point. This gives rise to the contusional changes described previously. Another factor giving rise to injury is that the brain will continue to move until it collides with the opposite side of the skull or its base. The result is a brain which can be injured in two places, with the site furthest from the impact being the most severely injured. This is known as a *contra coup injury*.

Acute intracranial haematoma

In the majority of cases, extradural haematomas (EDHs) develop in the temporoparietal area following a tear in the middle meningeal artery. However, a small number are due to tears in one of the venous sinuses inside the neurocranium. As the source of the haematoma is usually arterial, the EDH develops quickly and produces a rapid rise in the intracranial pressure.

The 'classic' presentation of an EDH (Fig. 2.9) only occurs in approximately one-third of patients. The remainder are either unconscious from the time of the impact or do not lose consciousness at the scene of the injury but go on to develop neurological signs. The most common clinical signs are a deterioration in the consciousness level and pupil-size changes.

Acute intradural haematoma (IDH)

This is a collective term used for both subdural (SDH) and intracerebral (ICH) haematomas. They frequently coexist, and are 3–4 times more common than EDHs. SDHs usually develop in the temporal lobe and can be bilateral. Following an inertial force, some of the bridging veins tear and blood collects in the subdural space.

- Transient loss of consciousness at the time of the injury from a momentary disruption of the reticular formation.

- Patient then regains consciousness for several hours, the lucid period.

- Localizing signs develop with neurological deficits, headache and eventually unconsciousness from the developing EDH, which causes the ICP to rise.

Fig 2.9 Classic history of an extradural haematoma (EDH).

Occasionally, a SDH develops with no accompanying ICH. Rarer still is the solitary presence of an ICH. When this occurs it is often found in the frontal lobes.

Small ICHs can also be produced by inertial forces, and their volume can increase over time. Depending on their location, ICHs may cause localizing signs or a rise in the intracranial pressure and a deterioration in the clinical state of the patient.

The forces needed to produce an IDH are greater than those needed to produce an EDH and an IDH is usually associated with cerebral contusion and cortical lacerations. Consequently, the patient commonly loses consciousness at the time of the injury. Fits (which are commonly focal), a deteriorating conscious level, contralateral hemiparesis and unilateral pupil dilatation are the usual signs. If a solitary SDH occurs, the patient may have a lucid period followed by a gradual deterioration in the neurological state. This takes longer to develop than in the case of an EDH, because the source of bleeding is venous rather than arterial. If only a few bridging veins are torn and there is plenty of intracranial space due to brain atrophy, then it can take several days for symptoms to develop.

Subarachnoid haemorrhage (SAH)

This can occasionally follow a head injury. The patient often develops severe headaches and photophobia, but other signs of meningism can occur. Any test for neck stiffness should not be done until injury to the cervical spine has been ruled out both radiologically and clinically (see Ch. 1).

PATHOPHYSIOLOGY OF SPINAL INJURIES

In the UK, 10–15 people per million of the population suffer spinal injuries each year (see Table 2.4). The commonest site is the cervical spine (55%), mainly because most people are injured following a road traffic accident (48%).

Primary neurological damage

This is a neurological injury resulting directly from the initial insult. It is usually due to blunt trauma which produces abnormal movement in the vertebral column. In severe cases this leads to ligamental rupture and fractures of the vertebrae. These movements reduce the space around the spinal canal and also allow bone and soft tissue to impinge directly on the cord. The potential space around the spinal cord may already be small, so the chance of neurological damage is increased.

Less commonly, the primary spinal damage is caused by penetrating trauma. A localized area of injury is the usual result of stabbings. Much more extensive areas of destruction and oedema occur when the spinal cord is subjected to a large force such as a gunshot.

Secondary neurological damage

This is deterioration of the spinal cord after the initial insult. The three common causes are mechanical disturbance of the back, hypoxia and poor spinal perfusion. These effects are additive.

Hypoxia can result from any of the causes mentioned above, but significant spinal injury on its own can also produce hypoxia. The reasons for this are listed in Table 2.5. The common underlying problem is usually a lack of respiratory muscle power following a high spinal lesion. Lesions above T12 will involve the intercostal muscles. Injuries above the level of C5 will also block the phrenic nerve and consequently paralyse the diaphragm.

Inadequate spinal perfusion results from either general hypovolaemia or a failure of the spinal cord to regulate its own blood supply. This failure in autoregulation can occur after cord injury. A fall in mean arterial pressure will therefore produce a reduction in spinal perfusion. Conversely, if the pressure is increased too much, then a spinal haemorrhagic infarct could develop.

Secondary damage leads to interstitial and intracellular oedema, which further aggravates the deficient spinal perfusion. As this oedema spreads, neurons are

Table 2.4	Sites of spinal injuries	
Site	Blunt trauma	Penetrating trauma
Cervical	55%	24%
Thoracic	35%	56%
Lumbar	10%	20%
Multiple	10%	

Table 2.5	Respiratory failure in spinal injury
Tetraplegic	Paraplegic
Intercostal paralysis	Intercostal paralysis
Phrenic nerve palsy	
Inability to expectorate	
V/Q mismatch	

squeezed and an ascending level of clinical deterioration is produced. With high spinal injuries, this process can lead to secondary respiratory deterioration.

Partial spinal cord injury

Anterior spinal cord injury

This is due to direct compression or obstruction of the anterior spinal artery. It affects the spinothalamic and corticospinal tracts (Fig. 2.10), resulting in a loss of coarse touch, pain and temperature sensation, and flaccid weakness. This type of injury is associated with fractures or dislocations in the vertebral column.

Central spinal cord injury

This is usually found in elderly patients with cervical spondylosis. Following a vascular event the corticospinal tracts are damaged, with flaccid weakness resulting. In view of the anatomical arrangement in the centre of the cord, the upper limbs are affected more than the legs and hands.

Sacral fibres in the spinothalamic tract are positioned laterally to corresponding fibres from other regions of the body (Fig. 2.10). It follows that anterior and central injuries, which are primarily affecting the midline of the spinal cord, may not affect the sacral fibres. This leads to the phenomenon of 'sacral sparing' in which sensation is lost below a certain level on the trunk but pinprick appreciation is retained over the sacral and perineal area.

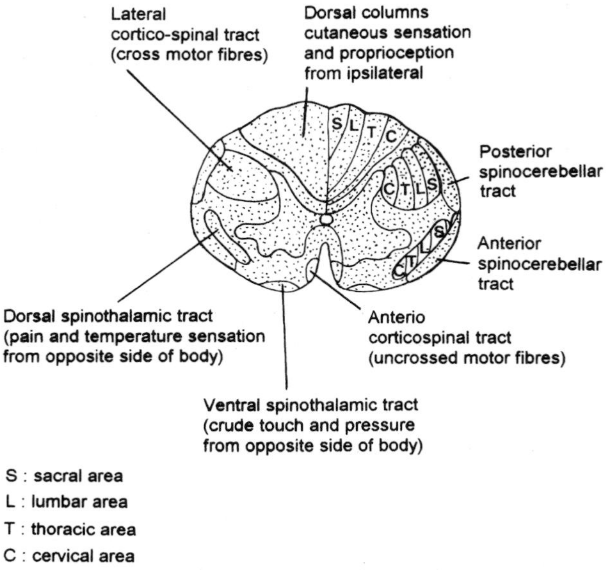
Lateral
cortico-spinal tract
(cross motor fibres)
Dorsal columns
cutaneous sensation
and proprioception
from ipsilateral
S L T C
C T L S
S L T C
Posterior
spinocerebellar
tract
Anterior
spinocerebellar
tract
Dorsal spinothalamic tract
(pain and temperature sensation
from opposite side of body)
Anterio
corticospinal tract
(uncrossed motor fibres)
Ventral spinothalamic tract
(crude touch and pressure
from opposite side of body)
S : sacral area
L : lumbar area
T : thoracic area
C : cervical area

Fig 2.10 Cross-section of the spinal cord demonstrating the longitudinal tracts. (With permission from Driscoll, P, Gwinnutt, C, Jimmerson, C, Goodall, O, from Trauma Resuscitation: The Team Approach, Macmillan Press Ltd).

Lateral (Brown-Séquard syndrome)

This results from penetrating trauma. On the side of the wound, at the level of the lesion, all sensory and motor modalities are disrupted. However, below this level there is a contralateral loss of pain and temperature sensation and an ipsilateral loss of muscle power and tone.

Posterior spinal cord injury

This is a rare condition. It results in a loss of vibration sensation and proprioception.

Spinal shock

This term refers to the totally functionless condition occasionally seen after spinal injury. The patient has generalized flaccid paralysis, diaphragmatic breathing, priapism, gastric dilatation and the autonomic dysfunction associated with neurogenic shock. Beevor's sign (movement of the umbilicus when the abdomen is stroked) may be present.

This state can last for days or weeks, but areas of the cord are still capable of a full recovery. Parts which are permanently damaged give rise to spasticity once the flaccid state resolves. Upper motor neuron reflexes will return, below the level of the lesion, if there has been a complete transection of the cord. This is seen as exaggerated responses to stimuli; however, there will be no sensation.

During this stage these patients are at risk of developing pressure sores, deep venous thrombosis, pulmonary emboli and acute peptic ulceration with either haematemesis or, occasionally, perforation.

FRACTURES

Following trauma. The fracture occurs in normal bone as a result of trauma. The type of fracture depends on the direction of the violence. For example, a twisting injury will cause a spiral or oblique fracture, whereas a direct blow usually causes a transverse fracture. Axial compression frequently results in a comminuted or burst fracture.

Stress fracture. The underlying bone is normal and the abnormal load placed on the bone would not be sufficient to cause a fracture on its own. However, the load is repetitive. This type of fracture is most frequently seen in individuals undertaking increased amounts of unaccustomed exercise, such as the 'march' metatarsal fracture in army recruits and dancers.

Pathological fracture. In this case the underlying bone is weak, perhaps as a result of metastatic cancer or metabolic bone disease, and gives way under minimal trauma.

Fracture repair

When a fracture occurs, not only is the bone broken, but the surrounding tissues are also damaged. Initially, the bone ends are surrounded by a haematoma which includes the surrounding injured tissues. Within hours, however, an aseptic inflammatory response develops, comprising polymorphonuclear leukocytes, lymphocytes, macrophages and blood vessels. Later, fibroblasts infiltrate the area.

Within this organized fracture haematoma, bone develops either directly or following the development of cartilage with endochondral ossification. At the same time osteoclasts develop and resorb the necrotic bone ends. The initial bone that is laid down (callus) consists of immature woven bone. This is gradually converted to stable lamellar bone with consolidation of the fracture. Resorption takes place within the bone trabeculae as recanalizing Haversian systems bridge the bone ends.

There are basically two types of callus. The first is the primary callus response, which is due to the proliferation of committed osteoprogenitor cells in periosteum and bone marrow. These cells produce directly membranous bone, and this response is a once-only phenomenon limited in duration. The second callus is inductive or external callus, which is derived from the surrounding tissues. This callus is formed by pluripotential cells. A variety of factors, including mechanical and humoral factors, may induce these mesenchymal cells to differentiate to cartilage or bone.

The mediators for callus formation are not fully understood, but it is likely that the fracture ends emit osteogenic substances such as bone morphogenetic protein into the surrounding haematoma. This is in addition to mediators such as interleukin-1 and growth factors which are released from the fracture haematoma. Angiogenic factors probably play an important role in the vascularization of the fracture haematoma. Movement of the fragments increases the fracture exudate. Consequently, rigid fixation minimizes the granulation tissue and external callus. It may also retard the release of morphogens and growth factors from the bone end. Reaming of the intramedullary canal may cause additional bone damage. Weight bearing stimulates growth factors and prostaglandins, which act as biochemical mediators.

PERIPHERAL NERVE INJURY

Blunt trauma to a nerve may produce a temporary block in the conduction of impulses, but leave intact the axonal transport system. The axon distal to the injury does not die, and complete functional recovery can be expected; this is called *neuropraxia*. More severe trauma will interrupt axonal transport and cause Wallerian degeneration: the distal axon dies, the myelin sheath disintegrates and the Schwann cells turn into scavenging macrophages which remove the debris. The cell body then embarks on a preprogrammed regenerative response which is usually known as *chromatolysis*, since it involves the disappearance of the Nissl granules which are the rough endoplasmic reticulum of the normal cell. An entire new set of ribosomes appear, dedicated to the task of reconstruction. By their efforts, axon sprouts emerge from the axon proximal to the lesion and grow distally. Injury of this severity is known as *axonotmesis*. It eventually produces a good functional result because the endoneurial tubes are intact and the regenerating axons are therefore guaranteed to reach the correct end organs.

Laceration or extreme traction produces neurotmesis, which also leads to Wallerian degeneration distally and chromatolysis proximally, followed by either cell death or axonal regeneration. In this case, however, the final functional result is bound to be much worse than in any injury which leaves the endoneurial tubes intact. Not only do the axon sprouts have to transverse a gap filled with organizing repair tissue, but they also need to grow down its original conduit at a rate of approximately 1 mm per day. Axons which fail to enter the distal stump may form a tender neuroma; the symptoms arising from this may be exceedingly troublesome. Progress may be monitored clinically by the Tinel sign (electric feelings in the territory of the nerve produced by light percussion over regenerating axon tips – described by the French neurologist Jules Tinel) whether in the distal portion of the nerve or in a neuroma.

Motor axons have the capacity to produce collateral sprouts once they enter muscle, leading to abnormally large motor units with relatively good return of strength. Sensory axons often fail to reinnervate the specialized receptors which form the basis for the sense of touch and this, together with the mismatching of axons with conduits, means that sensory recovery is invariably poor, except in the very young. In the hand this means a poor functional result.

COMPARTMENT SYNDROME

This specific type of neurovascular compromise can occur as part of any extremity injury, whether or not a fracture is present. It is defined as a progressive condition in which the elevated tissue pressure within a confined limb's myofascial compartment exceeds capillary pressure and ultimately compromises the circulation to the muscles and nerves. It can result from a variety of causes but the most common are fractures and soft tissue injuries:

Decrease in compartment size

- Constricting dressing or cast
- Closing fascial defects
- Third degree (i.e. full thickness) burns.

Increase in compartment contents

- Post ischaemic swelling
- Prolonged limb compression
- Haemorrhage following coagulopathy or vascular laceration
- Haemorrhage and oedema following fractures or soft tissue injuries.

The pressure required to produce these effects is estimated to be about 40 mmHg below the mean arterial pressure. If left untreated, fibrotic contractures may develop. Alternatively, areas of muscle may infarct giving rise to rhabdomyolysis, hypovolaemia, hyperkalaemia, hyperphosphataemia, high levels of uric acid and metabolic acidosis.

The four compartments of the lower leg are the most commonly involved areas, but it can occur in the shoulder, arm, forearm, hand, buttocks and thigh, lower leg, forearm, or foot. These sites must be continuously assessed for signs indicating that the compartment pressures are high:

- ↑ pain in the limb (Early)
- ↑ pain on passive movement of the distal joints (Early)
- ↑ Paraesthesia (Early)
- ↓ Distal sensation
- ↑ Compartment tension or swelling (Late)
- ↓ Muscle power (Late sign)
- ↓ Pulse pressure in the distal limb (Very Late sign).

> The presence of increasing pain in patients with limb injuries, especially when exacerbated by passive flexion and extension of the distal joints, is a good early sign of a compartment syndrome.

Diagnosis during this reversible stage is essential to prevent unnecessary morbidity. Though this is usually done clinically, special investigations are useful when dealing with certain types of patients where clinical assessment is difficult:

- Uncooperative or unreliable patients
- Patients unresponsive due to neurological injury or sedation
- Patients with nerve defects from other causes.

Direct monitoring of the compartments associated with a fractured long bone should therefore be considered in all unconscious patients because of their high risk of developing a compartment syndrome. However, absolute pressure values are unreliable because perfusion is dependent upon the difference between the mean arterial blood pressure and the compartmental pressure. A difference of less than 30–40 mmHg is associated with functional changes in muscles and nerves after 15 minutes and ischaemic necrosis after 4–8 hours. A fall in the distal pulse pressure is a very late sign and indicates imminent tissue ischaemia. Similarly, pulse oximetry is not a reliable help in diagnosing or monitoring impaired perfusion secondary to raised compartment pressure.

> The diagnosis of a compartment syndrome is made clinically. Pressure monitoring should be looked upon as an adjunct, not a replacement, for this.

CRUSH SYNDROME

Crush injuries occur in a variety of ways:

- Trapped under fallen masonry
- Trapped in a car following a road traffic accident
- Prolonged use of the pneumatic antishock garment
- Prolonged compression of an extremity by the patient's own body (typically where the patient's conscious level has been reduced for a prolonged period of time)
- Severe beatings.

Until the limb is released there is little systemic effect; however, once reperfusion starts, plasma and blood leak into the surrounding soft tissues for up to 60 hours. The extent is dependent upon the degree of tissue damage and in severe cases may cause hypovolaemia. In addition, there is often associated bone damage and the abnormal biochemical levels found with muscle infarction:

- Rising blood urea nitrogen concentration

- High serum potassium, phosphate and uric acid
- Metabolic acidosis with an increased anion gap
- Raised serum creatine kinase
- Raised packed cell volume
- Thrombocytopenia
- Myoglobinuria and raised plasma myoglobin.

The high serum potassium concentration, especially if associated with a low sodium, can lead to cardiac arrhythmias and arrest soon after the patient is released. In addition, hypovolaemic shock can occur due to associated blood loss as well as from reperfusion of the previously crushed areas of the body. The devitalized tissue is also at high risk of secondary infection with a further release of toxins systemically.

Several factors are considered important in the aetiology of acute renal failure following significant crush injuries. These include hypovolaemia and the release of vasomotor and nephrotoxic substances from the damaged muscle such as myoglobin, haemoglobin and tissue thromboplastins. When myoglobinuria is in high concentration it produces a red or smoky brown discolouration of the urine. It is important, therefore, to look for this when the patient is catheterized and to check the urine regularly.

FAT EMBOLISM SYNDROME

This has a reported incidence of 0.5–3% with single long bone or pelvic fractures and up to 30% in multiply injured patients.

In this condition, lipid globules are formed mainly from circulating plasma triglycerides, carried by very-low-density lipoproteins (VLDLs). In trauma, this is commonly a result of the release of lipid globules from damaged bone marrow adipocytes into the circulation. However, it can also occur with increased peripheral mobilization of fatty acids and increased hepatic synthesis of triglycerides or reduced peripheral uptake of plasma VLDLs (Fig. 2.11). It gives rise to thromboembolism of the microvasculature, with lipid globules and fibrin–platelet thrombi. In addition, the local release of free fatty acids can cause a severe inflammatory reaction which initiates the SIRS chemical cascade. The latter is thought to be responsible for the high association of fat emboli syndrome with both progressive anaemia and pyrexia (> 38.5°C).

As several organs can be affected, there is a wide range of possible clinical presentations. These usually begin 24–48 hours after the injury and classically involve two of the following:

- Pulmonary changes
- Neurological dysfunction
- Petechial rash.

Pulmonary changes include ventilation–perfusion (V/Q) mismatch, impaired alveolar surfactant activity and segmental hypoperfusion. Neurological changes occur as a result of hypoxia and/or the humoral and cellular factors released from the bone. The heart can also be affected such that there is a fall in mechanical performance and arrhythmias. Renal effects can lead to lipiduria with tubular damage and ischaemic glomerular–tubular dysfunction.

To diagnose this condition there has to be either: fat globules in body fluids (e.g. sputum, urine, or lipid emboli in retinal vessels on fundoscopy); or histological demonstration of intracellular and intravascular aggregation of lipid globules with Sudan black stain; or evidence of pulmonary and at least one other organ-system dysfunction.

PATHOPHYSIOLOGY OF WOUND HEALING

Soft-tissue injuries heal by a complex series of cellular events leading to connective-tissue formation and repair by scar formation. The process is continuous, but it is convenient to consider it in three phases.

Phase 1: inflammation

Tissue injury, with disruption of vessels, activates platelets and initiates the coagulation cascade, producing a clot in the wound and generating biologically active substances which cause vasodilatation, increased capillary permeability and oedema. These substances are also chemotactic to polymorphonucleocytes (PMNs) and monocytes, and act as potent growth factors for fibroblasts and endothelial cells.

PMNs are present in the wound within a few hours and their numbers increase during the first 24–48 hours. Macrophages, arising by local proliferation and from circulating blood monocytes, are present within 24 hours and both cell types act to remove cellular debris, foreign material and bacteria by phagocytosis. PMNs prevent infection and remove necrotic tissue, but their role is not essential to tissue repair as clean wounds will heal in the absence of PMNs. In contrast, macrophages are critical to wound healing and a reduction in their numbers will slow or stop wound healing. Part of this central role is due to the secretion by macrophages of growth factors which stimulate proliferation of fibroblasts, endothelial cells and smooth

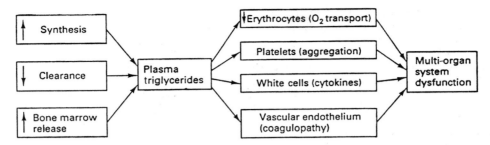

Fig 2.11 The mechanism of interaction between raised plasma triglycerides and the pathogenesis of multi-organ system dysfunction in fat embolism.

muscle cells and extracellular matrix deposition by fibroblasts. These processes start after 3–4 days and are characteristic of the second phase of wound healing.

Phase 2: cell proliferation and matrix formation

As tissue debris and clot are removed, fibroblasts migrate into the wound. Endothelial migration and proliferation produce new capillaries, and matrix synthesis of collagen, proteoglycans and glycoproteins occurs. Production of this granulation tissue occurs in all adult wound healing and is prominent in open wounds left to heal by secondary intention, but less obvious in incised, primarily repaired wounds. Epithelial migration and proliferation re-establishes epidermal continuity and the clot covering the surface of the wound is lost. As matrix production, and particularly collagen synthesis, continues, the mechanical strength of the wound increases, with approximately 50% of the normal strength of skin regained by 6 weeks after injury.

Phase 3: matrix remodelling

For practical purposes a wound is healed by the end of phase 2, but significant changes occur during phase 3. The latter is prolonged and in children may last 2 years or more. The scar becomes less vascular and less cellular, while collagen synthesis and degradation continue. Reorientation of collagen fibrils occurs and the tensile strength of the scar increases (although not to the level of undamaged tissue). However, the normal tissue structure is not restored and, because of its inelastic nature, the scar may cause long-term problems by restricting function and growth.

Wound contracture

In wounds where tissue loss has occurred, which are left to heal by secondary intention, contraction of granula-

tion tissue reduces the size of the tissue defect. There is some evidence that the cell responsible for this process is the myofibroblast, although the exact role of this cell is unresolved. Even though reducing the size of the tissue deficit is of benefit in wound healing, the distortion and scar formation produced by the process inhibit function in certain areas of the body (particularly on the face and around joints).

PATHOPHYSIOLOGY OF BURNS

> Three risk factors for death after burn injury have been identified: age more than 60 years, burn surface area of more than 40% and the presence of inhalational injury.

For the first 24–48 hours after a major burn there are fluid shifts. Leakage of intravascular water, salt and protein occurs through the porous capillary bed into the interstitial space. This, in turn, results in loss of circulating plasma volume, haemoconcentration and hypovolaemia, the severity of which increases with the severity of the burn. In a burn over 15% of the total body surface area (TBSA), the capillary leak may be systemic, causing generalized oedema and a significant fall in blood volume.

Shock associated with burn injuries

The effect on the circulation is directly related to the size and severity of the burn wound. The body compensates for this loss of plasma with an increase in peripheral vascular resistance, and the patient will appear cool, pale and clammy. However, this compensation will only be effective in maintaining circulation for a period of time, depending on the severity of the burn and the presence of other injuries. Ultimately, the patient will demonstrate signs of hypovolaemic shock as the cardiac output falls. During this time it is rarely possible to keep the circulating volume within normal limits. The end of the shock phase in the adequately resuscitated burn is usually marked by a diuresis. This occurs approximately 48 hours after the burn and is usually associated with fluid balance which is more like that of a normal patient.

A burn of greater than 25% TBSA almost always requires intravenous fluid administration to expand the depleted vascular volume. However, shock can occur with a burn involving as little as 15% TBSA, as a result of complicating factors such as age, pre-existing disease and other major injuries. In these circumstances, a burn of 25–40% becomes a potentially lethal injury.

Depth of burn and cause of burn

The diagnosis of the depth of burn is not always easy. If doubtful, it should be reassessed at 24 hours using only non-stick dressings between examinations.

First degree burns

First degree burns are characterized by erythema, pain and the absence of blisters. A typical example is sunburn. They are not life threatening and generally do not require fluid replacement. Superficial burns epithelialize in 14 days from the epithelial-producing elements (hair follicles and sweat glands) and from the edges of the wound. They heal with normal-quality skin, although there can be some pigmentation changes. Superficial burns include: scalds by non-boiling liquids; some chemical burns; and the edges of areas of flame burns and flash burns.

Second degree or partial-thickness burns

This is an important depth of burn to diagnose. They are pink but do not blanch on pressure (called the *zone of stasis*), they are associated with more swelling and blister formation. The surface may weep and in general they are painfully sensitive, even to air current. Healing is by epithelialization from the reduced number of epithelial-producing elements and from the edge of the wound. Therefore healing is often prolonged to 3–4 weeks. The final result of healing is dependent on the depth of the partial-thickness burn. If it is predominantly deep dermal then it results in poor-quality skin or occasionally hypertrophic scar formation. There is some degree of wound contraction and marked pigmentation change (either hyper- or hypopigmentation). Deep dermal burns can result from: scalds; contact burns; chemical burns; and flame burns.

Full-thickness burns

These are usually obvious and have no sensation to pin prick. The diagnosis between deep dermal and full-thickness burns can be difficult and sometimes is only made at surgery. They can only heal naturally by epithelialization from the wound edge and by wound contraction, leaving contracted poor-quality scars. In the acute situation, circumferential full-thickness burns around limbs and the chest can act as tourniquets, impeding the distal circulation and respiration respectively. Urgent escharotomy is required in these situations (see Ch. 25).

Full-thickness burns are caused by many scald injuries with near-boiling water, especially in the skin of the elderly or young patient. Even tea or coffee with milk can produce burns in the deep dermal and full-thickness range. Chemical burns such as those due to hydrofluoric acid, most flame burns, and virtually all electrical burns with a voltage of 220–240 V or above can also give rise to full-thickness burns. Most contact burns are full-thickness in unconscious patients (e.g. postepilepsy, or due to alcohol or drug intake). Similarly, they occur in denervated skin (e.g. diabetes and neuropathies). Burns below the deep fascia do occur, such as some contact burns, scalds in non-accidental injury in children and high-voltage electrical burns. The latter are particularly prone to destroy muscle groups.

Staphylococcal toxic shock syndrome

This can occur in children even with relatively small superficial burns. If a child with even a 1% burn becomes unwell, toxic shock syndrome must be considered and the specific treatment with fresh frozen plasma and antistaphylococcal antibiotics started immediately.

Response of the respiratory system to inhalation injury

The lungs themselves are rarely injured from 'burning', even with blast injuries that cause air to be inspired under pressure. Usually laryngeal spasm occurs from the heat of the inspired gases, thereby protecting the lower airway and lungs from exposure.

The upper airway may receive thermal burns and tissue swelling can develop very rapidly in these vascular tissues. The mouth and oropharynx in particular can cause acute respiratory obstruction. Oedema from these injuries may also involve the vocal cords. Dramatic changes in the patient's ability to maintain his airway have been observed over a short period of time following this type of injury. Soot and steam may carry heat to the lower airways resulting in significant distal thermal injury. The heat capacity of steam is approximately 4000 times that of dry air.

Smoke inhalational injury secondary to confinement in a house fire may be associated with a wide variety of concomitant chemical injuries; for example plastics in wire insulation, furniture and textiles will release hydrogen chloride which causes irritation to the eyes and throat and severe pulmonary oedema. Burning mattresses can produce nitrogen dioxide which is associated with a tri-phasic illness. The first phase is characterized by cough, wheeze and progressive dyspnoea. In the second phase there is progression to pulmonary oedema at approximately 24 hours. After 2–6 weeks bronchiolitis obliterans and chronic interstitial lung disease develop. Phosgene is produced from the burning of polyvinyl chloride and is associated with the development of significant pulmonary oedema. As fires can produce such a wide variety of chemicals, the resultant pulmonary damage may be multifactorial. This may result in necrosis of respiratory epithelium, inactivation of the respiratory cilia, and destruction of type-11 pneumocytes and alveolar macrophages. This leads to a decrease in lung compliance which is seen as an increase in the work of breathing and an impairment of diffusion through the alveolar membrane.

In view of the very large surface area of the lung, fluid requirements for resuscitation may increase by as much as 50% of the calculated values if a severe inhalation injury has been sustained. The severity of the injury will not be related to the TBSA burn size, but rather to the length of time and intensity of exposure to the inhalation. Accurate information from the prehospital-care providers relative to these conditions is vital in planning the patient's care and anticipating respiratory complications.

Carbon monoxide poisoning

Systemic absorption of inhaled toxins may also occur. Carbon monoxide is reported to be the leading toxicological cause of death. Burning any carbon-containing material can release CO, a by-product of incomplete combustion. The mechanisms of CO toxicity are multiple. CO competes with oxygen for binding with haemoglobin, myoglobin and cellular cytochrome oxidase. In addition, off-loading of oxygen to the tissues is impaired by the leftward shift of the oxygen-dissociation curve induced by carboxyhaemoglobinaemia. The result is profound hypoxia both in the intra- and extracellular environments. The areas most affected are those with a high metabolic rate: neurological and cardiovascular organ systems. Fetal tissue is also at significant risk.

The duration of the patient's exposure to carbon monoxide is significant, as short exposures to a high concentration may cause high carboxyhaemoglobin levels but not cause significant metabolic effects (usually acidosis with bicarbonate deficit). These are usually more severe in patients with low-level exposures of a longer duration. Carboxyhaemoglobin levels greater than 10% are significant and levels greater than 50% are generally lethal.

> Carbon monoxide intoxication is the biggest cause of death in people caught in house fires, or other types of closed-space fires.

Cyanide poisoning

When the polyurethane foam in modern furniture burns, a thick black smoke is produced. This not only contains carbon monoxide and the corrosive substances mentioned above but also cyanide gas. The latter is another metabolic poison which binds to the ferric moiety of mitochondrial cytochrome oxidase. This leads to inhibition of ATP production with rapid onset of profound cellular anoxia and death. Cyanide gas is difficult to measure but should be assumed to be present if the carbon monoxide level is greater than 10%.

TRAUMA SEVERITY SCORING

This allows the severity to be assessed, the prognosis to be estimated and comparisons to be made between treatment methods within a centre or between trauma centres. Such scores must be interpreted sensibly, especially in individual cases.

Injury Severity Score (ISS) describes the anatomical severity of an injury. The body is divided into six regions and the severity of injury is graded from 1 (minor) to 6 (unsurvivable). The highest grading scores, from three separate regions, are squared and added together to make the final score.

Revised Trauma Score (RTS) measures the physiological derangement. It combines the Glasgow Coma Scale score, the respiratory function score 0(nil)–4, and systolic blood pressure 0(nil)–4 (BP>89). The final score is calculated after weighting the individual scores, using a simple computer programme.

TRISS is a number derived from the ISS, RTS, the age of the patient and the mechanism of injury (i.e. blunt or penetrating). It enables the likely outcome to be predicted for an individual against a large database.

Summary

1. Trauma is an important clinical and economic problem because it is a major cause of mortality and morbidity.
2. In order to be effective in trauma care, the clinician needs a good understanding of the biomechanics of injury and how they relate to specific anatomical regions of the body.
3. The clinician also needs to be aware of both the physiological and pathophysiological response to trauma, as this has direct implications for optimum patient resuscitation.
4. These anatomical and physiological assessments can be used to quantify the severity of the trauma so that comparisons between treatment methods can be made.

ACKNOWLEDGEMENTS

Thanks are also due to Richard Cowie, Charles Galasko, Roop Kishen, Roderick Little, David Marsh, Mohamed Rady, Stewart Watson and David Whitby.

Further reading

Barton R (ed) 1985 Trauma and its metabolic problems. British Medical Bulletin 41(3) Barton R 1987 The neuroendocrinology of physical injury. Baillière's Clinical Endocrinology and Metabolism 13(2): 355–374

Barton R, Frayn K, Little R 1990 Trauma, burns and surgery. In: Cohen R, Lewis B, Alberti K, Denman A (eds) The metabolic and molecular basis of acquired disease. Baillière Tindall, London, pp 684–717

Beale R, Grover E, Smithies M, Bihari D 1993 Acute respiratory distress syndrome (ARDS): no more than a severe acute lung injury? British Medical Journal 307: 1335–1339

Bessey P, Wilmore D 1988 The burned patient. In: Kinney J, Jeejeebhoy K, Hill G, Owen O (eds) Nutrition and metabolism in patient care. W B Saunders, Philadelphia, pp 672–700

Bone R 1996 Toward a theory regarding the pathogenesis of the systemic inflammatory response syndrome: what we do and do not know about cytokine regulation. Crit Care Med 24: 163–172

Charlton J, Murphy M 1998 The health of adult Britain, 1841–1994. Volume 2. Office of National Statistics, London

Colucciello S 1995 The treacherous and complex spectrum of maxillofacial trauma: etiologies, evaluation and emergency stabilisation. Emergency Medicine Reports 16: 59–70

Cole R, Shakespeare P 1990 Toxic shock syndrome in scalded children. Burns 16: 221–224

Cuthbertson D 1980 Alterations in metabolism following injury: part 1. Injury 11: 175–189

Driscoll P, Duane L, Monsell F, Wardle T 1995 Optimal long bone fracture management – II. Emergency department assessment. International Journal of Orthopaedic Trauma 5: 110–117

Fong Y, Moldawer L, Shiners G, Lowry S 1990 The biologic characteristics of cytokines and their implication in surgical injury. Surgery, Gynecology and Obstetrics 170: 363–378

Frayn K 1986 Hormonal control of metabolism in trauma and sepsis. Clinical Endocrinology 24: 577–599

Gann D, Amaral J 1989 Endocrine and metabolic responses to injury. In: Schwartz S, Shires G, Spence F (eds) Principles of surgery, 5th edn. McGraw-Hill, New York, pp 1–68

Greenberg C, Sane D 1990 Coagulation problems in critical care medicine. Critical Care: State of the Art 11: 187–194

Grundy D, Swain A 1997 ABC of spinal cord injury, 3rd edn. British Medical Journal, London

Irving M, Stoner H 1987 Metabolism and nutrition in trauma. In: Carter D, Polk H (eds) Butterworths international medical reviews: trauma surgery 1. Butterworths, Oxford, pp 302–314

Johnson M, Lucas G 1996 Fat embolism syndrome. Orthopaedics International Edition 4: 59–68

Little R, Kirkman E, Driscoll P, Hanson J, Mackway-Jones K 1995 Preventable deaths after injury: why are traditional 'vital' signs poor indicators of blood loss? Journal of Accident and Emergency Medicine 12: 1–14

Matthay M 1990 The adult respiratory distress syndrome: definition and prognosis. Clinics in Chest Medicine 11 (4): 575–580

Moore J, Moore E, Thompson J 1980 Abdominal injuries associated with penetrating trauma in the lower chest. American Journal of Surgery 140: 724–730

Monsell F, Driscoll P, Wardle T, Southworth S, Kishen R 1995 Optimal long bone fracture management – III. Preoperative care in the accident and emergency department. International Journal of Orthopaedic Trauma 5: 158–166

Murphy P G, Jones J G 1991 Acute lung injury. British Journal of Intensive Care 1 (3): 110–117

Mubarak S, Hargens A 1983 Acute compartment syndromes. Surgical Clinics of North America 63: 539–565

Proctor J, Wright S 1995 Abdominal trauma: keys to rapid treatment. In: Bosker G (ed). Catastrophic emergencies. Diagnosis and management. American Health Consultants, Atlanta, GA, pp 65–74

Repine J 1992 Scientific perspective on adult respiratory distress syndrome. Lancet 339: 466–469

Schlag G, Redl H 1993 Pathophysiology of shock, sepsis and organ failure. Springer-Verlag, Berlin

Skinner D, Driscoll P, Earlam R 1996 ABC of major trauma. British Medical Journal, London

Stoner H 1986 Metabolism after trauma and in sepsis. Circulatory Shock 19: 75–87

Stoner H 1995 The metabolic and nutritional aspects of trauma – an historical introduction. International Journal of Orthopaedic Trauma 5: 60–68

ten Duis H 1997 The fat embolism syndrome. Injury 28: 77–85

Taylor R, Norwood S 1988 The adult respiratory distress syndrome. In: Civetta J, Taylor R, Kirby R (eds). Critical care. Lippincott, Philadelphia, pp 1057–1068

Wilmore D 1977 The metabolic management of the critically
ill. Plenum, New York

Wyatt J, Beard D, Gray A, Busuttil A, Robertson C 1995 The
time of death after trauma. British Medical Journal 310:
1502

Patient assessment

3

Clinical history and examination

R. M. Kirk

Objectives

- **Appreciate the paramount importance of history taking and examination.**
- **Remember that one of the most difficult clinical decisions is to state that there is no abnormality.**

Young child	Appendicitis
Young woman	Gynaecological
Young man	Hernia, appendicitis
Middle-aged woman	Gynaecological, diverticulosis coli
Middle-aged man	Diverticulosis coli
Elderly woman	Gynaecological, cancer colon
Elderly man	Cancer colon

Fig 3.1 The presenting patient prejudices the clinician. If you are seeing a patient with lower abdominal pain, the diagnoses that you first consider are influenced by the type of patient.

Should you read this chapter? Maybe you think you are already too experienced to need instruction. If you think so, then you are definitely lacking self-knowledge. Of all the skills you require in surgery and in medicine generally, taking a history, examining the patient and interpreting your findings are paramount. They form the base from which you work. If you take the wrong diagnostic path all the rest of your activities are misdirected.

HISTORY

Traditionally, surgeons have prided themselves on their ability to elicit physical signs and make accurate 'spot diagnoses'. We have, perhaps, not always sufficiently developed the skills of history-taking. Do not be in any doubt that a good history is vital. Many surgical diseases produce no physical signs. If you embark on surgical treatment after concentrating on a localized lesion you will be unprepared if complications develop.

As you first encounter the patient, take in every aspect of gender, age, dress, speech, gait and attitude. This prejudices your interpretation of what you are told. 'Prejudice' is often considered a pejorative term; it is reprehensible only if it is rigidly maintained against the evidence. By sensibly incorporating their impressions of the patient with the history, experienced clinicians often make a provisional diagnosis within a few seconds (Fig. 3.1). Treat such a diagnosis merely as a

working hypothesis, useful for the present, to be tested and abandoned at once if it is refuted.

> Ask 'open' questions whenever possible, e.g., 'Where is your pain?' not, 'Is your pain here?'

The next time you sit before a new patient, try to analyse the sequence of your questions, your motivation in asking them in that manner, and your interpretation of the answers. It is sometimes valuable to place a tape recorder on the table so that you can subsequently analyse the progression of your questions. Listen to others while they take a history; can you differentiate between the skilled and the unskilled? What is the difference?

There are two parts to taking the history – determining the cause of the complaint that has brought the patient to you, and determining the general state and feelings of the patient.

Presenting complaint

Do not passively listen and record the patient's words. The danger of this is that it leaves the direction of the discussion to the patient; you must control and lead the interview. This entails asking a question, letting the patient answer it, then cutting in at the correct moment to ask for clarification, ask a supplementary question, or change tack. Too early an interruption causes resentment but if the opportunity is missed the patient is likely to go off at a tangent and resist being brought back to your line of thought.

The object of questions about the presenting symptom is to determine the anatomical site of the lesion causing it. Does function of the suspect system affect the symptom, does the symptom affect the function of the system? The same line of questioning must be applied to all suspect systems. Your intention is that one system may be confidently implicated and the others are exonerated (Fig. 3.2).

Supplementary questions are intended to reveal a pattern of a group of features that 'run' together and form a syndrome (Greek: *syn* = together + *dromos* = a course). As a likely diagnosis enters your mind you will ask about other features that are usually associated with it.

As the origin of the presenting symptom is localized, determine its severity, duration, mode of onset, relieving factors and general effects.

General assessment

Having reached a provisional explanation for the presenting complaint, carefully assess each body system by means of questions about its function now and in the past. There are sets of fairly standard questions that may reveal malfunctions. If the patient answers 'Yes' to the question, 'Are you short of breath when climbing stairs?' the possibilities of cardiorespiratory disease and anaemia immediately spring to mind.

Ask what the patient thinks about the cause of the symptoms. The answers provide guidance in deciding how to explain the problem and give reassurance.

EXAMINATION

Where is the local lesion?

If there is a localized lesion, first determine exactly where it is. Remember the standardized progression:

Look, Feel, Percuss, Listen. Review the structures in the area and carry out tests to find out whether they lie over or under the lesion and whether it is attached to them. Examples are upward movement of a structure attached to the trachea when the patient swallows, and intra-abdominal tenderness to palpation that is allayed when the patient is asked to perform a manoeuvre that tenses the overlying abdominal muscles. If you know where the lesion is, and know the structures, you can usually deduce the likely diagnosis in this patient. Do not distress the patient by clumsy, painful palpation; except in some emergencies it is never necessary and is counterproductive because the patient guards against your examination, preventing you from gaining vital information.

> Be positive. If a structure is normal, say so. Do not avoid responsibility by stating, 'Query slight enlargement of ... e.g. spleen.'

What are the characteristics of a lump? You should already know the site. Now determine the size, shape, surface, consistency and special characteristics. For example, is it tender, hot, pulsatile, reducible, bilateral, fluctuant, coloured, translucent? Is there a cough impulse, overlying inflammation, oedema or vascularity? What is the effect of movement or function of the part?

Do not forget the simple principles of examination. For example, when you discover an enlarged lymph node in the neck, you should automatically remember to examine the drainage area of the gland and the remainder of the reticuloendothelial system. When you identify local vascular disease, examine the whole cardiovascular system. If one joint is diseased, look at the others.

Remarkably, we all miss diagnoses, not because they are obscure, but because we do not assiduously follow the routines that we learned at the beginning of clinical training.

General examination

Develop the skill to carry out a rapid but thorough examination of the patient. In this way you familiarize

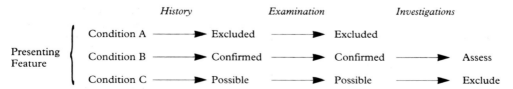

Fig 3.2   The presenting feature may suggest a number of diagnoses. Each step is intended to exclude or confirm each diagnosis. You hope to end with only one diagnosis, with the others confidently excluded.

yourself with the range of normality and can quickly and confidently detect abnormalities.

Thoughtless, repeated observation, palpation and other examinations are a waste of time and may be distressing for the patient. Try to examine everything once only, concentrating on the findings. A common fault is to 'go through the motions' of, for example, palpating lymph nodes, rather than to obtain accurate, crucial information at a single examination.

However, if a single examination is equivocal, be willing to repeat it after an interval. Physical signs often change rapidly, especially in acute conditions.

When you have completed the physical examination, ask yourself if there is anything you missed out and why you forgot it.

DIAGNOSIS

The mechanism of diagnosis is complex. Do not make your task more difficult by uncritically gathering vast amounts of irrelevant information. Medical students are often taught that if they listen to what the patient tells them, a diagnosis will emerge. This is not so. The clinician cannot then pick out the relevant, discriminating features from the confusing mass of accumulated facts. Medical and surgical diagnosis resembles scientific investigation. You must ask the right questions to obtain the correct answer.

You do not carry a ranked list of causes for each presenting feature in your head. In some cases it is pattern recognition. From your accumulated experience, reading, and listening to others, you develop associations in your mind. The overweight, multiparous woman with postprandial upper abdominal symptoms forms a pattern which triggers the possibility of gallstones or reflux oesophagitis. However, the discovery of an unexpected feature should warn you of the possibility of another diagnosis. Remember, also, that young, slim males may develop gallstones.

You now hope to have a reasonably confident diagnosis, you have eliminated other causes for the presenting features, and you have made an assessment of the physical and mental state of the patient.

Suitable investigations can now be ordered, to corroborate the working diagnosis, to exclude others more certainly, and to assess the severity, extent or anatomical site of an identified condition.

A firm diagnosis may not always be possible but sufficient information may be gained to plan a course of action. In a patient with an 'acute abdomen', the information often allows you to make a clinical decision to perform exploratory laparotomy, further investigation, medical treatment, to ask a specialist in another field, or

to observe the patient for a limited period and reassess the clinical features.

If you are still in doubt after taking a history and examining the patient, do not necessarily rush to order investigations in the hope that 'something will turn up'. Of course, intelligently selected investigations may be invaluable in confusing cases. All too often, however, they are instruments for vacillation. It is frequently more profitable and less time-consuming to go back to the beginning and retake the history, repeat the examination, or ask a colleague to do so with an open mind.

On many occasions the newly given history may differ markedly from the first, perhaps because you have misinterpreted what the patient has said, or allowed the patient to take charge and been led astray.

Some questions and signs have a high discriminatory value, others do not. A clinical feature or test may give a falsely positive prediction of the diagnosis. Two or three points that suggest one diagnosis may be of less value than one that has a high discriminatory capacity. For example, the diagnosis of acute, uncomplicated appendicitis is often mistakenly made because the pain is in the right iliac fossa, the patient has gastrointestinal symptoms and is tender in the right iliac fossa. However, if there is also tenderness in the left iliac fossa, this must either be complicated, i.e. perforated appendicitis, or another diagnosis must be considered. Localized tenderness over a localized organ is highly discriminatory.

When in doubt between the likely (i.e. the most common) diagnosis and a less frequent but important diagnosis, do not lightly pass over the important one. It is dangerous to miss a rarer but serious condition.

RECORD

All the effort you have put into elucidating the problem may be lost if you do not make a careful record that can be read and understood by others – and by yourself. Although various devices for recording are available, they sometimes fail. Even if you have dictated into a recording machine, write down the details as well.

Having recorded the findings in the history and the examination, state your conclusions, your policy and what emerged from your discussion with the patient. If you intend to arrange investigations, state what you have in mind. If you arrange treatment, state what monitoring procedures should be carried out.

THINK

Have you missed anything? Have you rushed to the wrong conclusion? Is there a vital question that you could ask, or a physical sign to test your provisional diagnosis?

Remember your obligations to the patient, not just to make a correct diagnosis but also to give reassurance that you have excluded a serious alternative condition. For example, the confident discovery that minimal haemorrhoids, which may not even warrant any treatment, are the cause of rectal bleeding, does not absolve you from carrying out sigmoidoscopy and any other tests to exclude large bowel cancer.

DISCUSS

In the past, informing the patient, discussing and explaining possible actions and their consequences were often casually performed. This is no longer tolerable. Listen to the patient and, if necessary, change your policy of management. Do not forget to inform relatives in appropriate circumstances.

EMERGENCY

You cannot obsessively stick to a routine in some situations. A patient may have airway obstruction or calamitous bleeding, or may be in excruciating pain, mentally disarranged, violent or unconscious. In each case you must quickly and accurately determine the cause of the emergency state, correct it and deal with lesser conditions as the opportunities occur. It is particularly important to record everything, otherwise some vital consideration may be missed when routines are broken. When the emergency condition is under control, meticulously carry out a thorough assessment.

We should all prefer to see patients one by one and complete our examination before seeing the next patient. Sometimes a number of patients present simultaneously or in rapid sequence. Do not obsessively continue examining a patient with a trivial complaint while keeping others waiting who have life-threatening or painful conditions.

When a number of emergencies present at the same time you must apply triage (French: *trier* = to pick out). In principle, this recognizes that loss of life is more important than loss of a limb.

Summary

1. The history is vital in directing you to the cause of the presenting features.
2. Recognizing what is normal demands extensive familiarity with the range of normality.
3. Do not fail to discuss the problems with the patient, or fail to respond to the patient's reactions.
4. Record what you asked, what you examined, what you found, what it means – and what actions you have taken, or will take.

4

Investigations

M. Pemberton, N. Cheshire, M. Pietroni

Objectives

- **To define the aims of investigation used in surgical practice.**
- **To understand the principles underlying selection of appropriate investigations.**
- **To determine the limitations of commonly used investigations.**
- **To consider appropriate sequences and timing of multiple investigations.**
- **To highlight those investigations most commonly used in clinical practice.**

INTRODUCTION

It should go without saying that the use of investigations in surgical practice is no substitute for clinical skill and that an investigation is only worthwhile when it is requested in order to answer a specific question, or confirm an important clinical impression prior to intervention. The ever expanding range of investigative modalities now available emphasizes this principle; the unwary surgeon who is clinically uncertain can easily find himself overwhelmed with information if too many poorly considered investigations are requested. Furthermore, many modern tests are expensive and the financial implications of any investigation must always be considered in today's cash limited health service. There are many other important issues that govern the effective use of special investigations, including their selection, timing and interpretation. The purpose of this chapter is to outline some of the principles that should be applied before investigations are requested in surgical practice, and to summarize the applications and limitations of those investigations most commonly used.

THE AIM OF INVESTIGATIONS

Investigations are performed for a number of different reasons but all should share the feature of directing management. The most common reasons for ordering investigations in surgical practice are outlined below.

Confirmation of diagnosis

Chronologically, the first use of investigations should be to confirm or refute a suspected clinical diagnosis as it is nowadays generally accepted best practice to confirm and define the extent of the suspected disease process before intervention is carried out – particularly in elective surgery (e.g. abdominal aortic aneurysm). Among other benefits, the use of investigations in this manner allows a full and informed discussion of the likely outcome to be undertaken with the patient and his family prior to surgery and optimizes the use of operating theatre time and equipment as well as minimizing the chances of the surgical team being presented with any unpleasant (or unprepared for) surprises during the operation.

Such preoperative confirmation is not always required, however, as there remain conditions for which clinical diagnostic acumen matches or exceeds the accuracy of any investigative tool (acute appendicitis), as well as conditions whose treatment uncontroversially confirms the diagnosis (ischiorectal abscess). None the less, even in these instances it is useful to confirm the clinical diagnosis made, usually histologically, to avoid missing an underlying condition (carcinoid as a cause of appendicitis, Crohn's disease leading to ischiorectal abscess formation).

Exclusion of alternative diagnoses

In addition to confirmation of the primary diagnosis, it is necessary sometimes to perform an investigation in order to exclude a specific important alternative or additional diagnosis (frequently malignancy), the presence of which may significantly alter management or the advice the clinician offers to the patient. In some specialities, most notably breast, this principle has become incorporated into standard practice and investigations are undertaken to exclude hepatic and skeletal metastases before management of the primary lesion in the breast. It is important, however, to remember resource and financial implications when planning investigations in this manner; a barium enema cannot be performed on all patients with irritable bowel syndrome, magnetic resonance imaging (MRI) cannot be performed on all patients with back-ache. In each individual consultation an attempt must be made to establish the degree of certainty appropriate to the clinical situation faced.

During the preoperative process of diagnostic confirmation, determination of the extent of disease and exclusion of specific alternative diagnoses, more than one special investigation may frequently need to be undertaken. In these circumstances thought must be given to determining the appropriate order of such investigations. If on liver ultrasound a patient with a lower oesophageal adenocarcinoma is found to have multiple metastases, investigation of local spread (endoluminal ultrasound, CT) becomes inappropriate as it will not contribute to management, which will be palliative.

Assessment of fitness for surgery

In patients in whom *major* surgery is required, an additional further aim of investigations is to assess fitness for anaesthesia. A patient with an asymptomatic aortic aneurysm typically presents with a history of smoking and widespread cardiovascular disease and requires particularly careful evaluation of cardiac and pulmonary function if informed advice about mortality and outcome are to be given to the patient preoperatively. Whilst in many cases a combination of the use of ECG, ECHO cardiography, lung function tests and blood gases can appropriately assess fitness for anaesthesia, these expensive and time-consuming tests cannot be undertaken on all patients and the clinical history is frequently not straightforward. Under such circumstances it is important to emphasize that a cardiological or respiratory opinion may be better than to request indiscriminate investigations in the domain of another speciality. Advance consultation with one's anaesthetist ahead of planned surgery may lead to fewer cancellations on the day of surgery.

Risk to others

Certain investigations may be appropriate in patients being prepared for surgery in order to determine risk to others. Thus in homosexual males and intravenous drug abusers, hepatitis B and HIV serology (with appropriate consent) should be performed. In vascular patients with leg ulcers, particularly those being transferred from another hospital, their MRSA status should be characterized and appropriate isolation procedures activated where necessary.

Postoperative investigations

After definitive surgical intervention, patients may also be investigated in order to screen for persistence or recurrence of disease. Once again such investigation is generally only appropriate in so far as it informs management. Thus while serial postoperative liver ultrasound may be worthwhile in patients who have undergone curative resection of colorectal cancer as resection of liver recurrence may be performed, in the case of upper gastrointestinal cancer such imaging would be relatively futile as curative resection of liver metastases is not possible. For vascular patients who have undergone lower limb bypass surgery, graft surveillance of vein bypasses to detect hyperplastic graft stenosis is worthwhile as it may allow an intervention to prolong the patency of the graft, but surveillance of prosthetic grafts is less beneficial as it may not effectively predict graft failure.

Medicolegal considerations

Finally, investigations are used to satisfy medicolegal considerations; their role in these circumstances may be quite different from their purely clinical application. While skull X-rays in patients with minor head injuries generally have little impact on their clinical management, the presence of a fracture may have significance in the criminal rather than the medical domain. In patients in whom a legal case is anticipated or impending, advice from colleagues (to produce a 'quorum opinion') or from those with experience in the medicolegal world is often invaluable. It is useful to remember, in these circumstances, that the confirmation or refutation of a diagnosis by an appropriate objective test may carry more weight with the court than a clinical impression; however, one should not blindly adopt a policy of over-investigation and defensive medicine without advice.

SELECTION OF APPROPRIATE INVESTIGATIONS

There is often more than one modality that may be used to answer the clinical question the surgeon is faced with, in which case consideration needs to be given to the selection of the most appropriate modality. Various factors should influence this choice:

The sensitivity of the investigation

If one test is known to be more sensitive than the alternative, this is obviously a good reason to choose it. Colonoscopy is more sensitive than barium enema for the detection of small polyps and is the investigation of choice with lower GI bleeding. If the test cannot answer the question asked, omit it. [123]I scintigraphy for investigation of thyroid nodules is hard to justify as only 10% low uptake nodules are subsequently shown to be malignant.

The simplicity of the investigation

If a plain X-ray confirms the clinical diagnosis of osteomyelitis in a diabetic foot and the management plan is clear, it is not necessary to order a bone scan or MR imaging.

The safety of the investigation

Endoscopy may provide useful information as to the cause of bowel perforation but it is not safe in this situation, nor is the use of barium-based contrast. Whilst a Tru-cut biopsy may confirm a diagnosis, it may also result in tumour seeding – ask the cyto/histopathologist whether a fine needle aspirate (FNA) may give sufficient information for management decisions to be made.

The cost of the investigation

If an ultrasound can show liver metastases and this is the only information you require to decide on appropriate management, then why order a CT scan which may be up to ten times more expensive.

The acceptability of the investigation to the patient

Whilst upper GI endoscopy may be the investigation of choice in your institution, if the patient with epigastric pain refuses the test, then a barium meal is required. In general the less invasive the investigation the more acceptable it is to the patient. A colour duplex scan may provide as much information as an arteriogram in patients with femoropopliteal occlusive disease with no discomfort and less risk. Acceptability to the patient is an especially important consideration in asymptomatic patients being screened for a particular disease. One of the limitations of the use of faecal occult blood testing as a screening investigation for colorectal cancer has been the relative unacceptability of this investigation to patients.

The availability of an investigation

An MRI scan may provide more information about the brain after injury or prior to neurovascular or neurosurgical intervention, but if the institution you are working in does not have an MR scanner and you need information rapidly you must make do with a CT scan.

THE LIMITATIONS OF INVESTIGATIONS

The most important limitation of an investigation is that the result it gives may be wrong and therefore misleading. If the result of any investigation conflicts with your clinical judgment, do not discard the clinical impression without considering the possibility that the test may be incorrect. Gaining sufficient confidence in your clinical ability to question the opinion of others is difficult but also essential if a safe and rewarding clinical practice is to be developed. Remember that in many circumstances you, as the surgeon, may be the only individual who has actually spoken to and examined the patient and therefore you are in a unique position to judge the likely accuracy of the investigation result you are presented with.

Any investigation can give a wrong answer for various reasons:

It was incorrectly performed. The blood test was taken from the same arm as normal saline was being infused. The bottle was incorrectly labelled. The bowel was inadequately prepared for the barium enema. The appropriate X-ray view for the fracture was not taken.

The investigation was wrongly interpreted. A polyp was mistaken as faecal residue. An air bubble was mistaken as a small gallstone.

The limited sensitivity of all tests. A breast FNA may have been technically well performed and correctly interpreted but still miss a carcinoma because of a sampling error of the lump assessed.

If an investigation does not support a firm clinical diagnosis, consider repeating it or choosing another test to answer the same question. Frequently, however, it is more helpful to discuss it with the person who performed the test to ensure that as much clinical information as possible has been passed on to the highly trained individual who is trying to give you a result. An inadequate report may have been based on inadequate information given on the request form. Providing the radiologist with more clinical information may change the interpretation of images obtained. To this end combined clinical meetings between the surgical team and radiologists, histopathologists, etc. are often the ideal forum for the exchange of information and ideas as well as an opportunity for you to discuss the best way forward in the investigation or management of complex patients. Remember also that an investigation may yield a false positive as well as false negative result.

> *Sensitivity* : number of cases of the condition detected by the test/total number of cases in population studied.
>
> *Specificity* : number of patients with condition/total number of positive results.

Complications of investigations

It is no less important than the above to remember that an investigation may be associated with a significant complication rate, an issue that may not only influence one's choice of its use, but also may have medicolegal implications if it has not been discussed at the time of consent. Is a selective carotid arteriogram really worth the 1% stroke rate when a duplex scan may give all the necessary information? Think whether this complication rate could be reduced or should be avoided altogether. Hydrate the patient with a raised creatinine intravenously before giving contrast to perform an arteriogram. Consider giving the older patient clean prep rather than picolax before a colonoscopy.

Financial implications

On a practical level, remember that resources are limited. Reassurance and certainty are purchased at a price. Moving from a position of 95% to 100% certainty is often very expensive. When using investigations it is vital to understand the need to manage risk while at the same time remaining accountable to the patient and to society for the way in which money is spent.

THE SEQUENCE AND TIMING OF INVESTIGATIONS

Whenever you are investigating a patient prior to surgery or during follow-up, do not collect data indiscriminately. Always organize the flow of information you require so that it follows a logical sequence which will culminate in you being able to discuss the patient's condition and management, with any attendant risks, in a fully informed manner and from a position of strength. Avoid the temptation to arrange all investigations at one sitting to prevent the patient having to come back repeatedly to the clinic. It is obviously inappropriate to arrange cardiology and pulmonary function tests to assess fitness for surgery at the same time as determining the primary disease and any spread. If the surgical problem turns out to be inoperable, then the other investigations undertaken have usually been a waste of time and resources as well as putting the patient at potential risk. Patients often understand the need for a logical sequence of investigations and the time this may require. Only when you have progressed through appropriate assessments will you be in a position to speak confidently to the complex patient with multisystem disorders who requires surgical intervention.

Once again, learning to investigate patients in this manner is difficult initially. You must constantly assess your skills and knowledge, explore your attitude and be aware of your constraints. You will usually work by pattern recognition and hypothesis testing rather than on a blank slate to which you gradually add data. During the diagnostic process you must always ask the vital questions such as, 'What is the likely cause here?' and 'What must I not miss?' In addition, learn to ask yourself, 'What is the urgency here? What management options (if any) are available for this patient if we reach a diagnosis? What is the most important complication of the investigation or management I am proposing (and can this be justified given the presenting symptoms)?'

Failure to ask these questions leads to inappropriate investigations in all the surgical specialities, especially when pursuing ill-defined abdominal pain (in general surgery), vague back pain (in orthopaedic surgery), 'cystitis' in young women (in gynaecology and urology), chronic catarrhal pharyngitis (in ear, nose and throat (ENT) surgery), ill-defined and long-standing headaches (in neurosurgery), and all the other chronic problems that overload the outpatient departments of all the surgical specialities.

The experienced surgeon facing a patient very quickly forms a working hypothesis while taking a history. The anatomical area of the problem, the physical process at play and the pathology are generally identified in that order. The purpose of investigations is to reduce the management options and to seek to obtain crucial information once, not repeatedly. Sometimes an impasse is reached. Reflect, reconsider, and perhaps postpone a decision for a while, using time as a diagnostic tool. If you rush to make a decision where there is no indication for urgency you will make mistakes. A high negative laparotomy rate in a surgeon usually indicates an unwillingness to use time in this way, perhaps because of organizational constraints. Avoid the temptation to do a laparotomy in the middle of the night just because of the difficulties you might encounter if the need for surgery emerges the next day.

THE PRACTICAL USE OF COMMON INVESTIGATIONS

General investigations

Blood tests

Haematology. Most laboratories use analysers that give all the common haematological indices when only a haemoglobin (Hb) estimation is required. Be careful to interpret these values in the light of the patient's general condition. For example, dehydrated patients have a high Hb and packed cell volume (PCV, haematocrit) because of haemoconcentration; a normal Hb in such patients may mask anaemia. Patients who are heavy smokers or who have chronic obstructive airways disease also have raised Hb levels. Do not be misled into overtransfusing patients. There are serious risks attached, especially in paediatrics and neurosurgery.

The Hb level by itself is insufficient to establish the transfusion requirements in acute blood loss. In the first few hours after blood loss it cannot answer the question: 'How much blood has been lost?' The body's physiological responses to shock produce a reduction in the capacity of the circulation. It is only after many hours that haemodilution produces a representative cellular/plasma ratio, when the PCV is a better guide.

The level of the white blood cell (WBC) count is a valuable indicator but not an accurate diagnostic tool. When raised it gives useful corroborative evidence of infection. When normal it does not exclude infection. By itself it cannot answer the questions: 'Has this patient got appendicitis?' and, 'Is there postoperative sepsis somewhere?' Remember that the WBC count is also raised in the presence of tissue necrosis (e.g. burns in plastic surgery) and need not necessarily imply infection.

In the presence of overwhelming sepsis, a low or normal WBC level indicates an inability of the patient's immune system to react to infection. Levels of $15-18 \times 10^9$ WBC per litre generally indicate intermediate degrees of infection, while levels over 20×10^9 WBC per litre suggest life-threatening sepsis. Trends can be more useful than absolute levels. A falling WBC count in a clinically improving patient suggests response to treatment.

Always seek the haematologist's help when analysing bleeding disorders and coagulopathies. In the presence of massive blood loss and whenever six or more units of blood have been transfused, check the platelet count, the prothrombin time (PT) and the kaolin cephalin clotting time (KCCT) to identify any prolonged bleeding tendency. The result may indicate the need to infuse platelets or fresh frozen plasma. In cases of suspected disseminated intravascular coagulopathy (DIC) the haematologist's help is essential. Measure fibrinogen degradation products and fibrinogen titres and measure the thrombin time. These results will assist in assessing the need for platelets, cryoprecipitate and fresh frozen plasma.

Patients with deep venous thrombosis (DVT) or pulmonary embolism (PE) require anticoagulation. Use the activated partial thromboplastin time (APTT) for heparin therapy and the PT for patients on warfarin. The laboratory results will usually be expressed as international normalized ratios (INR), to aid therapeutic adjustments. Once the patient has been stabilized, the frequency of testing can be gradually reduced to once weekly and eventually to once monthly. Sometimes there is a background predisposition to DVT and PE which may be congenital. Check on protein C, protein S, antithrombin III, lupus anticoagulant and anticardiolipin antibody, if you suspect this may be the case (recurrent DVT and PE, or if there is a family history).

Perform a sickle cell test on all patients from the Middle East, the Indian subcontinent and on those of African and Mediterranean extraction. Hypoxia and dehydration are especially dangerous in these patients as a sickle cell crisis may be so induced. When ordering blood for cross matching do not overestimate the need. Order blood grouping, saving the serum for operations of medium severity such as nephrectomy, cholecystectomy and thyroidectomy. The transfusion of blood postoperatively is rarely required here.

Discuss cases of suspected lymphoma with the haematologist. It may be that if the peripheral blood picture shows involvement (as in chronic lymphatic leukaemia), peripheral blood marker studies will lessen the need for lymph node biopsy. This will avoid the need for a general anaesthetic, and a bone marrow sample can be taken under local anaesthetic instead. If you do need a lymph node biopsy (see below), then do not forget that the haematologist can help as well as the histopathologist.

Biochemistry. As is the case for haematological assessment, modern biochemistry laboratories use an autoanalyser. All the common biochemical indices are measured even if only one has been requested. The results are expressed as concentrations per unit volume of blood. Blood loss, dehydration, infusion and transfusion will therefore affect the result. This is especially important when dextrose or lipids are being infused. Avoid a tourniquet if you want calcium levels.

Potassium leaches out of cells, so avoid delay in delivering the sample for analysis.

Remember you are sampling plasma. You are only indirectly discovering what is going on inside cells. Potassium levels, for instance, reflect poorly the intracellular potassium. The plasma amylase is only transiently raised in the plasma during pancreatitis. Hormone, enzyme and drug levels are affected by the levels of the plasma proteins, so allow for this when interpreting results.

You need information about electrolyte balance in patients with dehydration and intestinal obstruction. Sodium, potassium and bicarbonate levels will assist you in judging fluid and acid–base balance. The rate at which laboratory values change will dictate how often these tests should be performed. There is no need to repeat these tests on a daily basis if the changes are not clinically significant. The body's homoeostatic mechanisms are usually very good, but if the physiology of the lungs or kidneys is impaired then you will need information more often.

Be careful with dehydrated patients who have diabetes as well as intestinal obstruction. Use glucose and potassium levels as well as the electrolytes in gauging transfusion requirements. Keep an eye on the levels of urea and creatinine. Any element of renal failure in addition will make therapeutic judgements difficult.

In surgery the investigation of the jaundiced patient is now a radiological rather than a biochemical exercise. However, the balance between the levels of bilirubin, alkaline phosphatase and the transaminases will give valuable additional information. Obstruction is always characterized by high bilirubin and alkaline phosphatase levels. The latter often lag behind the bilirubin when the obstruction has been relieved. Hepatocellular damage is usually reflected more in the transaminases, which are then disproportionately raised.

Use hormone assays intelligently when investigating thyroid disease. There is scarcely ever a need for all the thyroid function tests to be performed. What do you want to know? Hypothyroidism is reflected in a low total thyroxine (T4) and high levels of thyroid-stimulating hormone (TSH), while hyperthyroidism will produce high levels of total T4 and tri-iodothyronine (T3). Measuring the levels of free T3 and T4 is not necessarily helpful unless the total levels are misleading in patients with protein abnormalities, the pregnant and the elderly. If your patient is on maintenance therapy, judge her control clinically. Do not be swayed by the biochemical levels. Thyrotoxic patients controlled with propranolol will still have abnormal biochemical levels even though they are well controlled clinically.

Microbiology

A pus swab only briefly contains a representative sample of organisms from an infected source. Organisms die because they are anaerobic (e.g. *Streptococcus faecalis*), because they are delicate (e.g. *Neisseria*), or because the other organisms in the sample proliferate faster and overwhelm them. Therefore lose no time between taking the swab and transferring it to an appropriate medium for culture. If pus is available then collect a quantity and send that, rather than a swab, to the microbiologist. Pus swabs (in appropriate transport medium) should be stored at 4°C when taken at night. Ensure that they are sent to the laboratory the next day. Remember that prior consultation with a microbiologist may increase the yield of relevant positive cultures obtained.

Taking swabs for culture without careful thought may cause you to miss the diagnosis. Make sure you ask the correct question in order to select the best method of answering it. The detection of amoebic dysentery is not accomplished by taking a swab for culture but by examining a fresh specimen immediately under the microscope. The positive identification of bacteria responsible for late vascular graft infections often requires special techniques (e.g. sonification) to separate the bacteria prior to culture and this requires all the clinical information to be passed on to the microbiologist prior to the arrival of the specimen.

Tell the microbiologist whether the urine specimen you send is a midstream specimen or a catheter specimen. Always interpret the culture report in the light of the microscopy report. More than 15 pus cells per microlitre of urine is generally taken as a significant result. Remember that tuberculosis may present as a sterile acid pyuria. Occasionally, pus cells are seen in great numbers in the absence of any growth on culture. This usually implies a recent operation (e.g. a transurethral resection of the prostate) or the presence of an antibiotic. Do let the microbiologist know about antibiotic therapy. This is especially important when taking blood cultures. Whenever possible, take blood before starting antibiotic therapy. If this is not possible, then let the microbiologist know: the addition of β-lactamase to the culture medium may neutralize the effect of penicillin or cephalosporin.

Always seek the help of the microbiologist whenever you deal with superadded infection, especially in transplant patients and in the immunocompromised (as in HIV infections or in patients on chemotherapy). *Pneumocystis carinii* is the commonest opportunistic infection here. The picture can, however, become quite complicated, partly because several infective agents can become involved (bacterial, viral or fungal) and partly because the picture may change from day to day.

Investigations in oncology

In the assessment of local and systemic spread of malignant disease remember that metastatic spread can only be demonstrated when the secondary lesion(s) is beyond a certain size. Local infiltration and nodal involvement is difficult to demonstrate in its early phases. Weight loss may abolish fat planes that allow CT scans in oesophageal and pancreatic cancer to show boundaries.

One way in which these investigative limitations have been met by improving technology is by taking the imaging modality closer to the site of disease. The use of endoluminal ultrasound (and indeed MR) probes for assessment of local spread of gastrointestinal malignancy exemplifies such developments, and in some centres is routinely used in the assessment of patients with oesophageal and rectal cancer before surgery.

The identification of specific serum tumour markers (CA125, CA19-9 α -fetoprotein, prostate specific antigen (PSA), carcinoembryonic antigen (CEA) represents another way of detecting subclinical recurrent disease. In such cases it is usually helpful to have a baseline measurement of the marker in order to be sure that the repeated measure is appropriate to the particular case. Preoperative measurement of tumour markers allows confirmation of the status of a tumour as a secretor and can also provide a measure of efficacy after intervention. Some markers are of interest for research but have less impact on clinical management at the present time. Once again, it is important to remember the limitations of these tests and their sensitivity and specificity; while oestrogen receptor status predicts the response rate of patients with breast cancer to tamoxifen, the fact that there is a significant response rate in patients who do not express oestrogen receptor means that this investigation may not influence the use of tamoxifen in breast cancer patients.

Gastrointestinal disease

The investigation of disease in the hollow organs of the gastrointestinal tract is traditionally accomplished using contrast media to outline the organ from within. Double-contrast studies using air enable fine mucosal details to be identified by coating the organ lining with the thinnest layer of the contrast agent. Use this form of examination when you wish to outline polyps, other mucosal abnormalities, malabsorption states and Crohn's disease in the small bowel and in determining the extent of colitis. Cancers of the stomach, colon and rectum can also be usefully outlined this way. Endoscopy, however, is usually a quicker and more certain way of establishing the diagnosis of GI malignancy, especially since the most common tumours are relatively accessible by flexible fibre-optic endoscopes and there is simultaneous access to biopsy. A negative endoscopy is usually more reliable than a negative contrast study, but remember that it is operator dependent and that subtle lesions may have been missed (ask about the seniority and experience of the operator if you did not perform the investigation yourself). It may need repeating in cases of doubt. The combination of brushings of suspicious lesions (80% accuracy alone) with biopsy increases accuracy to 90%.

In modern practice, most surgeons use barium studies to outline gross disease or for the small bowel, which is not generally accessible to endoscopy. Local factors in your hospital will determine whether upper gastrointestinal endoscopy and colonoscopy are easily obtained. If they are, then this facility is generally used in preference to barium studies. Of course, barium studies can be used in addition to endoscopy when there is difficulty or conflict between the clinical impression and the result obtained by endoscopy.

For the assessment of functional disease of a hollow organ, radiological contrast studies remain generally better than endoscopy. Better still, for motility disorders use oesophageal or rectal manometry. Barium, and especially cine-barium, studies of swallowing and defecation give good pictures of the functioning organ. Manometry will quantify the problem, as well as facilitate the selection of operative therapy. Thus a mean lower oesophageal sphincter pressure less than 6 mmHg is taken by some authors to be a necessary criterion of surgery for patients with reflux disease. Diagnosis and investigation of small bowel pathology is made more difficult by its relative (but not absolute) inaccessibility to endoscopic assessment. Alternative methods that have been employed here include radionuclide scanning (using the pertechnate anion) for Meckels, where the sensitivity is only 80%, and laparoscopy for the elusive diagnosis of Crohn's disease or small bowel obstruction. Clinical acumen remains at a premium, and a further opinion may often be more useful than asking for another investigation of limited sensitivity.

For screening studies (inflammatory bowel disease, Barrett's oesophagus), endoscopy is generally preferred. Take photographs, take multiple biopsies, take brushings to provide both the macro- and the micro-picture, and to reduce the risk of sampling errors.

Hepatobiliary disease

Ultrasound is frequently the first line imaging modality for patients with hepatobiliary disease. While it is useful for assessing the gallbladder wall and contained stones and for imaging the intrahepatic biliary tree, it is less reliable for imaging the bile duct. Although CT scanning is non-invasive, ask whether ERCP may be more worthwhile for the potential it offers to make an intervention; drainage of the bile duct in a patient with obstructive jaundice, or of the pancreatic duct in the patient with pancreatitis. But remember that even a straightforward diagnostic ERCP is associated with a significant rate of pancreatitis.

In the assessment of malignant disease, there has been considerable recent interest in the use of intraoperative ultrasound for the assessment of metastases. In conjunction with diagnostic laparoscopy, it may reduce the unnecessary laparotomy rate in patients under consideration for hepatectomy, pancreatectomy or other major cancer clearing surgery.

Other tests that have been used in the assessment of the biliary tract include oral and intravenous cholangiography and isotope scanning. These investigations are now considered constrained because of their relatively poor accuracy and are only occasionally indicated in current practice.

Breast disease

The initial assessment of a patient with a breast lump is based on the triad of clinical diagnosis, radiological imaging, and fine needle aspiration cytology (FNAC). Whilst each modality in turn may have an accuracy for diagnosis of malignancy of 80%, 95% and 90% respectively, their use in combination reduces the probability of missing a carcinoma. None the less, they do not provide 100% certainty and some patients may still require further evaluation before they can be safely discharged. Remember that young women (<35 years) have relatively dense breast tissue which makes mammography unsuitable. They are better assessed by ultrasound. If possible, imaging should be performed before performing FNAC, as radiological interpretation is made difficult by the presence of bruising. Otherwise wait for a week.

The debate about the optimum assessment of impalpable axillary nodes remains ongoing. Attempts to define risk of axillary involvement by the characterization of the 'sentinel node' using techniques such as radioscintigraphy remain in their infancy but may reduce the number of unnecessary axillary clearances performed.

In patients who have had previous surgery or with suspected tumour recurrence, for whom interpretation of mammograms or ultrasound is difficult, MRI is now recognized to be a useful diagnostic tool.

Vascular system

Doppler ultrasound

The use of a portable continuous wave Doppler probe remains a cornerstone in the assessment of a patient with vascular symptoms. Learn to use Doppler ultrasound on all your vascular patients. Do it yourself and get used to the problems of siting the probe accurately and using the correct angulation (30–60°). Do not press too hard, as this will occlude the vessel. Accustom yourself to the sound of the biphasic waveform of normal vessels. Obstructed vessels show a short duration waveform with delay before the next waveform. The hand-held Doppler ultrasound is an invaluable tool in the outpatient department, the ward and the operating theatre, and you should learn to diagnose problems by ear. Use Doppler ultrasound in conjunction with a proximally placed sphygmomanometer cuff to find the occluding pressure. The two lower-limb pressures can be compared with each other and with the pressure in the arm (Pressure index = Ankle pressure/Arm pressure). This gives important information about the severity of disease, although it should be remembered that in some patients, particularly those with diabetes and renal disease, the arteries may be incompressible due to vessel wall calcification, and spuriously high readings may be obtained. Remember also that Doppler assessment of flow with the hand-held device is essentially 'blind' and that you cannot confidently tell which vessel (or more importantly, a collateral) you are insonating.

As in other subspecialities, there has been a marked movement away from the use of invasive techniques in the assessment of vascular disease, facilitated by technological advances, particularly in the development of the duplex scanner which combines Doppler assessment of flow with the ability to ultrasonically determine which vessel you are measuring.

Apart from bleeding complications, intra-arterial angiography may cause other local arterial problems (false aneurysm formation, arterial dissection, thrombosis) as well as precipitate contrast-induced renal failure. Furthermore, arteriography is constrained in that it provides only an anatomic guide to disease without giving information as to the haemodynamic impact of an occlusive lesion. Because atheromatous disease is frequently eccentric, significant lesions may be missed altogether on arteriography unless oblique views are taken. For the lower limb this applies particularly to the iliac segment and to the origin of the profunda femoris artery. Digital subtraction imaging is now widely available and has the advantage of being operator-friendly as well as using smaller contrast loads, but in controlled studies has not been found to yield any more information than conventional plain film arteriography. Intravenous subtraction imaging has the advantage of avoiding the risks of arterial puncture, but cannot be reliably used below the level of the superficial femoral arteries due to lack of definition, particularly in patients with poor cardiac function. Importantly, and particularly in the presence of extensive proximal occlusion, even intra-arterial imaging may fail to show patent vessels below the popliteal trifurcation in over 30% of cases due to underfilling with contrast. Surgically reconstructable, critically ischaemic limbs may be inappropriately denied surgery if arteriography alone is depended on for assessment.

Colour duplex imaging has transformed the assessment of occlusive arterial and venous disease and in some centres has displaced arteriography as the primary imaging modality both in lower limb and carotid as well as venous practice. Colour duplex combines B mode ultrasound with pulsed Doppler, and computer-generated images show the vessel interrogated, along with the pattern of flow within, as different colours: at the site of a stenosis, the velocity increases (in proportion to the reduction in diameter) which projects as a colour change. Further waveform analysis at such sites can be performed to provide a more precise characterization of disease. In this way significant occlusive disease may be assessed not only in the lower limb, from aorta to pedal arch, but also in the visceral and carotid arteries. Transcranial Doppler ultrasound allows assessment of the circle of Willis and basilar system and is a useful non-invasive adjunct to carotid artery assessment in cerebrovascular cases.

Magnetic resonance arteriography (MRA) is an alternative non-invasive diagnostic tool for the assessment of occlusive disease and has proved useful particularly in the assessment of renovascular as well as lower limb arterial disease. It has the advantage of being relatively less operator-dependent than colour duplex imaging. Currently, great advances are occurring in software development which will probably result in MRA replacing much of diagnostic angiography in the near future.

Trauma

The successful management of the trauma patient requires a particularly well judged and continuous balance between diagnosis and management in which the correct use of investigative tools can be life-saving. Conversely their inappropriate use may result in dangerous delays in intervention. For major trauma patients, while primary attention should be focused on the ABC of airway, breathing and circulation, early X-rays of chest, cervical spine and pelvis should be organized. The fractured femur may be obvious, but a disrupted cervical spine in an unconscious patient may not be. Interpret blood results with caution (see above), but perform baseline tests anyway. For the initial man-

agement of the patient in shock, obtain large-bore cannula venous access – the insertion of a central line for measurement of CVP is a lesser priority; remember that most central lines do not have the capacity to pass large volumes quickly.

Skull X-rays are rarely of clinical value in trauma cases, but, in head-injured cases, CT scanning frequently is. Consult with a neurosurgeon if in doubt or if a transfer is pending, as transfer may be the overwhelming priority in the cardiovascularly stable patient.

Major chest injuries are usually self-evident. Have a high index of suspicion for an aortic dissection. A supine AP chest X-ray often gives a false positive result with apparent mediastinal widening: confirm or exclude the diagnosis with a contrast CT scan.

The early management of abdominal trauma is clinical. Remember that while ultrasound may be easily obtained, it is unreliable; a CT scan conversely is relatively more time-consuming, and requires transfer out of the resuscitation area. It may be safer to perform a diagnostic peritoneal lavage in borderline cases: but be wary where there is an old midline laparotomy scar or where there is a major pelvic fracture, and ensure that the bladder is emptied first. Think of retroperitoneal injuries or miss them. A simple IVU will demonstrate an intact renal tract; consider performing arteriography where there is complete failure of a kidney to take up contrast to define an arterial injury (has the patient got one kidney?). A CT scan will show major pancreatic injury; a contrast study may be helpful in defining the integrity of the duodenum.

Finally, remember to perform the secondary survey, in order to avoid missing less significant injuries. Have a low threshold for performing X-rays to exclude fractures. There is very often a legal aspect to trauma cases.

Summary

1. Remember that investigations are only worthwhile when they direct management.
2. Always question whether a particular investigation is the best one to answer the question asked.
3. Consider the timing of an investigation.
4. Be aware that all investigations have limitations, particularly with respect to accuracy, and often complications too.
5. Involve other clinicians when uncertain about the choice of an investigation or interpretation of a result.

5

Imaging techniques

S. W. T. Gould, N. Vaughan, T. Beale

Objectives

- Become familiar with the basic techniques and principles of radiological investigation.
- Be able to enumerate the different types of radiological modality, together with their advantages and limitations.
- Understand the principles of selection of the most appropriate radiological technique for a given clinical problem.
- Identify the key roles of radiology in the diagnosis and management of surgical disorders.

INTRODUCTION

Radiology is one of the most rapidly expanding specialities. This is due to continuing advances in both computer and machine technology. New imaging techniques, dramatically affecting patient assessment, are constantly being introduced. It is thus becoming increasingly difficult for the surgeon to keep up to date with all these advances. There must therefore be close communication between the surgeon and radiologist to ensure that the most appropriate imaging technique is utilized for each specific surgical problem. This should take the form of regular interdepartmental meetings and individual case discussions of the more problematic patients.

The correct imaging technique can only be chosen if all the facts are made available to the radiologist. To this end the appropriate clinical details must always be enumerated on the imaging request form.

The high cost and limited availability of some of the more sophisticated imaging techniques must be borne in mind when deciding how to image the patient. It should not be forgotten that the required information can often be obtained from plain X-rays and simple contrast studies.

RADIOLOGY AND SURGERY

No radiological technique can replace the skills of good history-taking and thorough clinical examination. Neither should clinical decision making be based on imaging findings alone; it should consider all the information available from the whole clinical scenario.

The old maxim, 'treat the patient and not the X-ray', still holds true. Nevertheless, the judicious use of imaging techniques is invaluable in all fields of surgery.

TYPES OF RADIOLOGICAL INVESTIGATION

The wide range of imaging techniques available includes plain film radiographs (X-rays), fluoroscopic screening, ultrasound, computed tomography (CT), magnetic resonance imaging (MRI) and nuclear medicine. Each of these will be described briefly.

Plain radiographs (X-rays)

X-rays were first demonstrated by W. K. Roentgen in 1895. He discovered, fortuitously, that X-rays expose photographic plates but are also absorbed to varying degrees by intervening structures which are projected onto the photographic plate as negative images. The clinical relevance of this discovery was immediately apparent as, for the first time, imaging of the living skeleton was possible enabling deformities, fractures and dislocations to be seen. To this day the indications for plain radiology have not changed, although X-ray imaging has now been used in every other system of the body. This has come about mainly due to the use of contrast agents. Plain radiographs are used to demonstrate contrast between tissues of different densities and, as such, obviously show the skeletal system well. However, they also demonstrate differences between gas and fluid and are therefore the most sensitive imaging technique for the detection of free intraperitoneal air after gastrointestinal perforation. With the use of radio-opaque contrast agents the diagnostic yield of plain radiography increases. For example, iodine-containing agents are excreted rapidly by the renal route and so will outline the kidneys, ureters and bladder with clarity. The same agents also delineate the internal characteristics of blood vessels in angiography.

Plain radiography is the most frequently requested examination. It is relatively cheap and simple to perform. These images can, however, be difficult to interpret (particularly soft tissue images), and of course ionizing radiation can be hazardous to health and to the developing fetus. The actual radiation dose to the patient varies greatly and depends on the density of the tissue through which the X-ray beam must pass. The greater the density of tissue, the more X-rays will be absorbed in the patient and fewer will reach the film cassette. Table 5.1 shows the relative dose of common surgical requests compared to the radiation dose of a chest X-ray. (The radiation dose of a chest X-ray is equivalent to 3 days of natural background radiation.)

Ultrasound

Ultrasound waves are created in a transducer by applying a momentary electric field to a piezoelectric crystal which vibrates like a cymbal. The transmitted waves interact with soft tissue interfaces and are reflected back, deflected or absorbed. Only the sound waves that are reflected are used to make the image. The greater the difference in density between two adjacent tissue planes, the greater the amount of reflected sound waves. For example when the sound waves reach a solid gallstone, a great deal of sound is reflected back resulting in a bright collection of echoes and an acoustic shadow deep to the stone. Ultrasound waves, however, are transmitted through the surrounding fluid bile, which appears black.

Ultrasound examinations are useful to visualize soft tissues. They easily demonstrate fluid collections in the subcutaneous tissues (e.g. breast cysts) and within the body cavities such as the chest and abdomen. Ultrasound has become the first line investigation in many conditions such as gallstone disease. Its use is limited by structures that obscure the passage of the ultrasound waves, so it cannot give images of, for example, the brain. Large amounts of bowel gas may prevent adequate examination of the abdominal cavity, and the retroperitoneum is often poorly visualized. It is highly operator dependent. It does, however, give dynamic, real time images and is safe to use in any patient, including those who are pregnant. It is relatively cheap and it is mobile. It is also useful for guiding diagnostic procedures such as aspiration cytology or needle biopsy (see below).

Fluoroscopic imaging

Many common requests to the radiology department involve the use of X-ray screening. These include all barium examinations, most interventional procedures (except those under ultrasound, CT or MRI guidance) and sinograms, cholangiograms, nephrostograms, etc. Each screening room has an image intensifier which converts the X-ray image into a light image, then to an electron image and finally back to a light image of increased brightness. Fluorescence (hence the term fluoroscopy) is the ability of crystals of certain organic salts (called phosphors) to emit light when excited by X-rays. This process is used both in film cassettes for plain radiographs and in an image intensifier.

Barium salts are used to delineate the mucosa of the gastrointestinal tract and are also used in dynamic studies to help define the function of this system (e.g. in barium swallow examinations).

Computed tomography (CT)

Some of the major advances in radiology in recent years have been in the field of cross-sectional imaging. Computed tomography (CT) and magnetic resonance imaging (MRI) have revolutionized the investigation of the central nervous system and other soft tissues.

The CT image is derived from computer integration of multiple exposures as an X-ray tube travels in a circle around a patient. The circular track is called the gantry. A fan shaped beam is produced by the X-ray tube(s); this is picked up by a row of sensitive detectors aligned directly opposite. The computer constructs the image by dividing the gantry into a grid. Each box in the grid

Table 5.1 Relative dose of common surgical requests	
Radiograph	Equivalent number of chest X-rays (approx.)
Chest PA	1
Abdomen AP	50
Pelvis AP	35
Lumbar spine AP and Lat	65
Barium meal	150
Barium enema	250
IVU	125
CT head	115
CT chest or abdomen	400

is called a voxel and has a length, width and depth (slice thickness). Each voxel is given a value representing the average density of the tissue in the box (the value is measured in Hounsfield units (HU) after the inventor of the CT scanner). Water has an HU of 0, air −1000, fat − 80–100, abdominal organs 30–80 and compact bone >250. Each voxel is assigned a shade of grey according to its HU. The window level (WL) is the HU number in the middle of the grey scale and the window width (WW) is the range of HUs over which the grey scale is spread. Both the WL and the WW can be adjusted to emphasize differences in soft tissue, lung or bony detail on the stored data. These figures are always seen on the printed film.

Computer processing of the images is now possible and impressive 3-dimensional reconstructions are useful, particularly to head, neck and facial surgeons.

Magnetic resonance imaging (MRI)

Each body proton can be thought of as a very small magnet. When the body is placed in a magnetic field these protons line up along the direction of that field. The images in MR are generated by the energy released from the protons when they realign with the magnetic field after the application of radiofrequency energy pulses. This electromagnetic energy is received by a 'coil' and converted to images by a computer. Scanning methods in MR are referred to as 'pulse sequences' and the images generated are often classified as T1-weighted or T2-weighted. In simple terms, in a T1-weighted image, fat will appear as a bright signal and water will appear dark, and in a T2-weighted image, water will appear as the brightest signal with fat appearing dark. There is therefore much scope for image manipulation by employing different pulse sequences during a single examination.

MR images give unparalled soft tissue resolution but are generally not as useful in examination of bony structures as other imaging modalities. MR has further inherent advantages over CT and other imaging techniques. Probably the most important is the lack of ionizing radiation. It has multiplanar capabilities, allowing imaging in any arbitrary plane, not just the orthogonal planes permitted by CT. It has great sensitivity to flow phenomena and unique sensitivity for temperature changes.

Its disadvantages include expense and availability. It is safe in the majority of patients but those with implanted magnetic devices or objects, such as certain intracranial aneurysm clips, indwelling pacemakers, cochlear implants or metallic intraocular foreign bodies, cannot be safely scanned. Most orthopaedic implants, however, are safe. Due to the physical con-straints of the machine, large or claustrophobic patients may be unsuitable for imaging by this technique.

Nuclear medicine

In nuclear medicine techniques a radionuclide is administered into the body by some route and subsequently undergoes radioactive decay. The commonest radionuclide used in medicine is technetium-99m (^{99m}Tc). The 'm' is placed after the mass number to indicate a metastable state, i.e. an intermediate species with a measurable half-life. ^{99m}Tc has a half-life of 6 hours and is a pure gamma emitter. This results in a relatively low dose of ionizing radiation delivered to the patient. The radionuclide is labelled so that it can be targeted to the tissue that is the object of the desired images. For example it may be labelled by attaching it to red or white blood cells or a variety of chelates. In the decay process gamma rays are given off. These are detected by a gamma scintillation camera and from them the image is formed.

Tomographic techniques, commonly used in X-ray and CT, have also been developed in nuclear medicine. (Greek: *tomo* = 'to cut'. This refers to the technique of 'cutting' the body into the required imaging planes.) An example is SPECT (single photon emission computed tomography) and involves gamma camera(s) rotating around a gantry as in X-ray CT. A volume of data can then be collected and transaxial images reconstructed.

HOW ARE RADIOLOGICAL TECHNIQUES USED IN SURGERY?

Radiological techniques are used in the management of surgical diseases in one of three main ways:

1. To aid in the diagnosis of a surgical disorder.
2. As an interventional technique to treat a surgical disorder or one of its complications.
3. To guide a surgical procedure.

Each of these main areas will be considered in turn, with a few specific examples.

AS AN AID IN THE DIAGNOSIS OF A SURGICAL DISORDER

This is of course the simplest and most well known application of radiological techniques to surgery. Examples include the use of an erect chest X-ray to detect free intraperitoneal gas and CT of the brain to detect intracranial bleeding following trauma. To this may be added the use of radiology in population screening exercises, such as mammography, and the use of protocol-based preoperative imaging (e.g. chest X-ray) in the preparation of patients for major surgery. Always prefer the simple (and hence cheaper) investigation before the complex (and hence costly) if the simpler investigation has a good chance of providing the diagnosis. Also, always consider non-invasive tests before invasive ones, or safer ones before those with a significant associated complication rate or inherent danger (for example, in pregnant women ultrasound techniques are safer than those using X-rays).

> All investigations, no matter how complex or invasive, have a given sensitivity and specificity and therefore there will always be a false negative and a false positive rate.

AS AN INTERVENTIONAL TECHNIQUE

The field of interventional radiology has developed into a speciality in its own right. There can be very few radiology departments that do not perform at least some interventional techniques. Interventional radiology may be defined as the performance of a procedure on some part of the anatomy whilst using a radiological modality to guide that procedure. Perhaps the simplest example is image-guided biopsy. This is commonly performed using ultrasound or CT guidance, although it is now possible to perform biopsies using the added advantage of MRI. In places this has replaced the need for an open surgical biopsy. A good example is stereotactic core biopsy of the breast guided by digital mammography. The placement of drainage catheters using ultrasound or CT has revolutionized the management of postoperative complications such as subphrenic abscess. Vascular surgery has been completely changed by the advent of interventional radiology techniques. These include not only angioplasty, catheter thrombolysis and stenting of aneurysmal or occlusive disease, but also novel techniques that replace the need for high-risk surgery (for example transjugular portosystemic shunting in portal hypertension).

This is a field that is likely to go on developing for some considerable time, given the rapid development and integration of computer technology into imaging methods, and the availability of new imaging systems (such as interventional MRI) and tissue destruction techniques (such as focused ultrasound and radio-frequency ablation systems).

IMAGE-GUIDED SURGERY

Image-guided surgery can be defined as the use of a radiological modality during a surgical procedure to give more information than is available by direct inspection of the surgical field. The information so gained is used to influence or guide the performance of the operation. There are many examples used in everyday surgical practice (Table 5.2). The best known are fracture manipulation using image intensification and intraoperative cholangiography during cholecystectomy to determine the presence of absence of gallstones within the main bile ducts. More advanced techniques include stereotactic CT-guided neurosurgery and the use of intraoperative ultrasound in hepatic and pancreatic surgery to determine resectability and to determine the anatomical location of vital structures as resection proceeds. This technique may be used in both open and laparoscopic procedures. It has recently become possible to perform surgical operations within interventional MRI units, harnessing the soft tissue and image manipulation power of MR to guide the procedure. There have been recent reports demonstrating the use of intraoperative MR to guide complete tumour resection in the brain (Moriarty et al 1996) and breast (Gould et al 1998). Much further work is required before the full potential of image-guided surgery is reached.

Finally, radiological data obtained preoperatively can be used to plan or guide the surgical procedure. The best examples are 3-dimensional CT reconstruction of the face or skull for surgical planning prior to major maxillofacial reconstructive surgery. However, this technique is now being used to plan the best

Table 5.2	Examples of image guided surgery
Modality	Procedure
X-ray	Fracture reduction
X-ray	Removal of foreign bodies
X-ray	Intraoperative cholangiography
X-ray	ERCP
X-ray	Retrograde ureterography
X-ray	Intraoperative arteriography
Ultrasound	Laparoscopic staging of pancreatic cancer
Ultrasound	Hepatic resection
Ultrasound	Complex anal fistula surgery
CT	Stereotactic neurosurgery
MRI	Neurosurgery
MRI	Breast surgery

approach for major hepatic surgery for trauma or tumour. A very exciting area of current investigation is the combination of the information obtained from a number of different radiological techniques, such as CT, and conventional and functional MRI to make a more complete preoperative model of a particular lesion and surrounding anatomical structures. Work is underway to 'register' this image to the patient during surgery, so that it may truly be used as an intraoperative guide.

References

Gould S, Lamb G, Lomax D, Gedroyc W, Darzi A 1998 Interventional MR-guided excisional biopsy of breast lesions. Journal of Magnetic Resonance Imaging 8: 26–30

Moriarty T, Kikinis R, Jolesz F, Alexander III, E 1996 Magnetic resonance imaging therapy. Neurosurgical Clinics of North America 7: 323–330

Royal College of Radiologists 1998 Making the best use of a department of clinical radiology 4th edn. Royal College of Radiologists, London

Summary

1. A wide variety of radiological imaging methods are currently available.
2. Consult the radiologist to ensure that the most relevant investigation is chosen.
3. The selection of the appropriate investigation for a given clinical problem is a balance between the aim of the investigation, effectiveness, cost and safety.
4. Radiological images must be used in conjunction with the rest of the available clinical information when planning treatment. They must not be used in isolation.
5. The three key areas in which radiological techniques are used in surgical practice are diagnosis, interventional radiology and for image guidance of surgical procedures.
6. Interventional radiology and image-guided surgery are rapidly expanding fields that are likely to have applications in all surgical specialities.

6

Histological techniques in surgical pathology

A. P. Dhillon

Objectives

- **Encourage surgeons to confer with pathologists to optimize the gathering from tissue specimens of information relevant to patient management.**
- **Understand the value of modern techniques in diagnosis and assessment of tissues.**
- **Appreciate the importance of care in handling, labelling, and fixing specimens.**

INTRODUCTION

Good communication is the secret of success both in life and in medicine in general, and in getting the best service from histopathology in particular. A request for a histopathological opinion is not a 'test' to be ordered like other machine-processed pathology tests. You are asking the histopathologist for a clinical opinion, subject to review in the light of further information such as the clinical course of the patient. As with requests for opinions from other specialist clinical colleagues, a full, relevant, clinical history is required. The opinion rendered depends on the experience of the histopathologist, so read the name at the bottom of the report. If the initial opinion does not fit with the overall clinical picture, politely question it and ask for a review.

Prior discussion is often helpful in cases of: lymphomas, endocrine tumours, tuberculosis, and metabolic disease. Frozen material should be kept in cases of lymphoma for immunophenotyping the tumour; endocrine tumours may need fixation in Bouin's fixative (which best preserves peptide antigens) and paraformaldehyde fixation (for investigation of mRNA expression), and a peptide hormone serum screen prior to removal of the tumour is helpful in characterizing the hormone profile of the tumour. Fresh, unfixed material from cases of

tuberculosis must be sent for microbiological examination, and fresh material from cases of metabolic disease may need biochemical investigation. There is benefit in electron microscopical examination of some tumours, metabolic and renal diseases, when glutaraldehyde fixation helps to optimize ultrastructural morphology.

Clinicians and histopathologists need to agree a trade-off between speed of reporting and accuracy. Frozen section and 'fast-track' techniques may preclude a firm or reliable opinion, if additional, better fixed material from these cases is not available. Histopathologists are worried by any errors in tumour diagnosis, and figures of 98% accuracy have been demonstrated in the best laboratories, with clinical follow-up information, while clinicians may consider speed to be more essential.

HISTOLOGICAL TECHNIQUES

1. The haematoxylin and eosin stain is the most widely used routine histochemical stain. It is used for the general examination of tissue structure prior to deciding which additional stains and techniques, if any, are necessary.

2. A wide variety of additional histochemical stains are used for further histological analysis. Histochemistry has a proud history which developed with the chemical and textile industries, together with the growth of histology since the time of Ehrlich. For example Alcian blue is used to identify mucus, van Gieson's stain is used to characterize connective tissue, Congo red is used to identify amyloid, Ziehl–Neelsen staining is used for mycobacteria, and silver stains are used to detect melanin and neuroendocrine granules. Many of these stains depend on the selectivity of dyes for certain tissue components. Some stains, such as Perls' Prussian blue reaction for ferric iron, have chemical specificity; others are biochemically specific, for example digestion of the red PAS reaction product by diastase proves the presence of glycogen.

3. Immunohistochemistry employs the specificity of antibodies for the relevant epitope. Practically any antibody–antigen system can be explored in histological sections, provided adequate epitope preservation has been achieved. Even when fixation is not optimal, sometimes, antigens can be 'retrieved' by novel methods such as heat or enzymatic techniques. The main problem in the use of immunohistochemistry lies in defining economical and pertinent questions which can be solved by these techniques, since so many can potentially be used. For example, in the case of an undifferentiated malignant tumour, immunostaining for cytokeratins and lymphoma markers will often help to decide the tumour immunophenotype, even when a morphological phenotype is lacking, thereby permitting important diagnostic decisions to be made.

4. Many other modern techniques are applicable to tissue sections. In situ hybridization invokes the specific affinity of nucleic acid for its complimentary sequence, so that both specific DNA and RNA sequences can be detected. PCR (polymerase chain reaction) techniques can be applied to tissue sections directly (in situ PCR), or nucleic acids can be extracted from tissues for more conventional PCR investigation. For example, invisible material such as viral nucleic acid can be identified by PCR to permit diagnosis of infections such as HCV. It is important to realize that a histological section is much more than a passive image. The tissue slice represents real biological material which can be explored with any of the molecular and other technologies of modern times.

5. Electron microscopy has been largely superseded in its diagnostic applications by immunohistochemistry and molecular methods. It is used routinely to characterize glomerulonephritis. Other new microscopical methods, such as confocal microscopy, have yet to be fully utilized in the diagnostic armamentarium.

THE CORRECT SPECIMEN:
HANDLING LABELLING AND FIXATION

1. Small biopsies (e.g. needle and endoscopy specimens) fix rapidly and an opinion can usually be given on the afternoon of the day after receipt. Larger specimens need to be fixed overnight before preparation of blocks, and reports on these cases will normally be written two days after receipt of the specimen. More complicated cases requiring special investigations may take several more days to report. If you require a rapid result contact a pathologist sooner rather than later.

2. Treat the tissue gently to retain morphological integrity, and avoid crushing or distorting it with forceps.

3. Mark specific points which need particular attention on the specimen with marker stitches, and provide a diagram to aid orientation. Include normal tissue as well as a representative amount of the lesion with incisional biopsies. Cautery and diathermy damage the tissues, and metallic staples damage microtome knives, so try to avoid these if possible in diagnostic biopsies. Send all (not part) of the tissue removed at operation or biopsy procedure. Use separate pots for multiple specimens and label the site of origin of each of these (one of several skin 'moles' may be a melanoma, and if these are put in the same pot, there is no way of knowing where it came from). Do not cram too much tissue into too small a container, with insufficient fixative, and do not use a narrow-necked container. If fixed infected material is submitted for histopathology, remember to send part of the unfixed specimen for microbiology and virology as a routine in addition, because fixed organisms will not grow in culture. Keep blood and body fluids inside the specimen pot and away from the outside of the pot, the bag containing the specimen pot, and the request form. The specimen is dissected, and 'tissue blocks' for microscopical examination are selected by the pathologist. If possible, present the specimen in a manner agreed with the pathologist (e.g. bowel with attached tissue and associated lymph nodes can be submitted fresh, or immersed in appropriate fixative, or opened and pinned out according to local protocol).

4. Accurately label the specimen and request form and give a contact number of a clinician familiar with the patient. Identify the clinical problem clearly.

5. If the specimen is really urgent, personally ensure it gets to the laboratory.

6. On receipt in the pathology department the specimen is assigned a sequential accession number, with time and date stamped as each specimen is received, proving receipt.

Summary

1. Plan beforehand and take advice from the pathologist.
2. Treat the specimen carefully and gently. Fix the specimen and label the container correctly.
3. Give a full and relevant clinical history, together with a clinical contact number on the request form.
4. Pathologists give the best service when they are treated as clinical colleagues.

Further reading

Hadfield G J, Hobsley M, Morson B C (eds) 1985. Pathology in surgical practice. Edward Arnold, London

Rosai J (ed) 1996 Ackerman's surgical pathology, 8th edn. General instructions: Chapters 1–3, and Appendices A, B, C, and G. For specific organs and diseases see relevant chapters. Mosby International, St Louis

7

Influence of coexisting disease

R. M. Jones, C. A. Marshall

Objectives

- **Recognize which coexisting disease processes are associated with increased morbidity.**
- **Understand which features of the patient's condition can be improved.**
- **Realize that a simple operation does not always mean an equally simple or risk-free anaesthetic.**
- **Understand that sick patients are best managed in daylight hours with fully trained staff.**
- **Recognize that in some circumstances it may be better to transfer a patient to another hospital preoperatively if there are inadequate facilities for his postoperative care.**

INTRODUCTION

About half of adult patients presenting to the surgeon will have a coexisting disease unrelated to the pathological process necessitating surgery. The proportion is increased in the elderly and patients presenting for emergency surgery. The morbidity and mortality associated with surgery and anaesthesia are increased in patients with coexisting disease and the more significant the coexisting disease the greater the risk (Buck et al 1987, Campling et al 1993). The medical diagnoses most commonly associated with an increase in surgical morbidity and mortality are:

- Ischaemic heart disease
- Congestive cardiac failure
- Arterial hypertension
- Chronic respiratory disease
- Diabetes mellitus
- Cardiac arrhythmias
- Anaemia.

It can be seen that pre-existing cardiac-related problems account for the most significant increase in operative risk.

Aims of management

- **To diagnose the presence of pre-existing medical disease and make an accurate assessment of the degree of the problem**
- **To ensure that the patient's medical condition is optimized before surgery**
- **To ensure that specialized postoperative care facilities are available if required**

The National Confidential Enquiry into Perioperative Deaths (NCEPOD) for 1990 (Campling et al 1992) emphasized the importance of discussion between surgeon and anaesthetist before a decision to proceed in a particular patient. All patients presenting for surgery should have a full clinical history and examination performed, including details of concurrent drug therapy, previous medical history and history of allergy. Depending on the nature of the coexisting medical disease and that of the planned surgery, additional specialized investigations may subsequently be needed. Young (<45 years), fit patients undergoing minor elective surgery do not need routine blood haematology or chemistry, a chest X-ray or an electrocardiogram (ECG).

The NCEPOD report for 1992/3 (Campling et al 1995) identified a substantial shortfall in critical care services, and a failure to anticipate the need for these services. Furthermore, it emphasized that the skills of the surgeon and the anaesthetist should be appropriate for the medical condition of the patient. These professionals would not always be doctors of the same grade.

Who Operates When (Campling et al 1997), an NCEPOD report into timing of operations, found that the patients who died were for the most part elderly and in poor preoperative health (82% suffered from at least one coexisting disease, of which cardiorespiratory disease was the most common, followed by malignancy). Preoperative management was criticized as sometimes poor and the rush to operate before adequate resuscitation contributed significantly to morbidity and mortality. Particular attention was drawn to the low use of intravenous fluids, infrequent use of objective cardiac assessment, and patchy application of thromboembolic prophylaxis.

CARDIOVASCULAR DISEASE

Coronary artery disease

Coronary atherosclerosis is the commonest type of cardiovascular disease; it is probably the single most common underlying factor in the production of operative morbidity and mortality (Aitkenhead et al 1989). the preoperative evaluation must include an assessment of diseases associated with the development of coronary atherosclerosis, e.g. systemic arterial hypertension, diabetes mellitus and smoking. The degree of activity that precipitates symptoms of myocardial ischaemia must be assessed and the presence or absence of congestive heart failure should be noted (does the patient also become breathless on exertion?). Patients with a degree of heart failure in addition to ischaemia have often had a previous myocardial infarction and may be taking digoxin. Concurrent drug therapy should be noted and, almost without exception, this should be continued until the time of surgery (see Concurrent drug therapy, p. 91). The drugs most frequently encountered are:

- Nitrates (e.g. glyceryl trinitrate)
- β-Adrenergic antagonists
- Calcium antagonists
- Angiotensin enzyme converting inhibitors
- Digoxin.

It is important to remember that the preoperative ECG is normal in 20–50% of patients with proven ischaemia. Smokers should be encouraged to stop smoking at least 12 hours before surgery in order to decrease the percentage of carboxyhaemoglobin present in the blood and to minimize the cardiovascular side-effects of nicotine. It is also important to differentiate chest pain of gastrointestinal origin (e.g. hiatus hernia) from ischaemic cardiac pain. This may necessitate a specialist opinion and subsequent investigations such as a thallium scan.

The basis of management depends on the fact that myocardial ischaemia will occur whenever the balance between myocardial oxygen supply and demand is disturbed such that demand exceeds supply. The major determinants of myocardial oxygen supply are:

- The coronary perfusion pressure (the aortic diastolic pressure minus the left ventricular end-diastolic pressure)
- Diastolic time.

The major determinants of myocardial oxygen demand are:

- Increasing heart rate
- Increasing inotropic state
- Afterload, which is the impedance to left ventricular ejection (the systemic arterial pressure is an approximate determinant of afterload)
- Preload, which is the left ventricular end-diastolic pressure.

In the perioperative period factors that decrease supply and/or increase demand must be avoided. It can be seen that an increase in heart rate and an increase in preload will be especially deleterious as they will increase myocardial oxygen demand and decrease myocardial oxygen supply. During the perioperative period a decrease in systemic arterial pressure to a significant degree (a decrease in diastolic pressure greater than 20% of the patient's normal resting diastolic pressure is a useful guide) must not be allowed to occur because this decreases coronary perfusion pressure, which is very poorly tolerated in patients with multiple sites of coronary artery narrowing. Good pain management postoperatively is essential, as the presence of pain will lead to hypertension and tachycardia. This may mean referring the patient to the hospital's acute-pain team. In addition, after major surgery, especially intra-abdominal or intrathoracic, supplemental oxygen should be administered for 24 hours and consideration given to providing supplemental oxygen overnight for the first 4 postoperative days.

Arterial hypertension

Moderate or marked, long-standing, untreated hypertension increases perioperative morbidity and mortality, and is a significant risk factor for the production of coronary atherosclerosis. Patients with sustained systemic arterial hypertension (systolic >160 mmHg, diastolic >110 mmHg) should be satisfactorily stabilized on antihypertensive therapy before elective surgery of any type or duration. The untreated or inadequately treated hypertensive responds in an exaggerated manner to the stress of surgery, with a resultant increase in operative morbidity and mortality. Patients with long-standing moderate to marked hypertension should be assumed to have coronary atherosclerosis, even in the absence of overt signs and/or symptoms of ischaemic heart disease, and managed appropriately. Antihypertensive therapy is associated with its own unique considerations for anaesthetic and surgical management, the specific issues depending upon the medication the patient is taking (see Concurrent drug therapy, p. 91).

Heart failure

This implies an inadequacy of heart muscle secondary to intrinsic disease or overloading. The latter may be due to an increase in volume (an increase in intravascular volume or valve incompetence) or pressure (systemic arterial hypertension or aortic stenosis). It is usual for one ventricle to fail before the other, but disorders that damage or overload the left ventricle are more common (e.g. ischaemic heart disease and systemic arterial hypertension), and hence symptoms attributable to pulmonary congestion are usually the presenting ones. Left ventricular failure is the most common cause of right ventricular failure and if this supervenes dyspnoea may actually decrease as right ventricular output decreases, leading to a reduction in pulmonary congestion. Conventionally, congestive heart failure refers to the combination of left and right ventricular failure with evidence of (and symptoms relating to) systemic and pulmonary venous hypertension. Physiologically, heart failure may be thought of as the failure of the heart to match its output in order to meet the body's metabolic needs. Treatment is aimed at normalizing this imbalance. Thus, cardiac output can be improved or metabolic needs decreased. Traditionally, digitalis glycosides have been thought of as mediating their beneficial effects by improving cardiac output. Their use has now been superseded by angiotensin converting enzyme (ACE) inhibitors, often combined with diuretics. Vasodilators can also be used to decrease peripheral demand. Digitalization is indicated in patients with atrial fibrillation or flutter.

Heart failure

- **Symptomatic heart failure must be managed by optimum medical therapy preoperatively in all but the direst of surgical emergencies.**
- **Surgery in the presence of decompensated heart failure is associated with a high mortality.**

The operative mortality and morbidity of patients with well-compensated heart failure is small. If the operation cannot be delayed, in a patient with decompensated heart failure, peri- and intraoperative haemo-

dynamic monitoring should be comprehensive. For major surgery this would indicate the use of a balloon-tipped pulmonary artery catheter; measurement of cardiac output and pulmonary capillary wedge pressure (a determinant of left ventricular preload) will allow the construction of ventricular function curves to guide in the selection of appropriate cardiovascular therapy. Postoperative admission to a high-dependency unit or an intensive-care facility (with the ability to measure and adjust preload, afterload and cardiac output) is indicated.

Congenital anomalies of the heart and cardiovascular system occur in 7–10 per 1000 live births (0.7–1%). It is the commonest form of congenital disease and accounts for approximately 30% of the total burden of congenital disease. In affected children 10–15% have associated anomalies of the skeletal, genitourinary or gastrointestinal system. Nine lesions comprise more than 80% of congenital heart disease; of these ventricular septal defect is by far the most frequent at 35%. Approximately 10–15% of patients with congenital heart disease may survive untreated to adulthood but the majority require some form of cardiac surgery as children.

A large cohort of patients with treated congenital heart disease is now surviving into adult life. Although these patients have traditionally returned to paediatric cardiac surgery centres for non-cardiac surgery as adults, this is not always possible.

Implications of adult congenital heart disease

- **This is a very high-risk group of patients, often with multiple anatomical and pathophysiological abnormalities**
- **They must be fully assessed preoperatively and receive perioperative care from individuals familiar with these problems**

It is not possible to review the subject comprehensively here, but the article by Findlow et al (See Further Reading) is recommended for further reading. In summary, however, the problems fall into four groups: arrhythmias, hypoxaemia, pulmonary disease, and ventricular dysfunction. Patients with Eisenmenger's syndrome (right to left shunt due to pulmonary hypertension) are very high risk patients. As well as circulatory failure, they run the risk of air embolism during surgery, postoperative deep vein thrombosis (DVT) and infective endocarditis. All patients with congenital heart disease should receive antibiotic prophylaxis, and care to avoid air in the tubing during the siting of intravenous lines.

Acquired valvular heart disease

Mitral stenosis

This is nearly always of rheumatic origin, but symptoms do not appear until the valve area is reduced to less than 2.5 cm², i.e. half the normal valve area. This may take 20 years following the episode of rheumatic fever. As valve area decreases below 2 cm², an increase in left atrial pressure is required at rest to maintain cardiac output. A valve area below 1 cm² is classified as severe mitral stenosis and is associated with a left atrial pressure in excess of 20 mmHg, and even at rest cardiac output may be barely adequate; there is pulmonary hypertension. Eventually right ventricular failure supervenes and atrial fibrillation is common. Patients with mild to moderate mitral stenosis and sinus rhythm tolerate surgery well. All patients should receive antibiotic prophylaxis. Fluid balance should be carefully monitored, as overtransfusion may precipitate pulmonary oedema whereas undertransfusion will compromise left ventricular filling. Similarly, changes in heart rate are poorly tolerated, and during surgery the anaesthetist will use a technique which minimizes changes in cardiac parameters. If major surgery is to be undertaken, with the possibility of large blood loss, consideration should be given to monitoring pulmonary capillary wedge pressure by means of a balloon-tipped flow-directed catheter. Unless the patient is taking oral anticoagulants, a local anaesthetic technique may be used for surgery, but a high spinal or epidural block may be associated with adverse cardiovascular effects (systemic arterial hypotension) and should be employed with caution.

Patients who are dyspnoeic at rest and have a fixed and reduced cardiac output present a significant risk during surgery. Digoxin should be continued up until the time of operation and plasma electrolytes checked, as hypokalaemia will increase the incidence of cardiac rhythm disturbances. These patients may have to be ventilated electively postoperatively.

Aortic stenosis

Valvular aortic stenosis is commonest in elderly males, although it may occur at any time of life. The aetiology is diverse and includes congenital, rheumatic, senile and mixed forms. It must be remembered that it is most common in patients in whom the incidence of ischaemic heart disease is also high. As in mitral stenosis, moderate degrees of stenosis of the aortic valve do not appreciably increase the risks of surgery. However, severe aortic stenosis is associated with an increased perioperative morbidity and mortality. These patients may be asymptomatic even with a large (>80 mmHg) gradient across the valve, if the left ventricle has not

failed. A preoperative echo and cardiac assessment is essential to determine the gradient, as the risk of surgery can be predicted from this. Systemic arterial hypotension must be avoided at all times, because it will compromise coronary perfusion. Thus peripheral vasodilatation, hypovolaemia and myocardial depression are all poorly tolerated. A change in cardiac rhythm is also poorly tolerated, as the atrial component to ventricular filling is essential to maintain normal cardiac output. For major procedures it is advisable to monitor left ventricular filling pressure, as higher than normal filling pressures are needed to maintain cardiac output.

Cardiomyopathies

Using echocardiography, three principal forms of cardiomyopathy are described:

1. Congestive or dilated cardiomyopathy: this may be associated with toxic, metabolic, neurological and inflammatory diseases. There is decrease in contractile force of the left or right ventricle, resulting in heart failure.
2. Hypertrophic or obstructive cardiomyopathy: this is an autosomal dominantly inherited condition in which there is hypertrophy and fibrosis; it mainly affects the interventricular septum but may involve the whole of the left ventricle.
3. Restrictive cardiomyopathy: this is a rare form of cardiomyopathy and the main feature is the loss of ventricular distensibility due to endocardial or myocardial disease. Restrictive cardiomyopathy in many ways resembles constrictive pericarditis, and the endocardial disease may produce thromboembolic problems.

Table 7.1 summarizes the treatment and management of these patients.

Disturbances of cardiac rhythm

Atrial fibrillation

This is the most commonly encountered disturbance of cardiac rhythm and it is important to define the disease processes causing the fibrillation. These are:

- Ischaemic heart disease
- Rheumatic heart disease, especially mitral stenosis
- Pulmonary embolism
- Bronchial carcinoma
- Thyrotoxicosis
- Thoracotomy
- Alcoholism.

If there appears to be no underlying cause, the rhythm disturbance is usually termed 'lone atrial fibrillation'.

Table 7.1 Cardiomyopathies: diagnosis and treatment

	Congestive (dilated)	Hypertrophic (obstructive)	Restrictive
Presenting signs/symptoms	Heart failure Rhythm disturbance Systemic emboli	Syncope Dyspnoea Angina Rhythm disturbance Systolic murmur appearing during long-standing hypertension	Heart failure Eosinophilia
Treatment	Diuretics Vasodilators Antiarrhythmics Anticoagulants	Antiarrhythmics β-Adrenergic antagonists Anticoagulants	Steroids Cytotoxic agents

The atrial discharge rate is usually between 400 and 600 impulses per minute, but the atrioventricular (AV) node cannot conduct all these impulses, so that some fail to reach the ventricle or only partially penetrate the node, and this results in a block or delay to succeeding impulses. Ventricular response is therefore irregular, but seldom more than 200 impulses per minute; the use of drugs or the presence of disease of the AV node often causes the response rate to be lower than this. The medical management of patients with atrial fibrillation must include the management of the underlying cause of the rhythm disturbance. It is important to ensure that the fibrillation is well controlled, i.e. that the response rate of the ventricle is not too rapid. Digitalis alkaloids remain the primary method of slowing AV nodal conduction, but if these fail to control the response rate, amiodarone is usually effective. Occasionally, cardioversion will restore sinus rhythm if the atrial fibrillation is of recent onset. The patient should be anticoagulated prior to this.

Atrial flutter

The causes of this disturbance of cardiac rhythm are similar to those of atrial fibrillation, and the perioperative considerations are principally those of the underlying disease process. Atrial flutter is less commonly seen than atrial fibrillation. Although control of ventricular rate is more difficult in flutter, unlike fibrillation cardioversion is often successful. The patient should be warfarinized prior to cardioversion. Second line therapy includes flecainide or digoxin. A bolus of adenosine may be used to aid in the differential diagnosis of atrial flutter versus paroxysmal supraventricular tachycardia (SVT).

Heart block

There are two basic types of heart block:

- Atrioventricular heart block
- Intraventricular conduction defects.

Atrioventricular heart block. This may be incomplete (first- or second-degree AV block) or complete (third-degree AV block). In first-degree heart block the PR interval of the ECG exceeds 0.21 seconds, but there are no dropped beats and the QRS complex is normal. It does not always imply significant underlying heart disease, but is seen in patients on digitalis therapy. It is important not to expose the patient to any drug in the perioperative period which will further decrease AV nodal conduction (e.g. halothane anaesthesia, β-adrenergic antagonists or verapamil).

There are two types of second-degree heart block: Mobitz types 1 and 2. Mobitz type 1 block is also known as the 'Wenckebach phenomenon' and this is usually associated with ischaemia of the AV node or the effects of digitalis. There is progressive increase in the length of the PR interval until the impulse fails to excite the ventricle and a beat is dropped. As a generalization, patients with this type of heart block do not require a pacemaker prior to surgery, and should it be necessary the administration of atropine will often establish normal AV conduction. Mobitz type 2 block is less common than type 1; it is a more serious form of conduction defect and may be a forerunner to complete AV block. The atrial rate is normal and the ventricular rate depends on the number of dropped beats, but it is commonly 35–50 beats per minute. The net result is that of an irregular pulse. The ECG indicates that there are more P waves than QRS complexes, but the PR interval, if present, is normal. It is probably acceptable to undertake minor surgery in patients with Mobitz type 2 block without the need for the insertion of a pro-phylactic pacemaker. However, in these circumstances drugs such as atropine and isoprenaline should be immediately at hand, and the means for temporary pacing should be available. Prophylactic pacemaker insertion is indicated for major surgery, especially if this is likely to result in significant blood loss and associated haemodynamic instability.

Third-degree heart block is also termed 'complete heart block'. It may result from conduction defects located within the AV node, bundle of His, or the bundle branch and Purkinje fibres. An escape pacemaker emerges at a site distal to the block (e.g. if the impulses are blocked within the AV node, the bundle of His usually emerges as the subsidiary pacemaker). In general, the more distal the site of the escape pacemaker, the more likely is the patient to suffer symptoms such as dyspnoea, syncope or congestive heart failure and to need permanent ventricular pacemaker therapy. Pacemaker therapy is always indicated before surgery, although in emergency situations (such as complete heart block appearing intraoperatively) various drugs may be tried to increase the heart rate. Atropine may be of value if the escape pacemaker is junctional. Isoprenaline may be of value if the escape pacemaker is more distal. A pacing Swann–Ganz catheter or a trans-oesophageal pacemaker can be inserted in an emergency and may be easier to place than a temporary wire.

Intraventricular conduction defects. Left bundle branch block is always associated with heart disease. The QRS complex is wide (>0.12 seconds). A hemi-block occurs if only one of the two major subdivisions (anterior and posterior) of the left bundle is blocked. The QRS complex is not prolonged in left hemiblocks. Left anterior or posterior hemiblock may occur with right bundle branch block and it is generally considered that left anterior plus right bundle branch block is not an indication for temporary pacemaker therapy before surgery, but that left posterior plus right bundle branch block is an indication for a pacemaker. The latter patients are at risk of developing complete heart block. Right bundle branch block is not invariably associated with underlying heart disease. The principal significance lies in its association with a left posterior hemi-block, as there is then a risk of complete heart block; in these patients a temporary pacemaker is indicated before surgery and anaesthesia.

Pacemakers

The patient with a pacemaker can safely undergo surgery and anaesthesia, but it is important to review the medical condition that gave rise to the need for pacemaker therapy. The usual indications for a pacemaker are:

- Congenital or acquired complete heart block
- Sick sinus syndrome
- Bradycardia, associated with syncope and/or hypotension.

Acquired complete heart block is probably the commonest indication, the underlying cause for this usually being ischaemic heart disease. The patient should be specifically asked about the return of symptoms such as syncope, which may indicate that the pacemaker is failing to capture the ventricle (or atria if an atrial pacemaker is present). The heart rate should be within a couple of beats per minute of the pacemaker's original setting. It is important to determine the type of pacemaker that has been implanted and the time when it was put in.

All patients with pacemakers are normally reviewed regularly in a pacemaker clinic. Whenever a pacemaker is in situ, atropine, adrenaline and isoprenaline should be available for use in the event of pacemaker failure. During surgery, diathermy is usually safe, but some precautions are needed (Simon 1977):

Precautions for the use of diathermy

- **The indifferent electrode of the diathermy should be placed on the same side as the operating site and as far away from the pacemaker as possible**
- **The use of diathermy should be limited to short bursts of 1–2 seconds at intervals not greater than every 10 seconds**
- **The anaesthetist should check the patient's pulse when the diathermy is used for inhibition of pacemaker function (Simon 1977, Aitkenhead & Barnett 1989).**

RESPIRATORY DISEASE

Asthma

Patients with asthma have bronchospasm, mucus plugging of airways and air trapping. These result in a mismatch of ventilation and perfusion and total effective ventilation may be severely impaired. A number of exogenous and endogenous stimuli may produce reversible airway obstruction. The most active chemical mediators are histamine and the leukotrienes. Expiration is prolonged, functional residual capacity and residual volumes are increased and vital capacity is decreased. Bronchospasm may be aggravated by anxiety, by instrumentation of the upper airway, by foreign material or irritants in the upper airway, by pain, and by drugs. The latter include morphine, papaveretum, unselective β-adrenergic antagonists, and various anaesthetic drugs including tubocurarine and anticholinesterases. In taking the clinical history, special attention should be paid to factors which precipitate an attack, and the patient's normal drug therapy should be reviewed. If possible, the timing of surgery should be arranged to coincide with a period of remission of symptoms. The patient's normal bronchodilator therapy should be continued up until the time of surgery, and consideration should be given to the provision of preoperative chest physiotherapy. It is important to allay preoperative anxiety, and suitable premedication should be prescribed. Diazepam, pethidine, promethazine and atropine are free from bronchospastic activity. If the patient is taking steroid therapy, additional doses may be needed during the perioperative period (see Concurrent drug therapy, p. 91). In the postoperative period, careful attention should be paid to pain management, together with the use of nebulized or intravenous bronchodilators if this is necessary. Local anaesthetic techniques are often suitable in the severe asthmatic undergoing suitable surgery and appropriate techniques can be used to provide postoperative analgesia (e.g. epidural blocks).

 Indications for the use of intermittent positive pressure ventilation in asthmatics

- **Distress and exhaustion**
- **Systemic arterial hypotension or significant disturbance of cardiac rhythm**
- **An arterial oxygen tension of less than 6.7 kPa or an arterial carbon dioxide tension of greater than 6.7 kPa, associated with an increasing metabolic acidosis in the face of maximum medical therapy.**

Chronic bronchitis and emphysema

A patient with chronic bronchitis will have had a cough with sputum production on most days for 3 months of the year for at least 2 years. The patient with emphysema will have destruction of alveoli distal to the terminal bronchioles and loss of pulmonary elastic tissue. Patients with chronic bronchitis are often smokers (see below), and have irritable airways leading to coughing and some degree of reversible airways obstruction in response to minimal stimulation. Patients with emphysema experience airway closure with air trapping and, therefore, inefficient gaseous exchange. Chronic bronchitis and emphysema commonly coexist in the same patient. Many of the considerations in the perioperative

period that apply to the asthmatic patient also apply to patients with chronic bronchitis and emphysema; there are, however, some additional points to note. These diseases are usually slowly progressive and may eventually result in a respiratory reserve which is so low that the patient is immobile and dyspnoeic at rest, and even speaking and eating may be difficult. It is important that elective surgery should take place during the months in which symptoms are least noticeable; this is usually during the summer. Every effort should be made to persuade smokers to quit their habit. If the patient requires major surgery, and if the disease is severe, elective tracheostomy and postoperative ventilation may be called for. These will facilitate the clearing of secretions, and thus gaseous exchange, during the postoperative period when diaphragmatic splinting and pain or respiratory depression may cause acute respiratory insufficiency.

Smoking

Smokers have about six times the incidence of postoperative respiratory complications compared with non-smokers.

Cigarette smoking has wide-ranging effects on the cardiorespiratory and immune systems and on haemostasis (Jones 1985).

Smokers may have arterial carbon monoxide concentrations in excess of 5%; the resultant carboxyhaemoglobin decreases the amount of haemoglobin available for combination with oxygen, and inhibits the ability of haemoglobin to give up oxygen (i.e. the oxygen dissociation curve is shifted to the left). Carbon monoxide also has a negative inotropic effect. Nicotine increases heart rate and systemic arterial blood pressure. Thus, carbon monoxide decreases oxygen supply, while nicotine increases oxygen demand and this is of particular significance in patients with ischaemic heart disease. In these patients, it is especially important that patients stop smoking for 12–24 hours before surgery; this will result in a significant improvement in cardiovascular function (the elimination half-lives of carbon monoxide and nicotine are a few hours).

However, the respiratory effect of smoking, especially mucus hypersecretion, impairment of tracheobronchial clearance, and small airway narrowing take at least 6 weeks before there is any improvement in function after smoking cessation. Similarly, the effects of smoking on immune function (smokers are more susceptible to postoperative infections) require at least 6 weeks before improvement occurs. Many smokers will complain that they find it difficult to clear their mucus if they stop smoking, and will use this as an excuse not to stop smoking before surgery; there may be some substance to this claim, but it does not outweigh the benefits of stopping. It is important that the risks of smoking are emphasized to smokers, and they should be encouraged to stop smoking for as long as possible before elective surgery.

ENDOCRINE DYSFUNCTION

Thyroid gland

Excluding diabetes, disorders involving the thyroid gland account for about 80% of endocrine disease. There are two practical issues for the surgeon and anaesthetist. Firstly, there are problems related to the local effects of a mass in the neck. These include airway problems and the potential for difficult tracheal intubation. Secondly, there are problems associated with the generalized effects of an excess or deficiency of hormone. Patients with hyperthyroidism must be made euthyroid and properly prepared before surgery. Propylthiouracil (average daily dose 300 mg) inhibits hormone synthesis and blocks the peripheral conversion of thyroxine to triiodothyronine. As a generalization, the larger the gland the longer it takes to achieve the euthyroid state. The vascularity of the gland can be considerably decreased by 7 days' treatment with potassium iodide solution. Propranolol is an alternative treatment to thiouracil, and 60–120 mg daily for 2 weeks may be the only treatment required, and is now routinely used at many centres.

The management of the properly prepared patient should cause few problems. An emergency operation in a poorly or non-prepared patient is associated with significant risk and should be avoided if possible. Cardiovascular complications are potentially life-threatening and intravenous esmolol should be considered before induction of anaesthesia (using increments every 5 minutes to decrease the resting heart rate by 10 beats per minute). Disturbances of cardiac rhythm, hypoxia and hyperthermia may all occur. If appropriate, a local anaesthetic technique may be the method of choice. Hypothyroidism is not uncommon, especially in elderly patients. Cardiac output is low and blood loss is poorly tolerated. However, blood transfusion must be given with caution in order to avoid overloading the circulation. It has been said that in hypothyroidism the respiratory centre is less responsive to hypoxia and hypercarbia, so that it may be necessary to ventilate patients electively in the postoperative period. These patients are especially sensitive to opioid analgesics and these should be used with caution in the perioperative period. The patient's temperature should be monitored and measures take to prevent hypothermia; hypother-

mia will aggravate the circulatory and respiratory depression.

Pituitary gland

In hypopituitarism, the varying involvement of the several hormones which the anterior pituitary produces leads to a variety of clinical presentations; amenorrhoea in females and impotence in males are common presenting features. If hypopituitarism is unrecognized, there is a greatly increased perioperative risk of hypoglycaemia, hypothermia, water intoxication and respiratory failure. If the diagnosis is known, planned substitution therapy is indicated before surgery. Oral hydrocortisone (15 mg twice daily) is administered. This is increased during the operative period; thyroxine is also given and the dose slowly increased to about 0.15 mg daily and the plasma thyroxine level is measured.

Acromegaly is caused by excessive production of pituitary growth hormone. This results in overgrowth of bone, leading to an enlarged jaw and kyphoscoliosis, as well as connective tissue and viscera. There is cardiomegaly, early atherosclerosis and systemic arterial hypertension, and diabetes mellitus is common. Management should include consideration of all associated conditions and the anaesthetist will carefully assess the patient, as tracheal intubation may be difficult.

Deficiency of antidiuretic hormone results in diabetes insipidus. A water deprivation test is used to differentiate diabetes insipidus from compulsive water drinking, and measurements are made of urine and plasma osmolality. When the plasma osmolality reaches about 295 mOsmol kg normal patients will concentrate their urine, but patients with diabetes insipidus cannot do so. If the syndrome is differentiated from compulsive water drinking, the operative management of these patients is usually uncomplicated. The patient should receive a bolus of 100 milliunits of vasopressin intravenously before surgery and during the operation 100 milliunits h^{-1} are administered by continuous infusion. Isotonic solutions, such as 0.9% sodium chloride, may then be administered with minimal risk of water depletion or hypernatraemia. Plasma osmolality should be monitored perioperatively (the normal range is 283–285 mOsmol kg).

Adrenal gland

Adrenocorticol insufficiency is known as Addison's disease. It may present in acute and chronic forms and may be due to disease of the gland itself or to disorders of the anterior pituitary or hypothalamus. A patient with adrenocortical insufficiency undergoing surgery presents a major problem. The cardiovascular status of the patient and the blood glucose and electrolytes must be measured. The patient is prepared by infusing isotonic sodium chloride and glucose solutions, in order to correct hypernatraemia and hypoglycaemia. The day before surgery, an intramuscular injection of 40 mg methylprednisolone is administered. Before induction of anaesthesia a further 100 mg hydrocortisone is administered, and for major surgery an infusion of hydrocortisone should be given during the operation. Hydrocortisone has approximately equal glucocorticoid and mineralocorticoid effects. Postoperatively, the dose of hydrocortisone is decreased from 100 mg twice daily to a replacement dose of about 50 mg daily.

Adrenocortical hyperfunction is commonly iatrogenic. Whatever the aetiology, these patients will have glucose intolerance manifest as hyperglycaemia or frank diabetes mellitus, systemic arterial hypertension (possibly associated with heart failure) and electrolyte disturbances, especially hypokalaemia and hypernatraemia. Protein breakdown leads to muscle weakness and osteoporosis. Muscle weakness will be aggravated by obesity, and respiratory function should be carefully assessed before surgery, as well as postoperatively. Osteoporosis may lead to vertebral compression fractures and patients should be positioned with great care during surgery. Prolonged immobilization after surgery will lead to further demineralization of bone, and hypercalcaemia may lead to the formation of renal calculi. Vitamin D therapy may therefore be needed in the postoperative period.

Aldosteronism may be primary (an adrenocortical adenoma – Conn's syndrome), or secondary, in which the condition is associated with an increase of plasma renin secretion (e.g. the nephrotic syndrome and cardiac failure). Patients will have hypokalaemia and hypernatraemia, which may be associated with systemic arterial hypertension. If the diagnosis is made before surgery, the administration of spironolactone (up to 300 mg daily) will reverse hypertension and hypokalaemia.

Phaeochromocytoma

These catecholamine-secreting tumours may produce sustained or intermittent arterial hypertension. During surgery, arterial hypertension and disturbances of cardiac rhythm are common, due to the release of adrenaline and noradrenaline into the circulation. Prolonged secretion of these produces not only arterial hypertension but also a contracted blood volume; α- and β-adrenergic blockade will help to reverse both these effects.

 Preoperative α-adrenergic blockade must not be complete because:

- **It may cause preoperative postural syncope**
- **It may cause difficulties in controlling the profound hypotension that sometimes occurs after tumour removal**
- **A rise in systemic blood pressure on tumour palpation is a useful sign in searching for small tumours or metastases**

Phenoxybenzamine is the agent usually used to induce partial α-adrenergic blockade. Careful preoperative preparation using α- and β-adrenergic blockade, as well as the introduction of anaesthetic techniques that promote cardiovascular stability, have greatly decreased the mortality of patients undergoing surgery for removal of a phaeochromocytoma, from 30–45% in the early 1950s to less than 5% recently.

Pancreas

Diabetes mellitus

Even minor surgery is associated with an increase in basal metabolic rate and protein breakdown with nitrogen loss and some degree of glucose intolerance. Thus, surgery in a patient with pre-existing glucose intolerance, whether this is known or not, will further exacerbate metabolic derangement. Diabetes is also a potent risk factor in the development of coronary artery disease and patients may have diabetic neuropathy which may cause autonomic nervous system dysfunction, leading to a lability in arterial blood pressure. Before surgery, the cardiovascular status of the patient should be carefully reviewed and the blood pressure taken both supine and erect to test for the possibility of autonomic neuropathy; the preoperative control of blood glucose is assessed and should be adequate. In the perioperative period it is important to monitor the patient by estimating blood glucose concentrations, rather than urinary glucose measurements, which are too insensitive for appropriate surgical patient management. It is important to treat ketoacidosis before surgery, including urgent surgery, if at all possible. Sepsis markedly increases insulin requirements. Patients undergoing cardiac bypass surgery may also have increased insulin requirements.

Table 7.2 summarizes the regimens suitable for minor and more major surgery in diabetics that are either controlled by diet alone, by oral hypoglycaemic agents, or with insulin.

Chlorpropamide is a sulphonylurea with a very long duration of action, and hypoglycaemia is a particular

Table 7.2 Severity of diabetes

	Type of surgery	
	Minor	Intermediate/major
Controlled by diet	No specific precautions	Measure blood glucose 4-hourly: if >12 mmol l⁻¹ start glucose-potassium-insulin sliding scale regimen
Controlled by oral agents	Omit medication on morning of operation and start when eating normally postoperatively	Omit medication and monitor blood glucose 1–2 hourly; if >12 mmol l⁻¹ start glucose-potassium-insulin sliding scale regimen
Controlled by insulin	Unless very minor procedure (omit insulin when nil by mouth) give glucose-potassium-insulin sliding scale regimen during surgery and until eating normally postoperatively	

concern in patients taking this agent; it should be stopped 48 hours before planned surgery and the blood sugar measured regularly after the patient becomes nil by mouth.

Patients taking long-acting insulin preparations should be converted to Actrapid insulin, and surgery should be scheduled for the early morning if possible. A number of regimens for blood sugar control have been described. But the following is easy to use:

Infuse 10% glucose 500 ml + 10 mmol potassium chloride (KCl) at 100 ml h⁻¹. Prepare a 50 ml syringe containing 50 units of Actrapid (short-acting) insulin in 50 ml normal saline (= 1 unit ml⁻¹) and connect via a 3-way tap to a glucose infusion. Adjust the rate of the syringe driver according to the following sliding scale:

Blood glucose (mmol l⁻¹)	Rate of syringe driver (ml h⁻¹)
<5	Switch off
5–7	1
7–10	2
10–20	3
>20	4

If two successive blood glucose values are > 20 mmol l⁻¹, leave instructions to consult the duty doctor.

The blood sugar is measured at least 2 hourly during surgery and the amount of insulin adjusted to maintain the blood sugar between 6 and 12 mmol l⁻¹. Following surgery blood sugar and plasma potassium are measured at least 4 hourly.

Postoperatively, as soon as the patient starts eating, those who are normally treated with oral hypoglycaemics may need subcutaneous insulin for a few days before oral therapy is recommenced. Patients normally treated with insulin can be converted to Actrapid insulin to a total equal to the normal preoperative dose. After 3 days the original regimen can usually be restarted (i.e. using long-acting insulins). In the perioperative period lactate-containing fluids (e.g. Hartmann's solution) should be avoided in diabetics. If oral feeding has not started within 72 hours of surgery, consideration should be given to the institution of parenteral nutrition.

Obesity

Life expectancy is decreased by obesity, and operative morbidity and mortality increase with increasing weight. In moderate obesity, the patient presenting for surgery should be instructed to decrease weight and given dietary advice appropriate to the patient's social and economic circumstances. They should also be examined carefully for the presence of conditions with which obesity is commonly associated; these include diabetes mellitus and systemic arterial hypertension. Patients who are double or more their ideal weight are usually termed 'morbidly obese'. These patients present a number of problems to both surgeon and anaesthetist. Their preoperative cardiorespiratory status should be assessed carefully and, as these patients are at an increased risk of inhalation of gastric contents, all should receive appropriate antacid therapy before surgery. Obesity is one of a number of conditions that will lead to an increase in postoperative deep vein thrombosis and associated thromboembolic phenomena; obese patients should receive appropriate preoperative prophylaxis for this. Transport and positioning of morbidly obese patients may cause difficulties, and occasionally two standard operating tables used side by side may be needed. Intravenous access may be difficult and non-invasive methods of monitoring arterial blood pressure may be inaccurate. Therefore, an intra-arterial line is indicated for all but the most minor procedures. This will also enable arterial blood gases to be monitored in the intra- and postoperative periods. Patients may need continued ventilatory support after surgery.

BLOOD DISORDERS

Primary blood disorders produce a wide range of clinical manifestations, which may affect any organ in the body. Conversely, there are nearly always some changes in the blood accompanying general medical and surgical disorders. Thus, haematological investigations form an important part of the assessment and subsequent monitoring of most disease processes.

Anaemia

This is defined clinically as a reduction in haemoglobin level below the normal range for the individual's age and sex. It becomes clinically apparent when the oxygen demand of the tissues cannot be met without the use of compensatory mechanisms. Although the level of haemoglobin at which elective surgery should be postponed will vary according to the precise medical status of the patient and the type of surgery planned, as a generalization a level of 10 g dl^{-1} is commonly accepted as one below which preoperative anaemia should be treated before surgery. It is important to realize that blood transfusion to raise the haematocrit should be carried out at least 48 hours before the operative procedure, as this period of time will allow full recovery of the stored erythrocytes' oxygen-carrying capacity. In order to minimize the risk of transmitting the human immunodeficiency virus (HIV), blood transfusion should be undertaken only if the urgency of surgery necessitates this. Tissue oxygenation appears to be maximal at around a haemoglobin concentration of 11 g dl^{-1} (tissue oxygenation depends upon cardiac output, peripheral vascular resistance, blood viscosity and blood oxygencarrying capacity). Patients with ischaemic heart disease are likely to suffer more from the consequences of decreased oxygen-carrying capacity from untreated anaemia, and it is especially important to treat preoperative anaemia in these patients.

Haemoglobinopathies

These are characterized by the presence of abnormal haemoglobins in the blood. Haemoglobin S is an abnormality in the amino acid sequence of the haemoglobin. When a deoxygenated haemoglobin molecule becomes distorted, this may lead to capillary occlusion and tissue hypoxia. The disease is inherited and it may be in the heterozygous or homozygous form. The former (HbAS) does not usually cause problems during surgery as the molecular distortion, known as 'sickling', only occurs at very low oxygen saturations. However, in the homozygous state (HbSS), there is a real risk of sickling during surgery and this may cause tissue infarction. Screening tests are available for the presence of haemoglobin S and electrophoresis is used to determine the exact nature of the abnormality. During surgery it is important to avoid low oxygen tensions and thus an elevated inspired oxygen concentration is used, and the patient is kept warm and well hydrated in order to maintain cardiac output and avoid circulatory stasis. If very major surgery is planned, where there is the possibility of perioperative hypoxia, for example pulmonary surgery, an exchange transfusion should be considered in an attempt to reduce the level of haemoglobin S to below 25%. Patients with haemoglobin C and haemoglobin SC should be managed in a similar way to those with haemoglobin SS.

Bleeding and coagulation disorders

As a generalization, purpura, epistaxis and prolonged bleeding from superficial cuts are suggestive of a platelet abnormality and bleeding into joints or muscle is suggestive of a coagulation defect. Both forms may be congenital or acquired and it may be possible to differentiate these from the patient's history, a recent onset being indicative of an acquired disorder. A family history should be sought but it must be remembered that the absence of other relatives with a positive history does not exclude an hereditary bleeding diathesis (one-third of haemophilia patients show no family history). Many systemic diseases may be complicated by bleeding, as may treatment with a number of drugs which can cause bone marrow depression leading to thrombocytopenia.

Platelet disorders

Thrombocytopenia arises from a number of causes:

- Failure of megakaryocyte maturation
- Excessive platelet consumption
- Hypersplenism.

Bone marrow disorders leading to failure of maturation may be due to hypoplasia or infiltration. Increased consumption occurs in disseminated intravascular coagulation, idiopathic thrombocytopenic purpura and certain viral infections. Sequestration in an enlarged spleen occurs in lymphomas and liver disease. Spontaneous bleeding does not usually occur until the platelet count has decreased to $30 \times 10^9 \ 1^{-1}$. Treatment has to be directed at the underlying disease, but thrombocytopenia resulting in clinically important bleeding necessitates a platelet transfusion. Ideally, the count should be increased to $100 \times 10^9 \ 1^{-1}$, but transfusing platelets until a clinically acceptable effect is attained is often performed. Routine major surgery should not be undertaken in the presence of an abnormal platelet count until the result is confirmed and the cause identified.

Haemophilia

Before surgery in patients with haemophilia A or B the concentration of the coagulation factors should be increased to a level that will minimize bleeding, and this concentration should be maintained until healing has occurred. It is important to seek specialist advice in determining the dosage of factors required. Cryoprecipitate and fresh frozen plasma or factor IX fraction are used to manage bleeding episodes, but the patients should be tested for antibodies to the products. If these are present, only life-saving operations should be contemplated. If cryoprecipitate or freeze-dried factor IX concentrate are administered, complications include viral hepatitis and allergy, and adrenaline and hydrocortisone should always be immediately at hand during their administration.

RENAL DISEASE

Chronic renal failure

This is said to be present when chronic renal impairment, from whatever cause, results in abnormalities of plasma biochemistry. Usually, this happens when the glomerular filtration rate (GFR) has fallen to less than 30 ml min^{-1}. Management before surgery depends on the severity of the renal failure. Patients in late and terminal degrees of the chronic renal failure (GFR < 10 ml min^{-1}) may already have commenced on dialysis. If not, dialysis should be performed before surgery if at all possible. Dialysis does not reverse all the adverse effects of chronic renal failure; for example, systemic arterial hypertension and pericarditis may still be present. In addition, patients who are dialysed very soon before surgery may have cardiovascular lability during anaesthesia and surgery because they may have a relatively contracted blood volume. These patients are also vulnerable to infection, anaemia, blood coagulation defects, electrolyte disturbances and psychological problems. It is important to define the degree of renal failure present before surgery, and review the dialysis regimen. Blood biochemistry, coagulation and haemoglobin must be checked. There should be a careful assessment of cardiorespiratory function and the patient's normal medication should be reviewed. The latter may well include antihypertensive drugs (see Concurrent drug therapy, p. 91). A careful search should be made for the presence of occult infection and all patients should have a preoperative chest X-ray. The susceptibility to infection is compounded in transplant patients by the administration of immunosuppressive drugs, and prophylactic antibiotics may be necessary preoperatively and postoperatively. Chest physiotherapy may also be needed. Procedures such as arterial or central venous cannulation must be carried out under strict aseptic conditions. Before, during and after surgery, fluid and electrolyte balance must be very carefully monitored.

The nephrotic syndrome

The clinical association of heavy proteinuria, hypoalbuminaemia and generalized oedema is usually referred to as the 'nephrotic syndrome'. The hypoalbuminaemia is the result of urinary albumin loss and the syndrome becomes apparent if more than 5 g of protein are lost per day, and the plasma albumin concentration falls to less than 30 g l^{-1}. It is important to define the underlying cause of the nephrotic syndrome. Before surgery, the plasma protein and electrolyte levels must be estimated and corrected as indicated. An albumin infusion (up to 50 g) will restore circulating blood volume and may in itself initiate a diuresis. An alteration in plasma proteins will cause changes in drug effect due to an alteration in drug binding. The anaesthetist may use more conservative doses of some drugs. Central venous cannulation is advisable for all but the most minor surgery.

LIVER DISEASE

Chronic liver disease is a continuum of pathophysiology from the patient with an abnormality of liver function tests with no adverse physiological consequences, to the patient with severe end-stage liver disease who represents an extreme surgical risk. Patients with liver disease were classified for general surgical risk by Child and Turcott in 1964 (see Table 7.3) and this is still valid today. The only important addition is the observa-

Table 7.3 Child's classification for hepatic functional reserve

	A (Minimal)	B (Moderate)	C (Advanced)
Serum bilirubin (mg d⁻¹)	<2.0	2.0–3.0	>3.0
Serum albumin (g d⁻¹)	>3.5	3.0–3.5	<3.0
Ascites controlled	None	Easily controlled	Poorly controlled
Neurological disorder	None	Minimal	Advanced 'coma'
Nutrition	Excellent	Good	Poor 'wasting'

tion that prothrombin time is the most significant preoperative predictor of mortality in patients undergoing surgery for variceal bleeding.

 Organ systems affected by cirrhosis

- **Cardiovascular system**
- **Lungs**
- **Kidneys**
- **Brain**
- **Gut**
- **Coagulation**
- **Immuno-competence**

A patient with moderate to severe cirrhosis has numerous pathophysiological changes affecting various organ systems and should always be managed by experienced personnel, both anaesthetic and surgical. Child and Turcott Grade C (even in the absence of coma) carries a very high perioperative mortality even for elective surgery. Although it is impossible to review the pathophysiology of end-stage liver disease in this text, concise reviews are available (see Further Reading).

Prior to surgery the patient's condition must be optimized. All patients should be screened routinely for Hepatitis B viral infection. They must be kept adequately hydrated to preserve renal function (although paradoxically they may be on diuretics to control ascites). Respiratory function may be poor due to basal atelectasis and/or intrapulmonary shunts. Ascitic drainage may improve the situation. If renal function deteriorates in the face of adequate filling, then a low dose dopamine infusion should be started. These patients are prone to sepsis and spontaneous bacterial peritonitis so body fluids should be cultured and strict aseptic precautions adhered to. Finally their coagulation will be deranged. In patients with predominantly cholestatic disease this may improve with vitamin K injection. Patients with hepatocellular disease are likely to have a combination of clotting factor deficiencies, chronic fibrinolysis and a low platelet count. The situation is best assessed and treated using a dynamic measure of clotting – thromboelastography (Mallett et al 1992).

These patients often lose large amounts of blood at operation due to a combination of surgical (varices) and medical (coagulopathy) causes; in addition they have a very high cardiac output, and low systemic vascular resistance circulation, which is often unresponsive to noradrenaline. It cannot be overemphasized that these are very high risk patients to operate on.

NEUROLOGICAL DISEASE

Multiple sclerosis

The aetiology of this disease of temperate-climates has become clearer in recent years. It appears that in genetically susceptible individuals activated T cells and macrophages responding to environmental triggers interact with type-1 astrocytes, causing a disruption of the blood–brain barrier and a leak of immune mediators into the nervous system. This causes demyelination. Patients may present for incidental surgery or surgery associated with alleviation of the complications, e.g. implantation of extradural stimulating electrodes. In order to decrease perioperative morbidity, careful preoperative examination is needed. Patients may have a labile autonomic nervous system associated with postural hypotension. Muscle atrophy may lead to significant kyphoscoliosis and this may result in a restrictive form of pulmonary disease. Urinary tract infections commonly occur, but the patient must be carefully examined to identify other infective foci. An elevation in temperature is the one definite factor known to precipitate an exacerbation of the disease, so that all but the most urgent surgery should be postponed until the patient is free from infection. Epilepsy is not uncommon in patients with multiple sclerosis.

Epilepsy

This term refers to a variety of types of recurrent seizure produced by paroxysmal neuronal discharge from various parts of the brain. Seizures may have a cerebral cause (e.g. tumour) or be due to a systemic disorder (e.g. uraemia or hypercalcaemia). The symptomatology is variable and seizures may cause total loss of consciousness or only a minimal alteration in awareness. The disease occurs in all age groups, with an incidence of about 1%. About 75% of patients have no recognizable underlying cause. If there is an underlying cause, the surgical management should take this into account. Otherwise management is usually uncomplicated; it is important that the patient's usual anticonvulsant medication be continued until the time of surgery and restarted as soon as possible postoperatively, if necessary using parenteral drug administration (see Concurrent drug therapy, p. 91). Anticonvulsant drugs such as phenytoin lead to induction of liver microsomal enzymes, and thus the patient's response to a variety of drugs that may be given during the perioperative period may be altered.

Myasthenia gravis

This is an autoimmune disease of the neuromuscular junction, involving the postjunctional acetylcholine receptors. Specific autoantibodies have been identified and microscopic changes in the membrane demonstrated. The disease is characterized by muscle weakness of fluctuating severity, most commonly affecting the ocular muscles. Facial and pharyngeal muscle weakness also occurs, leading to dysarthria and dysphagia. It can occur at any age in life, but is most frequently seen in the fourth decade. There is an association with thymic enlargement and thymomas, both benign and malignant. About two-thirds of patients without a thymic tumour will improve after thymectomy, although the outlook is less good for patients with tumour, whether this is excised or not. Inhibitors of the enzyme cholinesterase (e.g. edrophonium, neostigmine and pyridostigmine) are used in the treatment of myasthenia gravis, as are drugs which suppress the immunological response and eliminate circulating antibodies. The latter has now become the first line of treatment, and 90% of patients will benefit from the use of azathioprine or steroids.

Patients may present for thymectomy or incidental surgery, and the surgical management depends upon the nature of the operation and severity of the disease. As usual, the patient's normal medication must be continued up until the time of surgery. If the disease is severe, or major thoracic or upper abdominal surgery is planned, elective postoperative ventilation is advisable and, occasionally, a tracheostomy will be required, but this should only be needed if ventilation is prolonged and excess secretions are a problem. Respiratory failure in myasthenic patients may be secondary to either a myasthenic or a cholinergic crisis. Assisted ventilation should be instituted and anticholinesterase drug therapy stopped, and then cautiously reintroduced after testing with small doses of intravenous endrophonium (2–5 mg). Elective postoperative ventilation may also be advisable for lesser forms of surgery, including thymectomy, if the patient's preoperative vital capacity is less than 2 litres or there is a history of intercurrent respiratory problems. Following surgery, the requirements for anticholinesterase and other drug therapy may be changed and it is important to titrate drug dosage against clinical response. It should be remembered that overtreatment can cause weakness just as can undertreatment. Postoperatively, the adequacy of ventilation can best be assessed by repeated blood gas measurement and, therefore, before surgery there are advantages to the placement of an intra-arterial line. This will also facilitate accurate cardiovascular monitoring during surgery.

ALCOHOLISM AND DRUG ABUSE

Addiction is characterized by psychological dependence, change in tolerance and a specific withdrawal syndrome. Drugs including alcohol are used by susceptible individuals in order to obtain oblivion or excitement. Aetiological factors include psychiatric illness, personality disorders and social pressures. It should be remembered that many addicts abuse more than one drug. In general, it is advisable to maintain normal doses of the addict's usual drug in the immediate pre- and postoperative periods. The perioperative period is not the best time to attempt to wean a patient from an addiction and it may only serve to precipitate an acute withdrawal reaction. Addicts may not admit to their addiction and the first sign that there is a problem may be the appearance of a withdrawal syndrome.

Specific organ damage may result from drug addiction. Alcohol gives rise to liver damage and can progress to cirrhosis, and thus a change in protein synthesis, altered glycogen storage and susceptibility to hypoglycaemia. In addition, alcoholics are prone to bleeding, especially from the gastrointestinal tract, and there may be hypomagnesaemia. They may also have cardiomyopathy, and careful assessment of cardiovascular status is necessary in the alcoholic patient. Solvent or glue sniffers may have hepatic or renal damage and bone marrow suppression. Addicts to opioids will often have used contaminated needles and syringes, and there is a high incidence of hepatitis and liver damage and also of infection with the HIV virus (see below). If sudden hypotension occurs in the operative or postoperative period in a narcotic addict, and if other obvious causes are excluded, this may respond to the administration of intravenous morphine.

PSYCHIATRIC DISEASE

Anxiety and concern are a normal reaction of patients to forthcoming surgery and anaesthesia. A significant proportion of the population will suffer from an affective disorder at some time in their lives. A depressive illness is the commonest affective disorder and treatment may involve psychotherapy, antidepressant drug therapy or, if the disorder is severe, electroconvulsive therapy. It is important that the patient's preoperative drug therapy is continued, although both tricyclic antidepressants and monoaminoxidase inhibitors significantly interact with the drugs used during anaesthesia (see Concurrent drug therapy, p. 91). Before surgery both a psychiatrist and an anaesthetist should be consulted. Many anaesthetists would prefer that the drugs be continued up until the time of surgery, and their anaesthetic technique modified to take account of the potential for drug interactions. It should not be forgotten that severe affective disorders are accompanied by a very significant mortality rate in terms of suicide, and supportive drug therapy should not automatically be withdrawn before planned surgery unless there is a very good reason to do so. The postoperative course in patients with a depressive illness may be more prolonged and these patients should be treated with appropriate forbearance.

ACQUIRED IMMUNE DEFICIENCY SYNDROME (AIDS)

This is caused by infection with a retrovirus, the human immunodeficiency virus (HIV). Infection is most common in homosexual men and in users of drugs that are injected by needles which can be infected. However, it may also be seen in patients who have received infected blood products (e.g. haemophiliacs). The disease is not very infectious and is transmitted primarily in blood, and there is little evidence to support transmission via saliva or airborne transmission. It is thought that the risk of infection in medical and allied professions is low, unless accidental inoculation has occurred. The issue of routine preoperative screening is controversial.

THE PATIENT WITH A TRANSPLANTED ORGAN FOR NON-TRANSPLANT SURGERY

The era of transplant surgery dawned in the 1950s with the first kidney transplant (see Ch. 26). It is therefore not uncommon now to be faced with a patient with a transplanted organ presenting for non-transplant surgery.

Some aspects of management are common to all patients. It is essential to continue with their immunosuppressant regimen but consideration should be given to whether they are exhibiting signs of toxicity from the medication. These patients are all immunosuppressed. Apply strict aseptic precautions. Are they suffering from an infectious complication which may be due to an unusual pathogen such as a fungus? Have they developed a tumour as a consequence of the immunosuppression? The incidence of lymphomas is increased in these patients. Finally, are they displaying signs of rejection? This may be difficult to differentiate from infection in, for example, a lung graft.

Some specific considerations in a cardiac transplant recipient are: the heart is denervated; it will be pre-load dependent to achieve an adequate cardiac output. There will be a delayed heart rate response (e.g. to hypoxia) which will be generated by catecholamine secretion. These patients have accelerated coronary atherosclerosis but may not develop angina in response to myocardial ischaemia. The heart will have unusual responses to vasoactive drugs due to the denervation. Finally arrhythmias and a low cardiac output may be signs of rejection.

SURGERY IN THE ELDERLY

Although patients over the age of 65 years comprise only 22% of the surgical caseload, they are reported to account for 79% of perioperative deaths (Buck et al 1987). The mortality of surgery in elderly patients is significantly higher in those suffering from serious coexisting medical conditions. In a study of 100 000 surgical operations, the relative risk of dying within 7 days, comparing patients over 80 with those under 60 years, was 3, but the risk factor comparing patients having symptomatic medical disease with those having none was over 10 (Cohen et al 1988). Not only do elderly patients have an increased likelihood of coexisting disease, but physiological function in general decreases with age. As a generalization, many physiological functions (e.g. cardiac output, glomerular filtration rate and renal blood flow) decrease by about 1% per annum after the age of 30 years. Respiratory function also declines with age (maximum breathing capacity decreases from about 100 1 min^{-1} at 20 years to 30 1 min^{-1} at 80 years). The elderly are also more sensitive to the majority of drugs that might be used in the perioperative period (e.g. diazepam has a half-life measured in hours that is approximately equal to subject age in years). As in all other situations where a patient presents for surgery with a significant coexisting disease, the morbidity and mortality associated with surgery can be reduced to a minimum after careful preoperative evaluation and by optimizing the patient's condition.

CONCURRENT DRUG THERAPY

It is a general rule that any patients stabilized on long-term drug therapy should continue to take their normal medication until the time of surgery, and that this should be recommenced as soon as possible following surgery. If the patient is unable to take drugs by mouth, then appropriate parenteral administration is required. This is especially important for patients taking drugs such as antiepileptics, antiarrhythmics or antihypertensives. A thorough knowledge of the pharmacokinetic and pharmacodynamic profile of the individual drugs is needed, in order that the appropriate doses and interval between doses is arrived at for parenteral administration. A number of drugs (e.g. propranolol) undergo extensive first-pass liver metabolism after oral administration, and drugs such as this need much lower doses administered parenterally than they do orally. Admission to hospital for surgery gives the opportunity to review the appropriateness of long-term drug therapy and dosage; this may be especially important in elderly patients as they are more likely to suffer from toxic symptoms. The nature of some operations may mean that the need for continued drug therapy has to be reviewed postoperatively, or the dosage of the drugs may need to be altered. An example of this would be a myasthenic patient undergoing thymectomy. Although the majority of patients stabilized on long-term therapy should continue their normal drugs up until the time of surgery, there are a number of drugs whose administration or dosage will need to be modified before surgery (see Table 7.4 for the more important examples of these).

Summary

1. If there is a reversible feature to the patient's coexisting medical disease then elective surgery should be postponed until the patient is optimally treated.
2. It may be appropriate to delay even emergency surgery until the patient's condition is stabilized or improved.
3. A patient presenting for a minor surgical procedure may none the less require a high degree of anaesthetic expertise.

Table 7.4 Some important drugs, the administration or dosage of which needs to be modified before surgery

Oral contraceptives	Maintain for minor or peripheral procedures and institute prophylaxis against deep vein thrombosis, before surgery. Stop one complete monthly cycle before abdominal (especially pelvic) surgery
Anticoagulants	Stop oral agents several days before surgery and substitute heparin if continued anticoagulant is necessary. The action of heparin can be rapidly reversed with protamine
Agents used in diabetes	See section on diabetic management
Levodopa	Omit dose before surgery
Monamine oxidase inhibitors	Significant potential for drug interactions, causing severe physiological disturbance. Discuss with psychiatrist and anaesthetist and treat each case on its merits
Steroids	Supplement with hydrocortisone 100 mg i.v. 30 minutes before surgery, repeated 3-hourly during surgery, reducing slowly postoperatively to the patient's preoperative dose. Treat similarly if taking large dose regularly, any time during 3 months before surgery

References

Aitkenhead A R, Barnett D B 1989 Heart disease. In: Vickers M D, Jones R M (eds) Medicine for anaesthetists. Blackwell, London 1989

Buck N, Devlin H B, Lunn J N 1987 The report of a confidential enquiry into perioperative deaths. Nuffield Provincial Hospitals Trust, London

Campling E A, Devlin H B, Hoile R W, Lunn J N 1992 The report of the national confidential enquiry into perioperative deaths, 1990. King's Fund Publishing, London

Campling E A, Devlin H B, Hoile R W, Lunn J N 1993 The report of the national confidential enquiry into perioperative deaths, 1991/1992. King's Fund Publishing, London

Campling E A, Devlin H B, Hoile R W, Lunn J N 1995 The report of the national confidential enquiry into perioperative deaths 1992/1993. King's Fund Publishing, London

Child C G III, Turcotte J 1965 Surgery and Portal hypertension. In: Child C G III (ed) The liver and portal hypertension. Saunders, Philadelphia

Cohen M M, Duncan P G, Tate R B 1988 Does anaesthesia contribute to operative mortality? Journal of the American Medical Association 260: 2859–2863

Jones R M 1985 Smoking before surgery: the case for stopping. British Medical Journal 290: 1763–1764

Mallett S V, Cox D 1992 Thromboelastoplasty. British Journal of Anaesthesia 69: 307–313

Simon A 1977 Perioperative management of the pacemaker patient. Anesthesiology 16: 127–131

Further reading

Findlaw D, Doyle E 1997 Congenital heart disease in adults. British Journal of Anaesthesia 78: 416–430

McIntyre N, Benhamon J P, Bircher J et al 1991 Oxford textbook of clinical hepatology. (especially section 31: Surgery, anaesthesia and the liver.) Oxford University Press, Oxford

8

Immunity in surgery

P. L. Amlot, C. S. Gricks

Objectives

- **Appreciate the functions and complexity of the immune system.**
- **Recognize that disease processes are countered with minimal damage to the host.**
- **Understand the implications of immune processes in surgery.**

INTRODUCTION

The immune system evolved to protect the body from pathogens. In humans, specific and variable receptors of an adaptive immunity are linked to common effector pathways that provide an innate immunity.

INNATE IMMUNITY

Inborn immunity needs no prior contact with a pathogen to be activated. It reacts quantitatively but not qualitatively:

Lysozyme in saliva and tears digests peptidoglycan in bacterial cell walls. Susceptible bacteria are unable to invade the body.

The complement system consists of many proteins that can self-assemble to cause lysis of cells to which they are attached. Deficiency leads to susceptibility to infection by encapsulated bacteria or, surprisingly, to autoimmunity. Complement may be activated by:

- Classical pathway – initiated by antibody
- Alternative pathway – initiated directly by certain chemicals, such as sugars forming part of microbial cell walls.

Complement, C-reactive protein and mannose-binding protein can coat foreign particles, making them more easily digestible by phagocytes – '*opsonization.*'

Cellular: phagocytes – neutrophils, monocytes or tissue macrophages, possess a wide variety of receptors, capable of increasing in quantity but not of qualititive change. Deficiencies, which are usually iatrogenic, increase susceptibility to infection. Other, non-phagocytic cells may facilitate the immune response; stimulated mast cells release factors that increase vascular permeability, allowing more rapid access of other cells to sites of infection.

Natural killer (NK) lymphocytes, which lack receptors capable of qualitative change, are involved in the surveillance of altered cells, particularly against tumours and viruses. Activated NK cells are capable of lysing nucleated target cells, unless they are inhibited. On the membranes of NK cells are killer inhibitory receptors (KIRs) which bind to major histocompatibility complex (MHC) class I molecules of target cells protecting them from being killed. Both viruses and tumour cells interfere with, or eliminate, MHC class I on the surface of their transformed cells, making them susceptible to NK cells, since KIR now has nothing with which to bind and so no inhibitory signal is given.

ADAPTIVE IMMUNITY

In an adaptive response, exposure to infection leads to qualitative changes of specific receptors that are selected in a Darwinian fashion on the basis of their binding to pathogens. The structure that evokes a specific receptor is known as an *antigen*. This system has two collaborative branches, antibody immunity and cell mediated immunity.

Antibody mediated immunity

Antibodies belong to a class of proteins known as *immunoglobulins*. In man, antibody-producing B lymphocytes originate in the bone marrow and the B cell receptor is the membrane-bound form of antibody. Pathogens coated with antibody or complement are phagocytosed far more rapidly than uncoated pathogens. It is estimated that our B cell system can create more than 10^{11} unique antibody molecules but each B cell can produce antibody of but a single specificity. There is not enough DNA to encode all the possibilities and the mechanism of gene rearrangement allows the B cells to create antibodies with diverse specificities. This includes the possibility of creating antibodies that react with 'self', and can lead to *autoimmunity*.

Antibody binding region

Antibody in the B cell membrane acts as a receptor for antigen on its surface. The B cell may be stimulated by the binding of an antigen to undergo proliferation or differentiate into a plasma cell. B cell stimulation with antigen occurs mainly within lymphoid follicles (structures in which B cells aggregate) and stimulates the formation of germinal centres. A process known as somatic hypermutation now occurs which may reduce the ability of the antibody to bind to its specific antigen, but allows a few B cells to develop antibodies that bind with greater affinity. Within 2 weeks the affinity of the antibody increases by 10 to 100 times as the successfully mutated B cells outgrow others – *clonal expansion*.

Antibodies – structure and synthesis

One part of the antibody, the variable or V region, binds to the antigen. The other, the constant or C region, interacts with the invariable receptors of the common effector pathways. An antibody is composed of two heavy and two light chains of immunoglobulin linked together so that there are at least two antigen-binding sites per molecule (Fig. 8.1).

The constant domain. The major part of the antibody is largely invariable and so named the constant region which endows the antibody with different functional properties. There are five heavy chain genes giving rise to immunoglobulin (Ig)M, IgD, IgG, IgE, and IgA. Immature B cells usually express IgM but they can switch the constant region when stimulated by antigen. The switch is influenced by the environment and T helper cells. This is *isotype switching*.

IgM is so named because in its secreted form it is a macroglobin composed of five immunoglobulin molecules bound together. Because of its large size it is largely retained within the vascular system, where it is effective at complement fixation and in protection against blood borne infections. IgD is a largely membrane bound immunoglobulin of unknown function. *IgG* is the most abundant isotype in the blood and tissues. It is small enough to diffuse readily in the tissues

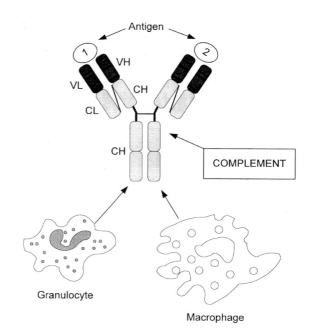

Fig 8.1 Antibody structure and effector relationships. VL – variable region of the light chain; VH – variable region of the heavy chain; CL – constant region of the light chain; CH – constant region of the heavy chain that consists of three domains. Note that there are two binding sites to the antibody molecule, each binding an identical antigen (1 and 2). Granulocytes and macrophages bind to antibody molecules via their Fc receptors (known as Fc because it is an old term for the constant region of the heavy chain of the antibody molecule). The complement system interacts with the constant region of the heavy chain and leads to lysis of cells.

and contains most of the high affinity antibody. There are several subclasses, each with different functional properties. Apart from coating pathogens for phagocytosis, they are also able to induce antibody dependent cellular cytotoxicity (ADCC) which may play a part in transplantation and tumour immunity. Because it can cross the placental barrier it provides the fetus with antibody protection. IgG and IgA are also provided in breast milk. *IgA* can be transported across mucosal epithelium, resists gastrointestinal digestion and is the principle isotype in respiratory and gastrointestinal secretions. It is thought to prevent adherence of microorganisms and toxins to receptors and so is sometimes termed 'antiseptic paint'. *IgE* is bound to receptors on blood basophils and mast cells, skin, mucosa, connective tissues and along blood vessels. Antigen binding causes degranulation of mast cells, which release mediators invoking coughing, sneezing, vomiting and diarrhoea. IgE protects against parasitation with worms but causes allergies such as hayfever, urticaria, asthma or anaphylaxis.

BACTERIAL INFECTIONS

Immunodeficiency is quite common and should be excluded in patients suffering repeated infections, especially those recurring rapidly following an adequate course of antibiotic therapy. Acquired immunodeficiency is most commonly iatrogenic but severe antibody deficiency occurs most frequently in common variable immunodeficiency (CVID) and in diseases affecting immunoglobulin production, such as lymphoma. Bacterial infection can be prevented in patients with hypogammaglobulinaemia by giving replacement immunoglobulin therapy fortnightly or monthly.

MONOCLONAL ANTIBODIES

In a normal immune response many B cells produce many different types of antibodies – a *polyclonal* response. A single B cell can produce but a single antibody; if it proliferates each daughter produces the same antibody – a *monoclonal* antibody. This is characteristic of B cell malignancy such as multiple myeloma. The monoclonal proteins can be detected by electrophoresis or immunofixation. Monoclonal antibodies have revolutionized diagnostic processes; they are developed by fusing a single B cell from a mouse or rat spleen to a myeloma cell line, allowing infinite production of a monoclonal antibody (Kohler and Milstein 1975).

T CELLS AND
CELL MEDIATED IMMUNITY

T lymphocytes have specialized membrane-bound T cell receptors (TCR) that are never secreted and always remain cell bound. T cells arise in the bone marrow but migrate to the thymus, a primary lymphoid organ, in order to differentiate. The thymus is a site of enormous cellular proliferation, like the germinal centres in B cell follicles; it is most active early in life and atrophies with age.

The T cell receptor, like immunoglobulin, is made up of two chains. It shows remarkable similarity to the heavy and light chains of immunoglobulin in that they undergo the same process of gene rearrangement producing a unique antigen-binding variable region, and a conserved constant region which is largely anchored in the T cell membrane.

T cell recognition of antigen

T cells recognize only protein antigens which have been broken down or 'processed' by another cell for interaction with the T cell receptor as part of specialized cell surface molecules that have been misnamed the major histocompatibility complex (MHC), because of the complications this region causes in transplanting tissues. The MHC is also known as HLA (human leukocyte antigens). The T cell receptor recognizes a combination of the major histocompatibility complex and the antigen which it 'presents', since the T-cell cannot recognize free antigen.

There are two major classes of MHC molecules, structurally related but differing in their expression on different tissues, the cellular compartment from which they bind peptides and in the way they bind and present fragments to different T cell populations.

MHC class I molecules are present on the majority of nucleated cells and bind endogenous peptides which originate in the cell cytoplasm. Cells degrade cytoplasmic proteins and transport fragments to the cell surface in MHC class I molecules where they are recognized by cytotoxic T cells, identified by the CD8 molecule (a surface antigen that can be detected with a specific antibody – CD = cluster designation). Cytotoxic T cells will kill the cell if the fragment is identified as foreign. In this way T cells recognize an MHC class I foreign peptide complex on the surface of a virally infected cell, and will kill it.

MHC class II molecules are located on B lymphocytes, macrophages and dendritic cells, collectively known as antigen presenting cells (APC). These cells can assimilate exogenous antigen from outside the cell by phagocytosis or receptor mediated endocytosis into vesicles within the cell. During the process of MHC class II synthesis it incorporates the peptides from the vesicles and transports it to the cell surface. The T cell receptor of T helper cells (identified by the CD4 molecule) is capable of binding to the antigen embedded in the MHC class II molecule. T helper and cytotoxic T cells are selected in the thymus (Fig. 8.2).

In both types of MHC a groove exists into which a peptide can fit, facilitating interaction with the T cell receptor, but limiting its interaction. A pathogen with a mutation that cannot fit is ignored. To counter this, the MHC gene cluster on chromosome 6 accommodates highly polymorphic genes; this benefits the population at the expense of the individual.

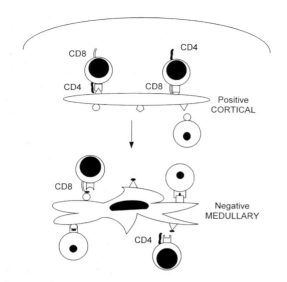

Fig 8.2 Thymic 'education' in T cell differentiation. CD4 = T helper cells; CD8 = cytotoxic T cells. During 'positive' selection T cells express both CD4 and CD8. Those cells capable of binding to MHC molecules on cortical epithelial cells are destined to survive. During 'negative' selection T cells express either CD4 or CD8 selected on the ability of the TCR to bind to MHC class II or class I respectively. During 'negative' selection, avid binding of TCR to MHC expressing self-antigens on medullary dendritic cells leads to the apoptotic death of such T cells, thus minimizing autoimmunity. Cells depicted with small nuclei represent apoptotic cells destined for elimination in the thymus. Binding ability of the TCR for MHC is depicted by the degree of 'fit' between the two molecules.

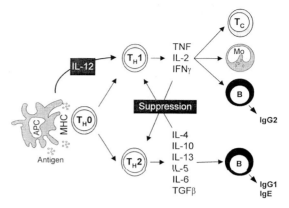

Fig 8.3 T helper cell (CD4) functions. APC – antigen presenting cell; MHC – major histocompatibility complex; IL – interleukin; TH0, TH1, TH2 – T helper cell subsets (CD4+); TNF – tumour necrosis factor; IFN – interferon; TGF – T cell growth factor; T_c – cytotoxic T cell (CD8+); Mo – monocyte/macrophage series; B – B cell.

T cell function

The T cell receptor detects MHC 'signatures' of non-self and in turn is linked to intracellular enzymic pathways that activate the T cell via a complex of molecules known as CD3. The activated T cell produces intercellular communicating *cytokines*, of which more than 50 have been identified, with many different effects. Most of them transmit between leukocytes and are therefore termed *interleukins* (IL), with attached numbers to indicate their intercommunications and actions. The immunosuppressive drug cyclosporin inhibits the secretion of IL-2.

The T cell response, directed by T helper cells, depends upon the microenvironment and may lead to a vigorous destructive cellular response including self-destruction of the target cell (apoptosis from Greek: *apo* = away + *ptosis* = a falling), or enhancement of antibody production (see Fig. 8.3). The T cell receptor is dependent on the major histocompatibility complex for recognizing antigen and self from non-self.

T cell depletion

Failure to develop a thymus results in complete absence of T cells. The human immunodeficiency virus (HIV) selectively infects T helper cells resulting in acquired immunodeficiency syndrome (AIDS) with consequent susceptibility to intracellular infections and virally mediated malignancies such as lymphomas and Kaposi's sarcoma.

AUTOIMMUNITY

Random generation of antigen binding sites in antibodies risks the development of autoimmune disease. One safeguard is that as immature B cells emerge from the bone marrow they bind to the abundant self proteins, leading to tolerance or death. Also, B cells require a number of growth factors (cytokines) derived from T cells and in their absence antibody production may fail. Autoimmunity arises in predisposed individuals, affecting both B and T cells. Antibody may bind to, and block, an important receptor such as the acetylcholine receptor in myasthenia gravis. Autoimmune antibody may lead to damage by complement fixation or antibody dependent cellular cytotoxicity (ADCC). Antibody may also form immune complexes that are deposited at the intimal surface of blood vessels and cause vasculitis.

SURGICAL ASPECTS

Immunity to infection

Significant natural protections against infection are the maintenance of intact skin and mucosal surfaces, and antibacterial secretions such as lysozyme and gastric acid. However, pathogens develop selective means of invading the body, so that mycobacteria are resistant to gastric acid. The cholera vibrio binds to a receptor in the gut to enter the body. Those that gain access may be ingested and killed by phagocytes but some pathogenic organisms inhibit phagocytosis and also release toxins. Antibodies are produced to neutralize the toxins and antibodies and complement are synergistic in opsonizing the organisms for ingestion by the phagocytes.

Immunodeficiency states

This may be primary but is more commonly secondary and often iatrogenic.

Primary

Neutrophils and monocytes may be defective and deficiencies can occur in the complement system. Both B cell, T cell and stem cell defects and deficiencies occur. B cell deficiencies are characterized by bacterial infection while T cell deficiencies more commonly lead to viral and opportunistic infection.

Secondary

This is much more common and results from many influences affecting or related to surgical treatment:

- Poor nutrition particularly affects cell-mediated immunity. Surgery carried out in countries where starvation is rife is likely to be complicated by infection.
- Malignant disease.
- Drugs, including anaesthetic drugs such as halothane.
- Infection, including viral effects on lymphoid cells.
- AIDS (acquired immunodeficiency syndrome) results from infection with the human immunodeficiency virus (HIV) which has primarily affected male homosexuals, intravenous drug users and haemophiliacs given factor VIII derived from pooled plasma in Europe and the United States of America. In Africa it is primarily a heterosexual disease. The virus attaches itself to the CD4 molecule on the helper T cell and the cytotoxic T cells are initially unaffected. It is particularly associated with susceptibility to opportunistic infections such as *Pneumocystis carinii*, cytomegalovirus, *Candida aspergillus*, and also to the development of Kaposi's sarcoma.
- Shock, trauma and burns have a profoundly immunosuppressive effect and result in increased susceptibility to infection.
- Surgery. Major operations with associated anaesthesia depress immune response so there is increased risk of infection.
- Radiotherapy for malignant disease produces lymphopenia, neutropenia, thrombocytopenia so that cellular and humoral immunity is depressed. However, the dose and rate of irradiation is such that marked cytopenias are rare and infection is not as common as with cytotoxic drugs.
- Chemotherapy to treat malignant disease is cytotoxic to neutrophils and leukocytes and is associated with increased bacterial and opportunistic infections.
- Steroids used in transplantation and in treatment of some diseases with an autoimmune basis.
- Immunosuppressant drugs such as azathioprine and cyclosporin A or tacrolimus used in transplantation.
- Specific diseases may have an effect. The small bowel is richly supplied with T, B and plasma cells and secretes the immunoglobulin IgA into the lumen. If it is diseased, it becomes susceptible to infection with, for example, *Giardia lamblia*. In Crohn's disease, which may have an autoimmune component but which is often treated with immune-suppressive drugs, coeliac disease and atrophic gastritis are all associated with immune deficiency. Remarkably, extensive bowel resection does not appear to have major immunological effects.
- Specific operations may have an effect. Splenectomy in children, particularly infants, increases their susceptibility to infection and they should be given long-term oral penicillins. There is a lesser risk in older children and adults and polyvalent pneumonococcus vaccine may be given to these, preferably before operation. Overwhelming post-splenectomy infection, usually with encapsulated bacteria (e.g. pneumococcus, haemophilus or meningococcus) occurs in 1–20% of splenectomized individuals; it is fatal in 50% of cases. Remarkably, thymectomy carried out for the treatment of myasthenia gravis does not appear to have severe effects on immunity.

TRANSPLANTATION

Autotransplantation (Greek: *autos* = self) of tissue, such as a skin graft, has no immunological consequences; nor does grafting between identical twins (isograft:

Greek: *isos* = equal). Non-vascularized allografts (Greek: *allos* = other) such as corneal grafts do not normally evoke a cellular rejection. Whole organ grafts include kidney, liver, heart, lung, pancreas, small bowel (see Ch. 26). They are mainly cadaveric organs although some are from related live donors. Rejection is predominantly acute and cell-mediated rather than as the result of antibodies, unless the recipient has had prior contact with the donor tissues, in which case a hyperacute rejection occurs. A chronic vascular rejection causing graft dysfunction and progressive graft loss is due to a variety of mechanisms including immune responses, physical effects, accelerated vasculopathy and immunosuppressive drug induced effects. Tubular structures, such as blood vessels and biliary ducts, are affected by this process.

Avoiding rejection

• Except when transplanting the cornea, the donor and recipient tissues are matched for ABO blood groups and as closely as possible for HLA (human leukocyte antigens). In addition the recipient's serum is cross matched with the donor lymphoid cells to exclude preformed cytotoxic antibodies.

• Except when transplanting between identical twins, the recipient is immunosuppressed, using a variety of drugs including steroids, azathioprine, mycophenolate mofetil, cyclosporine or tacrolimus. The anchors of current therapy are cyclosporine and tacrolimus, whose action prevents the development of cytotoxic T cells; however, both are nephrotoxic. Antilymphocytic globulin (ALG) or antithymocyte globulin (ATG) are polyclonal antibodies preferably raised in rabbits, and may be used to increase immunosuppression early in transplantation. Monoclonal antibodies such as OKT3 (CD3) or Campath 1 (CDw52) have been used to reverse acute rejection. Newer monoclonal antibodies reacting with the IL-2 receptor (CD25) are effective at prophylactically reducing acute rejection episodes.

• Graft versus host disease (GVHD) may develop if the graft contains competent T cells which react against the host cells that are incapable of rejecting them. This is most likely to develop following bone marrow transplantation. Graft versus host disease affects the skin, liver and gut predominantly.

CANCER IMMUNOLOGY

• The occasional but well documented spontaneous regression of tumours suggests that immunity may develop against them.

• Immunosuppressed patients have a higher than normal risk of malignancy, especially skin cancers and lymphoid tumours.

• Cancers are often infiltrated with lymphocytes and macrophages – this may be associated with an improved prognosis.

• Latent cancers, especially of the thyroid and prostate glands, are often disclosed at post mortem examination, suggesting that the tumours develop but lie dormant for many years without clinical disease. This has been attributed to immune mechanisms.

Tumour antigens

Specific antigens can be found on the surface of tumour cells, especially those that are virally induced, without being present on normal cells of this type. Some tumour cells express antigens normally found only in fetal tissue, such as α-fetoprotein (AFP) and carcinoembryonic antigen (CEA). These may be used as markers for some cancers or to monitor progress by measuring serum levels but there is little evidence that they act as targets for the immune system. Radiolabelled monoclonal antibody to CEA may be used to localize residual bowel tumour. Malignant cells may over-express proto-oncogenes on their surface that contribute to malignant behaviour, these were identified by antibodies developed for the recognition of specific tumour types.

Monoclonal antibodies that attach to receptors highly expressed in tumours can be labelled with isotopes such as ^{111}In and ^{99m}Tc. These can be identified by external scintigraphy. This is especially valuable in identifying residual tumour following treatment.

Immunotherapy

The identification of immune aspects of cancer has led to the search for therapeutic uses, especially for disseminated tumour cells beyond the scope of conventional treatment, or residual tumour following treatment. Antibodies alone are rarely cytotoxic to tumour cells and largely restricted to haemopoietic malignancy. Monoclonal antibodies can be conjugated to radioistopes, immunotoxins or enzymes. Radiolabelled antibodies can target highly expressed epidermal growth factor receptors (GFR) in lung and brain tumours and there is hope that monoclonal antibodies to GFR will be effective in treating tumours.

Summary

1. The immune system is composed of humoral and cellular elements. It is made up of innate and adaptive mechanisms.
2. Normally, the immune system recognizes self and non-self. In predisposed individuals autoimmunity may develop.
3. Immune deficiency arises from many causes, including surgery, and predisposes to surgical complications.
4. Except in specific circumstances, organ transplants must be protected from rejection by immunosuppressive drugs and other techniques.
5. There are immunological aspects of cancer that are becoming increasingly valuable in identifying, monitoring and treating malignancy.

Reference

Kohler G, Milstein C 1975 Continuous cultures of fused cells secreting antibody of predefined specificity. Nature 256(5517): 495–497

Further reading

Basic immunology
Janeway C A, Travers P 1997 Immunology. Harcourt Brace, Edinburgh

Clinical immunology
Stites D P, Terr A I, Parslow T G 1997 Medical immunology. Appleton and Lange, Connecticut

9

Haematological assessment and blood component therapy

A. B. Mehta

Objectives

- **Understand the need for preoperative detection of blood conditions (anaemia, easy bruising) which affect outcome of surgery and anaesthesia.**
- **Be aware of the range of blood components available for clinical use, understand their indications and the hazards associated with their use.**
- **Understand the underlying mechanisms and management of excessive intra- or postoperative blood loss due to a blood condition and not due to surgery.**

INTRODUCTION

This chapter outlines the management of surgical patients who have an abnormality of their blood count (anaemia, thrombocytopenia and, to a lesser extent, leucopenia) or an abnormality of blood plasma constituents, and focuses on replacement therapy. Anaemia and excessive bleeding are symptoms and not diagnoses. An accurate diagnosis is an essential initial step in the formulation of a management plan. In the majority of hospitals, a clinical haematologist will be available to advise you on optimum use of laboratory diagnostic facilities and interpretation of results. Make sure you discuss problems early, and take advice on the appropriate specimens to send and tests to order. If a result is puzzling, go and discuss it with the haematologist.

PREOPERATIVE ASSESSMENT

Growing pressure on hospital beds and increasing use of day surgery means that the preoperative assessment should, wherever possible, be performed prior to admission. The key aims are to assess a patient's fitness to undergo surgery and anaesthesia, anticipate complications, arrange for supportive therapy to be available perioperatively and to liaise with the appropriate specialist physician regarding non-surgical management. A full history and physical examination are mandatory. Laboratory evaluation begins by an assessment of the full blood count (FBC). This is performed by automated analysers and gives the haemoglobin concentration, red cell indices, white cell count, white cell differential and platelet count. If the FBC shows changes in more than one cell line (e.g. anaemia plus thrombocytopenia and/or leucopenia) or is in any other way indicative of intrinsic bone marrow disease (e.g. blood film showing leukaemic infiltration) surgery must be deferred pending a full haematological assessment.

Anaemia

Anaemia is defined as a reduction in haemoglobin concentration below the normal range after correction for age and sex (approximately 13–16 g dl^{-1} in males, 11.5–15 g dl^{-1} in females). A classification of anaemia is given below:

- *Decreased red cell production*
    - Haematinic deficiency:
      Iron, vitamin B$_{12}$, folic acid
    - Marrow failure:
      Aplastic anaemia
      Leukaemia
      Pure red cell aplasia
- *Abnormal red cell maturation*
    - Myelodysplasia
    - Sideroblastic anaemia
- *Increased red cell destruction*
    - Inherited haemolytic anaemia (e.g. sickle cell anaemia, thalassaemia)
    - Acquired haemolytic anaemia:
      Immune (e.g. autoimmune)
      Non-immune (e.g. microangiopathic haemolytic anaemia, disseminated intravascular coagulation)

- *Effects of disease in other organs*
  Anaemia of chronic disorder
  Renal, endocrine, liver disease.

Important clues regarding the cause of anaemia are gained from examination of red cell indices. The following alterations in red cell indices offer a clue to the cause of anaemia:

- *Lowered mean cell volume (MCV)/mean cell haemoglobin (MCH)*
  - Iron deficiency
  - Thalassaemia trait
  - Homozygous thalassaemia
  - Hyperthyroidism
- *Raised MCV*
  - Megaloblastic anaemia
  - Hypothyroidism
  - Liver disease
  - Reticulocytosis
  - Myelodysplasia
  - Aplastic anaemia
  - Paraproteinaemia
  - Alcohol abuse
- *Normochromic normocytic*
  - Anaemia of chronic disease
  - Renal failure
  - Bone marrow infiltration
  - Haemorrhage.

A reduction in MCV and MCH (microcytic hypochromic picture) is highly suggestive of iron deficiency, which in turn is most frequently due to haemorrhage. Nutritional deficiency leads to a well-compensated anaemia of gradual onset. A raised MCV is highly suggestive of megaloblastic anaemia and malabsorption (due to pernicious anaemia, coeliac disease, or after gastrectomy) or poor dietary intake are the commonest causes. Blood component therapy should be avoided wherever possible and the underlying cause of the anaemia should be specifically treated.

Haemoglobinopathies

These are a group of inherited disorders (autosomal recessive) of haemoglobin synthesis in which affected individuals (homozygotes) suffer a life-long haemolytic anaemia. They are the commonest inherited disorders of mankind.

The carriers (heterozygotes) have a small degree of protection against malaria; haemoglobinopathies are therefore common in all parts of the world where malaria is (or was) prevalent (Southern Europe, Asia, the Far East, Africa, South America and immigrant populations in Northern Europe and North America).

These carriers are asymptomatic and have a normal life expectancy, but may have a mild degree of anaemia. Haemoglobinopathies are divided into two types. In the structural haemoglobin variants, a single DNA base mutation leads to an amino acid substitution in haemoglobin to give rise to a variant haemoglobin, e.g. haemoglobin S (sickle haemoglobin, which leads to sickle cell anaemia). The variant haemoglobin may be functionally abnormal; thus, haemoglobin S tends to crystallize under conditions of low oxygen tension and this distorts red cell shape to cause 'sickling'. The second type of haemoglobinopathy is thalassaemia, where there is no change in the amino acid composition of the haemoglobin molecule but there is deficient synthesis of one of the globin chains (α or β) leading to imbalanced chain synthesis and anaemia.

It is important to detect carriers of some haemoglobinopathies (e.g. sickle cell) prior to surgery as anaesthesia and hypoxia can precipitate sickling. All patients of non Northern Europe origin should be screened prior to surgery (e.g. in the pre-admission clinic) by haemoglobin electrophoresis and/or a sickle solubility test. Affected individuals (homozygotes) usually present in childhood but occasional patients present incidentally. Patients with sickle cell disease (HbSS) should be managed jointly with a clinical haematologist. They require exchange transfusion prior to major surgery (e.g. hip replacement). This involves venesection of the patient together with transfusion of donor blood (6–8 units). This procedure can be performed manually or using a cell separator. Minor surgery (e.g. dental procedures) can be safely carried out without transfusion in the majority of patients. Intermediate procedures (e.g. cholecystectomy) can be performed following transfusion (2–3 units of packed red cells) to a haemoglobin level of 10 g dl^{-1} (Vichinsky et al 1995). Particular attention should be paid to the hydration of the patient and to oxygenation during anaesthesia. Patients with some haemoglobinopathies (e.g. HbSC disease) are at an increased risk of postoperative thrombosis.

Other inherited red cell disorders

Deficiency of the red cell enzyme glucose-6-phosphate dehydrogenase (G6PD) is a sex-linked disorder affecting more than 400 million people worldwide. It results in a reduced capacity of the red cell to withstand an oxidative stress. Patients are asymptomatic in the steady state and have a near normal FBC, but may suffer haemolysis of red cells in response to an oxidative challenge. Common precipitants are infection and drugs principally antimalarials (primaquine, pamaquine, and pentaquine but not usually chloroquine or mefloquine) and sulphonamide antibiotics (Mehta 1994).

Excessive bleeding

Preoperative assessment should allow us to anticipate problems. Many patients with an inherited or acquired defect of coagulation (Table 9.1) leading to peri- and postoperative complications cannot be detected preoperatively. However, a full history may reveal features such as excessive bleeding at times of previous surgery, bleeding while brushing teeth, nose bleeds, a family history of bleeding disorders, spontaneous bruising, a history of renal or liver disease and a relevant drug history. A coagulation screen (prothrombin time (PT), activated partial thromboplastin time (APTT), thrombin time (TT)) and platelet count should be done in any patient with a suspected bleeding disorder; however, disordered platelet function can be difficult to detect. A bleeding time is the time taken for firm clot formation following a standard skin incision (normal range 3–10 minutes) and is the best in vivo test of platelet function.

Table 9.1 Bleeding disorders associated with excessive bleeding which may cause peri- or postoperative complications

Disorder type	Cause
Congenital	
Clotting factors	Haemophilia A, B
	von Willebrand's syndrome
Platelets	Congenital platelet disorders
Vessel wall	Hereditary haemorrhagic telangiectasia
Acquired	
Clotting factors	Drugs (anticoagulants, antibiotics)
	Liver disease
	DIC* (in sepsis)
Platelets – function	Drugs (aspirin, NSAIDs*)
	Liver disease, renal disease, myeloproliferative disorders, paraproteinaemic disorders
Platelets – number	Autoimmune thrombocytopenia
	Hypersplenism
	Aplastic anaemia, myelodysplasia
Vessel wall	Drugs (steroids)
	Vasculitis
	Malnutrition

*DIC, disseminated intravascular coagulation; NSAIDs, non-steroidal anti-inflammatory drugs.

Anticoagulant therapy

The dose of oral anticoagulants (e.g. warfarin) is adjusted to maintain the international normalized ratio (INR, which is a measure of the ratio of the patient's PT to that of a control plasma) within a therapeutic range. The dose of heparin, which is a parenteral anticoagulant, is monitored by measurement of the ratio of the patient's APTT to that of control plasma. For elective surgery in patients on oral anticoagulants, the challenge is to balance the risk of haemorrhage if the INR is not reduced against the risk of thrombosis if the INR is reduced for too long or by too great an amount. For minor surgery (e.g. dental extraction) it is normally sufficient to stop the oral anticoagulant for 2 days prior to the procedure and restart with the usual maintenance dose immediately afterwards. For high-risk patients (e.g. those with prosthetic heart valves) or for patients undergoing more extensive procedures, it is necessary to stop warfarin and give heparin (either subcutaneously or by continuous intravenous infusion) under close haematological supervision to provide thrombosis prophylaxis. Patients on anticoagulants who present for emergency surgery or who have bled as a result of anticoagulant therapy may need reversal of the anticoagulant. This can be done with vitamin K in association with either fresh frozen plasma (FFP) or a concentrate of factors II, IX, X and VII.

ARRANGING INTRAOPERATIVE BLOOD COMPONENT SUPPORT

Elective surgery

For most surgical patients, *red cells* are best ordered as plasma reduced cells. Place your request at least 24 hours in advance; this allows the laboratory to establish the recipient's blood group and also to screen serum for the presence of atypical antibodies ('group and save' procedure). If no atypical antibodies are found, the subsequent cross match can be substantially simplified. Many hospitals now operate a 'maximum blood order schedule' (MBOS) (British Committee for Standards in Haematology 1990) which indicates the recommended number of units to be cross matched for the more common surgical procedures. For many procedures (e.g. appendicectomy and uncomplicated or laparoscopic cholecystectomy) analysis of blood usage indicates that blood does not have to be cross matched if a 'group and save' has been electively performed, as compatible blood can be issued, if required, within 10–15 minutes. The operation of a MBOS schedule improves efficiency within the blood bank and can also simplify ordering by junior doctors.

Other blood components should be discussed preoperatively with a clinical haematologist. Elective surgery in patients with thrombocytopenia or congenital and acquired disorders of coagulation should only be undertaken after careful preoperative assessment and transfusion therapy.

Preoperative autologous transfusion

Preoperative donation of 2–4 units of red cells (typically 1 unit per week) for autologous transfusion at or after operation is increasingly practised. Longer term storage of cryopreserved autologous units is reserved for patients with multiple red cell antibodies who are unable to receive standard donor blood. Directed donations from family or friends are not recommended in the UK, primarily because of confidence in the general safety of donor blood and concern that coercion may inhibit voluntary withdrawal of unsuitable donors. Autologous donations may not be given by patients with active infection, unstable angina, aortic stenosis and severe hypertension. A haemoglobin level of >10 g dl⁻¹ is maintained with oral iron supplements, and trials have failed to show a consistent advantage in using recombinant human erythropoietin (rhEPO) to accelerate haemopoiesis. Elective orthopaedic and gynaecological surgery are two areas where up to 20% of patients may be suitable for autologous donation.

A number of issues mitigate against the wider applicability of this procedure:

- Late cancellation of surgery can lead to waste
- Criteria for transfusion of donated units should be identical to those for ordinary units (they should not be used simply because they are available)
- Current UK guidelines (British Committee for Standards in Haematology 1993) stipulate that autologous units be tested for the same range of markers of transmissible disease as homologous donations, which increases costs and leads to ethical dilemmas if positive results are obtained
- Hospitals must operate secure laboratory and clinical protocols to ensure proper identification of autologous units and separation from homologous donation
- The practice is likely to be associated with increased cost, and benefits are difficult to quantify.

Emergency surgery

Patients who are in clinical shock (e.g. due to sepsis or haemorrhage) or actively bleeding require preoperative clinical and laboratory assessment and should be stabilized if possible prior to surgery. The aims in treating acute haemorrhage resulting in acute blood volume depletion are initially to maintain blood pressure, circulating volume and colloid osmotic pressure, and later to restore the haemoglobin level. Appropriate initial therapy is with a synthetic plasma substitute.

Whole blood is an appropriate form of replacement in acute haemorrhage as it will restore plasma volume as well as haemoglobin. It will not correct disordered coagulation or elevate the platelet count, and FFP and/or platelet transfusions may be indicated. Fully compatible blood is unlikely to be available in less than 1 hour. If blood is required sooner you may request group-compatible units (approximately 10 minutes). Non-cross-matched blood (group O, rhesus negative) can be made available in approximately 5 minutes, but always take a pretransfusion sample so that a retrospective cross match can be performed.

BLOOD COMPONENTS

The supply of whole blood and plasma in the UK is based on volunteer, healthy donors. Over 90% of donated blood is separated into its various constituents to allow prescription of individual components and preparation of pooled plasma from which specific blood products are manufactured (Table 9.2). The collection and processing of blood products is organized within the UK by the National Blood Authority (NBA). The hospital laboratory is primarily concerned with issuing appropriate components, compatibility testing and ensuring accurate documentation. These functions of a hospital transfusion laboratory require regulation and monitoring. Most hospitals have standard protocols which are issued to all medical staff and detail the range of components available, together with procedures and indications for their use. The Hospital Transfusion Committee provides a forum whereby clinical laboratory users meet with local transfusion specialists. The responsibilities of such a committee are to organize audit so that activity can be assessed against protocols, and to provide information on use of resources, the appropriateness of such use, and to provide a mechanism whereby the audit loop can be completed (i.e. to amend practice where it can be shown to deviate from protocol, or vice versa). Accurate documentation is of paramount importance, so that the ultimate fate of each component can be traced from donor to recipient.

BLOOD GROUPING AND COMPATIBILITY TESTING

Red cells carry antigens which are typically glycoproteins or glycolipids attached to the red cell membrane.

| Table 9.2 Blood constituents available for clinical use |

Whole blood*

Blood components*	Red cells – plasma reduced
	– leukocyte poor
	– frozen
	– phenotyped
	Platelets
	White cells (buffy coat)
	Fresh frozen plasma
	Cryoprecipitate
Plasma products	Human albumin solution
	Coagulation factor concentrate
	Immunoglobulin
	– specific
	– standard human

*These products are not heat treated, and all may transmit microbial infection.

Antibodies to the ABO antigens are naturally occurring. Antibodies to other red-cell antigens (e.g. rhesus, Kell and Duffy) appear only after sensitization by transfusion or pregnancy and may cause haemolytic transfusion reactions and haemolytic disease of the fetus and newborn.

Naturally occurring antibodies are principally of the immunoglobulin M (IgM) type and are detectable by suspension of cells with diluted antibody at room temperature. They are therefore termed 'complete' antibodies. Immunoglobulin G (IgG) antibodies are termed 'incomplete' as their reactions can only be demonstrated using special techniques (e.g. enzyme treatment of red cells, addition of albumin to reaction mixture, use of antihuman globulin, and microscopical examination for agglutination). Compatibility testing entails suspension of group-compatible red cells from a donor pack with recipient serum, incubation (at room temperature and at 37°C) to allow reactions to occur, and examination for agglutination to ensure that no reaction has occurred. Atypical 'incomplete' (IgG) antibodies in recipient serum will coat incubated donor red cells and their presence is demonstrated by adding antihuman globulin, which leads to agglutination (antihuman globulin or Coomb's test). Many hospitals now use less labour-intensive solid-phase techniques in which reagents are provided already suspended in plastic tubes; donor red cells are added, followed by incubation, centrifugation and non-microscopic examination for reactions.

RED CELL TRANSFUSION

Major indications are haemorrhage, anaemia (once the cause has been established) and bone marrow failure.

Whole blood (1 unit usually contains 450 ml) is available for the treatment of acute haemorrhage with hypovolaemia. Fresh whole blood (<5 days after collection) is preferable for neonates and may have value in patients with haemostatic defects. However, accurate diagnosis of the haemostatic defect and correction by drugs or blood and its components (e.g. FFP or platelets) is preferred. Granulocytes and platelets lose function, many coagulation factors lose activity and aggregates of aged platelets, leukocytes, fibrin strands and cellular debris are formed.

Plasma-reduced red cells are whole blood from which plasma has been removed to allow the use of plasma for the preparation of other blood components. The red cells are usually suspended in optimum additive solution (OAS), e.g. SAG-M (sodium chloride, adenine, glucose and mannitol), to give a total volume of 350 ml. These preparations have a shelf-life of 35 days when stored at 4°C. During storage the concentration of the red cell 2,3-diphosphoglycerate (2,3-DPG) gradually falls, which increases their oxygen affinity and reduces the amount of oxygen they can deliver to tissues. Red cells in OAS are generally considered unsuitable for neonates.

Leukocyte-depleted red cells have been passed through a bedside leukocyte filter to remove contaminating white cells. They are given to patients who are sensitized to HLA, granulocyte and platelet antigens (e.g. multiply transfused patients) who experience febrile reactions during transfusion. Leukocyte depletion reduces the theoretical risk of transmission of viral and prion diseases, and is therefore likely to become widely adopted within the UK (Barbara & Flanagan 1998).

Phenotyped red cells correspond as closely as possible to the red cells of the recipient. *Frozen red cells* are only available from NBA Transfusion Centres, and may be useful in rare patients with multiple antibodies.

PLATELET TRANSFUSIONS

Platelet concentrates are available as pooled platelets (usually equivalent to 5 single units each prepared from 1 unit of whole blood within a few hours of collection) or as platelets collected using a cell separator. The standard adult dose is one pooled donation which contains approximately 25×10^{10} platelets in 150–200 ml of fresh plasma and, when stored at room temperature in a platelet agitator, has a shelf-life of 4–6 days. Group compatible (but not cross matched) units are given.

Indications

Indications for platelet transfusion are:

1. Thrombocytopenia ($<50 \times 10^9$ 1^{-1}) in the presence of significant bleeding or prior to an invasive procedure. The count should be raised to 100×10^9 1^{-1} prior to surgery on critical areas (e.g. the eyes). Such transfusions are only rarely required if platelet destruction is antibody mediated.

2. Prophylactic transfusions in patients after chemotherapy or with failure of marrow production. In clinically stable patients with no fever or coagulopathy the count can safely be allowed to fall to 10×10^9 1^{-1}.

3. Others, including platelet function defects (in the presence of bleeding or prior to surgery), DIC, dilutional thrombocytopenia following massive transfusion and following cardiopulmonary bypass (CPB) surgery (see below).

White cell transfusions are now rarely used as there are few data demonstrating clinical efficacy.

FRESH FROZEN PLASMA (FFP)

FFP is prepared by centrifugation of donor whole blood within 6 hours of collection and frozen at $-30°C$. It may be stored for up to 12 months and is thawed prior to administration. It has a volume of approximately 200 ml. It is a source of all coagulation and other plasma proteins. Compatibility testing is not required, but group-compatible units are used. FFP from group AB donors may be used if the recipient blood group is unknown. Although 2–4 units are usually administered, the volume and frequency of administration should be assessed separately for each patient. FFP is not heat sterilized and the possibility of viral transmission must be borne in mind. Virus inactivated plasma (VIP) from pooled and single donations is currently under evaluation.

Indications

Indications for FFP transfusion are:

1. Coagulation factor replacement: coagulation tests and a platelet count must be performed prior to use. Patients with disseminated intravascular coagulation (DIC), who have undergone massive transfusion or CPB, who are at risk of bleeding or have coagulation abnormalities may benefit.

2. Liver disease: in the presence of bleeding or prior to invasive procedures, together with vitamin K.

3. Haemolytic uraemic syndrome (HUS) or thrombotic thrombocytopenic purpura (TTP): FFP replacement, often in conjunction with plasma exchange, is indicated. Cryoprecipitate-poor FFP is also available and is useful in this setting.

4. Reversal of oral anticoagulation or thrombolytic therapy.

Cryoprecipitate is prepared from FFP, is rich in fibrinogen, fibronectin and factor VIII, is stored at $-30°C$ for up to 12 months and thawed prior to infusion. Its low volume makes it useful in patients with DIC following massive transfusion, and occasionally in liver or renal disease.

PLASMA PRODUCTS

The following products are derived from pooled human plasma, but have undergone a manufacturing process designed to concentrate the component and to sterilize it, thus markedly reducing the risk of viral infection.

There is, however, a theoretical risk that they could transmit prion proteins which are implicated as a transmissible cause of new variant Creutzfeld–Jakob disease (nv CJD) (Flanagan & Barbara 1996). They are increasingly produced from plasma sourced from countries which do not have clusters of cases of nv CJD.

Albumin solution

This is available as 5%, 20% and 20% salt-poor formulations in a variety of dose units. It does not contain coagulation factors. Indications for 5% albumin are replacement of plasma proteins and expansion of plasma volume, as in hypoproteinaemia following burns (after the first 24 hours) and as a part of the replacement fluid in large-volume plasma exchange. Albumin solutions may play a role in restoration of circulatory volume in haemorrhage, shock and multiple organ failure, but the view that administration of colloid and crystalloid solutions is preferable (it is certainly cheaper) is gaining popularity. The indications for 20% albumin are: replacement of plasma proteins in severe hypoproteinaemia in renal or liver disease, after large-volume paracentesis, following massive liver resection and in some cases of Gram-negative septicaemia.

Coagulation factor concentrates

For patients with congenital bleeding disorders, recombinant factor VIII and factor IX are now widely used. Concentrates are also manufactured from pooled fractionated human plasma. They are available as freeze-dried powder which is reconstituted prior to use.

Prothrombin complex concentrate contains factors IX, X and II and is used for treatment of bleeding complications in inherited deficiencies of these factors. Given with vitamin K, it is also used in treatment of oral anticoagulant overdose, and in severe liver failure. Its use carries a risk of provoking thrombosis and DIC. Other concentrates include the naturally occurring anticoagulant factors protein C and antithrombin (see below), and factors VII, XI and XIII; they are used in the corresponding congenital deficiencies.

Immunoglobulins

These are prepared from pooled donor plasma by fractionation and sterile filtration. Specific immunoglobulins include hepatitis B and herpes zoster and can provide passive immune protection. Standard human immunoglobulin for intramuscular injection is used for prophylaxis against hepatitis A, rubella and measles, whereas hyperimmune globulin is prepared from donors with high titres of the relevant antibodies for prophylaxis of tetanus, hepatitis A, diphtheria, rabies, mumps, measles, rubella, cytomegalovirus and *Pseudomonas* infections. Intravenous immunoglobulin is used as replacement therapy in patients with congenital or acquired immune deficiency and in autoimmune disorders (e.g. idiopathic thrombocytopenic purpura).

PLASMA SUBSTITUTES

These include products based on hydroxyethyl starch (HES), dextran (a branch-chained polysaccharide composed of glucose units) and modified gelatin. Such components remain in the circulation longer than crystalloid solutions (up to 6 hours for modified gelatin and up to 24 hours for some high molecular weight starch-based products). Other advantages are that they are relatively non-toxic, inexpensive, can be stored at room temperature, do not require compatibility testing and do not transmit infection. Adverse effects include anaphylaxis, fever and rash, such effects being more frequent with starch-based products. Dextran can also impair coagulation and platelet function and can interfere with compatibility testing, so that samples for this must be taken prior to therapy. The maximum dose of synthetic plasma expanders is approximately 20–30 ml kg^{-1}. Patients receiving larger volumes or with significant evidence of other organ failure (e.g. pulmonary or renal disease, or a bleeding diathesis) may be given albumin.

ADVERSE CONSEQUENCES OF BLOOD TRANSFUSION

In general, transfusion of blood and blood products is a safe and effective mode of treatment. Avoid administrative and clerical errors by rigorous adherence to procedures for checking, and rigorous documentation when ordering, prescribing, issuing and administering blood and blood components.

The safe administration of blood components is a deceptively complex process involving phlebotomists, clerical staff, junior doctors, porters, nurses as well as transfusion laboratory staff (Williamson et al 1996). A recent survey in the UK (McClelland & Phillips 1994) suggests that a 'wrong blood in patient' incident occurs approximately once per 30 000 units of red cells transfused. By far the commonest cause is a failure at the bedside of pre-transfusion identity checking procedures, either at the time of phlebotomy or while setting up the actual transfusion.

> Pay rigorous attention to all administrative and clerical aspects of blood component therapy; they are overwhelmingly the commonest cause of fatal errors.

IMMUNE COMPLICATIONS

ABO-incompatible red cell transfusions will lead to life-threatening intravascular haemolysis of transfused cells, manifesting as fever, rigors, haemoglobinuria, hypotension and renal failure (immediate haemolytic transfusion reaction (HTR)). In the anaesthetized patient, persistent hypotension and unexplained oozing from the wound may be the only signs.

Atypical antibodies arising from previous transfusions or pregnancy may cause intravascular haemolysis, but more commonly lead to extravascular haemolysis in liver and spleen and may be delayed for 1–3 weeks (delayed HTR). Typical manifestations are jaundice, progressive anaemia, fever, arthralgia and myalgia. Diagnosis is easily established by a positive direct antiglobulin test (DAT) and a positive antibody screen. Non-haemolytic febrile transfusion reaction (NHFTR) usually occurs within hours of transfusion in multi-transfused patients with antibodies against HLA antigens or granulocyte-specific antibodies. The reaction is due to pyrogens, released from granulocytes damaged by complement in an antigen–antibody reaction. It presents as a rise in temperature with flushing, palpitations and tachycardia, followed by headache and rigors. Hypersensitivity reactions to plasma components may cause urticaria, wheezing, facial oedema and pyrexia, but can cause anaphylactic shock (e.g. in patients with congenital IgA deficiency who have anti-IgA antibodies following previous sensitization).

Treatment

Stop the transfusion immediately in all cases except for the appearance of a mild pyrexia in a multiply transfused patient. Check clerical details and send samples from the donor unit and recipient for analysis for compatibility and haemolysis. Recipient serum is analysed for the presence of atypical red cell, leukocyte, HLA and plasma protein antibodies. Treat severe haemolytic transfusion reactions with support care to maintain blood pressure and renal function, to promote diuresis and treat shock. Intravenous steroids and antihistamines may be needed, with the use of adrenaline in severe cases. Management of NHFTR consists of administration of antipyretics (e.g. paracetamol) and, for severe symptoms, 100 mg of hydrocortisone intravenously can also be given. Prevent NHFTR by administering blood filtered through one of the specific leukocyte-depletion filters (e.g. Sepacell R-500 and Pall RC-100).

TRANSMISSION OF INFECTION

Blood transfusion is an important mode of transmission of a range of protozoal, bacterial and viral infections. There is also a theoretical risk of transmitting infections mediated by prion proteins such as new variant CJD (Barbara & Flanagan 1998, Flanagan & Barbara 1996), though no proven or even probable instances of such transmissions have ever been identified. It should be emphasized that the safety of blood components and plasma fractionated products has improved greatly in recent years. Bacterial infections can occur through failure of sterile technique at the time of collection or due to bacteraemia in the donor (especially if organisms such as *Yersinia*, which can survive at 4°C, are incriminated). Donors at risk of malaria are not eligible to donate. Transmission of syphilis is now very rare.

Viral infection

Transmission of viruses may occur in spite of mandatory screening because: serological tests may not have had time to become positive in a potentially infectious individual; the virus may not have been identified; or the most sensitive serological tests may not be routinely performed. The risk of transmission is much lower, although still present, for those blood products which have undergone a manufacturing and sterilization process.

Viruses that are transmissible by blood transfusion are:

- *Plasma-borne viruses*
  - Hepatitis B and its variants
  - Hepatitis A (rarely)
  - Hepatitis C
  - Hepatitis G
  - Other unidentified hepatitis viruses
  - HIV-1 and HIV-2 (also cellular)
  - Parvovirus
- *Cell-associated viruses*
  - Cytomegalovirus
  - Epstein–Barr virus
  - HTLV-I and HTLV-II.

Hepatitis B vaccine should be given to hepatitis B virus negative recipients of pooled plasma products or repeated red cell transfusion.

> The perceived risk of viral transmission is high: the actual risk in the UK is very low – less than 1 in 2.5 million for HIV and 1 in 200 000 for hepatitis C (Williamson et al 1996).

OTHER COMPLICATIONS

There is increasing evidence that transfusion of blood components can cause immunosuppression in the recipient. This may lead to earlier relapse or recurrence of malignant disease after surgical removal of malignant tumours (shortened disease-free interval) as well as an increased incidence of postoperative infection. These effects are probably due to defective cell-mediated immunity and are reduced by the use of leukocyte-depleted components. Circulatory overload may result from the infusion of large volumes in patients with incipient heart failure. Iron overload occurs in patients who have received repeated red cell transfusions and these patients require iron chelation therapy. Graft-versus-host disease may be caused by transfusion of T-lymphocytes into severely immunosuppressed hosts, and cellular components should be irradiated prior to transfusion to severely immunodeficient patients.

INTRAOPERATIVE ASSESSMENT

Rapid bleeding confined to one site is usually due to a surgical problem. Suspect haemostatic failure in a high-risk patient with multiple sites of bleeding or an unusual bleeding pattern and confirm it by appropriate laboratory tests. The following tests are useful in assessing the degree of blood loss and should serve as a guide for determining need for replacement therapy:

- *Oxygen-carrying capacity of blood*
  - Haemoglobin concentration
  - Pulse oximetry
- *Haemostatic function*
  - Coagulation screen:
    prothrombin time (PT)
    activated partial thromboplastin time (APTT)
    thrombin time (TT)
    platelet count
  - Thromboelastography.

Quantification of intraoperative blood loss is imprecise. Clinical evaluation must be accompanied by laboratory tests (Table 9.3) and many of the latter cannot be performed outside the main laboratory. Thromboelastography is a useful and rapid test whereby a graphical recording is produced of in vitro blood clot formation and dissolution, and provides a global test of coagulation and fibrinolysis which can be performed rapidly within the operating suite in high-risk patients.

Intraoperative autologous transfusion

Normovolaemic haemodilution involves removal of 1–2 units of whole blood during induction of anaesthesia, with replacement by crystalloid, reducing the haematocrit to 25–30%. Surgery is usually well tolerated, the collected blood can be returned later during the operation, and there is no need to undertake virological testing of the unit (Williamson 1994).

Salvage of blood lost during an operation (British Committee for Standards in Haematology 1997) is accomplished using a simple device (e.g. Solcotrans) or a cell saver (e.g. Haemonetics Cell Saver IV). Blood shed into the thoracic or abdominal cavity is aspirated and mixed with anticoagulant. It can then be returned to the patient (Solcotrans) or the red cells can be washed, suspended in saline and transfused to the patient (Haemonetics Cell Saver IV). The use of a cell saver may considerably reduce the number of units required for transfusion. Contraindications for the use of the blood-salvage procedure is exposure of blood to a site of infection or the possibility of contamination with malignant cells.

Methods of reducing intraoperative blood loss

Meticulous surgical technique clearly plays a major role, but there is increasing interest in the use of pharmacological agents to improve haemostasis. Desmopressin (DDAVP) improves platelet function by increasing plasma concentrations of von Willebrand factor, but has not been convincingly shown to reduce blood loss in cardiac surgery. Aprotinin is a serine protease inhibitor which inhibits fibrinolysis and has been shown to reduce blood loss and operative morbidity in cardiac surgery (particularly in repeat procedures) and major hepatic surgery (e.g. liver transplantation) (Hunt 1991).

SPECIAL SITUATIONS

Massive blood transfusion

This is defined as transfusion of a volume of blood greater than the recipient's blood volume in less than

Table 9.3 Results of laboratory tests as an aid in differential diagnosis of excessive bleeding

Cause of bleeding	Laboratory test				
	PT	APTT	TT without protamine	TT with protamine	Platelet count
Loss of platelets	N	N	N	N	↓↓
Lack of coagulation factors	↑↑	↑↑	N	N	N or ↓
Excess of heparin	↑	↑↑	↑	N	N or ↓
Hyperfibrinolysis	↑	↑	↑↑	↑↑	N or ↓
DIC	↑↑	↑↑	↑↑	↑↑	↓↓
Massive blood transfusion	↑	↑	N	N	↓
Vitamin K deficiency	↑↑	↑	N	N	N

Key: N, normal; ↑↑, markedly raised; ↑, mildly raised; ↓↓, markedly decreased; ↓, mildly decreased.

24 hours. Blood-group-specific, compatible whole blood or red cell preparations can be transfused, usually using an in-line microaggregate filter. A pressure infusor or a pump and blood warmer will provide more rapid administration. FFP and platelet concentrates (from the same blood group as the red cells) may also be required.

Complications include:

1. Cardiac abnormalities (ventricular extrasystoles, ventricular fibrillation (rarely) and cardiac arrest) due to the combined effect of low temperature, high potassium concentration and excess citrate with low calcium concentration. They can be prevented by using a blood warmer and a slower rate of transfusion, particularly in patients with hepatic or renal failure. Routine administration of calcium gluconate is unnecessary and may even be dangerous unless the ionized calcium concentration in the plasma can be monitored.

2. Acidosis in the patient with severe renal or liver disease may be aggravated by the low pH of stored blood.

3. Failure of haemostasis manifests as local oozing and, infrequently, as a generalized bleeding tendency due to the lack of coagulation factors and platelets in stored blood. Laboratory assessment is essential (see above). FFP (1–2 units) corrects the abnormalities of coagulation and should be given prophylactically after every 10 units of blood. Platelet transfusion may be required when the platelet count is lower than 50×10^9 l^{-1}, particularly if the patient is bleeding.

4. Adult respiratory distress syndrome (ARDS), also called non-cardiogenic pulmonary oedema, occurs in severely ill patients after major trauma and/or surgery. Clinical features include progressive respiratory distress, decreased lung compliance, acute hypoxaemia and diffuse radiographic opacification of the lungs. The mortality is high; post-mortem studies show widespread macroscopic and microscopic thrombosis in the pulmonary arteries. Local disseminated intravascular coagulation, microvascular fluid leakage and embolization of leukocyte aggregates and microaggregates from stored blood all contribute to pathogenesis. Management consists of stopping the transfusion, administering corticosteroids and providing supportive treatment to combat pulmonary oedema and hypoxia by using oxygen and positive-pressure ventilation.

Transfusion in open heart surgery

This requires cardiopulmonary bypass (CPB) for maintaining the circulation with oxygenated blood. In adults blood is not required for priming of the heart–lung machine, but it is needed in neonates and small children. Usually 4 units of blood (ideally less than 5 days old) are initially cross matched (6–8 units for repeat procedures). The use of albumin solutions either for priming the heart–lung machine or postoperatively is unnecessary.

Bleeding associated with CPB is due to activation and loss of platelets and coagulation factors in the extracorporeal circulation, failure of heparin neutralization by the first dose of protamine, activation of fibrinolysis in the oxygenator and pump, and/or disseminated intravascular coagulation in patients with poor cardiac output and long perfusion times. Management requires: administration of 1–2 pools of platelet concentrate when the platelet count is less than 30×10^9 l^{-1}; transfusion of 2–4 units of fresh frozen plasma to correct the loss of coagulation factors; neutralization of excess heparin by protamine (1 mg of protamine neutralizes approximately 100 IU of heparin); administration of tranexamic acid (or a similar antifibrinolytic agent) when hyperfibrinolysis is confirmed by laboratory testing; treatment of disseminated intravascular coagulation, in the first instance by correcting the underlying cause (e.g. poor perfusion, oligaemic shock, acidosis or infection) and then by transfusion of FFP and platelet concentrate, as required.

Prostatic surgery

This may be followed by excessive urinary bleeding due to local fibrinolysis related to the release of high concentrations of urokinase. Antifibrinolytic agents, which include ε-aminocaproic acid (EACA) and tranexamic acid are often helpful in reducing clot dissolution, but should be used cautiously as fibrinolytic inhibition can lead to ureteric obstruction in patients with upper urinary tract bleeding.

Liver disease

This warrants special mention as the liver is an important site of manufacture of the components as well as the regulatory factors of the coagulation and fibrinolytic pathways (Mehta and McIntyre 1998). Vitamin K is required for hepatic synthesis of the coagulation factors II, VII, IX and X as well as the coagulation inhibitors proteins C and S. Impaired vitamin K absorption can occur in biliary obstruction and patients should receive 10 mg vitamin K by intramuscular injection preoperatively. The liver is also the site of manufacture of factor V and fibrinogen (factor 1), the regulatory factors antithrombin and α_2-antiplasmin, and defects of both platelet function and number (e.g. thrombocytopenia due to complicating hypersplenism) can occur. These patients are at increased risk of DIC and renal failure, and require assessment by a gastroenterologist as well as a haematologist.

POSTOPERATIVE ASSESSMENT

Anaemia, coagulopathy and excessive bleeding in the immediate postoperative period are often due to the operation or its complications. Blood component therapy commenced intraoperatively for the management of special situations (see above) must be continued postoperatively.

Patients with excessive bleeding and clinical evidence of haemostatic failure require laboratory assessment (Table 9.3). The trauma of surgery triggers both the coagulation and fibrinolytic pathways and places patients at increased risk of DIC. Do not routinely use red cell transfusions to correct postoperative anaemia (e.g. to maintain the haemoglobin concentration arbitrarily greater than 10 g dl^{-1}) as this practice has not been shown to improve wound healing or aid surgical recovery. Thromboprophylaxis is an important aspect of postoperative care (see Ch. 36).

FUTURE DIRECTIONS

The field of transfusion medicine is rapidly developing and there is increasing awareness of the risks of homologous blood. The advent of recombinant DNA technology has already led to use of recombinant erythropoietin, but granulocyte and granulocyte–monocyte colony stimulating factors are in routine use to elevate the white cell count in leukopenic patients. Recombinant thrombopoietin is now available and will revolutionize platelet transfusion therapy. Synthetic oxygen carriers ('artificial blood') have been under development for many years (Ogden 1995). Perfluorocarbons dissolve oxygen but function only in high concentrations of ambient oxygen and are only useful for short-term perfusion in the intensive care unit setting (e.g. following coronary angioplasty). Recombinant haemoglobin solutions and liposomal haemoglobin are under active development.

Summary

1. Pre-operative haematological assessment is essential to identify any inherited or acquired factors (anaemia, haemoglobinopathy, excessive tendency to bleed) which may affect outcome of surgery and anaesthesia.

Summary (contd.)

2. A range of blood components and plasma products are available for intra- and postoperative use. There are specific indications for, and risks associated with their use.
3. Pre-deposit and intraoperative autologous transfusion are increasingly used.
4. The perceived risks of transmission of infection are greater than the actual risks, and dwarfed by the risks of failure to comply rigorously with administrative and clerical procedures.
5. You should always seek the advice of the clinical and scientific staff of the haematology department when planning the perioperative care of patients with inherited or acquired haematological conditions and in special situations (e.g. massive transfusion).
6. You should be aware of written policies and procedures in your institution which govern the ordering, prescription, administration and documentation of blood components and plasma product therapy.

References

Barbara J, Flanagan P 1998 Blood transfusion risk: protecting against the unknown. British Medical Journal 316: 717–718

British Committee for Standards in Haematology 1990 Guidelines for implementation of a maximum surgical blood order schedule. Clinical and Laboratory Haematology 12: 321–327

British Committee for Standards in Haematology, Blood Transfusion Task Force 1993 Guidelines for autologous transfusion: 1: Pre-operative autologous donation. Transfusion Medicine 3: 307–316

British Committee for Standards in Haematology, Blood Transfusion Task Force 1997 Guidelines for autologous transfusion: II: Perioperative haemodilution and cell salvage. British Journal of Anaesthesia 78: 768–771

Flanagan P, Barbara J 1996 Prior disease and blood transfusion. Transfusion Medicine 6: 213–215

Hunt B J 1991 Modifying perioperative blood loss. Blood Reviews 5: 168–176

McClelland DBL, Phillips P 1994 Errors in blood transfusion in Britain: survey of hospital haematology departments. British Medical Journal 308: 1205–1206

Mehta A B 1994 Glucose-6-phosphate dehydrogenase deficiency. Prescribers Journal 34: 178–182

Mehta A B, McIntyre N 1998 Haematological changes in liver disease. Trends in Experimental and Clinical Medicine 8: 8–25

Ogden J E, MacDonald S L 1995 Haemoglobin-based red cell substitutes: current status. Vox Sanguines 69: 302–308

Vichinsky E P, Haberkern C M, Neumayr L et al 1995 A comparison of conservative and aggressive transfusion regimens in the perioperative management of sickle cell disease. New England Journal of Medicine 333: 206–213

Williamson L 1994 Homologous blood transfusion: the risks and alternatives. British Journal of Haematology 88: 451–458

Williamson L M, Heptonstall J, Soldan K 1996 A SHOT in the arm for safer blood transfusion. British Medical Journal 313: 1221–1222

Further reading

American Association of Blood Banks 1993 Blood transfusion therapy: a physician's handbook, 4th edn. AABB, Virginia

Contreras M (ed) 1990 ABC of transfusion. British Medical Journal, London

McClelland DBL (ed) 1989 Handbook of transfusion medicine. HMSO, London

McClelland DBL (ed) 1995 Clinical resources and audit group: optimal use of donor blood. Scottish Office, Edinburgh.

10

Fluid, electrolyte and acid–base balance

W. Aveling, C. Hamilton-Davies

> ### Objectives
>
> Understand:
> - **The physiology of fluid distribution throughout the body.**
> - **Methods of detecting hypovolaemia.**
> - **Managing fluid balance.**
> - **Principles of acid–base balance.**
> - **Interpretation of arterial blood gas results.**

INTRODUCTION

To be able to manage the surgical patient optimally it is essential that all tissues are perfused with oxygenated blood throughout the course of the operation and the postoperative recovery period. To do this well it is necessary to understand the basics of fluid balance in the healthy person and then be able to apply this knowledge, along with that of basic physiology, to the surgical patient. Understanding the results provided by both arterial blood gas analysis and modern monitoring systems, including their limitations, will help us to achieve optimal tissue perfusion. This has been shown to result in reduced morbidity and length of hospital stay.

FLUID COMPARTMENTS

Every medical student knows that man is mostly water. For the surgeon the key to fluid and electrolyte balance is a knowledge of the various fluid compartments. An adult male is 60% water; a female, having more fat, is 55% water; newborn infants are 75% water. The most important compartments are the intracellular fluid (ICF) – 55% of body water – and the extracellular fluid (ECF) – 45%. ECF is further subdivided into the plasma (part of the intravascular space), the interstitial fluid, the transcellular water (e.g. fluid in the

gastrointestinal tract, the cerebrospinal fluid (CSF) and aqueous humour) and water associated with bone and dense connective tissue which is less readily exchangeable and of much less importance. The partitioning of the total body water (TBW) with average values for a 70 kg male, who would contain 42 litres of water, is shown in Figure 10.1 (Edelman & Leibman 1959).

To understand fluid balance one needs to know from which compartment or compartments fluid is being lost in various situations, and in which compartments fluids will end up when administered to the patient. For practical purposes we need only consider the plasma, the interstitial space, the intracellular space and the barriers between them.

The capillary membrane

The barrier between the plasma and interstitium is the capillary endothelium, which allows the free passage of water and electrolytes (small particles) but restricts the passage of larger molecules such as proteins (the colloids). Although no one has demonstrated holes in the membrane, capillaries behave as if they had pores of 4–5 nm in most tissues. Kidney and liver have larger pores, and brain capillaries are relatively impermeable. The osmotic pressure generated by the presence of colloids on one side of a membrane which is impermeable to them is known as the colloid osmotic pressure (COP). Only a small quantity of albumin (mol. wt. 69 000) crosses the membrane and it is mainly responsible for the difference in COP between the plasma and the interstitium. The COP is normally about 25 mmHg and tends to draw fluid into the capillary, while the hydrostatic pressure difference between capillary and interstitium tends to push fluid out. This balance was first described by Starling (1896).

Staverman (1952) introduced the concept that different molecules will be 'reflected' to a different extent by the membrane. This term, the reflection coefficient, varies between zero (all molecules passing through the

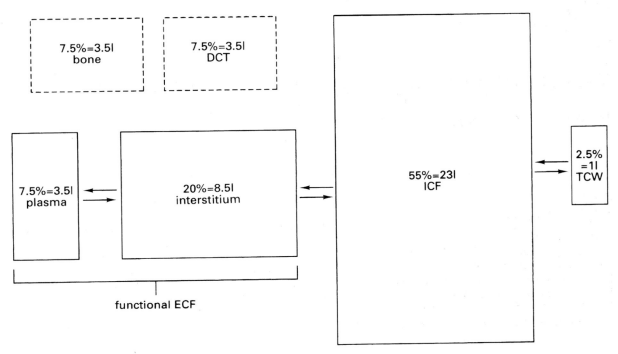

Fig 10.1 Distribution of total body water in a 70 kg man. ECF, extracellular fluid; ICF, intracellular fluid; DCT, dense connective tissue; TCW, transcellular water.

membrane) and +1 (all molecules reflected). In disease states when the capillary membrane becomes leaky the reflection coefficient will fall. Flow across the membrane is represented by the equation:

$$V = K_f S[P_c - P_{IF}] - \sigma (\pi p - \pi_{IF})]$$

where V is the rate of movement of water, K_f is the capillary filtration coefficient, S is the surface area; P_c and P_{IF} are the capillary and interstitial hydrostatic pressures, πp and π_{IF} are the plasma and interstitial oncotic pressures, and σ is the reflection coefficient.

The cell membrane

The barrier between the extracellular and intracellular space is the cell membrane. This is freely permeable to water but not to sodium ions, which are actively pumped out of cells. Sodium is therefore mainly an extracellular cation, while potassium is the main intracellular cation. Water will move across the cell membrane in either direction if there is any difference in osmolality between the two sides. Osmolality expresses the osmotic pressure across a selectively permeable membrane and depends on the number of particles in the solution, not their size. Normal osmolality of ECF is 280–295 mOsm kg^{-1}. Since each cation is balanced by an anion, an estimate of plasma or ECF osmolality can be obtained from the formula:*

$$\text{Osmolality (mOsm kg}^{-1}) = 2 (Na^+ + K^+) + \text{Glucose} + \text{Urea (mmol l}^{-1})$$

Note that the colloids contribute very little to total osmolality as the number of particles is small, although, as we saw above, they play an important role in fluid movement across the capillaries.

Movement of water between compartments

Consider what happens when a patient takes in water, either by drinking or in the form of a 5% glucose infusion, the glucose in which is soon metabolized. It will rapidly distribute throughout the ECF with a resultant fall in ECF osmolality. Since osmolality must be the same inside and outside cells, water will move from ECF to ICF until the osmolalities are the same. Thus 1 litre of water or 5% glucose given to a patient will distribute itself throughout the body water. In spite of

---

*Osmolality is expressed per kilogram of solvent (usually water), whereas osmolarity is expressed per litre of solution. The presence of significant amounts of protein in the solution, as in plasma, means that the osmolality and osmolarity will not be the same.

being infused into the intravascular compartment (3.5 litres) it will be distributed throughout the body water space (42 litres) of which only 3.5/42, approximately 7.5%, is intravascular. For this reason approximately 13 litres of 5% glucose will need to be infused to increase the plasma volume by 1 litre. By a converse argument we can see that someone marooned on a life raft with no water will lose water from all compartments.

Normal saline (0.9%) contains Na^+ and Cl^- at concentrations of 150 mmol l^{-1}. If this is infused into a patient it will stay in the ECF because the water tends to follow the sodium ion and osmolality matches that inside the cells, thus there is no net movement of water into the cells. Thus a volume of normal saline given intravascularly will tend to distribute throughout the extracellular space. The extracellular fluid makes up approximately 45% of the body water with the plasma volume being approximately 7.5%, and therefore 1/6 will remain intravascular and 6 litres will need to be given to increase the plasma volume by 1 litre. Equally, a patient losing electrolytes and water together, as in severe diarrhoea, loses the fluid from the ECF and not the ICF.

Finally, consider the infusion of colloid solutions (e.g. albumin, starch solutions and gelatins). The capillary membrane is impermeable to colloid and thus the solution stays in the plasma compartment (there are, of course, circumstances in which it can leak out). A burned patient losing plasma loses it from the vascular compartment and initially there is no shift of fluid from the interstitial space. As blood pressure falls, hydrostatic pressure in the capillary falls, and if colloid osmotic pressure is maintained the Starling forces will draw water and electrolytes into the vascular compartment from the interstitium. Because there are only 3.5 litres of plasma, losses from this compartment lead to hypoperfusion and reduced oxygen transport to tissues and are potentially life-threatening. The use of hypertonic saline as a resuscitation fluid has become topical lately with reports of improved survival (Mattox et al 1991), the mechanism being the transfer of water into the intravascular space in the short term, leading to better tissue perfusion.

Since the plasma is part of the ECF, any loss of ECF results in a corresponding decrease in circulating volume and is potentially much more serious than loss of an equivalent volume from the total body water. For example, compare a man losing 1 litre a day of water because he is marooned on a life raft with a man losing 1 litre a day of water and electrolytes due to a bowel obstruction. The man on the life raft will lose 7 litres in a week from his total of 42 litres body water, i.e. a 17% loss. The plasma volume will fall by 17%, which is sur-

vivable. The man with a bowel obstruction, on the other hand, loses his 7 litres from the functional ECF of 12 litres, i.e. a 58% loss. Losing more than half of the plasma volume is not compatible with life.

NORMAL WATER AND ELECTROLYTE BALANCE

We take in water as food and drink and also make about 350 ml per day as a result of the oxidization of carbohydrates to water and carbon dioxide, known as the metabolic water. This has to balance the output. Water is lost through the skin and from the lungs; these insensible losses amount to about 1 litre a day. Urine and faeces account for the rest. A typical balance is shown in Table 10.1.

The precise water requirements of a particular patient depend on size, age and temperature. Surface area (1.5 l H_2O/m^2 daily) is the most accurate guide, but it is more practical to use weight, giving adults 30–40 ml kg^{-1}. Children require relatively more water than adults, as set out in Table 10.2. Requirements for the first 10 kg should be added to the requirements for the next 10 kg and likewise added to subsequent weight. Therefore, for a 25 kg child the basal requirements per hour should be $(10 \times 4) + (10 \times 2) + (5 \times 1) = 65$ ml h^{-1}.

Table 10.1 Average daily water balance for a sedentary adult in temperate conditions

Input (ml)		Output (ml)	
Drink	1500	Urine	1500
Food	750	Faeces	100
Metabolic	350	Lungs	400
		Skin	600
Total	2600	Total	2600

Table 10.2 Daily water requirements by body weight in children

Weight (kg)	Water requirements
0–10	4 ml kg^{-1} h^{-1}
10–20	40 ml h^{-1} + 2 ml kg^{-1} h^{-1} for each kg >10 kg
>20	60 ml h^{-1} + 1 ml kg^{-1} h^{-1} for each kg >20 kg

The average requirements of sodium and potassium are 1 mmol kg^{-1} day^{-1} of each. Humans are very efficient at conserving sodium and can tolerate much lower sodium intakes, but they are less good at conserving potassium. There is an obligatory loss of potassium in urine and faeces and patients who are not given potassium will become hypokalaemic. As potassium is mainly an intracellular cation there may be a considerable fall in total body potassium before the plasma potassium falls.

PRESCRIBING FLUID REGIMENS

In prescribing fluid regimens for patients, we need to consider three things:

- Basal requirements
- Continuing abnormal losses over and above basal requirements
- Pre-existing dehydration and electrolyte loss.

Intraoperative fluid balance needs special consideration, as all three of the above apply. Normally nourished patients who are nil by mouth for a few days during surgery do not in general need feeding intravenously, although some work has shown early feeding to lead to better postoperative recovery. Only in special circumstances is intravenous feeding required; this topic is outside the scope of this chapter.

Basal requirements

We have seen above the daily requirements of water and electrolytes. If we look now at the various crystalloid solutions that are available (Table 10.3), we can design fluid regimens for basal requirements. Normal saline, Hartmann's, 5% dextrose and dextrose saline are the most commonly used. Note that their osmolalities are similar to that of ECF, i.e. they are isotonic with plasma. The purpose of the glucose is to make the solution isotonic, not to provide calories, although a small amount of glucose does have a protein sparing effect during the catabolism that follows major surgery and trauma. Our standard 70 kg patient can be provided with the 24-hour basal requirements of 30–40 ml kg^{-1} of

Table 10.3 Content of crystalloid solutions

Name	Known as	Na^+	Cl^-	K^+ (mmol l^{-1})	HCO_3^-	Ca^{2+}	Calculated (mOsm l^{-1})
Sodium chloride 0.9%	Normal saline .	150	150				300
Sodium chloride 0.9%, potassium chloride 0.3%	Normal saline + KCl	150	190	40			380
Sodium chloride 0.9%, potassium chloride 0.15%	Normal saline + KCl	150	170	20			340
Ringer's lactate	Hartmann's	131	111	5	29 (as lactate)		280
Glucose 5%	5% dextrose						280
Glucose 5%, potassium chloride 0.3%	5% dextrose + KCl			40	40		360
Glucose 5%, potassium chloride 0.15%	5% dextrose + KCl			20	20		320
Glucose 4%, sodium chloride 0.18%	Dextrose saline	30	30				286
Glucose 4%, sodium chloride 0.18%, potassium chloride 0.3%	Dextrose saline + KCl	30	70	40			366
Glucose 4%, sodium chloride 0.18%, potassium chloride 0.15%	Dextrose saline + KCl	30	50	20			326
Sodium chloride 0.45%	Half normal saline	75	75				150
Sodium chloride 1.8%	Twice normal saline	300	300				600
Sodium bicarbonate 8.4%	–	1000			1000		2000
Sodium bicarbonate 1.4%	–	167			167		334

water and 1 mmol kg^{-1} of sodium in any of the ways shown in Table 10.4.

Potassium

None of these regimens supply significant amounts of potassium. Potassium chloride can be added to the bags and is supplied as ampoules of 20 mmol in 10 ml or 1 g (=13.5 mmol) in 5 ml. Bags of crystalloid are available with potassium already added and this is safer than adding ampoules. It cannot be stressed enough that potassium can be very dangerous because hyperkalaemia causes cardiac arrhythmias and asystole. It should never be injected as a bolus. There have been a number of tragedies reported to the medical defence societies in which potassium chloride ampoules were mistaken for sodium chloride and used as 'flush', with fatal consequences. Hyperkalaemia may also occur if potassium supplements are given to anuric patients. For this reason, you should usually wait until you are certain of reasonable urine output before adding potassium to the regimen postoperatively. Safe rules for giving potassium are:

- Urine output at least 40 ml h^{-1}
- Not more than 40 mmol added to 1 litre
- No faster than 40 mmol h^{-1}.

Continuing loss

Patients with continuing losses above the basal requirements need extra fluid. The commonest example in anaesthetic and surgical practice is the patient with bowel obstruction. Fluid can be aspirated by a nasogastric tube to assess both volume and electrolyte content. Saline with added potassium should be given to replace it. Dextrose saline is not an appropriate fluid for this purpose because it only contains Na 30 mmol l^{-1}, and 5% glucose is even worse. Hyponatraemia will result if these solutions are used to replace bowel loss.

Table 10.4 Basal water and sodium regimens for a 70-kg patient on intravenous fluids

Solution	Volume (ml)	Na$^+$ (mmol)	K$^+$ (mmol)
5% glucose	2000	–	
0.9% saline	500	75	
5% glucose	2000	–	–
Hartmann's	500	65.5	2.5
4% glucose	2500	75	–
0.18% saline			

To keep track of the fluids, a fluid balance chart should be kept. This records all fluid in (oral and intravenous) and all fluid out (urine, drainage, vomit, etc.). Every 24 hours these are totalled, an allowance is made for insensible losses and the balance, positive or negative, is recorded. Any patient on intravenous fluids should have a daily balance, daily electrolyte measurements and a new regimen prescribed every day. The instruction 'and repeat' should never be used in fluid management and has led to disasters in the past.

Correction of pre-existing dehydration

Patients who arrive in a dehydrated state clearly need to be resuscitated with fluid over and above their basal requirements. Usually this will be done intravenously. The problems are:

- To identify which compartment or compartments the fluid has been lost from
- To assess the extent of the dehydration.

The fluid used to resuscitate the patient should be similar in composition and volume to that which has been lost. From what we know about the movement of fluid between compartments (see above) and the patient's history, we can usually decide where the losses are coming from. As we have seen, bowel losses come from the ECF, while pure water losses are from the total body water. Protein-containing fluid is lost from the plasma and there may sometimes be a combination of all three types of loss.

Assessment of deficit

> Occult untreated intraoperative hypovolaemia may lead to organ failure and death long after the operative period.

In estimating the extent of the losses, the patient's history, clinical examination, measurement and laboratory tests all play a part. A dehydrated patient may be thirsty, have dry mucous membranes, sunken eyes (and in infants fontanelles) and cheeks, loss of skin elasticity and weight loss. They will feel weak and, in severe cases, will be mentally confused. The cardiovascular system responds with tachycardia and peripheral vasoconstriction, so that the patient feels cold. Prior to the fall in blood pressure seen in continuing haemorrhage, there is evidence that other organs (e.g. gut), can suffer from occult hypoperfusion. A recent study by Hamilton-Davies et al (1997) showed that in progressive haemorrhage, gastrointestinal tonometry demonstrated gut mucosal hypoperfusion greatly in advance of blood pressure, heart rate or arterial blood gas changes. Next follow decreases in stroke volume, which up until this point have been maintained by a decrease in the capacitance of the vascular system. Cardiac output falls, causing a compensatory rise in heart rate and, eventually, a fall in blood pressure. At this point the protective autoregulation of blood flow to the brain, heart and kidneys may fail and clouding of consciousness and oliguria are signs of severe dehydration. Weight, pulse, blood pressure and urine output are essential and simple measurements in the assessment and treatment of fluid loss, although these may be misleading as sympathetic drive from the nervous system may maintain blood pressure until very late.

Venous pressure. Equally important is the measurement of central venous pressure (CVP). An intravenous catheter is inserted into a central vein. The tip should lie within the thorax, usually in the superior vena cava. In this position, blood can be aspirated freely and there is a swing in pressure with respiration. The pressure is usually measured by an electronic transducer but can be done quite simply by connecting the patient to an open-ended column of fluid and measuring the height above zero with a ruler.

The zero point for measuring CVP is the fifth rib in the mid-axillary line with the patient supine (this corresponds to the position of the left atrium). The normal range for CVP is 3–8 cmH$_2$O (1 mmHg = 1.36 cmH$_2$O). A low reading, particularly a negative value, confirms dehydration, but the converse is not true. A high or normal CVP does not mean an adequately filled vascular system. For example a patient on a noradrenaline infusion or with a high intrinsic sympathetic tone may have a high CVP in spite of a low-volume, high-resistance vascular system. CVP measurements are of more use as a guide to the adequacy of treatment. The response of the CVP to a fluid challenge of 200 ml colloid tells you more about the state of the circulation than a single reading. A dehydrated patient's CVP will rise in response to the challenge but then fall to the original value as the circulation vasodilates to accommodate the fluid. If the response to the challenge is a sustained rise (5 minutes after the challenge) of 2–4 cmH$_2$O, this indicates a well-filled patient. If the CVP rises by greater than 4 cmH$_2$O and does not fall again, this indicates overfilling or a failing myocardium.

The CVP reflects the function of the right ventricle which usually parallels left ventricular function. In cardiac disease, either primary or secondary to systemic illness, there may be disparity between the function of the two ventricles. The left ventricular function can be assessed by the use of a balloon-tipped catheter (Swan–Ganz) in a branch of the pulmonary artery. When the balloon is blown up to occlude the vessel, the pressure measured distally gives a good guide to the left atrial pressure. This is called the pulmonary capillary wedge pressure (PCWP) and is normally 5–12 mmHg. In certain circumstances the CVP may be high when the PCWP is low, which then indicates that although the right atrium may be well filled, the filling state of the systemic circulation is low. Here, as with the fluid challenge of the CVP, management of the filling status of the patient should be by means of fluid challenging the PCWP. Similar changes in level apply.

Key points

- **Elderly patients have poor cardiovascular system compliance**
- **Consider frequent small volume fluid challenges**
- **Left ventricular failure does not equate to hypervolaemia**

Work performed by Shoemaker et al (1988) demonstrated that the Swan–Ganz catheter could be used to treat patients to oxygen delivery/consumption goals when undergoing high-risk surgery. They found that those who achieved goals of:

- Oxygen delivery* > 600 ml min^{-1} m^{-2}
- Oxygen consumption† > 170 ml min^{-1} m^{-2}
- Cardiac index > 4.5 l min^{-1} m^{-2}

demonstrated an improved outcome. However, one argument is that these patients are self-selecting and that they would have had a good outcome anyway as they are able to achieve these goals thus demonstrating better cardiovascular function.

Boyd et al (1993) also demonstrated an improvement in outcome in patients treated with dopexamine to achieve these goals, but again the same arguments apply. It has been shown that if critically ill patients are subjected to a similar style of management by driving their cardiovascular systems to achieve these goals with inotropes, then this group fare worse than a control group (Hayes et al 1994).

In summary, it would seem to be a reasonable form of management to attempt to achieve delivery/consumption goals in the cardiovascularly fit subject undergoing high-risk surgery. However, in patients with

---

*Oxygen delivery = Cardiac output × Hb × Arterial saturation × 1.34.
†Oxygen consumption = Cardiac output × Hb × (Arterial – Mixed venous saturations) × 1.34.

cardiovascular disease these goals should probably be sought only with the use of fluid and agents that offload the left ventricle, such as glyceryl trinitrate, thus reducing myocardial work. This should be performed under Swan–Ganz monitoring of cardiac function or the more recent non-invasive Doppler cardiac output monitor.

For those patients in whom these goals are non-attainable, attention should be turned to ensuring an otherwise meticulous perioperative course.

One other recent measure of occult hypovolaemia has been the measurement of gut intramucosal pH (pHi). This has been demonstrated to be the area that first suffers during haemorrhagic blood loss (Price et al 1966) and thus possibly the first to develop an acidosis due to anaerobic metabolism. Assessment can be made of this by means of a saline-filled balloon passed into the gut lumen which equilibrates with the CO_2 generated in the gut mucosa. From this, intramucosal pH can be derived. This value again has been related to outcome following high-risk surgery (Mythen et al 1993) and studies are currently being devised to investigate the effects of resuscitating patients to a pHi end-point. The technology has recently been extended to an automated air-filled balloon in combination with an end-tidal CO_2 monitor (Tonocap©), thus eliminating user bias due to sampling technique differences. Current trials with this device are ongoing.

Quantification of plasma and ECF loss

If plasma is lost from the circulation, the plasma remaining still has the same albumin concentration, although the volume is diminished. Since no red cells are lost they become concentrated, resulting in a rise in haematocrit. Plasma is, of course, part of the ECF, so that losses of fluid and electrolytes without protein loss will cause a rise in haematocrit but also a rise in plasma protein concentration (Fig. 10.2). Changes in plasma albumin and haematocrit thus provide a good guide to ECF losses, while only haematocrit is of use in monitoring plasma loss (Robarts et al 1979).

In ECF depletion, the total amount of albumin stays the same although its concentration goes up. If Pr_1 is the initial albumin concentration and Pr_2 is the concentration after dehydration, it can be shown that:

$$\% \text{ Fall in ECF volume} = \left(1 - \frac{Pr_1}{Pr_2}\right) \times 100$$

For example, if the albumin rises from 35 to 45 g l^{-1}

$$\% \text{ Fall in ECF volume} = \left(1 - \frac{35}{45}\right) \times 100 = 22\%$$

By a similar argument one can calculate the fall in plasma volume as follows:

$$\% \text{ Fall in plasma volume} = 100 \left[1 - \left(\frac{Hct_1}{100 - Hct_1} \times \frac{100 - Hct_2}{Hct_2}\right)\right]$$

For example, if the haematocrit (Hct) rises from 40% to 50%:

$$\% \text{ Fall in plasma volume} = 100 \left[1 - \left(\frac{40}{60} \times \frac{50}{50}\right)\right] = 33\%$$

Haematocrit and plasma albumin are thus very useful in the assessment of ECF and plasma losses; much more so than the sodium which, though being lost, does not change in concentration.

A practical application of this from the paper by Robarts et al (1979) is shown in Figures 10.3 and 10.4. Figure 10.3 shows the results in a patient with acute pancreatitis. The plasma volume has fallen 30% (as determined by a rise in haematocrit), but the rest of the ECF volume is unchanged as there was no change in plasma protein concentration. After giving 1.5 litres of plasma, the plasma volume has been restored. By contrast, Figure 10.4 illustrates a patient who had lost ECF through the bowel; both the haematocrit and the plasma protein estimations show a 25% fall in plasma, and hence ECF, volume. As saline is administered, the values return to normal. Table 10.5 summarizes the changes in volume and composition of various compartments in (1) isotonic fluid loss, (2) loss of water in excess of electrolytes, and (3) loss of sodium in excess of water. The corresponding expansion of compartments is also shown. It is a useful exercise to work through the various boxes predicting what change, if any, will occur. In the case of water loss (from both ECF and ICF) remember that the red cells are part of the ICF, so when water is lost from both compartments the haematocrit may not change. Similarly, when there is hypotonic expansion, red cells increase in volume as part of the ICF and with the simultaneous expansion of ECF there may again be no change in haematocrit.

Water and electrolyte replacement

Having assessed the amount of deficit, as discussed above, we come to the question of what to give to restore the situation. A look at the composition of various body fluids (Table 10.6) shows us that ECF losses of water and electrolytes should be replaced with either normal saline or Ringer's lactate with added potassium (see Basal requirements, p. 115). The only hypotonic secretions are saliva and sweat. The sodium content of sweat varies and responds to aldosterone. Gastric secretion, though having a sodium content of only 50 mmol l^{-1}, is isotonic with ECF because of the hydrogen it contains. Where the losses are primarily of

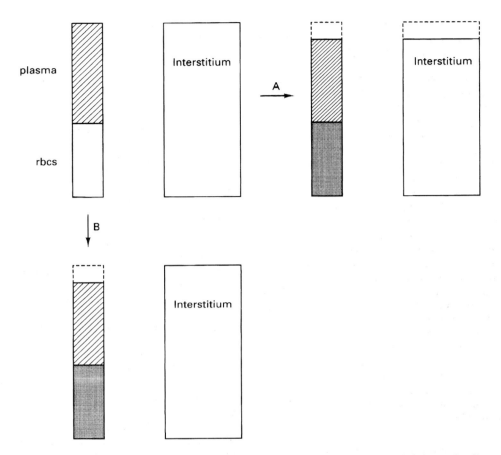

Fig 10.2 **A** Loss of ECF leading to a rise in albumin concentration and haematocrit. **B** Loss of plasma leading to a rise in haematocrit but no change in albumin concentration.

gastric secretion, e.g. pyloric stenosis, one might think it necessary to supply hydrogen ions. In fact, the kidney compensates by retaining hydrogen and excreting sodium and bicarbonate, so that the net effect is a loss of sodium and chloride. Normal saline with potassium should therefore be used in rehydration.

Plasma replacement and plasma substitutes

When we need to replace lost plasma there is a choice between giving plasma prepared from donated blood or one of the synthetic plasma substitutes. Human plasma protein fraction (HPPF) or human albumin solution (HAS) is prepared by separating red cells from donated blood. A bottle contains plasma from several donors and has been pasteurized to prevent the transmission of disease (e.g. hepatitis or human immunodeficiency virus (HIV)). It contains 4.5% albumin, has no clotting factors and is stable at room temperature. The main

disadvantage is its cost (£40 in the UK, 1991), which reflects its limited availability. A number of solutions containing molecules large enough to stay within the capillaries and generate colloid osmotic pressure are available as plasma substitutes (Table 10.7).

Dextrans. The dextrans are glucose polymers available in preparations of different molecular weights. There is a large range of molecular weights in the solution. Dextran 70 is so called because the average molecular weight is supposed to be 70 000. In fact, the number-average molecular weight, which is much more relevant to the colloid osmotic pressure, is 38 000 (see footnote to Table 10.7) (Webb et al 1989). Dextran 40 has smaller molecules and can be nephrotoxic. Dextran 110 has larger molecules. Neither of these will be considered further. Dextran 70 is quite a good plasma substitute, but its use has declined in popularity because of its adverse effects on coagulation and cross-matching and the relatively high incidence of allergic reactions.

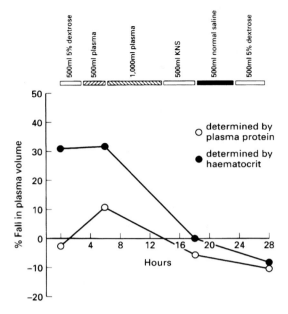

Fig 10.3 Changes in plasma volume as determined by changes in plasma protein and haematocrit, during treatment of acute pancreatitis (see text).

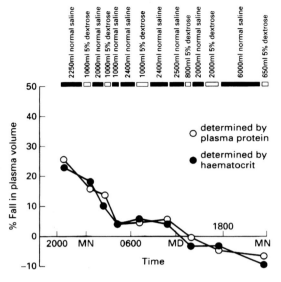

Fig 10.4 Changes in plasma volume as determined by changes in plasma protein and haematocrit during treatment of bowel obstruction (see text).

Table 10.5 Changes resulting from three kinds of expansion and contraction of body fluids

Acute change	Example	Change in ECF vol	Change in ICF vol	Change in [Na]	Change in [Hct]	Change in [protein]
Loss H_2O + NaCl	Cholera	↓	→	→	↑	↑
Loss H_2O > Na	Excess sweating	↓	↓	↑	→	↑
Loss Na > H_2O	Addison's	↓	↑	↓	↑	↑
Isotonic expansion	Saline infusion	↑	→	→	↓	↓
Hypertonic expansion	2 × normal saline	↑	↓	↑	↓	↓
Hypotonic expansion	5% glucose infusion	↑	↑	↓	→	↓

Table 10.6 Electrolyte content and daily volume of body secretions

	Na	K (mmol l⁻¹)	Cl	Volume (litres daily)
Saliva	15	19	40	1.5
Stomach	50	15	140	2.5
Bile, pancreas, small bowel	130–145	5–12	70–100	4.2
Insensible sweat	12	10	12	0.6
Sensible sweat	50	10	50	Variable

Table 10.7 Characteristics of colloid solutions

Name	Brand name	No. average* mol. wt.	Mol. wt. range	Na⁺ K⁺ Ca²⁺ (mmol l⁻¹)	$t_{1/2}$ in plasm	Adverse reactions (%)		Effect on coagulation	Cost (UK 1998)
						Mild	Severe		
Human plasma protein fraction	HPPF	69 000	69 000	150 5 2	20 days	0.02	0.004	None	£40
Dextran 70 in saline 0.9% or glucose 5%	Macrodex Lomodex 70 Gentran 70	38 000	<10 000→250 000	150	12 h	0.7	0.02	Inhibit platelet aggregation Factor VIII↓ Interfere with cross-match	£4.78
Polygeline (degraded gelatin)	Haemaccel	24 500	<5 000→50 000	145 5 6.25	2.5 h	0.12	0.04	None	£3.71
Succinylated gelatin	Gelofusin	22 600	<10 000→140 000	154 0.4 0.4	4 h	0.12	0.04	None	£4.63
Hydroxyethyl starch 6% in saline (Hetastarch)	Hespan	70 000	<10 000→10⁶	154	25 h	0.09	0.006	>1.5 g kg⁻¹ day⁻¹ can cause coagulopathy	£16.25

*Number-average molecular weight should not be confused with weight-average molecular weight, which is usually quoted by the manufacturers. No average molecular weight is more appropriate.

Gelatins. Gelatin solutions are prepared by the hydrolysis of bovine collagen. They have the advantage over dextrans of not affecting coagulation and having a low incidence of allergic reactions. Being of smaller average particle size they stay in the intravascular space for a shorter time. Haemaccel contains potassium and calcium ions, which can cause coagulation if mixed with citrated blood in a giving set. Haemaccel stays a shorter time in the circulation, 30% of the molecules being dispersed to the interstitial tissues in 30 minutes. Gelofusin is probably preferable from this point of view.

Hetastarch. In the last few years, 6% hetastarch in saline has become available. It has the largest average molecular weight of any of the plasma substitutes and therefore stays in the circulation longer. The dose should be limited to 1500 ml/70 kg; more can cause coagulation problems. About 30% of a dose is taken up by the reticuloendothelial system without apparent detriment to its function. Smaller molecules (mol. wt. <50 000 Da) are filtered by the kidneys. Larger ones are broken down by plasma amylase until small enough for real excretion.

Electrolyte balanced colloid solutions (e.g. Hextend®) represent a new area of fluid development and it is possible that these solutions offer increased benefit over currently used colloids due to provision of a more favourable physiological milieu.

Choice of solution for plasma expansion. The intravascular space can be expanded by the use of crystalloid solutions, e.g. saline, but because the fluid spreads throughout the ECF, 6 litres of crystalloid are needed to expand the plasma by 1 litre. In an emergency, crystalloid is useful. All the battle casualties in the Falklands War were resuscitated in the field with Hartmann's solution.

Five per cent glucose should not be used from choice as it is distributed throughout both ECF and ICF compartments; thus 13 litres are needed to increase the intravascular space by 1 litre. For most patients with acute hypovolaemia, the best combination of advantages at low cost is offered by succinylated gelatin (Gelofusin). Being relatively short acting it is particularly useful as a holding measure until blood becomes available.

In continuing hypovolaemia, hetastarch gives more prolonged expansion and its larger molecules are better retained in the circulation when the capillaries are leaky, e.g. in septicaemic shock.

Blood loss and blood transfusion

So far we have talked about plasma loss and plasma expansion. Most of what has been said about the assessment and replacement of plasma volume applies to blood loss. Transfusion of donated blood is possible in most circumstances, but has several disadvantages to be weighed against the fact that only haemoglobin carries oxygen. With a haemoglobin of 14 g dl⁻¹, evolution has equipped us with spare capacity as far as oxygen-carrying capacity is concerned. Indeed, as haematocrit falls, the decrease in oxygen carrying is compensated by better tissue perfusion due to reduced blood viscosity. It has been shown that the best balance between oxygen carrying and viscosity occurs around a haematocrit of 30%. It is also suspected that blood transfusion at the time of surgery for certain cancers leads to immunological suppression and poorer long-term survival. On the other hand, blood transfusion prior to transplant procedures improves graft survival. Since the AIDS scare, and with a lack of knowledge of mechanisms of prion transfer relating to bovine sclerosing encephalitis (BSE), there is greater reluctance on the part of the public to accept blood transfusion. For all these reasons, as well as the hazards of blood transfusion listed in Box 10.1, the expense of blood and rarity of some blood groups, one is reluctant to transfuse blood. In practical terms, operative blood loss up to 500 ml can be replaced with saline, remembering that six times as much will be needed (see above), or plasma substitutes. Only if more than 1 litre of blood has been lost in a healthy adult should one consider giving blood.

Rather than supply whole blood, it is more efficient for the transfusion service to separate it into components as listed in Box 10.2. Blood cross-matched for patients undergoing surgery usually comes as plasma-

---

Box 10.1   The hazards of blood transfusion

Any transfusion

- Transmission of disease, e.g. AIDS, malaria (donor blood screened for HIV, hepatitis, syphilis)
- Bacterial contamination
- Pyrogenic reactions (antibodies to white cells)
- Incompatibility reactions
- ± Haemolysis (clerical error commonest cause)

Massive transfusion

- Hypothermia
- Hyperkalaemia
- Citrate toxicity
- Acidosis
- Microaggregate embolism, 'shock lung'
- Dilution and consumption of clotting factors

Box 10.2 Blood products

- Plasma-reduced blood (packed cells)
- Washed red cells: if transfusion reaction a problem
- Plasma protein fraction (HPPF)
- Fresh frozen plasma (FFP): contains clotting factors more dilute than the concentrates below
- Cryoprecipitate: rich in factor VIII
- Factor VIII concentrate: even richer in VIII
- Factors II, VII, IX and X concentrate
- Factor XI concentrate
- Fibrinogen
- Platelet concentrate

reduced blood ('packed cells'). This is more viscous than whole blood and needs to be given with appropriate amounts of crystalloid or colloid solution to restore the volume.

The quantity of blood lost is assessed clinically as outlined above, and at operation by watching the suction bottle and weighing swabs, but this generally underestimates the loss. In operations such as transurethral resection of prostate, measurement of haemoglobin in the irrigating fluid gives an accurate measure of blood loss. In acute blood loss, haematocrit and haemoglobin concentrations do not change until the blood remaining in the patient has been diluted by shift of fluid from the interstitial space or intravenous infusion. Plasma-reduced blood and whole blood more than 1 day old (which it almost always is) contain no viable platelets and a few clotting factors. The same applies to plasma protein fraction. In massive transfusion both dilution and consumption of clotting factors make it necessary to send blood for a clotting screen and give platelets and fresh frozen plasma (FFP) according to the results. As a rule, one gives a unit of FFP for every 4–6 units of stored blood transfused.

As stored blood is generally collected into citrate containing bags it is important to remember that exogenous calcium may be required after massive blood transfusion, to ensure both adequate haemostasis and a normal vascular response to inotropes.

Intraoperative fluid balance

During an operation, everything we have discussed so far may be going on at the same time. The patient is starved for 6–12 hours, there may be blood loss, plasma loss, ECF loss and evaporation of water from exposed bowel. As part of the stress response to surgery the patient retains water and sodium. The importance of careful monitoring in major surgery will be obvious; this includes accurate assessment of blood loss, haemodynamic variables and urine output.

As a rule of thumb, in intra-abdominal surgery Hartmann's solution 5 ml kg^{-1} h^{-1} may be given up to 2 litres. This will compensate for starvation, ECF loss, evaporation and some blood loss. Blood or colloids may have to be given in addition. If the patient is being treated in an attempt to achieve oxygen delivery/consumption goals, then continually fluid challenging the CVP in cardiovascularly healthy patients, or the PCWP in those with cardiac dysfunction, should be performed to maintain an optimal haemodynamic state.

For the first 36 hours postoperatively there is water retention, and there is sodium retention lasting 3–5 days. Obligatory potassium loss of 50–100 mmol per day continues. If additional sodium is given it is simply retained, although the urine may show an increase in sodium output. Provided that intraoperative losses have been replaced by the end of the operation, one should give the basal requirements (30–40 ml kg^{-1} day^{-1} H$_2$O + 1 mmol kg^{-1} day^{-1} Na$^+$ and K$^+$) plus additional blood or colloid if there is significant wound drainage. Remember not to start potassium until urine output is established; the operation of inadvertent bilateral ureteric ligation is not unknown.

ACID–BASE BALANCE

Claude Bernard was the first to recognize that to function effectively the body needs a stable *milieu interieur*. The hydrogen ion concentration is the most important contribution to this. An acid is a hydrogen ion (proton) donor and a base accepts hydrogen ions. Throughout life the body produces hydrogen ions and they must be excreted or buffered to keep the internal environment constant.

Terminology and definitions

Hydrogen ion activity

Hydrogen ion activity is traditionally expressed in pH units, pH being the negative log$_{10}$ of the hydrogen ion concentration:

$$pH = -\log [H^+] = \log \frac{1}{[H^+]}$$

Hydrogen ion concentration can also be expressed directly in nanomoles per litre (Table 10.8). Note that the pH is a log scale, so that each 0.3 unit fall in pH represents a doubling of hydrogen ion concentration.

Table 10.8 Conversion table for pH units and hydrogen ion concentration

pH unit	H^+ (nmol l^{-1})
8.00	10
7.70	20
7.44	36
7.40	40
7.36	44
7.10	80
7.00	100

Acidosis and alkalosis

The normal ECF pH is 7.36–7.44 (44–36 nmol l^{-1}). Acidaemia is a blood pH below this range and alkalaemia a pH above it. Acidosis is a condition that leads to acidaemia, or would do if no compensation occurred, but the terms 'acidosis' and 'acidaemia' are often used loosely to mean the same thing, which is not strictly correct. Alkalosis and alkalaemia are defined in a similar way.

Respiratory acidosis. A fall in pH resulting from a rise in the $P\text{CO}_2$ is a respiratory acidosis, e.g. opiate overdose leading to hypoventilation causes a rise in $P\text{CO}_2$.

Respiratory alkalosis. This is a rise in pH due to a lowering of the $P\text{CO}_2$, such as occurs in hyperventilation.

Metabolic acidosis. This is a fall in pH due to anything other than carbon dioxide (sometimes referred to as non-respiratory acidosis). There is a primary gain of acid or loss of bicarbonate from ECF.

Metabolic alkalosis. This is a rise in pH from non-respiratory causes. There is either a gain in bicarbonate or a loss of acid from the ECF.

Compensatory changes. If the initial problem is respiratory, the result is called a *primary respiratory acidosis* or alkalosis. If the respiratory problem persists for more than a few hours the kidney will excrete or retain bicarbonate to try and compensate for the respiratory disturbance. This is referred to as *secondary* or *compensatory metabolic acidosis* or alkalosis.

Thus a primary respiratory acidosis may be accompanied by a secondary metabolic alkalosis. For example, chronic obstructive airways disease leads to a rise in the $P\text{CO}_2$: primary respiratory acidosis. To compensate for this the kidney retains bicarbonate, leading to a rise in ECF bicarbonate: secondary or compensatory metabolic alkalosis.

In the same way primary respiratory alkalosis (e.g. the hyperventilation that occurs at high altitude) will be compensated by a secondary metabolic acidosis. Where the first disturbance is metabolic, e.g. the build-up of acid in diabetic ketoacidosis, the primary metabolic acidosis will cause hyperventilation (secondary respiratory alkalosis), which will tend to restore the pH to normal. This respiratory compensation for a metabolic change happens much more rapidly than the metabolic compensation for a respiratory problem.

The fourth possible combination of changes is to have a metabolic alkalosis (e.g. loss of H^+ ions in pyloric stenosis) compensated by a respiratory acidosis. However, hypoventilation (respiratory acidosis) leads to a fall in $P\text{O}_2$, which stimulates ventilation so that in practice compensatory respiratory acidosis is not usually seen.

In deciding which is the primary and which is the secondary change it is important to realize that the compensatory changes do not bring the pH back to normal; they bring it back *towards* the normal range. In other words, even after compensation the measured pH is altered in the direction of the primary problem (acidosis or alkalosis). Compensatory mechanisms merely make the disturbance in pH less than it otherwise would have been. It is also important to consider the history. Examiners may give candidates blood gas results to interpret, but in real life blood gases come from patients. Knowing that a patient is an unconscious diabetic breathing spontaneously, rather than an anaesthetized patient on a ventilator, certainly helps one's interpretation.

Buffers

Buffers are substances which by their presence in solution minimize the change in pH for a given addition of acid or alkali. Three-quarters of the buffering power of the body is within the cells; the rest is in the ECF. Proteins, haemoglobin, phosphates and the bicarbonate system are all important buffers. The particular importance of the bicarbonate system is that carbon dioxide is excreted in the lungs and can be regulated by changes in ventilation. Bicarbonate excretion in the kidney can also be regulated. The lungs are responsible for the excretion of 16 000 mmol per day of acid and the kidneys for only 40–80 mmol per day. The formation of carbonic acid from carbon dioxide and water is catalysed by carbonic anhydrase (present in red cells). The reaction may go in either direction:

$$H^+ + HCO_3^- \Leftrightarrow H_2CO_3 \Leftrightarrow H_2O + CO_2$$

The Henderson–Hasselbalch equation is derived from this and expresses the relationship between the bicarbonate concentration, the carbon dioxide and the pH:

$$pH = pK + \log \frac{[HCO_3]}{[H_2CO_3]}$$

The carbonic acid can be expressed in terms of carbon dioxide, so that a more useful form of the equation is:

$$pH = pK + \log \frac{[HCO_3]}{0.03\ P_{CO_2}}$$

As this is a buffer system which minimizes changes in pH, we can see that if the carbon dioxide rises so will the bicarbonate, to keep $[HCO_3]/P_{CO_2}$ constant. Similarly a fall in bicarbonate will be accompanied by a fall in P_{CO_2} to prevent a change in pH.

Interpretation of acid–base changes

As the patient's acid–base status varies, three things are changing at once: pH, $[HCO_3^-]$ and P_{CO_2}. Blood gas machines measure P_{O_2}, pH and P_{CO_2} directly. The actual bicarbonate $[HCO_3^-]$ is calculated from the Henderson–Hasselbalch equation. Blood gas machines also derive other variables which help in the interpretation of the acid–base status. These are as follows:

Standard bicarbonate (SBC)

This is the concentration of bicarbonate in the plasma of fully oxygenated blood at 37°C at a P_{CO_2} of 5.3 kPa (40 mmHg). In other words, it tells you what the bicarbonate would be if there was no respiratory disturbance. Looking at the standard bicarbonate therefore tells you what is going on on the metabolic side. Normal standard bicarbonate is 22–26 mmol l^{-1}. Values above this indicate metabolic alkalosis and those below, metabolic acidosis.

Base excess (BE)

This is the amount of strong base or acid that would need to be added to whole blood to titrate the pH back to 7.4 at a P_{CO_2} of 5.3 kPa and 37°C. It tells you the same thing as standard bicarbonate, namely the metabolic status of the patient. Normal base excess is obviously zero (±2 mmol l^{-1}). Positive base excess occurs in metabolic alkalosis, and negative base excess (sometimes called base deficit) indicates metabolic acidosis. The base excess is an in vitro determination in whole blood. It is also known as the actual base excess (ABE) or the base excess (blood) (BE b).

Standard base excess (SBE)

This is an estimate of the in vivo base excess and takes into account the difference in buffering capacity between the patient's ECF and the blood that was put in the blood gas machine. Interstitial fluid, having less protein and no haemoglobin, has a lower buffering capacity than blood. SBE is therefore 1–2 mmol l^{-1} greater than BE, but this makes very little difference in practice. SBE is sometimes called base excess (e.c.f.).

Total carbon dioxide (Tco_2)

This is the total concentration of carbon dioxide in the plasma as bicarbonate and dissolved carbon dioxide.

$$T_{CO_2} = [HCO_3^-] + (P_{CO_2} \times \text{Solubility})$$

Oxygen saturation (O$_2$ sat.)

The percentage saturation of haemoglobin by oxygen is derived from the haemoglobin oxygen dissociation curve and the measured P_{O_2}. The normal value is >95%. This value should not be relied upon to be accurate, as other forms of haemoglobin such as carboxyhaemoglobin will be included as oxyhaemoglobin. If this is suspected (e.g. in burns patients) then a co-oximeter should be used to determine the level of oxyhaemoglobin.

PO$_2$ and inspired oxygen (F$_I$O$_2$)

To interpret the P_{O_2} one needs to know the age of the patient and the F_IO_2. Normal arterial P_{O_2} declines with age. Roughly speaking $P_{O_2} = 100 - $ age in years/3 mmHg or $13.3 - 0.044 \times$ Age kPa.

The expected alveolar P_{O_2} (P_AO_2) can be predicted from the inspired oxygen by the simplified alveolar gas equation: $P_AO_2 = P_IO_2 - P_ACO_2/R$, where R is the respiratory exchange ratio (normally 0.8). In dry gas P_IO_2 (in kPa) = Fractional inspired oxygen (F_IO_2)%. Alveolar gas is saturated with water vapour (6.3 kPa), for which allowance must be made. If the $F_IO_2 = 40\%$ and the $P_{CO_2} = 5.3$:

$$P_AO_2 = \left(40 - \frac{40 \times 6.3}{100}\right) - \frac{5.3}{0.8} = 30.85 \text{ kPa}$$

As an approximate rule of thumb one can deduct 10 from the F_IO_2% to give the expected P_AO_2 in kPa (e.g. if $F_IO_2 = 50\%$ then P_AO_2 is approximately 40 kPa). The difference between the estimated P_AO_2 and the measured arterial P_{O_2} is called the (A–a) P_{O_2} gradient. It is normally 0.5–3 kPa.

Without considering the inspired oxygen it is not possible to comment sensibly on the observed P_AO_2. A rough calculation of the (A–a) P_{O_2} gradient should be made when commenting on blood gas results. Some machines even calculate this for you as well!

A blood gas machine usually prints out the variables shown in Table 10.9. There is often a haemoglobin

Table 10.9 Printout from a blood gas machine with normal values

Temp	37°C
pH	7.36–7.44 (44–36 nmol l⁻¹)
$P\text{CO}_2$	4.6–5.6 kPa (35–42 mmHg)
$P\text{O}_2$	10.0–13.3 kPa (75–100 mmHg)
HCO_3^-	22–26 mmol l⁻¹
$T\text{CO}_2$	24–28 mmol l⁻¹
SBC	22–26 mmol l⁻¹
BE	–2 to +2 mmol l⁻¹
SBE	–3 to +3 mmol l⁻¹
O_2 sat.	>95%
Hb	11.5–16.5 g dl⁻¹

measurement and the temperature of measurement (37°C) is quoted.

Temperature correction

The blood gas machine operates at 37°C. Because gases are more soluble in liquid at lower temperatures (as drinkers of cold lager will know) the blood gases would be different if measured at another temperature. Blood gas machines are programmed to correct the gases if you tell the machine the patient's actual temperature. However, there has been much debate as to whether it is appropriate to correct for temperature. Suffice it to say that the protagonists of not correcting for temperature (the alpha stat theory) hold sway and one should probably act on the blood gases as measured at 37°C and not the temperature-corrected values.

The anion gap

For electrochemical neutrality of the ECF the number of anions must equal the number of cations. The main cations are sodium and potassium and the main anions are chloride, bicarbonate, proteins, phosphates, sulphates and organic acids.

Normally, only Na^+, K^+, HCO_3^- and Cl^- are measured in the laboratory. Thus, when we add the normal values for these they do not balance:

Cations		Anions	
Na^+	140	Cl^-	105
K^+	5	HCO_3^-	25
Total	145	Total	130

The difference is known as the *anion gap* and represents the other anions not usually measured. Anion gap = $(Na^+ + K^+) - (HCO_3^- + Cl^-) = 11$–$19$ mmol l⁻¹. Its signif-

icance is that in certain metabolic acidoses (e.g. ketoacidosis or lactic acidosis) the anion gap will be increased by the presence of organic anions. However, in metabolic acidosis in which chloride replaces bicarbonate (e.g. bicarbonate loss due to diarrhoea), the anion gap will be normal.

Plan for interpreting blood gases

1. Check for internal consistency. Remember that the machine only measures pH, $P\text{CO}_2$ and $P\text{O}_2$. If it measures any of these wrongly, which is not infrequent, the derived variables will be wildly abnormal too. If the results do not fit with the clinical picture, suspect the machine. Example: a patient on a ventilator in theatre with an end-tidal carbon dioxide of 5% has the following gases:

$P\text{O}_2$	13.0
pH	7.64
$P\text{CO}_2$	5.1
HCO_3^-	37.5
$T\text{CO}_2$	38.5
SBC	39.0
BE	+15
SBE	+16
O_2 sat.	99%

It is much more likely that the pH has been measured wrongly than that the patient has a gross metabolic alkalosis.

2. Look at the pH. Remember the pH change is always in the direction of the primary problem acidosis or alkalosis.

3. Look at the $P\text{CO}_2$. Abnormality of the $P\text{CO}_2$ indicates the respiratory component.

4. Look at the base excess or standard bicarbonate. Both give the same information, i.e. the metabolic acid–base status after correcting for the $P\text{CO}_2$.

5. Calculate the anion gap.

6. Look at the $P\text{O}_2$ and calculate the A–a gradient.

Examples of abnormal blood gases

pH	7.51	The alkalaemia is due to primary
$P\text{CO}_2$	3.7	respiratory alkalosis (low $P\text{CO}_2$).
$P\text{O}_2$	29	There is no metabolic
HCO_3^-	22.1	compensation (normal base
$T\text{CO}_2$	23.6	excess). The $P\text{O}_2$ would be
SBC	25	expected if breathing 40%
BE	+1.1	oxygen $P_1\text{O}_2 - 10 = (40 - 10) =$
SBE	+2	30. The patient is
O_2 sat.	100%	hyperventilating.
($F_1\text{O}_2$ 40%)		

pH	7.28	A respiratory acidosis with high
P_{CO_2}	7.33	P_{CO_2} due to hypoventilation.
P_{O_2}	9.21	Again no metabolic
HCO_3^-	25.2	compensation (normal SBC and
T_{CO_2}	28.4	BE). Low P_{O_2} due to
SBC	22.3	hypoventilation.
BE	−1.9	
SBE	−2.5	
O_2 sat.	91%	
(F_IO_2 air)		

pH	7.35	Again a respiratory acidosis
P_{CO_2}	9.33	(high P_{CO_2}) but this time
P_{O_2}	7.11	compensated by metabolic
HCO_3^-	39.1	alkalosis (high SBC and positive
T_{CO_2}	41.2	base excess). This is typical of
SBC	32.4	chronic obstructive airways
BE	+8.2	disease with renal
SBE	+9.1	compensation.
O_2 sat.	85%	
(F_IO_2 air)		

pH	7.21	The acidaemia (low pH) is
P_{CO_2}	4.0	primarily due to a metabolic
P_{O_2}	13.3	acidosis (low SBC, base excess
HCO_3^-	11.5	−15). Compensatory
T_{CO_2}	12.8	respiratory alkalosis (low P_{CO_2}),
SBC	9.3	does not return the pH to
BE	−15.2	normal. P_{O_2} normal.
SBE	−16.4	
O_2 sat.	99%	
(F_IO_2 air)		

pH	7.36	The pH is in the normal range
P_{CO_2}	4.21	despite low P_{CO_2} (respiratory
P_{O_2}	10.49	alkalosis) and low standard
HCO_3^-	17.6	bicarbonate (metabolic
T_{CO_2}	18.5	acidosis). The important thing
SBC	17.8	here is the P_{O_2}. It is apparently
BE	−6.2	in the normal range but not
SBE	−6.9	when breathing 60% oxygen.
O_2 sat.	96%	The (A–a) P_{O_2} gradient is
(F_IO_2 60%)		roughly 40 kPa. These gases are
		typical of a patient with adult
		respiratory distress syndrome.

TREATMENT OF ACID–BASE DISTURBANCES

As in any other field of medicine, treatment should be directed at the underlying cause. Correcting the P_{CO_2} is usually possible by taking over the patient's ventilation and adjusting the minute volume to give the desired P_{CO_2}.

Treatment of a metabolic acidosis is more controversial. It was traditional to treat a metabolic acidosis by giving sodium bicarbonate according to the formula (Base excess × Body weight in kg/3) mmol starting by giving half the dose; 8.4% sodium bicarbonate contains 1 mmol ml^{-1}.

It is now argued that, particularly in a hypoxic state such as exists at cardiac arrests, bicarbonate administration may do more harm than good (Graf & Arieff 1986). The bicarbonate generates carbon dioxide which crosses easily into cells, making the intracellular acidosis worse. If ventilation is impaired the carbon dioxide generated is unable to escape via the lungs. The traditional practice of giving 50–100 mmol bicarbonate at a cardiac arrest is probably unjustified. In metabolic acidosis due to poor perfusion of tissues the best way to manage this is to correct the perfusion defect which may be achieved, in some instances, by improving oxygen delivery using fluids, vasodilators or inotropes. This may involve the use of invasive monitoring such as Swan–Ganz catheterization in order to guide therapy. Treatment of the metabolic acidosis due to sepsis is controversial and, even though goal-directed therapy may not be universally accepted, most will still try to achieve reasonably high oxygen delivery targets. In sepsis, however, this does not give the anticipated rise in oxygen consumption after allowing for the rise in oxygen consumption due to increased myocardial work required to achieve the delivery. Sepsis appears to involve a defect in tissue oxygen uptake/utilization.

There is still a place for bicarbonate therapy in acidosis due to diarrhoea, renal tubular acidosis and uraemic acidosis. As outlined above, the base excess is used to calculate the dose; 8.4% sodium bicarbonate is hyperosmolar and must be given into a large central vein. Accidental subcutaneous administration can cause tissue necrosis. One must also bear in mind that each millimole of HCO_3^- is accompanied by Na+ and it is easy to overload the patient with sodium. Frequent blood gas and electrolyte analyses must be made during treatment with bicarbonate.

Summary

1. Ensure an adequate knowledge of basic fluid physiology.
2. Visible fluid deficit is only the tip of the iceberg.
3. Occult intraoperative hypovolaemia leads to increased postoperative morbidity.
4. Monitor patients thoroughly to gain maximal information about their fluid status.
5. Suspect hypovolaemia as the most common cause of an intraoperative metabolic acidosis.

References

Boyd O, Grounds R M, Bennett E D 1993 A randomised clinical trial of the effect of deliberate peri-operative increase of oxygen delivery on mortality in high-risk surgical patients. Journal of the American Medical Association 270: 2699–2707

Edelman I S, Leibman J 1959 Anatomy of body water and electrolytes. American Journal of Medicine 27: 256, 277

Graf H, Arieff A I 1986 Use of sodium bicarbonate in the therapy of organic acidosis. Intensive Care Medicine 12: 285–288

Hamilton-Davies C, Mythen M G, Salmon J B, Jacobson D, Shukla A, Webb A R 1997 Comparison of commonly used clinical indicators of hypovolaemia with gastrointestinal tonometry. Intensive Care Medicine 23: 276–281

Hayes M A, Timmins A C, Yau E H 1994 Elevation of systemic oxygen delivery in the treatment of critically ill patients. New England Journal of Medicine 330: 1717–1722

Mattox K L, Maningas P A, Moore E E 1991 Prehospital hypertonic saline/dextran infusion for post-traumatic hypotension. Annals of Surgery 213: 482–491

Mythen M G, Purdy G, Mackie I J 1993 Post-operative multiple organ dysfunction syndrome associated with gut mucosal hypoperfusion, increased neutrophil degranulation and C-1-esterase inhibitor depletion. British Journal of Anaesthesia 71: 858–863

Price H L, Deutsch S, Marshall B E 1966 Haemodynamic and metabolic effects of haemorrhage in man with particular reference to the splanchnic circulation. Circulation Research 18: 469–474

Robarts W M, Parkin J V, Hobsley M 1979 A simple clinical approach to quantifying losses from the extracellular and plasma compartments. Annals of the Royal College of Surgeons of England 61: 142–145

Shoemaker W C, Appel P L, Kram H B 1988 Prospective trial of supranormal values of survivors as therapeutic goals in high-risk surgical patients. Chest 94: 1176–1186

Starling E H 1896 On the absorption of fluids from the connective spaces. Journal of Physiology 19: 312–326

Staverman A 1952 Apparent osmotic pressure of solutions of heterodisperse polymers. Rec Trav Chim 71: 623–633

Webb A R, Barclay S A, Bennett E D 1989 In vitro colloid pressure of commonly used plasma expanders and substitutes. Intensive Care Medicine 15: 116–120

11

Nutrition support

J. J. Payne-James

Objectives

- Be aware of the incidence and causes of protein energy malnutrition in surgical patients.
- Be aware of the effects of protein energy malnutrition.
- Understand the need for documentation and how to assess nutritional status.
- Understand when to initiate nutrition support.
- Understand when to use oral, enteral or parenteral nutrition support.
- Be aware of methods and complications of nutrition support techniques.

INTRODUCTION

The metabolic response to injury – such as multiple trauma, major surgery and sepsis – is synonymous with increased demands for nitrogen and energy. Failure to match these increased demands with appropriate intake will result in protein-energy malnutrition (PEM). Oral feeding is the optimum method of administering additional nutrients to a nutritionally compromised patient with increased needs. Sip feeds and oral diet supplementation are important ways of increasing nutrient intake and are therefore widely used in hospitals and community practice (Keel et al 1997). Palatability is an essential part of the use of such supplements, and the range of flavours (sweet/savoury, milky/fruit) is now extensive.

Many hospitalized patients, however, will not be appropriate for oral or supplemental feeding, either because they are physically incapable, or lack the motivation or desire. For these patients other routes of administration must be sought. Artificial nutrition support (provision of nutrient substrates by other than the oral route) is therefore indicated for many critically ill patients such as those in the postoperative period.

It is still often noted with surprise that malnutrition can be considered a problem in hospitals. Hill et al (1977) and Bistrian et al (1976) showed over 2 decades ago incidences of malnutrition of up to 60% of hospital patients, and these data were replicated in all patient groups. Despite increasing awareness of the problem and increased sophistication in the practice of clinical nutrition, McWhirter & Pennington showed in 1994 that up to 40% of patients were undernourished at the time of admission to hospital, and over half of those patients had no nutritional data documented in their case notes. Protein energy malnutrition is still a significant (and often unrecognized) problem in hospitals. The aim of nutrition support should therefore be to identify the malnourished (or potentially malnourished) patient, and to correct or improve the nutritional status such that morbidity and mortality are minimized. Patients require nutrition support because studies have demonstrated poorer outcomes of treatment in patients who are malnourished. Worse outcome caused by impairment and eventual failure of physiological protein-dependent functions may be manifested as increased infection rates (e.g. chest, urinary or wound), slower healing, wound breakdown and dehiscence, and death.

ASSESSMENT

Identification of the patients suffering from protein energy malnutrition (PEM) is not always straightforward. Some assessment of the nutritionally compromised patient is possible by measuring a variety of parameters, including biochemical (e.g. serum albumin, transferrin and retinol-binding protein), anthropometric (e.g. triceps skin-fold thickness (TSF) and midarm muscle circumference (MAMC)), immunological (e.g. lymphocyte count and delayed hypersensitivity skin-testing) and dynamometric (e.g. hand-grip strength). However, these markers may have poor sensitivity or specificity when used alone. In the absence of a single specific measure of nutritional state it is necessary for the practising clinician to identify and define groups of patients for whom nutritional support is indicated.

INDICATIONS FOR NUTRITION SUPPORT

> All patients admitted to hospital, even for elective procedures, should have a nutritional assessment, the results of which should be recorded clearly in the notes, with the decision made about whether nutrition support is required (King's Fund 1992).

The routine history and clinical examination of a patient should enable patients to be placed in one of the following four groups:

1. Obvious severe malnutrition (recent or long term) (>10% recent weight loss; serum albumin <30 g l^{-1}; gross muscle wasting and peripheral oedema)
2. Moderate malnutrition (some nutritional parameters suggestive of depletion; dietary history shows impaired nutrient intake in preceding 2–4 weeks or more; there may be no obvious physical evidence of malnutrition)
3. Normal or near-normal nutritional status (but underlying pathology is likely to result in malnutrition if nutritional support withheld, e.g. trauma patients, ventilated patients)
4. Normal nutritional status which is unlikely to be affected by illness.

There are specific aspects of bedside clinical assessment which assist with this nutritional classification (Payne-James & Wicks 1994). Height and weight must be recorded and compared with standardized charts. Protein and energy balance may be estimated from the dietary history and from the assumption that the maximum requirements of protein and energy for hospitalized patients are 1.5 g kg^{-1} per 24 h and 40 kcal kg^{-1} per 24 h, respectively. Body composition can be assessed clinically. Hill (1992) has described the 'positive finger–thumb test' when the dermis can be felt between finger and thumb when pinching triceps and biceps skinfolds. Body composition studies suggest that, when positive, the body mass is composed of <10% fat. Hill has also described the 'positive tendon–bone test' when tendons are prominent to palpation and bony promi-

nences of the scapula are apparent – at which point patients have lost >30% of body protein stores. Additionally, look for and record other signs of PEM; these include loss of muscle power, peripheral oedema, skin rashes, angular stomatitis, gingivitis, nail abnormalities, glossitis, paraesthesia and neuropathy.

Once the patient has been classified into one of the above four groups, a decision can be made as to whether nutritional support is indicated. If it is considered that nutritional support is required, the best route of administration must be chosen. Figure 11.1 illustrates the decision-making process. These routes are explored in more detail below.

> Use the enteral route as the technique of choice in all patients with a normal or near-normal functioning, accessible gastrointestinal tract.

ENTERAL AND PARENTERAL NUTRITION FOR SURGICAL PATIENTS

Until recently, the gut has been considered to be an unimportant organ during critical illness caused by injury or infection. In the last few years the metabolic role of the gastrointestinal (GI) tract in both fasting and stressed states has been elucidated. It is now accepted that the GI tract is frequently a reservoir for bacteria that may cause systemic infections by allowing bacterial translocation across the gut wall. Gut-derived endotoxin may therefore be the link between GI failure and multiple organ failure in patients without overt clinical evidence of infection. The relationship between GI bacteria, systemic host defences and injury in the development of bacterial translocation is represented in simplified form in Figure 11.2. In summary, enteral nutrition may improve antibacterial host defences, blunt the hypermetabolic response to trauma, maintain gut mucosal mass, maintain gut barrier function and prevent disruption of gut flora. These effects may relate in part to the maintenance of splanchnic blood flow and the direct provision of nutrients for enterocytes.

Research continues to determine whether dietary manipulation (e.g. provision of glutamine or fibre) can prevent bowel atrophy and maintain intestinal mass and thus impact on clinical outcome in terms of reduced morbidity and mortality (Braga et al 1996). However, for the majority of critically ill patients (including those after surgery) the GI tract is an appropriate and desirable route for nutrition support, as long as there is no evidence of bowel dysfunction, such as abdominal distension, vomiting and large volume

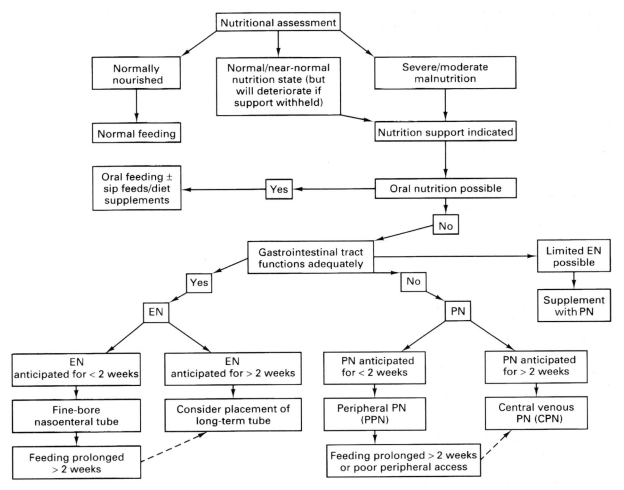

Fig 11.1   Flow chart of options when nutrition support is required. CPN, central venous parenteral nutrition EN, enteral nutrition; PN, parenteral nutrition; PPN, peripheral parenteral nutrition.

nasoenteral aspirates. Small intestinal function is maintained postoperatively (as the main sites of 'ileus' are the stomach and colon), and enteral nutrition (EN) may be delivered safely into the small bowel immediately after intra-abdominal surgery (including major aortic reconstruction). It is sometimes suggested that bowel anastomosis is a contraindication to EN in the early postoperative period, but studies have confirmed its safety. EN should be considered the first choice for feeding patients with severe head injuries, and should be commenced early as aggressive nutrition support confers benefit on outcome.

Landmark studies have shown the beneficial effects of EN on patients who would previously have been considered solely appropriate for parenteral (intravenous) nutrition (PN). Kudsk et al (1992) undertook a prospective study investigating 98 trauma patients with an Abdominal Trauma Index (ATI) of >15 who were randomized to receive either EN or PN feeding within 24 hours of injury. The aim of the study was to examine the effects of the two regimens on outcome in the first 15 days of hospitalization. All patients had laparotomy for management of intra-abdominal injuries and had a needle catheter jejunostomy placed at that time. The EN group had significantly fewer episodes of pneumonia, intra-abdominal abscess and line spesis. EN patients with penetrating injuries had significantly fewer infections, and this was also observed in those needing >20 units of blood, in those with an ATI >40 and in those requiring reoperation within 72 hours.

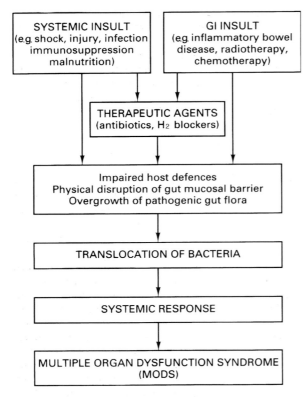

Fig 11.2 Simplified mechanism of bacterial translocation and multiple organ failure.

Thus there was a significantly lower incidence of septic morbidity in EN-fed patients (compared with PN-fed patients) after blunt and penetrating trauma, and this difference was enhanced with the most severely injured patients. In a meta-analysis which included data from eight previously published randomized trials comparing the outcome of high-risk surgical patients fed either by early EN or PN, only 18% of EN patients, compared with 35% of PN patients, developed postoperative septic complications (Moore et al 1992).

PERIOPERATIVE NUTRITION

The way in which nutrition support (including supplementation and EN) should be used in the preoperative period is summarized in Box 11.1. The length of preoperative nutritional support should not be such that the patient's primary condition can deteriorate as a result of progression of the disease, so operative intervention will take priority over nutrition support in particular patients.

Box 11.1 Recommendations for preoperative nutrition support

1. If a patient is severely malnourished (e.g. > 10% weight loss), give at least 10 days of:
   - dietary supplementation *or*, if not possible
   - give enteral nutrition *or*, if not possible
   - give parenteral nutrition, unless early surgery is clinically indicated.
2. If a patient is borderline or mildly malnourished, operation should not be delayed solely for nutrition support.

Postoperative nutrition should be considered for any patient who fails to have an adequate oral intake (as assessed by a dietitian) 5 days after surgery. Postoperative PN should be considered when oral or enteral nutrition is not anticipated within 7–10 days in previously well-nourished patients or within 5–7 days in previously malnourished or critically ill patients. For some patients it may be clear at the time of operation that adequate oral intake will not be possible (for example after major oropharyngeal/maxillofacial surgery) for some time postoperatively, or that normal gut function will take more than a few days to recover (major upper GI resection). In cases such as these it may be advisable to gain access to the GI tract (e.g. via gastrostomy, jejunostomy or central venous lines) while the patient is still in the operating theatre and still anaesthetized. If unexpectedly rapid recovery ensues, these may be removed; but, if they are required, the patient is not then subject to, and the surgeon does not have to arrange, placement at a later date.

These are all general principles and each case must be assessed individually. The reason for operation, the degree of malnutrition and expected postoperative course are all important in making this decision. Extreme examples are: a severely malnourished elderly patient who is a smoker, requiring oesophagectomy, would be a candidate for preoperative nutritional support; a patient with a prolonged exacerbation of inflammatory bowel disease unresponsive to medical management who presents with a perforated viscus requires surgery first and nutritional support later.

ENERGY AND NITROGEN REQUIREMENTS

Most surgical patients in need of nutrition support are metabolically stressed, septic or have been subject to trauma (accident or operation). These patients (particularly those with burns or head injuries) are likely to be hypermetabolic as a result of the normal neuroendocrinological response to injury. Specific energy requirements may be determined from indirect calorimetry, but this is not practical for most clinicians. In general, energy requirements are very rarely more that 2200–2400 kcal per 24 hours for surgical patients to achieve positive energy balance. Thus 35–40 kcal kg^{-1} per 24 hours will be appropriate for most patients, and this will be supplied as a mixture of carbohydrate and fat. Nitrogen requirements are often considerably greater than normal, and in hypermetabolic, stressed and injured patients nitrogen balance may be impossible to achieve until the primary pathology has been treated. The amount of nitrogen administered should ideally: minimize net losses without wasting administered nitrogen; permit maintenance of the patient's lean body mass, allowing an adequate supply of nitrogen for repair; and allow active repletion of lean body mass in the previously compromised patient. For most adult patients, 14–16 g nitrogen will be appropriate. Those patients with increased energy needs will require increased nitrogen and amounts of up to 0.4 g kg^{-1} per 24 hours have been suggested.

Monitoring

The main parameters used to monitor a patient receiving nutrition support are:

- Diet charts
- Weight
- Haematology
- Biochemistry.

Diet charts (for patients on enteral nutrition) enable an accurate record of the patient's actual versus prescribed intake to be kept, and the charts will allow prompt recognition of inadequacies of nutrient intake. These charts are also of importance during the changeover from enteral feeding to oral nutrition. Weighing is the simplest but most valuable way to ensure that the nutrition regimen prescribed for a particular patient is satisfactory. A steady increase in weight of 1–2 kg per week suggests adequate nutrition in those requiring body mass repletion. Remember, however, that weight gain may result from water retention. Basic haematological and biochemical parameters should be measured at the commencement of nutrition. Initially, close monitoring of the plasma potassium, phosphate and glucose are important, particularly in the severely malnourished patient. In patients on long-term feeding, vitamin levels or trace-element levels may be required if clinically indicated. The plasma proteins albumin, transferrin

and thyroid binding pre-albumin can all be useful markers for indicating a response to nutrition support over a period of time.

Anthropometric and dynamometric measurements are often considered as research tools, but they can offer sensitive and effective measurement of the efficacy of nutrition support over a period of time, and where available should be used.

Nitrogen balance

Nitrogen balance is frequently used as an assessment technique for monitoring day-to-day progress of nutrition support. One of the aims of nutrition support should be to place the patient in positive nitrogen balance. This is often difficult or impossible to achieve in the very stressed or catabolic patient. The components of nitrogen balance are those of whole-body protein turnover, which represents the difference between whole-body protein synthesis and breakdown. It is a measure of metabolic state rather than nutritional status. In most patients nitrogen balance can be calculated from urinary and faecal nitrogen losses and, whenever possible, 24-hour collections of urine should be undertaken on all patients receiving nutrition support. Faecal output is often negligible. There is a reasonable correlation between urinary urea excretion and total urinary nitrogen, with urea accounting for about 80%. Adjustments must be made for plasma urea levels and a figure of 2–3 g allowed for other routes of loss, including faeces. These figures are not appropriate for the severely ill patient, where the urinary urea may represent considerably less than 80% of the total nitrogen because of excessive excretion of ammonium and other non-urea nitrogenous compounds. In many centres total urinary nitrogen is measured routinely by chemiluminescence, obviating the need to estimate output from urea values.

ENTERAL NUTRITION (EN)

Types of enteral diet

There are three main types of nutritionally complete enteral diet appropriate for the surgical patient: polymeric, predigested (or elemental), and disease specific.

Polymeric diets are indicated for the vast majority of patients with normal or near-normal GI function. They contain whole protein as a nitrogen source, energy is derived from triglycerides and glucose polymers, while electrolytes, trace elements and vitamins are included in standardized amounts. Generally, one of two polymeric diets, a standard or an energy (nitrogen dense) diet, is prescribed. The standard polymeric diets contain approximately 6 g nitrogen per litre with an energy density of 1 kcal ml^{-1}. The energy (nitrogen dense) diets contain between 8 and 10 g nitrogen per litre and an energy density of 1–1.5 kcal ml^{-1}. Polymeric diets are suitable for over 90% of patients with normal or near-normal GI function. In a few patients with very severe exocrine pancreatic insufficiency or with intestinal failure because of short bowel syndrome, intraluminal hydrolysis may be severely impaired, thereby limiting diet assimilation. In such cases a predigested or elemental diet may be indicated.

Predigested or elemental diet. These diets have a nitrogen source derived from free amino acids or oligopeptides. Energy is derived from glucose polymer mixture predominating with polymers of chain length >10 glucose molecules. The fat source consists of a combination of long- and medium-chain triglycerides. A recent study has shown the benefit of one such peptide-based enteral diet on the course of patients with acute pancreatitis when compared with standard treatment with parenteral nutrition (McClave et al 1997).

Disease-specific diets. Specially formulated disease-specific diets have been developed for patients with disorders such as encephalopathy associated with chronic liver disease, and respiratory failure. Malnourished patients with cirrhosis who present with encephalopathy, or who have a previous history of episodes of encephalopathy, present a difficult problem of nutritional management. Branched-chain amino acid enriched diets have been advocated to normalize plasma amino acid profiles with the aim of improving nutritional state and preventing worsening of encephalopathy. Patients with respiratory failure on ventilators are adversely affected by diets with high carbohydrate loads which increase carbon dioxide production. Diets with higher fat energy component allow earlier weaning from a ventilator as a result of decreased carbon dioxide production and reduced respiratory quotient. Much research is being undertaken on the use of nutrition substrates or supplements designed to modify or modulate the metabolic response to stress and the immune response – immune-enhancing diets (IED). Such substrates include n-3 fatty acids, arginine, glutamine and nucleotides. Clinical studies have been undertaken in a number of areas, including the critically injured (Mendez et al 1997), major abdominal surgery (Braga et al 1996) and burns patients (Saffle et al 1997) but no clear recommendations can yet be made.

Route of administration

Most patients will require nutrition support for less than a month. For these patients the best method of enteral delivery is via a fine-bore nasogastric feeding tube. The most frequent complication (less than 5% of patients) is tube malposition at insertion, generally into the trachea and bronchi. This complication occurs most commonly in patients with altered swallowing, diminished gag reflex or those who have had upper airway or pharyngeal surgery. In patients who are alert and orientated, tube positioning may be confirmed by aspiration of gastric contents and auscultation of the epigastrium.

> Confirm the position of the enteral tube by X-rays routinely in all patients with altered consciousness, or altered cough or gag reflex, and those who are mechanically ventilated or who have had upper airway surgery.

In some patents nasogastric delivery of nutrients may not be appropriate because of an increased risk of regurgitation and/or pulmonary aspiration of feed (Box 11.1).

All patients in the groups indicated in Box 11.2 and those with gastric atony or paresis for any reason should at least be considered for postpyloric nasoduodenal or nasojejunal feeding to reduce the risk of regurgitation or aspiration. Accurate siting of fine-bore tubes beyond the pylorus remains a problem. Techniques using metoclopramide, manipulation of the tube at the bedside or under fluoroscopic control are used with varying success. For the surgical patient in whom postoperative feeding is anticipated, placement at laparotomy is advised. In other cases a fine-bore tube of appropriate length may be introduced pernasally, and if spontaneous passage has not occurred after 12–24 hours, endoscopic or fluoroscopic positioning is undertaken. For some patients other routes of administration may be more appropriate than, or preferable to the nasoenteral route.

> **Box 11.2 Patient groups/diseases with risk of gastric atony or paresis**
>
> - Critically ill
> - Diabetes with neuropathy
> - Head injury
> - Hypothyroidism
> - Neuromotor deglutition disorders
> - Postabdominal surgery
> - Recumbent patients
> - Intensive care unit/ventilated patients.

Pharyngostomy and oesophagostomy are used by a few surgeons. Percutaneous endoscopically placed gastrostomies (PEG) are the technique of choice for long-term administration of enteral nutrition. PEG placement has a lower morbidity and mortality compared with the conventional surgical placement. The technique of needle catheter jejunostomy (NCJ), whereby a fine catheter is inserted either as a separate surgical procedure or concurrently at the time of abdominal surgery, may be used for:

- Patients who are malnourished at the time of surgery
- Patients undergoing major upper GI surgery
- Patients who may receive adjuvant radiotherapy or chemotherapy after surgery
- Patients undergoing laparotomy after major trauma.

Reservoirs and giving sets

Enteral diets may be dispensed from different sized containers ranging from 500 ml to 2 litres in volume. The policy of using larger reservoirs improves the ratio of administered diet/prescribed diet and reduces the amount of handling time needed. Increasing attention is now paid to the risks of bacterial contamination and enteral nutrition, and sterile closed systems are the choice of enteral diet reservoir, particularly in the immunosuppressed and critically ill. Giving sets and reservoirs should be changed every 24 hours.

Infusion versus bolus administration

Compared with continuous infusion, bolus feeding of enteral diets has greater incidence of side-effects such as bloating and diarrhoea, in addition to which a considerable amount of nursing time is required and feeds may often be accidentally omitted. A continuous infusion either by gravity feed or by using a peristaltic pump is therefore the method of choice.

Starter regimens

Starter regimens (diluting the feed or reducing the volume) results in limited intake of diet in the first few days of feeding, thereby prolonging the length of negative nitrogen balance. Undiluted, full-volume diet does not, as is commonly thought, increase the incidence of GI side-effects in patients with normal bowel, or those with inflammatory bowel disease, when used to commence enteral nutrition. Therefore, in general, starter regimens should not be used.

Commencing enteral feeding

In most adult patients with no other metabolic or fluid balance problems, 2–2.5 litres of diet are prescribed on a daily basis. This volume is infused from day one.

Complications

The potential complications of enteral nutrition are summarized in Box 11.3.

Tube blockage most commonly occurs after the giving set is disconnected from the feeding tube, and the residual diet solidifies. This complication may be prevented by flushing the tube with water after disconnection. An obstructed tube may occasionally be unblocked by instilling pancreatic enzyme or cola.

Diarrhoea occurs in about 10% of patients. Its aetiology is multifactorial with a strong association with concomitant antibiotic therapy. Hypoalbuminaemia may play a role. Symptomatic treatment (with antidiarrhoeals such as codeine phosphate or loperamide) is appropriate, and only rarely does enteral feeding have to be discontinued. Antibiotics that are no longer clinically indicated should be stopped. Drug charts should be frequently reviewed.

Nausea and vomiting rarely occur due to enteral feeding but may result from slowed gastric emptying. Antiemetics may be of benefit. The symptoms of bloating, abdominal distension and cramps most commonly occur following inadvertent too rapid administration of feed, and are very similar to the symptoms described in association with bolus-type feeding.

Enteral diets will interact with enterally administered drugs (e.g. theophylline, warfarin, methyldopa and digoxin). Failure of drug therapy in previously stable

---

Box 11.3   Complications of enteral nutrition

Feeding tube related
- Malposition
- Unwanted removal
- Blockage.

Diet and diet-administration related
- Diarrhoea
- Bloating
- Nausea
- Cramps
- Regurgitation
- Pulmonary aspiration
- Vitamin, mineral, trace element deficiencies
- Drug interactions.

Metabolic/biochemical

Infective
- Diets
- Reservoirs
- Giving sets.

patients receiving EN support must be assumed to be feed related until proved otherwise.

PARENTERAL NUTRITION (PN)

The successful use of intravenous nutrition (parenteral nutrition) in maintaining body weight and allowing growth to progress normally was first demonstrated by Dudrick et al (1968) 3 decades ago. The term total parenteral nutrition (TPN) has been commonly used, but as any patient solely receiving nutrition via the parenteral route will be receiving total parenteral nutrition, the term parenteral nutrition (PN) is now superseding it. PN plays an essential role in the management of some acutely ill patients, although, as a result of the increasing use of EN in preference to PN, the range of patients is perhaps more limited than previously. Up to 25% of patients in hospital requiring nutrition support need it administered via the parenteral route (Payne-James et al 1995). PN can be considered for all malnourished or potentially malnourished patients with non-functioning and/or non-accessible GI tract. Four main areas need to be considered when providing PN for a patient (see Box 11.4).

Access

Historically, PN solutions generally have high osmolalities which, if administered into peripheral veins, can result in rapid development of thrombophlebits and line failure. This problem was overcome by using central venous catheters to deliver PN solutions into large veins such as the superior vena cava (SVC), most commonly via the subclavian or internal jugular veins. Getting access to, and the presence of central venous catheters within these veins give rise to certain complications, the most well recognized of which are listed in Box 11.5. These catheter insertion complications repre-

---

Box 11.4   Considerations for PN

- Access route (peripheral or central)
  - techniques
  - complications
  - delivery
- Nutrients
- Monitoring
- Complications
  - metabolic
  - catheter-related.

Box 11.5   Central venous catheter complications

Insertion-related
- Air embolism
- Arterial puncture
- Cardiac arrhythmia's
- Catheter embolus
- Chylothorax
- Haemopericardium
- Haematoma
- Haemothorax
- Hydro/TPN-thorax
- Malposition
- Neurological injury
- Pneumothorax.

Late complications
- Catheter infection, or sepsis
- Catheter displacement
- Central venous thrombosis
- Luminal occlusion.

---

sent most of the serious complications associated with PN.

The majority of catheters used for PN in the UK are single-lumen central venous catheters. Most of these are inserted with a short subcutaneous tunnel fashioned to allow the catheter to exit away from the point of vein penetration. Strict catheter care protocols should be followed and monitored by an infection-control or specialist nutrition nurse to minimize the incidence of catheter-related sepsis. If a patient on PN develops a pyrexia and leucocytosis in the absence of any other focus of infection, then the central venous catheter should be considered the source of infection. However, all other possible sources of infection should be considered and culture of sputum, urine, wound and other sites is mandatory.

The current widespread use of lower energy regimens with lipid providing a larger percentage of calories is one reason for the increase in use of PN administered by the peripheral route (peripheral parenteral nutrition (PPN)). A number of other factors have been identified which can reduce the incidence of peripheral vein thrombophlebitis, including the use of heparin, in-line filtration, cortisol, buffering, locally applied glyceryl trinitrate patches and using fine-bore cannulas. These factors, and the reduction of osmolality by modifying the parenteral nutrition formulations, allow PPN to be given routinely. Thrombophlebitis cannot be totally abolished, however, but as most courses of hospital-based PN rarely last more than 10–14 days

(Payne-James et al 1995) this is no longer a limiting factor. Thus PPN should now be routinely considered if it is anticipated that nutrition support will be needed for less than 2 weeks. In this manner the risks associated with placement of central venous catheters are avoided. PPN is now widely used in many centres in the UK.

PN nutrients

PN solutions require macronutrients and micronutrients. Macronutrients consist of energy sources, nowadays consisting of carbohydrate (glucose) and lipid emulsions. Most regimens consist of a combination in proportions up to 50% : 50%. Nitrogen sources are most commonly L-amino acids. Novel substrates for better nitrogen retention and protein synthesis, and for modifying immune responses are continually being evaluated (Rohovsky et al 1997).

Micronutrients are electrolytes, trace elements and vitamins, deficiencies of which may present complex and obscure clinical problems. Commercial sterile solutions of the parenteral nutrition requirements are now generally provided as all-in-one bags (AIO) (all appropriate macro- and micronutrients mixed together), the contents of which can be infused safely over a given period (12–24 hours). AIO bags are used widely in clinical practice, and solutions can be compounded and stored for several weeks without deleterious effect. Compatibilities of solutions vary, and if in doubt manufacturers should be consulted for advice.

Monitoring

It is important that an accurate record of the administration of parenteral nutrition (PN) is maintained. PN should be administered using infusion pumps or flow-control devices. In the first week of PN administration, blood glucose should be measured 6 hourly, as many patients will develop some degree of insulin resistance because of their underlying pathology and may require exogenous insulin administered by injection/infusion, or occasionally incorporated in the PN regimen. Electrolytes should be measured daily to allow correction of initial electrolyte imbalance and fluctuations, and to detect changes before severe metabolic/biochemical changes can affect the patient's clinical status. Monitor liver function tests to observe changes in serum albumin, and to detect PN-related hepatobiliary dysfunction, which occurs inevitably in many patients fed parenterally.

Metabolic complications

A wide variety of metabolic complications can occur with PN, and the results of a study documenting complications in order of frequency are listed in Box 11.6.

Box 11.6 Metabolic complications of PN in decreasing order of frequency

- Hyperglycaemia
- Hypoglycaemia
- Hypophosphataemia
- Hypercalcaemia
- Hyperkalaemia
- Hypokalaemia
- Hypernatraemia
- Hyponatraemia
- Other (particularly after long-term feeding): deficiencies of folate, zinc, magnesium, other trace elements, vitamins and essential fatty acids.

Although wide ranging, these complications only occurred in under 5% of patients, the majority of whom were in intensive care. A specific complication of PN of multifactorial aetiology is the development of hepatic dysfunction. This is characterized by elevated hepatic enzymes, intrahepatic cholestasis and fatty infiltration of the liver. This is generally self-limiting and hepatic function returns to normal after cessation of PN.

NUTRITION SUPPORT TEAM

A multidisciplinary nutrition support team is the best way of optimizing the nutritional care of hospitalized patients. The different members of the team can provide expert advice within their own speciality. Input to the team should come from clinicians, dietitians, pharmacists, nurses, chemical pathologist and microbiologists. The multidisciplinary approach ensures the most appropriate administration of nutrition support, and minimizes complications.

Summary

1. Malnutrition in is prevalent in surgical patients.
2. Malnutrition affects the outcome of surgical patients.
3. Appropriate nutrition assessment is essential in all patients.
4. Certain patient groups require nutrition support.
5. Nutrition support may be given by the oral, enteral or parenteral routes.

Summary (contd.)

6. Enteral nutrition is appropriate with a functioning gut.
7. Parenteral nutrition is appropriate with intestinal failure or a non-accessible gut.
8. Peripheral administration of PN is appropriate for many patients.
9. Nutrition support is best managed by a nutrition support team.

References

Bistrian B R, Blackburn G L, Vitale J, Cochran D, Naylor J 1976 Prevalence of malnutrition in general medical patients. Journal of the American Medical Association 235: 1567–1570

Braga M, Vignali A, Gianotti L et al 1996 Immune and nutritional effects of early enteral nutrition after major abdominal operations. Eur J Surg 162: 105–112

Dudrick S J, Wilmore D W, Vars H M, Rhoads J E 1968 Long-term total parenteral nutrition with growth, development and positive nitrogen balance. Surgery 64: 134–142

Hill G L 1992 Body composition research: implications for the practice of clinical nutrition. Journal of Parental and Enteral Nutrition 16: 197–218

Hill G L, Blackett R L, Pickford I et al 1977 Malnutrition in surgical patients. Lancet i: 689–692

Keel A M, Bray M J, Emery P W, Duncan H D, Silk D B A 1997 Two phased randomised controlled clinical trial of post-operative oral dietary supplements in surgical patients. Gut 40: 393–399

King's Fund 1992 A positive approach to nutrition support. King's Fund, London

Kudsk K A, Croce M A, Fabian T C et al 1992 Enteral versus parenteral feeding. Effects on septic morbidity after blunt and penetrating abdominal trauma. Annals of Surgery 215: 503–513

McClave S A, Green L M, Snide H L et al 1997 Comparison of the safety of early enteral vs parenteral nutrition in mild acute pancreatitis. Journal of Parenteral and Enteral Nutrition 21: 14–20

McWhirter J P, Pennington C R 1994 Incidence and recognition of malnutrition in hospital. British Medical Journal 308: 945–948

Mendez C, Jurkovich G J, Garcia I et al 1997 Effects of an immune-enhancing diet in critically injured patients. J Trauma 42: 933–945

Moore F A, Feliciano D V, Andrassy R J et al 1992 Early enteral feeding, compared with parenteral, reduces postoperative septic complications. The results of a meta-analysis. Annals of Surgery 216: 172–183

Payne-James J J, Wicks C 1994 Key facts in clinical nutrition. Churchill Livingstone, London

Payne-James J J, de Gara C K, Grimble G K, Silk D B A 1995 Artificial nutrition support in hospitals in the United Kingdom, 1994: third national survey. Clinical Nutrition 14: 329–335

Rohovsky S A, Babineau T J, Bistrian B R 1997 Total parenteral nutrition. Curr Opin Gastroenterol 13: 146–152

Saffle J R, Wiebke G, Jennings K et al 1997 Randomised trial of immune-enhancing enteral nutrition in burn patients. J Trauma 42: 793–800

Further reading

Payne-James J J, Grimble G K, Silk D B A (eds) 1999 Artificial nutrition support in clinical practice, 2nd edn. Greenwich Medial Media, London

12

Clinical pharmacology

M. Schachter

INTRODUCTION

Over a decade ago an eminent professor of clinical pharmacology could foresee a time when every district general hospital would have its own clinical pharmacologist. This obviously has not happened and does not seem imminent. Indeed, many clinicians have reservations about the role of clinical pharmacology as a speciality, except perhaps within the pharmaceutical industry. In fact, clinical pharmacologists themselves have very divergent views on their role. They have their own subspecialities and no one person can pretend to have comprehensive knowledge of all medicines – probably not even in their own field. However, clinical pharmacology does provide a framework of principles for evaluating the effectiveness and dangers of new drugs, for comparing them with established agents, for detecting and sometimes predicting both wanted and unwanted interactions, and for defining the ways in which drugs are handled in the body. It is also involved in understanding the effects of age, pregnancy and intercurrent disease on the use of drugs. This role is increasingly reinforced by the drug information services within hospital pharmacies, with access to databases of many kinds, and also of course by access to information on the Internet (there will be more on this at the end of the chapter).

Surgeons are, sometimes reluctantly, major prescribers of drugs of all kinds from analgesics to antibiotics. It is hoped that this chapter will provide reminders of some practically useful principles of clinical pharmacology.

Pharmacokinetics

It can hardly be claimed that pharmacokinetics is popular among most clinicians, or even some clinical pharmacologists. In fact, most doctors need to know very little about the mathematics of pharmacokinetics but should understand some basic concepts. These are defined in Box 12.1.

DRUGS IN THE YOUNG AND OLD

Neonates, infants and children

Babies cannot be regarded simply as small adults. Every aspect of drug handling is different in neonates and infants, as compared to adults. Some of these differences are summarized below:

- The adult body has a lower water content than the neonate's (about 60% compared to 75%).
- Fat represents 12–15% of body weight in the neonate and 18–20% in most adults (much more in some, of course!).
- Renal function is initially poor in neonates, with a glomerular filtration rate only 5–10% of that in the adult. However, adult values are reached in 3–6 months. Tubular function is also immature in the very young.
- Hepatic function presents a more complex picture. Some enzyme systems are grossly underdeveloped

Box 12.1 Basic concepts in pharmacokinetics

Half-life (t$_{1/2}$)
This is a measure of how quickly the body as a whole removes a drug. It is usually fairly easy to estimate from plasma drug concentrations (see Fig. 12.1). It will take a drug about 5 half-lives to reach steady state if it is given at a constant rate, whether continuously or intermittently.

Clearance (Cl)
This is a reflection of the relationship between drug concentration and its rate of elimination. It can be thought of as the volume of plasma totally cleared of a drug per unit time (hour or minute).

Volume of distribution (V$_d$)
This relates the amount of drug in the whole body to that in plasma at a given time,. It can be calculated from assuming a concentration (C$_0$) at time 0. Although this is not real it can be derived from a graph such as Figure 12.2, which represents the equation:

$$V_d = Dose/C_0$$

Very high values of V$_d$ may be seen with highly lipid-soluble drugs. These may seem impossible but just mean that the drug binds to solid components of tissue such as membranes.

Bioavailability
If a drug is given intravenously the whole dose enters the systemic circulation and its bioavailability is defined as 100% (see Fig. 12.3). Drugs given by oral or other routes usually have lower bioavailability because of poor absorption or breakdown of the drug in the gut wall or the liver (*first-pass metabolism*).

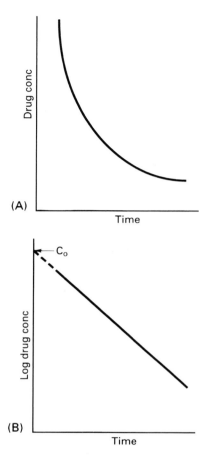

Fig 12.1 Simplified representation of change in drug concentration with time: (A) linear concentration scale; (B) logarithmic scale. C$_0$ is the theoretical concentration at time zero used in calculating the volume of distribution.

in neonates (chloramphenicol glucuronidation is a notorious example), but other processes are fully active (most sulphation for instance). Oxidative systems are not fully mature and this can be of clinical importance, for instance with anticonvulsants.

• Gastric acidity increases with age. Higher pH leads to increased absorption of some drugs, such as amoxycillin. Gastric emptying is also impaired in the neonate.

• The blood–brain barrier is relatively permeable in the very young. This can have serious consequences both in disease (kernicterus) and after drug administration, as in the case of the antidiarrhoeal opiate loperamide, which can cause dangerous central nervous system (CNS) depression in infants.

All this emphasizes the importance of using the minimum number of drugs at the lowest possible doses: no different from any other patient, in fact.

In children the principal difficulty lies in the calculation of the appropriate dose. Several approaches are possible, and none is ideal. Adjusting dose to surface area is considered the most appropriate method for neonates, but may not be accurate enough in premature babies. In these, weight may be a more reliable guide, and this is sometimes also used in older children. Another system matches the age to a fixed percentage of the adult dose: for example, 12.5% at 1 month, 25%

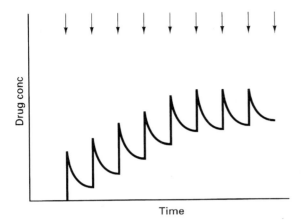

Fig 12.2 Diagram of step-wise increase in plasma drug concentration when a drug is administered (arrows) at intervals of approximately one half-life. Steady-state concentration is reached in about 5.5 half-lives: note that this is not necessarily a *therapeutic* level.

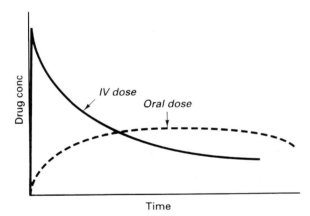

Fig 12.3 Diagram to illustrate the calculation of bioavailability: the ratio of the area under the oral administration curve to that under the intravenous curve over a specified period.

at 1 year, 50% at 7 years, 75% at 12 years. This is safe with relatively non-toxic drugs with a high therapeutic index, but is too approximate for more dangerous substances.

Drugs and the elderly

The clinical pharmacology of the elderly has become a subspeciality in its own right. This is very welcome and hardly surprising. The number of patients over the age

of 65 and even 80 or 90 years is rising rapidly in all developed countries. In parallel, the number of available drugs is also increasing. This section summarizes some of the most important considerations in prescribing for the elderly:

• It is safer to assume that elderly patients will show, increased sensitivity to the therapeutic and adverse effects of most drugs. Some of this can be explained by pharmacokinetic changes which are relatively easy to measure. However, there are also many examples where there seem to be alterations in pharmacodynamic responsiveness. These are usually poorly understood, but are often more important.

• CNS depressants, such as benzodiazepines, have an enhanced effect in the elderly: there is more prolonged sedation, often accompanied by confusion, disorientation or even hallucinations. For many benzodiazepines, including lorazepam and nitrazepam, pharmacokinetic measure differ little in the elderly and in young adults. The exaggerated response is often attributed to 'hypoxia', but the evidence for this is poor.

• Warfarin often produces a disproportionate fall in clotting factor synthesis in the old, again with unchanged pharmacokinetics.

• There is the increased likelihood of diuretic-induced hypokalaemia.

• In the elderly there is a generalized reduction in cardiovascular β_1-adrenoceptor number. The efficacy of both β-agonists and β-antagonists (in angina and hypertension) is likely to be impaired.

• The frequency and severity of drug-induced hypotension is greater in elderly patients, possibly due to impaired baroreceptor reflexes.

Much more is known about the altered pharmacokinetics characteristic of the elderly:

• Drug absorption is little changed, in the absence of specific gastrointestinal disease.

• Body composition is significantly different, with reduced muscle mass and total body weight, and a relative reduction in body water. There is a compensatory increase in the percentage of bodily fat, though this may be drastically reversed in the very old. Increased body fat can mean that there is prolonged action of fat-soluble drugs, such as the tricyclic antidepressants.

• Plasma albumin concentration is often reduced, but this is rarely of practical importance.

• Renal function declines with age. This is true both of glomerular filtration rate and of tubular function, though the former is usually of greater clinical relevance. Many important drugs are affected, including digoxin, the aminoglycoside antibiotics, tetracycline and lithium. Tetracyclines (except doxycycline and minocycline) should be avoided if there is significant renal impairment. Plasma levels of the other drugs can be monitored where possible. Some drugs (methyldopa and methotrexate are examples) are cleared by both renal and non-renal routes, and therapeutic monitoring is not usually available. If these drugs cannot be avoided doses can be reduced according to plasma creatinine levels or, preferably, creatinine clearance.

• Changes in hepatic metabolism are more complex and are less often of clinical importance. There is usually a reduction in hepatic blood flow, reflecting diminished cardiac output, and this leads to reduced clearance of some highly metabolized drugs, such as propranolol and (probably) lignocaine. On the other hand, the clearance of other extensively metabolized drugs, including warfarin and ethanol, hardly changes with ageing.

From the clinician's point of view these are not necessarily the most relevant problems in prescribing for the aged. The real difficulties can be summarized as follows:

1. The elderly often have multiple illnesses, and tend to be prescribed many drugs – often far too many. This inevitably leads to additive side-effects and great potential for drug interactions.
2. There is a high incidence of non-compliance amongst the elderly, for a variety of reasons, including failure to understand the prescriber's instructions and unwillingness (sometimes justified) to take medication.
3. Patients may be taking non-prescribed medication, often of unknown composition.
4. Patients may have other illnesses than those for which they are receiving treatment (see below).

DRUGS IN PREGNANCY

Unfortunately, prescribing is often unavoidable in pregnancy as, sometimes, is surgical intervention. Although there are considerable changes in drug handling (increased plasma volume and glomerular filtration rate, decreased plasma albumin) this is rarely clinically important. The overriding anxiety is the possibility of toxic (teratogenic) effects on the fetus. Some of the most important teratogens and other drugs with potentially adverse actions are listed in the Box 12.2.

DRUG USAGE IN DISEASE

Drugs in renal disease

It has already been pointed out that renal impairment almost always accompanies ageing. Although this is

---

> **Box 12.2   Drugs to be avoided in pregnancy**
>
> **In early pregnancy – potentially teratogenic**
> • Cytotoxic drugs
> • Sex steroids
> • Warfarin
> • Retinoids
> • Anticonvulsants (most) (risks of drug withdrawal may outweigh possible teratogenic effect)
> • Tetracyclines
>
> **In later pregnancy – fetal and perinatal effects**
> • Sex steroids
> • Warfarin
> • Tetracyclines
> • Sulphonamides
> • Chloramphenicol
> • Alcohol
> • Tobacco
> • Non-steroidal anti-inflammatory drugs
> • Sulphonylureas
>
> **May be used if essential but *caution***
> • Any CNS depressant
> • Lithium (probable teratogen, only use in first trimester if withdrawal considered dangerous)
> • Antithyroid drugs
> • Corticosteroids (probably teratogenic, but may be essential, e.g. in severe asthma)

---

significant it is rarely very severe. However, in many cases much more abnormal renal function has to be taken into account when using drugs. Naturally, renal elimination of many drugs and their metabolites is impaired, but there are also changes in drug distribution. The plasma protein binding of many drugs, particularly acidic drugs such as phenytoin, warfarin and salicylates, is reduced. The reduction is proportional to the severity of renal failure, and may have several causes. The importance of these changes should not be overemphasized, as they often have been, but for drugs that are affected it will mean a higher free unbound fraction in plasma: since this is the active component of the drug it will effectively lower the therapeutic range of the drug. However, the increased free fraction will also increase the clearance.

Many drugs will require dosage adjustment in the presence of renal failure: a few (discussed below) should be avoided altogether. In cases where a drug is used in reduced dosage, the target blood level can be achieved in two ways: by reducing the unit dose, or by increasing the dosage interval. Both approaches are used in practice. Digoxin is produced in a low-dose for-mulation (0.0625 mg against the standard dose of 0.25 mg) specifically for use in the elderly or in other patients with renal impairment. Occasionally, the stan-dard dose unit is used at 2- or 3-day intervals, but pro-longed dosage intervals tend to cause problems with patient compliance. By contrast, the aminoglycosides tend to be administered at prolonged intervals, but at standard unit doses. These drugs are classical examples of the usefulness of therapeutic plasma drug level mon-itoring to minimize toxicity where drug clearance may be abnormal. Nomograms have been constructed which allow reasonable estimates of desirable dosages even if drug assays are not available. The nomograms are based on creatinine clearance or, if this is not known, on plasma creatinine. However, measurement of plasma drug levels is always preferable. For most other drugs this degree of monitoring is not available and dosage adjustment must be based on known renal function. Important examples of such drugs are:

- Atenolol, sotalol
- Cephalosporins (most)
- Lithium – *always monitor*
- Cimetidine, ranitidine (less significant).

Box 12.3 lists some drugs that should be avoided in renal failure.

Drugs in liver disease

Given the central role of the liver in drug handling, it is to be expected that liver disease would have a dramatic impact on drug usage. This is true, but in fact most of the problems arise from abnormal responses to drugs rather than from pharmacokinetic changes. These can be very complex, for several reasons. Firstly, severe liver disease is often accompanied by some degree of renal failure. Secondly, plasma albumin levels may be very low because of diminished synthesis. Thirdly, cirrhosis is often associated with an increase in total liver blood flow, which can lead to increased flow to metabolically inactive areas. The overall effect can be very difficult to predict, but can lead to increased bioavailability and possible tox-icity of several important drugs such as metoprolol, pro-pranolol, labetalol and chlormethiazole. Predictably, the clearance of many extensively metabolized drugs is reduced. These include theophylline, phenytoin, vera-pamil, chloramphenicol and most benzodiazepines.

The following are among the more important drugs to avoid in severe liver disease:

1. *All CNS depressants*, including benzodiazepines and opiate analgesics. These may precipitate or aggravate hepatic encephalopathy.

> **Box 12.3** Drugs to be avoided in severe renal impairment (glomerular filtration rate <10 ml min^{-1})
>
> - Amiloride
> - Spironolactone
> - Thiazides
> - Nalidixic acid
> - Nitrofurantoin
> - Tetracyclines (except doxycycline, minocycline)
> - Methotrexate
> - Pancuronium
> - Chlorpropamide
> - Aspirin

2. *Diuretics*, which may cause hyponatraemia and hypokalaemia and increase the likelihood of encephalopathy. However, the aldosterone antagonist spironolactone is widely used in cirrhosis-associated ascites.
3. *Warfarin and other oral anticoagulants*, since there is already decreased synthesis of clotting factors.
4. *Potentially hepatotoxic drugs*, such as rifampicin and tetracyclines.

Drugs in heart failure

Severe heart failure can have far-reaching effects on drug disposition. Reduced cardiac blood flow will lead to diminished perfusion of gut, liver and kidneys. The absorption of some drugs (for example, hydrochloro-thiazide and frusemide) is therefore impaired. Reduced perfusion of the liver will diminish clearance of some extensively metabolized drugs: lignocaine may be par-ticularly important in this context, with potentially seri-ous toxicity. Altered renal blood flow will naturally result in reduced glomerular filtration rate and there-fore reduced clearance of drugs such as digoxin.

DRUG INTERACTIONS

The number of possible drug interactions is astronomical, and lists of even the more important can fill large volumes. Usually, but not always, these interactions are unwanted. They can be considered under three major headings: *phar-maceutical*, *pharmacodynamic* and *pharmacokinetic*.

Pharmaceutical interactions

These interactions occur outside the body, usually involving intravenous drugs which are incompatible with one another on the basis of chemical and physical reactions. Well-known examples include calcium salts and sodium bicarbonate, dopamine and sodium bicarbonate and amiodarone and sodium chloride. The *British National Formulary* includes a very comprehensive list of safe and incompatible intravenous mixtures and additives.

Pharmacodynamic interactions

Two main types of interaction are possible under this heading. Drugs may have an additive or even synergistic effect, or they may antagonize each other's actions. The best-known example of the first type is the action of CNS depressants, which usually potentiate one another, generally acting through different mechanisms. Alcohol is very frequently one of the drugs involved, while others may be antidepressants, benzodiazepines, opioids or antihistamines. This interaction is potentially very serious and even fatal in overdose. A less well-known example, potentially of importance in anaesthetics, is the enhancement of the effect of non-depolarizing muscle relaxants by aminoglycoside antibiotics. Finally, β-blockers and some calcium antagonists (notably verapamil and diltiazem) can each produce bradycardia and worsen atrioventricular block. In combination they can produce *severe* bradycardia, which may be associated with hypotension and heart failure. The latter might be further worsened by the negative inotropic action of both types of drug. Of all the above examples there is action at a common receptor only in the case of neuromuscular blockade.

Pharmacokinetic interactions

This heading includes many different varieties of drug interactions, most of which are listed here:

1. Drugs may interfere with each other's *absorption*. Well-known examples involve the tetracyclines, which bind metal ions such as iron, aluminium and calcium. Iron supplements and antacids may therefore prevent absorption of tetracyclines, and the latter block the absorption of iron. Anticholinergics, including tricyclic antidepressants, and opiates, slow gastric emptying and, therefore, the rate of absorption of many drugs such as paracetamol, levodopa and diazepam.

2. The *displacement of drugs from binding sites on plasma albumin* is well known, but its importance has been greatly overemphasized, as has already been mentioned. Some genuine examples include, as ever, warfarin, together with tolbutamide (now little used) and salicylates. Any drug that is genuinely involved must be over 95% protein bound, in fact probably about 99%.

3. There are many well-documented examples of *changes in drug metabolizing systems*. Enzyme inducers include most of the common anticonvulsants (phenytoin, carbamazepine, primidone and phenobarbitone), rifampicin and the antifungal griseofulvin. The list of target drugs is much longer and includes these drugs themselves as well as oral anticoagulants, oral contraceptives, corticosteroids and opiates. There are many other examples. In most instances drug effects are significantly reduced.

A specific case of metabolic inhibition concerns monoamine oxidase inhibitors, which prevent the breakdown of amines such as levodopa and tyramine, potentially causing a hypertensive crisis. On the other hand, tricyclic antidepressants and pethidine can cause hypotension in combination with monoamine oxidase inhibitors. Another special interaction is the prevention of alcohol breakdown by disulfiram, metronidazole and some cephalosporins.

Other drugs inhibit more general drug oxidizing enzymes (the cytochrome P-450 system): for instance, cimetidine, ketoconazole, erythromycin and isoniazid. The target drugs include phenytoin, warfarin, theophylline and most benzodiazepines. As expected, this can produce drug accumulation, prolonged action and toxicity.

4. Finally, interactions can occur at the level of *drug excretion*. Urinary pH can alter the rate of drug clearance: alkaline urine enhances the elimination of salicylates, while acidification increases the excretion of amphetamines. There are some important examples of tubular interactions: probenecid inhibits the excretion of acidic drugs such as penicillin, salicylates and indomethacin. On the other hand, salicylates reduce the elimination of methotrexate, increasing the latter's toxicity. Finally, there is a very important and potentially lethal interaction between lithium and thiazide diuretics. The diuretics promote the excretion of sodium ions at the expense of lithium, rapidly leading to toxic plasma levels of the ion.

PHARMACOGENETICS

The genetic basis of variations in the handling of drugs, and in responses to them, is an area of growing interest. Apart from the well-investigated examples, some of which are described below, it is clear that there are many potentially more important variations. For example, people of Chinese and Japanese origin appear to be more susceptible to the effect of β-blockers. This has far-reaching implications for drug usage, and for drug testing. For instance, Japanese licensing authorities in fact insist that clinical trials should be performed locally. This type of variability is poorly understood. Most of the well-known pharmacogenetic variations are based on alterations at a single gene. One of the earliest examples, and of particular relevance to surgeons and anaesthetists, is suxamethonium apnoea. The duration of action of the muscle relaxant suxamethonium is abnormally prolonged, because the serum enzyme that hydrolyses the drug (pseudocholinesterase) is abnormal or even totally inactive. Many abnormal alleles of the gene have now been identified. Mild forms of the syndrome are relatively common and affect up to 4% of the population. The severe forms are extremely rare (1 in 100 000) or less. Another well-defined genetic variation concerns the metabolism, by acetylation, of hydralazine, procainamide and isoniazid. The minority of so-called 'slow acetylators', about a third or less of the population in the UK, have a greater likelihood of developing a systemic lupus erythematosus-like syndrome. However, a given dose of these drugs may also have greater efficacy in poor metabolizers.

A much more important genetic anomaly is the sex-linked *deficiency of the red cell enzyme glucose-6-phosphate dehydrogenase*. This plays a vital role in the protection of the erythrocyte from oxidants, including many drugs. There are at least two major variants of this syndrome, with up to 100 rarer forms. These syndromes have a very wide geographical distribution among Africans, Chinese and several ethnic groups around the Mediterranean: each of these groups has one or more abnormal variants of the enzyme. The more severe, Mediterranean, forms of this syndrome have a mild chronic anaemia with severe haemolysis on drug challenge. The African variant may not cause chronic anaemia. The drugs to be avoided include aspirin, sulphonamides, chloramphenicol, nitrofurantoin and, notoriously, the fava bean. It is interesting that antimalarial drugs, including quinine, chloroquine and primaquine, can also precipitate haemolysis, since it is thought that the enzyme deficiency confers some protection to the red cell against malarial parasites.

Finally, a much rarer group of conditions must be mentioned, not all of them genetically determined. These are the *porphyrias*, of which the best known is the autosomal dominant acute intermittent porphyria which can cause severe abdominal pain, peripheral neuropathy, psychiatric disturbance and even death. Variegate porphyria is similar in manifestations and inheritance pattern, while a somewhat milder form may accompany acquired liver disease such as cirrhosis. The biochemical abnormalities are very complex and the pathogenesis is very poorly understood. In general, it is necessary to avoid drugs which stimulate porphyrin synthesis. This is an extensive list. Among the most important are the enzyme inducers already described, but also the short-acting barbiturates, chlordiazepoxide, chlorpropamide, methyldopa, chloroquine, chloramphenicol, the contraceptive pill, and other oestrogens. It is essential to consider all potentially active drugs in patients with definite or suspected porphyria.

CONCLUSION

This chapter may provide a brief guide to some practical aspects of clinical pharmacology and therapeutics. One further area which must be mentioned is that of adverse drug reactions. The monitoring system in this country relies entirely on voluntary reporting to the Committee on Safety of Medicines, using the 'yellow cards'. It is therefore very susceptible to doctors' apathy, or to the feeling that a particular adverse reaction is too well known to need further reporting. Often this is true, but it must be emphasized that *all* suspected adverse reactions must be reported for new drugs, marked with a black triangle in the *British National Formulary* or in *MIMS*. Even well-known reactions should be reported if they are serious or potentially life-threatening.

No original references have been cited in this chapter. Instead, there is a short list of more or less comprehensive books which deal with all the above topics, and more, in far greater detail. Of course all books are out of date to some extent and become more so daily. Fortunately, there are many sources of information which are regularly updated. The *British National Formulary* is an obvious example, as is the *Drug and Therapeutics Bulletin*. There are also commercially published magazines (e.g. *Prescriber*) which provide valuable information on newly introduced drugs and put them in context. Some semi-official publications also provide data of this kind (for instance, from the Merseyside Resources Centre, MEREC). As mentioned earlier, hospital and regional drug information centres can answer many questions relating to drug usage. Finally, it is occasionally worth talking to a clinical pharmacologist, if you happen to find one.

Summary

1. Understanding basic clinical pharmacology is essential for the effective and safe use of drugs.

Summary (contd.)

2. Drug use has particular problems in pregnancy, the very young and elderly. In pregnancy, prescribe as few drugs as possible (preferably none).

3. In general, prescribe as few drugs as possible to minimize adverse effects and interactions. Always think about possible interactions when prescribing additional drugs.

4. Drug handling and response are altered in many diseases, particularly if liver or renal function is impaired.

5. Look for and report adverse drug reactions, especially with new drugs.

6. Be aware of sources of information, whether from books, journals, pharmacies or electronic databases: remember how quickly information becomes out-dated in this field.

Further reading

Denham M J, George C E (eds) 1990 Drugs in old age: new perspectives. British Medical Bulletin 46 (1)

Dukes M N G 1997 Meyler's side effects of drugs, 13th edn. Elsevier, Amsterdam (also Side Effects of Drugs Annual from same publisher)

Hardman J G, Limbird Lem Molinoff P B, Ruddon R W, Gilman A G 1996 Goodman and Gilman's pharmacological basis of therapeutics, 9th edn. Pergamon Press, New York

Grahame-Smith D G, Aronson J K 1992 Oxford textbook of clinical pharmacology and drug therapy, 2nd edn. Oxford University Press, Oxford (new edition in preparation)

Ritter J M, Lewis L D, Mant T G K 1995 A textbook of clinical pharmacology, 3rd edn. Edward Arnold, London (new edition in preparation)

Speight T M, Holford N H G 1997 Avery's drug treatment, 4th edn. ADIS International, Auckland

There are an enormous number of pharmacology and therapeutics based sites on the Internet. Many of these can be accessed through links in the following site: http://www.medfarm.unito.it/pharmaco/pharmaco.html

Another very useful site which includes up-to-date information on pharmacotherapy (and much else in medicine and surgery) is Medscape: http://www.medscape.com/

13

Evidence-based practice

J. W. McClenahan

Objectives

Understand the purpose and nature of valid, important and applicable evidence to augment personal experience.

- **Recognize the factors that help and hinder more widespread application of 'evidence-based practice' to surgery.**
- **Identify some suggestions for action that you or your colleagues could take.**

PURPOSE: LEARNING TO BECOME EVEN BETTER SURGEONS

You already use evidence of many kinds in your surgical practice. The more systematically you can do that, the better a surgeon you can become. The encouragement given to evidence-based practice (EBP) seeks to enhance the role that systematic, critical review of valid, reliable and applicable evidence can play in enabling you to:

- Perform more appropriate surgery
- Inform patients better about the probable benefits and risks of surgery for their condition – both in general, and in relation to their own personal circumstances
- Enlarge the range of surgical interventions that have been *reliably* shown to be worthwhile, by participation in higher quality research.

WHAT IS 'EVIDENCE-BASED PRACTICE'?

Definition

Different authors will give varying definitions of what the phrase means, or even limit it to evidence-based medicine (excluding other clinical professions such as nursing or therapies).

The following definition from McKibbon et al (1995) is the one I prefer:

> **Evidence-based practice: a definition**
>
> An approach to health care that promotes:
> - the collection, interpretation and integration [into clinical practice] of
> - valid, important, and applicable
>   - patient reported
>   - clinician observed, and
>   - research derived evidence.

There are several points of note about this definition. It is an *inclusive* approach to health care as a whole, not a narrow limitation to research-derived evidence, let alone just to evidence from randomized controlled trials (RCTs). It acknowledges the potential validity of patient perceptions and the clinician's own observations, and the use of judgement to integrate the different sorts of evidence. However, RCTs remain the 'gold standard' of evidence. They will be applicable if the types of patients included in them adequately match the real world of your clinical practice.

The definition also emphasizes the importance of building the use of evidence into your routine clinical practice, not just seeing it as an 'off-line' educational or research activity done by others. Furthermore, it implies the development of skills and judgement to decide what is valid, important, and applicable, both to the individual patient you are considering now, and the whole range of patients you are or should be treating.

The intellectual revolution in medicine

It is probably not much of an exaggeration to say that evidence-based practice constitutes an intellectual revolution in the practice of medicine (in the broadest sense – i.e., what doctors of all kinds, including surgeons, do). It has been fuelled in the last decade or so particularly by five interrelated factors:

1. The *knowledge explosion* – the exponential growth in published research and knowledge.

2. The particular technique of *meta-analysis* – pooling the results of multiple clinical trials to derive more robust conclusions than any one alone can support.

3. The rapid evolution of *systematic review* – now a formalized, thorough, and reproducible (but resource-intensive) method of finding virtually all evidence on a topic, grading it by quality and relevance, and summarizing the results in a form able to be peer reviewed, and used by busy clinicians.

4. The organization of the *International Cochrane Collaboration*. This links researchers, information analysts, and practising clinicians world wide. In the UK, two centres of particular importance are the Cochrane Centre in Oxford, and the Centre for Reviews and Dissemination in York. The collaboration helps to resource systematic reviews and engages with others in doing so world-wide.

5. Technological developments in *knowledge distribution* – particularly CD-Rom and the Internet – which make knowledge widely accessible easily and relatively cheaply. Increasingly, this means in the ward, operating theatre, diagnostic department, outpatient clinic, clinical staff's own offices, and GP surgeries, as well as in libraries, post-graduate centres, and people's own homes.

Clinical effectiveness

Evidence-based practice aims to improve clinical effectiveness – doing the right things for the right people at the right time in the best known way in routine practice. This means translating the findings of research which demonstrated *efficacy* – that there was a difference in a controlled trial in favour of one intervention over another – into *effective use* for a real population of patients.

Achieving clinical effectiveness requires:

- Professional staff who have up-to-date knowledge and skills, together with appropriate attitudes
- Working together in a cohesive and coordinated fashion within clinical teams
- The support of managers to meet both patient needs and strategic needs of the organization. (Batstone & Edwards 1997)

For surgeons, this can mean some significant personal changes or even challenges. Only those with strong individual egos seem to become surgeons, and surgery has a competitive culture. Acknowledging the importance of teamwork is perhaps easier now than allowing that managers have a valid role to play, but both run counter to many stereotypes if not the reality of modern surgery. Some of your behaviours may have to be unlearned!

Weren't we doing it anyway?

No conscientious medical practitioner I know wants to perform badly, and most make strenuous efforts to keep up to date. So it hurts to be told that your practice could be improved if you were to change the way you approach the use of evidence. You think that you already do the best you can with your limited time and, with help from your colleagues, you already use evidence – you were taught to do so by your professors or consultants or you have been challenged by your up-and-coming juniors. Well, yes ... up to a point.

The reality, as opposed to the aspiration, is that there are often long delays between the production of convincing research evidence and its widespread adoption. The proponents of evidence-based practice believe, often with justification, that these delays could and should be shortened.

Things are getting better, however. A historical perspective illustrates the point. Prevention of scurvy took roughly 2 centuries between the first evidence of efficacy in 1601 (James Lancaster) and its routine adoption by the British Navy from 1775–1814. In this century, thrombolytic therapy post-MI, and *H. pylori* eradication therapy took about 2 decades (from the 1970s to the 1990s) to be acknowledged as appropriate, and gain general acceptance as what ought to be done (even if its application is still uneven) (see for example Antman et al 1992). Surfactants for neonates were adopted even more quickly – in part because their effects were obvious and dramatic, and in part because they went 'with the grain' of clinical culture and experience.

What EBP is not, but is feared to be

Just cost-cutting, or being banned from doing certain procedures?

Many doctors fear that EBP is just an attempt to reduce costs. They therefore react negatively. However, careful interpretation of the evidence may suggest that *different* things be done, some of which may cost more, some less, and some about the same. Part of the senior surgeon's task is about balancing the many competing demands on resources, and evidence of effectiveness should play a bigger part in such decisions in future.

Another reduction in clinical freedom, or 'cook-book' medicine?

Appropriate integration of research evidence into clinical practice poses no threat to clinical freedom (using the McKibbon et al definition), except to help you avoid unnecessary or indefensible mistakes. Is that the freedom you want to retain?

How the evidence is used, and how guidelines, protocols, or 'the way we do things here' are established and used locally will determine the nature and extent of clinical freedom you retain. By establishing more clearly your own and your colleagues' understanding of what is known with reasonable certainty, based on research evidence, experience, and patient feedback, you can make commonplace practice more consistent, and higher quality easier to deliver, audit, and sustain. The result should be to leave more, not less, freedom and time to use your judgement in areas where the circumstances are not routine, the research-based evidence is absent or equivocal, or the patient's individual preferences are uniquely out of the ordinary.

Just for doctors, or just for clinical staff?

Evidence-based practice is just as relevant for patients and their families or carers, and for managers, as it is for clinical staff. Media attention and the Internet now make much more of the evidence widely available.

WHO IS EBP FOR?

At least five major groups of people have a use for EBP:

- Patients (who want better informed discussions with their surgeon about options and risks)
- Professionals (who can improve their practice)
- Providers (who seek greater effectiveness for their organizations)
- Purchasers (now Commissioners – alas the alliterative loss!) (who want to get the best quality service they can afford)
- Public (who want assurance that all of the above is happening properly in their interests).

HOW CAN EVIDENCE MAKE A DIFFERENCE?

Different nature of availability of evidence

Evidence can impact practice in several different ways, and what needs to be done to improve things depends on the nature of the evidence, and what sort of barriers prevent its use. Examples (not exhaustive) are shown in Table 13.1.

Table 13.1 Examples and issues

Nature of evidence	Examples	Issues
Evidence convincing, widely accepted, but not universally applied	Early thrombolytic therapy for AMI	(Often mistaken) belief that 'we already do it here' – local and national audits often show otherwise Achieving organizational change to allow it
Evidence readily available but not sought	Which surgical patients benefit from DVT prophylaxis Whom should we treat for atrial fibrillation?	Shifting professional attitudes to seeking evidence CPD (continuous professional development) Interpretive skills (critical appraisal training)
Evidence sought, but not locally accessible at the relevant time or place	As above, and ... Adjuvant therapy following surgical removal of cancers	Organizational and technical infrastructure Information and library facilities and staffing Technical skills training
Evidence actively sought, not found, equivocal or disputed	When should we remove catheters after paediatric cardiac surgery?	Establishing effective local guidelines, and local audit or research projects Feedback to national R&D priority setting or local academic centre

Perceived power of vision	x	Perceived pain of present	x	Perceived feasibility of first steps	>	Perceived pain of change

Fig 13.1 Beckhard's change equation

What helps or hinders change?

The 'change equation' (adapted from Beckhard & Harris 1987) is shown in Figure 13.1.

You need to pay attention to all four boxes to maximize the likelihood of successful use of evidence to change practice. You also need to acknowledge that you may be able to work on the *perception* that others have of the proposed changes as well as the 'real' content of the change, since for them, their perception *is* the reality.

This means:

- Presenting a clear and persuasive view of how things might be (the vision) in terms relevant to the intended audience
- Showing the drawbacks of the present (perhaps unsatisfactory or even dangerous) state of affairs, and making sure that other people become as uncomfortable with it as you are yourself
- Devising some initial changes that people see as feasible to get started (so make them as easy to adopt as possible)
- Minimizing the discomfort of the change as it will be *perceived* by individuals or groups affected.

Changing clinical practice is a multi-stage process

Change does not happen all at once, and different influences work at different stages of people's readiness for change. It is a mistake to presume that a rational argument, clearly and forcefully presented, will of itself predispose people to change, especially if they are not yet emotionally ready even to believe it is necessary at all.

Figure 13.2 shows one model of individual change (based on Prochaska & DiClemente 1984) that may be helpful in understanding where you and your colleagues stand. It is crucial to acknowledge the importance of the early stages – initial awareness of the possibility of change, and recognition of a need to change. This can often take time (months, or occasionally years, in some cases) to work through.

Where the major personal block is an emotional one, restating the rational case ever more forcefully to someone is positively unhelpful. Ask rather than tell, and try to find out what emotion is being triggered by your proposal (or your own reaction to others' proposals) and seek to deal with *that* first.

Organizational change is a slower process than you expect – be patient

You may be used in your surgical team to making decisions and seeing them implemented very quickly or even instantly, if the power to change lies wholly within the surgical team. However, much of the improvement in clinical practice suggested by research evidence requires change on a broader organizational front. Many people with different professions, personal backgrounds, beliefs and values may have to be persuaded. Evaluation of change 'in the field' in response to evidence suggests four major hindrances to change at a scale larger than a single clinical team:

1. *Getting momentum going* – raising awareness and recognition of the need to change takes time, patience, and repeated application as the 'cast of characters' is constantly changing in the hectic pace of NHS reorganization.
2. *Staff turnover* – original sponsors of change may leave the organization.
3. *Action* – getting guidelines agreed and accepted is more difficult than most people initially believe is possible.
4. *Implementation and maintenance* – if you think getting guidelines agreed is the hard part, think again. After that is when the most difficult (but ultimately rewarding) part really starts. To engage others more widely beyond the enthusiasts, you or a small group around you will need yet more patience, careful planning, wide consultation and listening, and adequate resource to see your proposals into widespread and sustained use. Grol (1997) has a useful review of the different types of approach that could be adopted, and the evidence for their effectiveness.

You need other sorts of information as well as the research and clinical evidence

In addition to the research and clinical evidence which will be a familiar requirement, you will find that engaging others will require other sorts of information. You

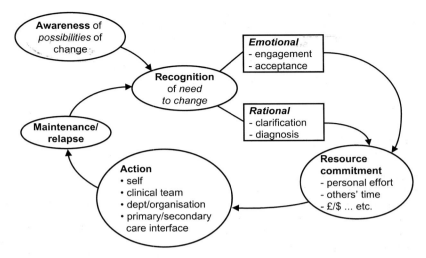

Fig 13.2   A model of individual change

need to know many other things too, some relatively obvious, others perhaps unexpected:

- Local demographics and prevalence of the disease or condition of interest. How many people does it affect? How seriously?
- Actual local practice. Audit of current practice, and open discussion with colleagues may reveal unexpected differences between what you believe *should* happen or *think* is already happening, and what actually *does* happen.
- Patients' and service users' views. Have you asked them, or looked for previous evidence of their views, rather than what you think their views are, or ought to be?
- Understanding of the organizational context. How does the diagnostic, treatment and care process actually work at present, and who would be affected by proposed changes? How are referral decisions influenced? How could you change that?
- Local 'political insight'. Who has a stake in this process? What do they think about the issues? What else is on their agenda that may help, or hinder, progress in the direction you want?
- Knowledge of where resources might be obtainable. As the change is unlikely to be completely neutral in resource terms, you will at least need to know where resources (e.g. time, energy, money, facilities) might be freed up to pump prime change, or where additional resources might be sought with some chance of success.

WHAT SEEMS TO HELP?

In our own research into the process of implementing evidence-led change in North Thames region, six factors seem to make progress more likely (Smith & McClenahan 1997, 1998):

- Support from both managers and clinicians at a senior level
- Adequate resourcing in relation to the scale of ambition
- A project management approach, with clarity about lead roles, and clarity of objectives for the change process on a realistic scale (neither over-ambitious nor too modest)
- Having, or putting in place, the right organizational infrastructure to support clinical service improvements
- An understanding of change management as a process
- Closing the loop properly – auditing whether clinical *processes* have changed to match those associated with efficacy in a research environment. It is usually not possible or necessary to audit outcomes themselves – that was what the research was about.

SOME SUGGESTIONS FOR ACTION

Depending on your present level of seniority and influence, you might want to consider some of the following ways of making a difference:

- Consider your own attitude to the possibility of improvement to your own practice. Talk it over with colleagues. Analyse your emotional reactions as well as the practical and rational ones.
- Make sure you get access to information sources (particularly the Cochrane database (CD-Rom),

Medline, CINAHL, and the Internet) and learn how to make use of them. Encourage *all* staff whom you manage to learn to use them. Get help from others with the relevant skills.

- Seek local training (if you have not already had some) in *critical appraisal* – the process of reviewing published research evidence to assess its quality and relevance to your own patients' circumstances. Continue to practise it in your routine work.
- Try to make or reinforce connections between the clinical effectiveness committee (or its local equivalent) and its sub groups; clinical audit; library and information services; multi-disciplinary team working; education and training; Continuous Professional Development/Continuing Medical Education; guideline development; and patient information provision.
- Seek management support for implementing desired change processes: in your own team; across departments; for common clinical conditions; and across organizational boundaries with primary and tertiary care.
- For the real enthusiast: take part in a systematic review of an area of practice you are interested in.

References

Antman E M, Lau J, Kupelnick B, Mosteller F, Chalmers T C 1992 A comparison of results of meta-analyses of randomized control trials and recommendations of clinical experts. Treatments for myocardial infarction. Journal of the American Medical Association 268: 240–248

Batstone G Edwards M 1997 Challenges in promoting clinical effectiveness and the use of evidence. In: Harrison A (ed) Health care UK, 1996/7. Kings Fund Policy Institute, Kings Fund, London

Beckhard R, Harris R T 1987 Organizational transitions: managing complex change (2nd edn). Addison Wesley, Reading, Massachusetts

Grol R 1997 Beliefs and evidence in changing clinical practice. British Medical Journal 315: 418–421

McKibbon K, Wilczynski N, Hayward R S, Walker-Dilks C, Haynes R B 1995. The medical literature as a resource for evidence based care. Internet only: http://hiru.mcmaster.ca/hiru/medline/mdl-ebc.htm

Prochaska J, DiClemente C 1984 The transtheoretical approach: crossing traditional boundaries of therapy. Dow Jones–Irwin, Homewood, Illinois

Smith L, McClenahan J W 1997 Putting practitioners through the paces: initial findings in our evaluation of putting evidence into practice. King's Fund and North Thames R&D division, London

Smith L, McClenahan J W 1998 Snakes and ladders: levers, obstacles and solutions to putting evidence into practice. King's Fund and North Thames R&D division, London

14

Decision making

R. M. Kirk

Objectives

- **Understand why opinions differ between surgeons faced with similar problems.**
- **Recognize that decisions require the best available information – and are valid only at the time they are made.**
- **In decision making there is a trade-off between accuracy and simplicity. Identify the discriminating features.**

INTRODUCTION

Surgical practice varies remarkably. A patient with a particular condition may be treated expectantly by one surgeon and operated upon by another. In theory, once the diagnosis of a common condition is made, it should be possible to determine the best action from previous trials. However, many important surgical and other decisions cannot be made with mathematical precision. In collecting and analysing information we are all selective in what we dismiss and what we accept as valid. When we have the information we interpret it idiosyncratically (Greek: *idios* = one's own + *syn* = together + *krasis* = a mixing; hence, according to one's own constitution or temperament).

Our characters, philosophy and previous experience colour our judgement. We often cannot logically justify why we made a particular decision, any more than we can give the real reasons why we studied medicine, chose a surgical career, or chose a particular life partner.

Attempts to apply reason may be thwarted because the problem is too complex, with too many imponderables. Often the aspects that can be tested objectively are unimportant while the crucial aspects are not amenable to objective testing in our present state of knowledge. This should not deter us from attempting to deduce the implications of different courses of action. Some surgeons appear to get better results than others; perhaps they have exceptional inborn technical skills, but more often they make a higher percentage of decisions that prove to be correct. Spencer taught that good surgery required 75% decision making and 25% dexterity (Spencer 1979).

PROCESSING INFORMATION

Personal and acquired experience

In the distant past clinicians based their decisions on their own experience, supplemented by advice from those colleagues with whom they came into contact. With the availability of written treatises they were given access to wider experience. We are fortunate in being able to survey the accumulated experience of our colleagues throughout the world. However, it remains our own responsibility to view critically what we read. The validity of a report must be judged on the clarity and logic of the investigation and the soundness of the interpretation. It is not always necessary to be statistically competent to detect flaws in the construction of an experiment or the conclusions drawn from the findings (See Chs 44, 45).

Incomplete data

Decision making is facilitated if all the required information is available. However, in surgical practice we never have a complete knowledge of the physical and psychological state of the patient and of the extent and severity of the condition we are treating. Moreover, it is often necessary to take some action even before all the available information reaches us.

Discriminating features

A frequent cause of failure, especially among inexperienced clinicians, is indiscriminate over-collection of information, resulting in confusion. Long lists can be composed of the presenting features of recognized conditions but if all the features are given equal 'weight' the possible interpretations are multiplied. Identify the cardinal features (Latin *cardinis* = a hinge, i.e. on which the diagnosis hinges), and base decisions on them.

Oversimplification

Because so many factors affect clinical diagnosis and impinge on treatment decisions, it is sometimes convenient to identify those aspects that can be set aside or ignored, in order to focus on fewer determinants. This method is applied when trials of differing treatments are planned; limits are placed on the range of age, sex, general condition and certain features of the disease under study. Provided these are fulfilled, patients can be entered into the trial. There may, however, be so many factors having an effect on outcome that some have to be excluded from consideration. If the process is taken too far, the problem becomes oversimplified. Numerical probabilities are calculated that are not valid in real life. As the American writer, H L Mencken is said to have stated, 'To every complex problem, there is a simple – and usually wrong – answer.'

A similar oversimplification may mar judgement of individual cases so that important factors are brushed aside.

Distracting pressures

It is rare to have but a single patient on whom to concentrate. Other patients and other activities need attention. Rank these demands in order of priority, remembering that this order is not static.

In battles and major disasters the urgency of the calls may be overwhelming. Doctors then need to select those whose lives can be saved by quick action, setting aside for the moment those requiring too much time and those whose lives are not endangered. This often agonizing series of decisions is called 'triage' (Old French: *trier* = to pick, select).

Processing information

- **All facts are not of equal importance**
- **Identify discriminating features**
- **Critically read the literature. Trials are designed for 'black or white' situations; most clinical decisions involve various shades of grey**

AIDS TO DECISION MAKING

In some cases repeated experience has shown that particular attitudes to 'set' circumstances produce the best results. These responses are formalized in various recommendations (Greep & Siezenis 1989).

Algorithms (Ar. al-Khwarazmi, modern Khiva in Uzbekistan). In this city lived the 9th-century mathematician Abu Ja'far Mohammed ben Musa, who developed a rule for solving a problem in a finite number of steps, hence a step by step method for progressing through a fairly straightforward clinical decision (See Ch. 3, Fig. 3.2). The sequential steps are followed automatically, since the algorithms incorporate standard practice.

Protocol (Greek: *protos* = first + *kolla* = glue; a glued-on first leaf of a manuscript). Among other things it is a set of rules, or uniform method, of approaching a problem. It is sometimes displayed as a *flow chart* (See Ch. 11, Fig. 11.1) with alternative pathways to treat differing circumstances or outcomes.

Guidelines When outcomes from differing treatments have not been statistically determined, a particular view may be given the approval of an authoritative person or body. The issuing of guidelines has become a contentious issue in recent years because those who, for good reason, do not follow the guidelines, may feel vulnerable to criticism if the outcome in a particular case is poor.

Decision trees

Reliable information exists on outcomes in some well defined circumstances, allowing comparisons of differing treatments (Clarke 1989, Debsky et al, 1991). For example, a malignant condition is amenable to treatment by either operation or radiotherapy. If reliable reports are available on outcome with each method, a decision tree can be constructed with probability of the patient being better, the same, or worse after a defined interval. All the probable outcomes for a particular course of action should add up to 1 (Fig. 14.1). In addition to the objective outcome measure, there is also a subjective value – what the patient sees as acceptable, called a 'utility' (Royal College of Physicians 1975). A high utility value indicates a desirable result to the patient, a low value indicates an undesirable result. The utility is multiplied by the probability to produce an 'expected utility'. The sums of the expected utilities for each or all the possible courses of action can be compared. The course gaining the highest expected utility should be the preferred one (Fig. 14.2).

Objective evidence that can be constructed in this way may be difficult to accumulate. However, the considerations that go into the construction of a decision tree make a worthwhile exercise when trying to decide between courses of action. The patient's view of 'utility' may differ from yours, and must be included in the equation.

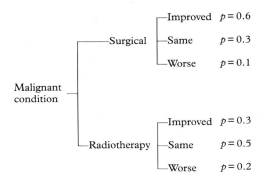

Fig 14.1 A simple decision tree comparing the probability (p) of outcomes for two methods of treating a malignant condition.

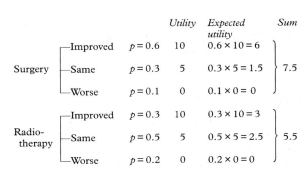

Fig 14.2 The utility (subjective benefit or disability) resulting from the outcome is graded from 10 (good) to 0 (bad). The product of probability (p) and utility is the 'expected utility'. Finally, the sum of the expected utilities for each decision can be compared. The course scoring the highest mark is the preferred one, in this case, surgery.

Deferment

The solution to a puzzle often appears apparently spontaneously as the result of a shift in the way that the problem is viewed. For this reason, when time permits, put aside the decision when an impasse is reached and reconsider it later.

Ask advice

This has two advantages. An often overlooked virtue is that in laying out the problem to some one else, you clarify your own thoughts, placing the facts in a manageable order. The second advantage, provided you choose someone who is not involved in the problem, is that the advice is free of the 'baggage' of emotional commitment. We tend to feel that if a great deal of effort has already been invested in a particular aspect, this somehow has a value of its own, so that we are reluctant to abandon it and cut our losses.

ACTING ON YOUR DECISION

> If you decide to act unconventionally, contrary to authorized teaching, first consider how you will face your patient, your peers, and your own conscience, if disaster follows.

Preparation

Standard reactions are appropriate in certain conditions. Examples are external haemorrhage, respiratory obstruction and cardiac arrest. Of course, following standardized algorithms, protocols and guidelines will not save everyone and indeed may, rarely, be inappropriate. Nevertheless, such routines are likely to save the greatest number of lives. Whenever you can identify a routine reaction that is safe and acceptable, learn it and practise using it. Regrettably, many medical practitioners prove to be inexpert when tested in procedures such as administering cardiac resuscitation.

Anticipation

Actively look for predictable features that will affect your decisions. After selecting a course of action, do not totally reject the ones you have passed over. Consider the ill-effects your action may produce if you have misjudged the condition, and be ready to change it if necessary. Your management may, of itself, produce predictable effects that should be anticipated, recognized, and corrected if necessary.

Provisional decisions

All decisions must be provisional. They rest on incomplete knowledge and on the interpretation of events at the time they are made. The situation may alter rapidly from progression of the presenting condition and from the effects of your response. The initial plan may be called the strategy (adapted from Greek: *stratos* = army + *agein* = to lead; hence, the battle plan). You monitor the situation as it is played out and should respond as necessary by altering the tactics (again, adapted from Greek: *taktos* = ordered; in warfare = manoeuvring in the presence of the enemy). Too often, initially good management fails because it is not reviewed and revised in the light of subsequent changes. Decide what needs to be monitored as an indication of deterioration and recovery (Fig. 14.3). Be willing to accept that your actions are incorrect early, and change tactics. Most people find the admission of error to be painful and a few will not, for this reason, accept that they have made a mistake and so doggedly refuse to respond to changed circumstances. Such people should not pursue a surgical career.

Acting on your decision

- **Prepare**
- **Anticipate likely or possible developments**
- **All decisions are provisional**

PERSONAL AUDIT

Whether or not others review your results, make sure that you look back on your successes and failures. A successful outcome does not necessarily signify that you have acted wisely, nor does failure necessarily denote that your actions were at fault. Sometimes you conclude that the patient has recovered in spite of errors in your management. At other times your may console yourself that your decisions were correct but the problems were overwhelming or there were factors that you

could not be aware of. Identify, admit and learn from your mistakes. Some people, claiming to be experienced, have merely repeated the same mistakes over a long period. Remember the statement of the novelist, Thomas Hardy, 'Experience is as to intensity, not as to duration.'

Summary

1. Identify the discriminating features which override less reliable, perhaps contradictory features.
2. Do not be obsessed with your personal, perhaps limited, experience, which may not be typical.
3. Critically read the surgical literature to determine the best action to take in standard circumstances. Keep up to date, since evidence gathered at one time is not necessarily of permanent value, as fresh assessments are made.
4. If you make a decision to act, do not continue doggedly with it if circumstances change. The decision is only for the time that it was made.
5. Constantly monitor the condition of the patient to note the effect of the action and be ready to change course if necessary.
6. Whenever you have a difficult decision to make, ask yourself, 'If my selected course of management fails, can I justify it to the patient, to my peers, and most importantly to myself?'
7. Ask advice. Outlining the problem clarifies your own thoughts. Choose a confidant with no responsibility for the problem.
8. Carefully record and audit your results. Learn from your mistakes – and your successes.

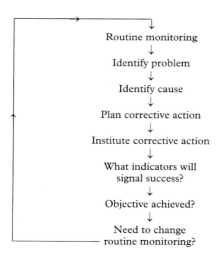

Routine monitoring
↓
Identify problem
↓
Identify cause
↓
Plan corrective action
↓
Institute corrective action
↓
What indicators will signal success?
↓
Objective achieved?
↓
Need to change routine monitoring?

Fig 14.3 The essential part played by planned monitoring after taking a decision and acting on it. There is no point at which this can be relaxed until the patient is fully recovered. As the circumstances change and effective action is taken, the response must be checked and, when correction is achieved, routine monitoring must be continued.

References

Clarke J 1989 Decision making in surgical practice. World Journal of Surgery 13: 245–257

Debsky A S, Naglie G, Krahn M D, Naimark D, Redelmeier D A 1991 Primer on medical decision analysis. Part I: Getting started. Medical Decision Making 17: 123–125

Greep J M, Siezenis L M L C 1989 Methods of decision analysis: protocols, decision trees and algorithms in medicine. World Journal of Surgery 13: 240–244

Royal College of Physicians 1975 The role of utility in decision making. Journal of the Royal College of Physicians of London 9: 225–230

Spencer F C 1979 Competence and compassion; two qualities of surgical excellence. Bulletin of the American College of Surgeons 64: 15–22

 Further reading

Balla J I, Elstein A S, Christensen C 1989 Obstacles to acceptance of clinical decision analysis. British Medical Journal 298: 579–582

Eisman B, Anderson B 1989 Surgical decision making – introduction. World Journal of Surgery 13: 2392

Elstein A S, Bordage G 1988 Psychology of clinical reasoning. In: Dowie J, Elstein A S (eds) Professional judgement. A reader in clinical decision making. Cambridge University Press, Cambridge, pp 109–129

Philips C (ed.) 1988 Logic in medicine. British Medical Journal, London

Thornton J G, Lilford R J, Johnson N 1992 Decision analysis in medicine. British Medical Journal 304: 1099–1103

Weinstein M C, Fineberg H V (eds) 1980 Clinical decision analysis. Saunders, Philadelphia

Preparations for surgery

15

Consent for surgical treatment

L. Doyal

Objectives

- **Recognize the need to establish trust and confidence in patients under your care.**
- **Understand that a signature on a consent form is not legal proof that informed consent has been given.**
- **Realise that you must warn patients of the hazards as well as the benefits of surgical treatment.**
- **Identify and deal appropriately with difficulties in gaining consent. Respect the confidentiality of your dealings with patients.**

For surgery to be successful, there must be a relationship of trust and confidence between surgeon and patient. Otherwise, patients will be reticent to present themselves for treatment or to divulge the detailed personal information required for recording accurate case histories and making successful diagnoses. Aside from the belief that their care will conform to a high clinical standard, the trust of patients also depends on their belief that their autonomy will be respected – that they will have the right to decide their own medical destiny, whatever anyone else may think.

Moral rights are like that. They indicate claims that individuals can legitimately make against others who have corresponding duties to respect those claims. To the degree that we believe that the right to make such a claim exists, then those on whom it is properly made must respect it and act accordingly, irrespective of their preferences. Examples of often-cited moral rights emphasize the entitlement of individuals to self-determination – to be able to pursue life goals and perceived interests in ways in which the individual has chosen – provided that others are not harmed in the process. Moral rights might or might not be backed up by the

force of law. For example, the legal right of women to choose to have an abortion under certain circumstances is regarded as immoral by those who believe that a fetus has the rights of a born child. In short, our beliefs about who has a right to what inform our decisions about how we should act toward others if our actions are to be deemed morally, and perhaps legally, acceptable.

The general right of surgical patients to self-determination can be subdivided into three further rights: to informed consent, to the truth and to confidentiality. The latter two clearly follow from the first. Choices cannot be properly informed on the basis of deception and cannot be respected if what patients deem private is made public. Therefore, it is the principle of informed consent itself which is fundamental and on which both the mortality and the legality of good surgical practice partly depend.

THE MORAL IMPORTANCE OF INFORMED CONSENT

The moral unacceptability of anyone exercising unlimited power over others is at the heart of many of our liberal values. It is our capacity for rational choice that differentiates humans from other creatures. Respect for this capacity – especially our right to be the informed gatekeepers of our own bodies – is an indication of the seriousness with which we respect the humanity and dignity of others.

What is informed consent?

For patients to give their informed consent to surgery – to be able to make a considered choice about what is in their personal interests – they must receive sufficient accurate information about their illness, the proposed treatment and its prognosis. For this to be more than a moral abstraction, the surgeon must complete four general tasks. Firstly, the procedure itself must be described, including information about its practical implications and probable prognosis. Secondly, the probability of specific associated risks or complications should be revealed. Thirdly, it should not be assumed that the patient already knows the risks of other aspects of the proposed surgical procedure, such as the complications that might result from a general anaesthetic, bed rest, intravenous fluids or a catheter. Finally, other surgical or medical alternatives to the proposed treatment – including non-treatment – should be outlined, along with their general advantages and disadvantages.

Ideally, the amount of such information should be that which mentally competent patients require to make their informed choice a realistic possibility. Competence should be thought of here as the ability to understand, retain and deliberate about such information and to accept its applicability to themselves. Surgeons should remember that the amount of information they are obligated to divulge may well change depending on what they should know about their patients as individuals. For example, it may not be necessary for a manual labourer to be told of an extremely small operative risk of minor stiffness in one finger. This would obviously not be true of a concert pianist, underlining the importance of recording the patient's employment in case notes and referring to it in the presentation of case histories.

Good consenting practice

As much as possible, the physical surroundings during the discussion between surgeon and patient should be conducive to easy, quiet conversation. Ideally, the place should be private and free of disturbances and interruptions by junior staff or medical students following in retinue on a busy Nightingale ward. The surgeon should not stand threateningly over a patient in bed and should avoid giving the appearance of being rushed by other duties. Empathy with the patient will be crucial.

The language with which the surgeon communicates should be as simple as possible, avoiding needless technicalities. When serious matters are being discussed, it is often helpful for a relative or friend to be present – always assuming that patients have given their permission. This is both for support and to help ensure that the patient really does understand – both at the time the information is given and later when the patient returns home. In the hospital ward, nurses with whom the patient is familiar can often fulfill this role very effectively. Appropriate leaflets or booklets can be of great help, and innovative work is also being done with audio recording of interviews with patients who are encouraged to take the recording home to discuss with others.

Having attempted to provide clear information, it is then important to try to determine whether or not the patient has actually understood it. No doubt there will be time constraints on doing both. However, it is clear that the surgeon is morally responsible for attempting to achieve both to an acceptable standard. There are a variety of ways in which this might be done – asking patients to go back over what has been said in their own terms, for example, and asking them at various times if they have any questions. The more confident surgeons become in exercising these skills, the less time it will take to obtain effective consent.

Surgeons have often limited the amount of information given to patients on the grounds of the potential distress that might result. This is unacceptable, if the long-term aim is to keep the patient in ignorance. All competent individuals have a right to decide what is and is not in their best interests, even if what they decide is not endorsed by their professional advisors. It would not be morally acceptable for a solicitor or accountant to delude their clients on the grounds that they did not want to distress them about the possibility of losing a court action or of going bankrupt. Why should the moral obligations of the surgeon be any different?

The consent form

In principle, the consent form which patients should sign before having surgery is a public and permanent affirmation that they have indeed agreed to it. All competent patients who are 16 years or older should sign the form for all surgical procedures involving a general anaesthetic. A form should also be signed by the patient for procedures under local anaesthetic if there might be significant sequelae – for example, an excision of skin lesions. Clinicians obtaining the consent should also sign the form to indicate that, to the best of their knowledge, the patient has both been given and understands the information necessary to make a considered judgement.

This being said, two things should be remembered about the consent form. Firstly, it is not necessary for competent patients to sign it for all surgical interventions. Simple investigative procedures (e.g. venepuncture) which involve minimal risk of harm can be undertaken on the basis of a verbal explanation of what they physically entail. Explicit verbal consent should then be requested, although consent can be assumed to be implied if the patient then accepts the procedure. Secondly, the consent form is not legal proof that consent has been given – something that should always be borne in mind when there is a temptation to cut corners as regards good consenting practice. At most, it is only one piece of evidence that some attempt was made to obtain informed consent, not that it was a morally or legally satisfactory attempt.

THE LEGAL IMPORTANCE OF INFORMED CONSENT

Aside from its general moral and clinical importance, doctors also have a legal obligation to respect the patient's right to consent to treatment.

Battery

In principle, battery is a violation of the civil law which forbids intentionally touching other persons without their consent. For example, a woman won damages in the UK for this reason because she was given a sterilization to which she did not agree in the aftermath of a gynaecological operation for another problem. In Canada, a woman who made it clear that she wanted to be injected in one arm successfully sued when she received the injection in the other! The harm resulting from battery is not necessarily physical. In law, a battery can be deemed to have occurred without such harm having taken place. Here harm should be construed as the violation of the right of persons to exercise autonomous control over their own bodies.

Of course, in many situations involving minor surgical procedures or tests, it will not be possible or advisable specifically to ask for the consent of patients every time they are touched. Were this the case, surgery would become practically impossible. But it does not follow that even here the consent of patients is legally irrelevant. Rather, as we have just seen, they can be said to have given their implied consent by virtue of the fact that they have presented themselves for treatment and have accepted what is offered. A man once argued in the USA, for example, that a ship's surgeon had committed a battery because he was vaccinated without having given specific verbal permission for the injection to be administered. He lost on the grounds that his consent was implied since he was in a queue of people who were clearly waiting to be injected and he held out his arm when his turn came!

Clearly, there will be many situations which are much less clear-cut. For example, is there a risk of battery if patients claim that had they been given more information before surgery, they would have refused it? If the patients are informed in broad terms of the general nature of their conditions and the surgery proposed to try to correct them, if they are not deliberately deceived about this information, if they give no indication of desiring not to proceed by asking for more information, and if they sign the appropriate consent form then the answer is probably no. Of course, this presupposes that the surgeon has not deprived the patient of information that has been specifically requested, or,

returning to our example of an unwanted hysterectomy, has usurped a clinical choice now commonly regarded as remaining with the patient.

Negligence

Battery is not the only legal action surgeons risk for inadequately respecting their patients' right to informed consent. In an important case, Mrs Sidaway suffered paralysis resulting from spinal surgery to relieve pressure on a nerve root without being told that the operation carried a small risk of paralysis. Here, it was judged that she had not been a victim of battery because, again, she had given her general consent to the surgery in question. However, her solicitors then claimed negligence, the legal action now recommended in such cases. The negligence concerns the professional duty of surgeons properly to advise patients not just about the proposed surgery but also about its potential hazards. In such cases, patients argue that, had they known the risks in question, they would not have proceeded with the surgery.

It would again be wrong to assume that in these circumstances surgeons are protected from such accusations by a signed consent form for treatment. Patients might still successfully argue that even though they had signed the form, they were not given enough relevant information to make an informed decision before they signed and/or that they were unaware of the significance of the form. There is no escaping the general duty of surgeons to disclose information about potentially harmful side-effects and to do so in a way that the patient can understand in principle. For example, in all cases other than those of acute emergencies, care must be taken to provide translations for non-English-speaking patients.

How are we to establish whether or not compliance with this duty has been sufficient – whether or not enough information has been disclosed about risks so that the rights of patients are respected? Legal judgments concerning negligent standards of adequate disclosure in the UK are still primarily determined by the profession itself. Suppose that expert witnesses for the defence are regarded by the court as constituting a recognized body of professional opinion. If they agree that they would have communicated the same amount of information in similar circumstances as the defendant then this should be sufficient to ensure that the plaintiff will lose the legal action. In other words, in such actions the judge does not decide which expert witnesses are right – those for the plaintiff or defendant. All that is required to exonerate the latter is for a responsible body of professional opinion to endorse the action in dispute even if the endorsement does not represent the views of the majority of members of the profession.

Recent legal developments have underlined this 'professional standard' in the determination of what constitutes negligent informed consent. In the Sidaway case, for example, a majority of appellate judges in the House of Lords agreed with this approach to determining negligence, as have other judges since. However, many have also warned of the dangers of completely equating the right of patients to information with standards set by the profession. Indeed, in the Sidaway case, one judge stated in a minority opinion that there will be some information about surgery, for example serious hazards, which any 'prudent' patient would wish to know before giving consent to proceed. A similar legal standard of negligence as regards informed consent is found in North America and is increasingly becoming accepted good practice by the medical profession in the UK.

Therefore, surgeons should not look to the law for advice for how much information about risks and side-effects is morally required by the right of their patients to informed consent. They should ask what a resonable person would want to know under similar circumstances, especially in the context of any other personal information they have about the patient and their public and private interests. They should disclose the same amount of information about risks to their patients as they would wish to be communicated to their close friends and relatives. The fact that an adequate amount of information for informed consent may be legally acceptable does not entail that this should be regarded as professionally or morally acceptable.

The unconscious adult patient

Suppose that a surgeon in the accident and emergency (A&E) department is confronted with the victim of an automobile accident who requires an immediate operation to save life or to prevent permanent and serious disability. Here there is a clear duty to treat, despite the fact that it is impossible to obtain the patient's consent, and there would be no risk of battery if surgery proceeded. This is not because the surgeon becomes the proxy of the patient and makes a substituted judgement on his behalf, one which attempts to second guess what the choice of the patient would have been. It is because it is the surgeon's moral and legal responsibility to act in the patient's best interests – to do what is 'necessary' since there is no way of knowing for certain what the patient might choose.

Indeed, no adult in the UK can legally consent to surgery on behalf of another, including close relatives. Relatives should not be asked to sign consent forms on behalf of unconscious or otherwise incompetent adults. It would be both a misrepresentation of the law and a

liability risk: if the surgical outcome is poor, the relatives may inappropriately and harmfully blame themselves.

Therefore, the only circumstance that could justify surgery without consent is the dramatic need of patients coupled with their inability to give consent. Again, inconvenience will not suffice. For example, the arrest of a life-threatening haemorrhage in an otherwise healthy patient would clearly be in order, while the same could not be said of the repair of a hernia. Of course, if patients are conscious and evidently capable of rational judgement, then even in an emergency they should be advised about their condition and the proposed treatment. If it is physically possible, a patient should also sign a consent form, as would be the case in normal circumstances. Verbal consent is adequate if the patient's condition precludes giving written consent. However, in these circumstances it is advisable, if possible, for another health worker to act as a witness and to record the verbal consent in the notes.

Children

Ordinarily, consent for elective surgery on young children must always be obtained from someone – usually the parent – deemed competent to make informed choices about the child's best interests. This is not, however, to suggest that surgeons must always be guided solely by parental wishes. If such decisions are believed to be necessary to save the life of the child then they can be overriden. If there is time, the court should provide the appropriate order; if not, the surgeon can still proceed. If parents are proposing long-term treatment or non-treatment options which are regarded as similarly inconsistent with the best interests of the child, these wishes can again be overriden by an appropriate court order.

Generally speaking, the legal age for medical consent is 16. However, it is legally acceptable for surgeons to treat adolescents under the age of 16 years without parental consent, just as it is for GPs to prescribe contraceptives. If this is considered, care must be taken to ensure that the young person is competent – again, mature enough to understand, retain and deliberate about information concerning the nature of the illness, the prognosis, proposed treatment and any important associated risks. Such patients should also be able to believe that this information applies personally to them. Equally, before proceeding without parental consent, the surgeon should encourage the young person to discuss the proposed treatment with their parents and be assured that the treatment is in the best interests of the child.

This said, treatment without parental consent should be regarded as the exception and not the rule.

Unless the adolescent has specifically refused permission, attempts should be made if possible to find and consult parents who are not already on site. In the case of life-threatening illness, even young people below the age of 18 years do not have the right to reject treatment on their own which might save their lives. Only those with parental responsibility can exercise such judgement, in agreement with the responsible clinician. Paradoxically, the law appears to be that the right of a competent adolescent to consent to life-saving treatment does not entail the right to refuse it. As regards elective surgery which is not life saving or will not prevent serious and permanent injury, the law is the same. Morally, however, the wishes of the competent young person not to proceed should be and are commonly respected – even where the parent disagrees. If surgical treatment is forced upon such patients without consent then it might undermine the relationship of trust and the willingness to comply with future treatment, both of which will be important for sustained clinical success. Such force can be argued not to be in the best clinical interests of the child.

Certainly, quite young children often have a good grasp of their prospects and treatment, especially when they have already experienced distressing surgical therapy for an illness which they have had for some time. In such circumstances, before further surgery is undertaken, attempts should be made to consult such children about their wishes. Where there is disagreement between parent and child about the best course of action, especially in instances of potentially terminal disease, both should be counselled about what appears clinically to be in the child's best interests. Such counselling will be particularly important in situations where there is disagreement between the surgeon and parent about the most appropriate way to proceed. Again, in the unusual event that a surgeon believes parental choice dramatically conflicts with the medical interests of the child, the court should be approached for a judgment.

Mental handicap and psychiatric illness

In the case of adults who are judged incompetent to choose for themselves, we have seen that no one may legally act as a proxy for this purpose. However, decisions about incompetence are complex. For example, incompetence to consent to surgery does not follow from severe psychiatric illness. Just because individuals may be incompetent in one respect due to illness does not mean that they are incompetent in all respects. People may be detained under the 1983 Mental Health Act on the grounds that, because of the seriousness of their psychiatric illness, they are a potential danger to themselves or others. As a result they may be given psychiatric treatment without their consent. However, this does not hold for ordinary surgical treatment. In such circumstances, attempts must therefore be made to obtain the patient's consent, even when communication is difficult and certainty of understanding not assured. For example, in a recent legal case in Britain, a judge accepted that a detained patient suffering from schizophrenia was competent to refuse to have a foot amputated if it became terminally gangrenous.

With the exception of specific and extreme interventions such as psychosurgery, there are circumstances where surgical treatment can be given to detained psychiatric patients who cannot consent due to extreme illness. There are two conditions: the treatment must be deemed necessary to protect life or to avoid permanent and serious disability, and patients must be diagnosed as unable to give informed consent as a direct result of their psychiatric illness. As a consequence of psychotic delusion, for example, they might believe that their surgeon is going to kill them and that the diagnosis of a life-threatening condition is a sinister plot. Here, necessary treatment can proceed, provided that the surgeon and the relevant psychiatric team agree that it is in the best interests of the patient. Note that this exception to the consent requirement would not ordinarily apply to elective surgical care since the assumption should be that there will be time for patients to make up their own minds when their competence to do so is no longer being impaired by their illness.

Some patients in need of surgery will suffer not from psychiatric illness but from permanent mental disability. This may severely impair their competence to give informed consent for either life-saving or elective surgery. The fact remains, however, that in such circumstances, no adult can act as a legal proxy for another as regards the provision of such consent. The only person who can make the decision that surgery is in the best interests of severely mentally handicapped patients is their surgeon in consultation with their principal carers, including close relatives. Yet great care must be taken. As regards elective surgery, responsibility for promoting the interests of mentally handicapped patients can be a heavy burden, especially if there is dispute among carers about what these actually are. The sensitivity of these issues is witnessed by the fact that the courts sometimes refuse to permit the sterilization of mentally handicapped women under the age of 16 years, even if a surgeon has agreed to perform the procedure.

TWO PRACTICAL PROBLEMS

The general obligation to disclose information about both proposed surgery and its hazards is not open to debate. However, putting this moral and legal imperative into practice does involve discretion and is not always easy for two reasons.

1. Limitations on the understanding of patients

It is sometimes unclear whether or not consent has really been obtained, even if the surgeon has taken care to explain the proposed procedure and its potential hazards. The comprehension of competent patients can be compromised by their illness, their educational and social background and by other aspects of their personalities which may make them overly anxious or unwilling to listen. Yet difficult as such instances of impaired autonomy can be, especially for patients facing acute and complex surgery, surgeons should still be able to show that they have disclosed adequate information for proper consent to be possible.

Practically speaking, therefore, how should surgeons demonstrate to themselves (and, if necessary, a judge) that they have done their best in this regard? Most important of all, they need to work constantly to improve their ability to communicate. Both the General Medical Council (GMC) and the British Medical Association stress this point, and its importance is underlined by the increasing emphasis placed on communication skills within medical education. Surgeons can do no more than their best. However, it follows from the moral importance of informed consent that they should always attempt to optimize their ability to communicate well.

Furthermore, it is important to keep a written record in the case notes of the main points about treatment which have been communicated prior to the signing of the consent form. If one follows the model of the reasonable patient outlined above, information should certainly be given on what will be done and why, along with significant risks of mortality and other hazards to bodily functions relevant to normal social participation: swallowing, speaking, continence, mobility, pain and sexual performance, for example. A brief indication in the notes that each of these variables has been mentioned should not be too onerous a task and will provide surgeons with evidence which could be useful if the fact is denied by the patient in a context of medicolegal dispute. This approach can be reinforced by giving all patients written information about their proposed treatment and possible side-effects.

Even after they have followed good practice in obtaining consent, surgeons may conclude that patients still cannot be said properly to have given consent to treatment. Here, life-saving emergencies aside, the most appropriate choice is to postpone therapy until better communication has been achieved. This may be inconvenient, but it is necessary if the rights of patients are to be protected and if surgeons are to be able to demonstrate that they have taken their moral and legal duties to do so seriously.

2. Limitations on the right of patients to consent

The right of patients to consent to surgery does not entail their right to demand and receive it. There is no professional duty to provide surgery which is requested by patients who have no need for it. The same can be said for surgery which will be futile no matter how much patients may want it. But what if patients clearly need surgery but do not want it? Here respect for the autonomy of patients may well conflict with the surgeon's other moral obligation to protect their life and health. This conflict is most acute when, in considered and unambiguous terms, patients refuse surgery which will save their lives.

The moral and legal emphasis on respect for autonomy within surgery is so strong that, even in such circumstances, treatment must not be undertaken without consent, again assuming that the patient is conscious and competent. This fact is sometimes obscured because patients who are terminally ill and do not wish further treatment are reticent to refuse it. Where it becomes very clear, however, is in the case, say, of Jehovah's Witnesses who will only proceed with surgery on the understanding that if they haemorrhage they will not be transfused. Legally, competent patients have every right to make such a demand. A surgeon who proceeds to the contrary risks on action for battery.

It is not being suggested that surgeons have to operate on patients who place stipulations on the types of life-saving treatment which they will accept. In principle, and assuming that there is time, surgeons may refer them to others who are more sympathetic and willing to undergo the stress which such restrictions inevitably carry. Equally, we have already seen that if a patient is unconscious or incompetent for some other reason the surgeon must do what is necessary to try to save life. However, even this is changing in the face of so-called 'advance directives' or 'living wills' which are now regarded by expert opinion in the UK as having legal force. Thus any competent adult can draft a document specifying in advance which life-saving treatments they do and do not consent to if they become incompetent and contract specific types of illnesses. Ideally, an advance directive should be witnessed and should be acted upon. Such documents are common in North America and will eventually be so in the UK.

After consultation with their surgeons, competent

patients may, therefore, decide that further treatment is pointless, given the irreversible and terminal character of their particular disease. Complying with such a request to omit or to stop treatment can be argued to be neither actively killing nor aiding and abetting suicide. It is reasoned that, unlike the potential suicide, competent patients may well want desperately to live but not at any cost to their quality of life. Furthermore, as we have seen, to treat them against their will constitutes a battery. Whatever the correctness of these arguments, what patients cannot expect is for active steps to be taken to end their lives, although they do at times request this as well.

Yet to go along with a patient's refusal of surgery when it is clear that the consequence will be death is a very serious moral and legal matter. Great care must be taken to ensure that the patient fully understands the implications of refusing life-saving treatment and is competent to make an informed judgement, especially if the refusal is followed by a lapse into unconsciousness. Here a mistake either about the patient's understanding or wishes cannot be corrected. Therefore, prior refusal should be respected only if it is judged to be an autonomous decision intended to apply in the circumstances that have arisen. For example, a young adult woman in the UK refused a blood transfusion on the grounds of her acceptance of the doctrine of the Jehovah's Witnesses, despite the fact that she was not a Witness herself. She lost consciousness and the court overruled her refusal on the grounds that she had been unduly influenced by her mother and that her decision was based upon a false impression of her prognosis.

INFORMED CONSENT AND SURGICAL RESEARCH

The availability of surgical options is dependent on the experimental research which makes them possible. Yet researchers must be careful. Without enthusiasm and conviction about the importance of their work, they will not have the commitment that successful research requires. However, such commitment can lead to an underestimation of the risks or discomfort of experiments. Research can be either therapeutic and to the potential benefit of participants, or non-therapeutic with no such promise. Participants in the former will be patients and in the latter either patients or healthy volunteers.

Focusing for the moment on research involving patients, they have a right to informed consent for the same reasons described above. Furthermore, allowing them to make an informed evaluation for themselves is one of the best ways of regulating experimental zeal, a factor which has unquestionably led to moral abuses in the past. A clear example is the notorious and needless experiments inflicted by some Nazi doctors and surgeons on Jewish prisoners. However, there have been more recent illustrations involving patients, some of whom have died as a result of their participation in research.

The Nuremburg Code, which was adopted internationally as a result, declared that 'the voluntary consent of a patient is essential' in any medical research. The later Declaration of Helsinki is also explicit. It states: 'In any research, each potential subject must be adequately informed of the aims, methods and anticipated benefits and potential hazards of the study and the discomfort it may entail.' And after this, their consent must be obtained.

The enforcement of the Helsinki Declaration in the UK is entrusted to research ethics committees. These are administered by health authorities and are responsible for evaluating all surgical research involving humans wherever it might be undertaken. Under no circumstances should research proceed without the approval of the appropriate ethics committee, and academic journals will usually not publish the results unless such approval has been given. In principle, research ethics committees are supposed to ensure that the proposed protocol makes good scientific sense and poses no further risks than those of the best available treatment. Only then should patients be asked to consent to participate, on the basis of being given appropriate information about the research which the committee has also approved.

There is, however, one significant problem concerning surgical research and informed consent which remains. As a result of differing ability and willingness to understand and to question medical authority, we have seen that patients vary in their ability to assimilate the details of clinical information. Consequently, enthusiastic researchers are in a position, wittingly or not, to manipulate patients to subject themselves to procedures that might not be proposed in ordinary treatment. Patients may be encouraged to agree to participate in the development of surgical procedures, for example, without realizing how experimental they are. Here the general guidelines concerning informed consent should be followed with extra vigilance. For example, care must be taken to identify surgical procedures that might not be regarded as standard professional practice and to proceed only when the patient gives informed and written consent with the knowledge that this is the case. When in doubt about whether or not a procedure is standard, the research ethics committee should be consulted.

In non-therapeutic research with patients or healthy volunteers, it is equally important to avoid confusing agreement to participate with informed consent to do so. The researcher must try to ensure that the moral legitimacy of the consent of the volunteer is not obtained under financial, social or professional duress. In the UK, for example, the difficulty of doing so has led to surgical research not ordinarily taking place among the prison population.

INFORMED CONSENT AND CONFIDENTIALITY

As a corollary of their right to informed consent, patients have the right to control access to information which they give to surgeons for the purposes of treatment. The GMC supports this right through the importance it attaches to the principle of confidentiality – of obtaining the permission of patients before revealing clinical information about them to others. Few acts can more quickly lead to a surgeon being professionally disciplined than a proven breach of confidence in unwarranted circumstances.

There are two types of justification for this emphasis. First, the right to be the moral gatekeeper of one's own body extends to information divulged in clinical consultations. Second, if patients are frightened that their confidence might be breached, they may not be willing to provide the honest information on which successful diagnosis depends or even to turn up for treatment at all. This can pose a severe danger to them and possibly to the general public.

But it is in the area of potential conflict between the freedom of the individual and the interest of the public that circumstances may arise in which the surgeon either must or might divulge information otherwise regarded as private. The same professional codes which stress the importance of confidentiality – the 'Duties of a Doctor' of the GMC, for example – also outline the exceptions to the rule. These fall into two general categories.

The public interest

Suppose that in a clinical consultation in A&E a surgeon discovers that a highly agitated patient is armed, has committed a robbery and has killed a bank clerk and a customer as a result. Here, it seems straightforward that the confidence should be broken and the police informed. The patient might strike again. Indeed, it is legally mandatory to breach confidentiality where patients are suspected of involvement in terror-ism within the UK or where they are found to be suffering from a highly infectious and notifiable disease.

But how serious must a risk to the public actually be to breach confidentiality legitimately? For example, should a surgeon be just as willing to turn someone in who confessed in confidence that they had stolen a badly needed winter coat? It is not always easy to balance the interests of the patient against those of the public. This can create difficult dilemmas for surgeons when the two seem in direct conflict and when, as is often the case, there is considerable professional discretion as to how morally to proceed. Debates about HIV and AIDS have recently underlined these issues.

Two things are clear. Firstly, it does not follow from a claim that the public interest demands a breach of confidence that it actually does. For example, the police have no right to disclosure or to access to clinical records which may provide evidence of a crime. A judge may issue a warrant legally authorizing such access or a subpoena demanding disclosure in court. However, even this does not make it morally mandatory. Some clinicians have felt so strongly about the immorality of breaking a patient's confidence that they have risked being charged with contempt of court for refusing to do so. Again, the law and morality should not be conflated, even though they often do overlap.

Secondly, patients have no right to harm others through the exercise of their right to confidentiality. There is an obvious link between this right and the right of individuals to control the use of their private property. Yet just as the legitimate exercise of this property right stops at the point at which the safety of others is threatened, the same can be said about clinical information. Therefore, if a surgeon discovers that maintaining confidentiality will lead to the threat of serious harm to another known individual – just the suspicion of a general threat is not sufficient – then a breach of confidence may be warranted. For example, although the legal precedent does not apply in the UK, a psychiatrist in the USA was successfully sued for negligence for not informing a young woman that he had clearly been told by a patient that he was going to kill her. He did.

The interest of the individual patient

Breaches of confidence may not just be in the public interest. They may also be necessary in order to obtain information vital for successful treatment. Because of the physical or psychological effects of their illness, some patients are unable to communicate clearly about their medical history. Under such circumstances, relatives or friends may have to be consulted, especially in emergencies.

This said, strong attempts should still be made to obtain the patient's consent and to verify the identity of any others from whom information is sought. No more information about the patient's condition should be revealed than is necessary for the clinical purposes at hand. Knowledge about prognosis and treatment, for example, should remain confidential, remembering how its unwarranted spread might drastically affect the patient's private and public life. Certainly, clinical information should never be communicated over the phone to those not involved in treatment, unless it is with the patient's prior consent and there is a reliable way of identifying the person to whom the information is given.

The interests of patients are also served if the surgeons to whom they reveal clinical information share it with colleagues whose assistance they require. Patients are presumed to consent to such revelations by virtue of their general agreement to treatment. Given the complexity of its division of labour, surgery is an essentially cooperative exercise and its success depends on the free flow of relevant information. This said, only those professionals involved should have access to the information, something which requires caution, especially on open wards.

MORAL INDETERMINACY, INFORMED CONSENT AND OPEN COMMUNICATION

Thus far, we have examined the general principles governing informed consent which are endorsed by the profession of surgery and which are reinforced by statute and case law. Yet, clear as these are, their correct interpretation may be much more obscure in practice. Such rules do not interpret themselves: individual surgeons interpret them when faced with the complexities of specific cases.

In the majority of cases there will be a consensus among the surgical team about the most appropriate interpretation. It will be reasonably clear, for example, how much information should be communicated to knowledgeable patients about the hazards of a particular treatment and whether or not they have understood enough of it to warrant proceeding. Yet in some situations, such agreement will not exist and interpretations will conflict. Here reference to the facts of the case themselves cannot solve the problem. Their openness to conflicting interpretation is what poses it.

Suppose, for example, that despite careful attempts to communicate the considerable risks of an urgently needed operative procedure there is still disagreement among a surgical team about whether or not the patient has fully understood. Here, and against the background of the necessity to come to a quick decision, there may be no 'right' interpretation as to how ethically to proceed. Another illustration might be conflicting beliefs about whether or not urgently to operate on a Jehovah's Witness who refuses a blood transfusion but seems partly to be doing so under pressure from family or congregation.

What is crucial in such circumstances is that, despite their disagreements, individual members of the surgical team accept that the final decision about how to proceed is reached after an open and reasoned discussion where everyone has the chance to present their arguments. As a result, clinicians will be much more willing to cooperate in the search for a common view, even when it involves a degree of what they may perceive as moral compromise. Open communication does not have to conflict with the recognition that it is the senior clinician who must take responsibility for the final choice. Surgeons in authority should always try to create space for such discussions, a practice which is increasingly common in the face of taxing moral dilemmas which have to be resolved in short periods of time – for example, those concerning non-treatment.

Summary

1. Respect the right of patients to give or with-hold consent to surgical treatment.
2. Provide patients with sufficient information to make informed choice possible.
3. Even in surgical emergencies, do not override the right of conscious and capable patients to decide on treatment.
4. Ensure that you continue to respect the rights of all patients, including children, and those who are unconscious, mentally handicapped, or psychiatrically ill.

ACKNOWLEDGEMENTS

Many thanks to John Cochrane, Robert Cohen, Lesley Doyal, John Dickenson, Arlene Klotzko, Alastair McDonald, Rosanne Lord, Paul Lear, Norman Williams, Daniel Wilsher, Christopher Wood and Richard Wood. Special thanks to Ian Kennedy.

Further reading

Alderson P 1993 Children's consent to surgery. Open University Press, Buckingham

Appelbaum P, Lidz C, Meisel A 1987 Informed consent. Oxford University Press, New York

Beauchamp T, Childress J 1994 Principles of biomedical ethics. Oxford University Press, New York

Brazier M 1992 Medicine, patients and the law. Penguin, Harmondsworth

Buchanan A, Brock D 1989 Deciding for others: the ethics of surrogate decision making. Cambridge University Press, Cambridge

Davis H, Fallowfield L 1991 Counselling and communication in health care. Wiley, London p. 140

Faden R, Beauchamp T 1986 A history and theory of informed consent. Oxford University Press, Oxford

Harris J 1985 The value of life. Routledge, London

Kennedy I 1988 Treat me right. Oxford University Press, Oxford

Kennedy I, Grubb A 1994 Medical law – text and materials. Butterworths, London

McHale J, Fox M 1997 Health care law—text and materials. Sweet and Maxwell, London

McLean S 1989 A patient's right to know: information disclosure, the doctor and the law. Dartmouth, Aldershot

Mason J, McCall Smith R 1994 Law and medical ethics. Butterworths, London

Montgomery J 1997 Healthcare law. Oxford University Press, Oxford

Royal College of Surgeons 1997 The Surgeon's duty of care. Royal College of Surgeons, London

Wear S 1993 Informed consent. Kluwer, Dordrecht

16

Preoperative preparation for surgery

B. R. Davidson, S. Bhattacharya

Objectives

- **Understand the general principles of preoperative preparation.**
- **Appreciate how, in high-risk patients, preoperative preparation may lower the risk.**
- **Understand the principles of preparation for specific types of operations.**
- **Appreciate the value of protocols and routines, and the importance of adhering to them, even in emergency situations.**

To obtain satisfactory results in general surgery requires a careful approach to the preoperative preparation of patients. The importance of this preparation becomes more evident as the surgical procedure performed becomes more complex. Attention to detail is the key to success.

ROUTINE PREOPERATIVE PREPARATION

- **Take a full history (especially medications and allergies) and do a clinical examination**
- **Decide what investigations are required**
- **Follow a standard protocol appropriate to your clinical firm**

History and examination

Confirm that the planned operative procedure is appropriate and exclude any significant medical problems (Ch. 7). Take a full history and carry out a thorough clinical examination on all patients being admitted for a surgical procedure. Check clinical signs against the planned surgical procedure, in particular noting the side involved. Take a full drug history with specific enquiry regarding allergic responses to drugs and skin allergies. Continue medication over the perioperative period, especially drugs for hypertension, ischaemic heart disease and bronchodilators. Patients on oral steroid therapy should be given intravenous hydrocortisone and those anticoagulated with oral warfarin should have this stopped at least 48 hours preoperatively. Warfarinized patients who have had a life-threatening thrombotic episode (e.g. pulmonary embolus) within the previous 3 months should be heparinized intravenously until 6 hours prior to surgery. Stop drugs over the perioperative period which may interfere with anaesthetic agents, including monoamine oxidase inhibitors, lithium, tricyclic antidepressants and phenothiazines. If possible, stop the oral contraceptive pill 4 weeks prior to any major surgery. Post-menopausal patients on hormone replacement therapy do not need to have their medication stopped before an operation.

Preoperative tests

Young and fit patients undergoing minor procedures do not require any preoperative investigations. In older patients or those with significant medical problems, standard investigation would include a full blood count, urea and electrolytes, chest X-ray and electrocardiogram. For a critical evaluation of routine preoperative investigations see Velanovich (1994).

Some abnormality is noted on routine biochemical testing in approximately 5% of patients; the majority of these relate to elevated blood sugar levels or urea. Elevated urea and creatinine levels in asymptomatic patients are mainly detected in patients over 50 years of age; under this age, therefore, it may be argued that no routine biochemical testing is necessary in asymptomatic patients, if urine analysis has excluded glycosuria. The full blood count is unnecessary in young asymptomatic patients undergoing minor surgery. In other patients it is necessary to exclude anaemia and poly-cythaemia. Test black African patients for the presence of sickle cell anaemia and patients from Mediterranean countries to exclude thalassaemia. Take blood for grouping if transfusion is possible and cross-match blood if it is likely to be needed. The number of units depend on the procedure being performed.

Some radiological abnormality is present in one-third of patients over 60 years of age, but the majority of these abnormalities are of no clinical significance. A respiratory history and clinical examination are of more importance than radiological findings in predicting perioperative respiratory complications. The preoperative chest X-ray is important in patients with new respiratory symptoms, as a baseline for those undergoing major surgery, and in older patients (>50 years).

Routine testing for viral hepatitis or HIV is not performed in the UK. Any patient with a history of jaundice should, however, have serological testing for hepatitis B and C. Ask patients at high risk for HIV (intravenous drug abuse, homosexuals, or patients from high-risk areas) if they are willing to undergo testing, and counsel them. Most hospitals are progressing towards universal precautions, where all patients undergoing surgery are considered as potentially infectious, and all operating room staff are therefore adequately gloved, instruments and sharps are handled very carefully, and disposable equipment is used wherever possible.

Patients with no history or clinical findings to suggest ischaemic heart disease who are under 40 years of age do not require a preoperative electrocardiogram (ECG). The main reasons for performing an ECG preoperatively is to detect arrhythmias or conduction defects, evidence of myocardial ischaemia or previous infarction or evidence of left ventricular hypertrophy.

Routine preoperative measures

Each clinical firm evolves a standard protocol for preoperative preparation appropriate for its patients.

Adhere to the protocol followed by your firm. Use a checklist – these are very useful in ensuring that you have not left out an important step. Keep adult patients nil by mouth for solids for 6 hours (children for 4 hours) prior to an elective general anaesthetic. The operation site must be prepared by the removal of hair, if this is necessary for access, using a depilatory cream. Shaving or clipping hair from the operation site increases the risk of infection, unless the skin preparation is carried out immediately prior to surgery. Mark the operation site on the skin with an indelible marker pen. Explain to the patient or guardian the procedure and any likely complications, answer any questions or clarifications, then have them sign the consent form. If you are out of your depth in answering the questions of a patient, involve a senior colleague. Antibiotic administration is guided by the surgical procedure involved and is discussed below, as is prophylaxis against deep vein thrombosis. If specific services such as frozen section histopathology or intraoperative radiography are likely to be required during the operation, organize these in advance.

THE USE OF ANTIBIOTICS

Antibiotic use depends on whether it is going to be a clean or a contaminated operation, and the type of flora likely to cause infection.

Patients with clinical infection should be treated with systemic antibiotics prior to undergoing surgery. With elective surgery, antibiotic prophylaxis depends on the procedure being performed (Table 16.1). Clean procedures (e.g. varicose vein surgery) do not need antibiotic prophylaxis. Abdominal surgery which is not associated with significant contamination (e.g. cholecystectomy)

Table 16.1 The risk of infection

Type of wound	Description	Incidence of infection (%)
Clean	No violation of mucosa No inflammation No drains	2
Clean–contaminated	Incision of mucosa but no spillage *or* Clean procedure in immunocompromised	10
Contaminated	Pre-existing infection Spillage of viscus contents	20–40

requires only a single-dose prophylaxis given on induction of anaesthesia. Procedures with a contaminated field (e.g. appendicitis) should be treated with a preoperative dose and two postoperative doses. This regimen would also be satisfactory for the majority of other procedures in the gastrointestinal tract (e.g. gastric surgery and colonic surgery with prepared bowel). The choice of antibiotic prophylaxis is determined by the surgical procedure itself. Operations which may be contaminated by skin flora should have prophylaxis against staphylococcal infection with flucloxacillin 500 mg intravenously. Procedures involving the bowel require broad-spectrum cover for Gram-positive and Gram-negative organisms and anaerobes. Commonly used regimens include co-amoxiclav or a cephalosporin with metronidazole. Biliary tract procedures rarely involve a flora of anaerobes, and satisfactory prophylaxis would be obtained from a cephalosporin alone. For a review of antimicrobial prophylaxis see Paluzzi (1993).

PROPHYLAXIS AGAINST DEEP VEIN THROMBOSIS AND PULMONARY EMBOLI

Pulmonary emboli are a major cause of mortality for surgical patients. In the UK they account for 10% of inpatient deaths. Recent surgery, immobilization and trauma were responsible for 50% of deep vein thrombosis (DVT) in a review by Cogo et al (1994), but there are other important predisposing factors, such as the oral contraceptive pill (when it has a high oestrogen content) and significant obesity (see Table 16.2). Many of the risk factors cannot be avoided, but measures should be taken to avoid propagation of any thrombosis. These measures include the use of pre- and postoperative subcutaneous heparin administration, graduated compression stockings and intraoperative intermittent pneumatic calf compression. Subcutaneous heparin may reduce the incidence of DVTs by 50%; it is generally well tolerated but very occasionally thrombocytopenia may result. The systemic anticoagulation effects of low-dose subcutaneous heparin are minimal and should not produce any risk for impaired haemostasis during surgical procedures. The newly introduced low-molecular-weight heparins are as effective as standard heparin and have the convenience of a once daily dosage. They are more expensive. For a summary of recent advances in DVT prophylaxis, see Wheatley & Veitch (1997). For a discussion of risk factors for thromboembolism see also Thromboembolic Risk Factors Consensus Group (1992).

Table 16.2 Risk factors for deep vein thrombosis*
Recent surgery
Immobilization
Trauma
Oral contraceptive pill
Obesity
Heart failure
Arteriopathy
Cancer
Age > 60 years
*Adapted from Cogo et al (1994)

ASSESSMENT OF RISK FOR SURGERY

Unfortunately, there are few patients who have no risk factors for surgery. It is important to quantify the risks involved so they can be discussed with the patient. Risk scores may also be used to compare different forms of treatment and their effectiveness in different risk groups. The two main prognostic scoring systems which are in current use are the Acute Physiology and Chronic Health Evaluation (APACHE) system and the American Society of Anesthesiologists (ASA) system. These systems were initially introduced to predict the outcome of patients admitted to the intensive care unit and have subsequently been applied to patients undergoing surgery. With the APACHE II system (Knaus et al 1985) 12 acute physiological variables, the patients' age and their chronic health are individually scored and added to give a final figure that provides risk stratification for an acutely ill patient. Many computer programs are available to instantly calculate these variables (summarized in Box 16.1). Recently the APACHE III system (Knaus et al 1991) has been introduced, which includes five more physiologic variables (blood urea nitrogen, urine output, serum albumin, bilirubin and glucose) and a modified version of the Glasgow Coma Score. The ASA assessment is very simple and has therefore been widely adopted (Table 16.3).

MANAGEMENT OF THE HIGH-RISK PATIENT

Key point

Identify the high-risk patient and seek specialist help sooner rather than later

---

Box 16.1   Apache II classification

Apache II score is A + B + C

A Acute Physiology Score (APS)
1. Rectal temperature (°C)
2. Mean blood pressure (mmHg)
3. Heart rate (beats per minute)
4. Respiratory rate (breaths per minute)
5. Alveolar–arterial oxygen gradient if $FiO_2 > 0.5$ or P_aO_2 if $Fio_2 < 0.5$
6. Arterial pH
7. Serum Na^+ (mmol l^{-1})
8. Serum K^+ (mmol l^{-1})
9. Serum creatinine (mg/100 ml)
10. Haematocrit (%)
11. Leucocyte count (cells mm^3)
12. Glasgow Coma Score (GCS)

B Age points graded from <44 to >75 years

C Chronic health points
2 points for elective postoperative admission
5 points for: emergency operation
                 nonoperative admission
                 immunocompromised patient
                 chronic liver, cardiovascular,
                 respiratory or renal disease.

Table 16.3   American Society for Anesthesiologists (ASA) status

Category	Description
I	Healthy patient
II	Mild systemic disease – no functional limitations
III	Severe systemic disease – definite functional limitation
IV	Severe systemic disease that is a constant threat to life
V	Moribund patient not expected to survive 24 hours with or without surgery

---

Patients with major medical problems are at a high risk from surgery and should be identified early in the preoperative period. This allows prior discussion with the anaesthetists and booking of intensive care unit beds if necessary. Also, specialist opinion can be sought and effective treatment commenced or precautions taken to minimize risk.

Assessment of cardiovascular risk

The major determinants of perioperative cardiac complications are recent myocardial infarction and clinical heart failure. Systemic hypertension and a history of arrhythmias may also be risk factors, but are of lesser significance. The risk of sustaining a further myocardial infarct in the perioperative period varies with the time period post infarct. The major risk period is within the first 3 months where the risk may be of the order of 30%. The risk, however, decreases rapidly thereafter and elective surgery could be considered at 6 months post infarct in a patient with no persisting cardiac symptoms or signs. Seek the opinion of an experienced cardiologist in patients with ischaemic heart disease who require a surgical procedure. Patients with a history suggestive of ischaemic heart disease, but no evidence of infarction on ECG, should proceed to an exercise or stress ECG. A coronary angiogram and angioplasty or coronary artery bypass grafting may then be considered. Patients with a history or clinical signs to suggest congestive cardiac failure can have their left ventricular function assessed by echocardiography. Systemic hypertension is a common problem in the general population and is a significant risk factor unless satisfactorily controlled. All patients found to be hypertensive at the time of assessment for elective surgery should have their surgery delayed until they are established on antihypertensive drugs. For further information on assessing cardiovascular risk see Goldman et al (1977).

Assessment of respiratory problems

The most common conditions found during preoperative assessment are chronic obstructive airways disease (COAD) and bronchial asthma. The severity of these conditions can largely be predicted from a careful history, but further objective evidence of the extent of their airway disease can be obtained from respiratory function tests. Commonly measured parameters are the peak expiratory flow rate (PEFR), vital capacity (VC) and forced expiratory volume in 1 second (FEV_1). The measurements can be used to assess the response to bronchodilators as well as acting as a baseline for subsequent testing in the postoperative period. Arterial blood gas analysis is also a useful baseline in patients undergoing major surgery or those expected to have significant postoperative respiratory complications. The combination of a painful incision from upper abdominal surgery and significant lung disease is of considerable concern and is best treated by the use of epidural analgesia in the intra- and postoperative period. Discuss epidural catheters with the anaesthetist and the patient before the operation, and ensure that the ward nurses are trained to manage epidural catheters. Guidance should be given preoperatively on breathing exercises to allow expansion of the lung bases and for holding the abdominal incision to produce adequate expectoration in a less painful manner. Introduce the patient to the physiotherapists before the operation, and ensure regular chest physiotherapy in the early postoperative period. Give antibiotics (guided by culture and sensitivity) to patients with infected sputum, who are at increased risk of postoperative chest infection. Seek the expert opinion of a chest physician whenever you foresee major respiratory problems.

Management of preoperative renal dysfunction

The most common disorder which would be diagnosed preoperatively in an elective surgical patient would be a degree of chronic renal failure as demonstrated by an elevated urea and creatinine on routine electrolyte estimations. Moderate elevation of urea and creatinine would be expected in elderly patients with significant atherosclerosis. Such patients may develop acute renal failure if exposed to a period of intraoperative hypotension. Unexplained renal impairment in a young patient should be investigated prior to any elective surgery. Patients in established renal failure on dialysis require to be dialysed prior to any surgical procedure to ensure a good fluid balance and to correct any hyperkalaemia. Patients with functioning renal transplants require to have their immunosuppression continued over the perioperative period and to avoid any periods of operative hypotension. Always consult a nephrologist to discuss perioperative management of such patients. In elderly, frail or acutely ill patients, ensure adequate hydration to avoid precipitating pre-renal failure.

Nutritional assessment

There is a clear and well-established correlation between malnutrition in the preoperative period and an increased morbidity and mortality from surgery. Nutritional assessment can be based on total body weight loss, anthropomorphic measurements such as skin-fold thickness to assess the amount of subcutaneous fat, or biochemical tests which reflect protein deficiency such as the measurement of serum albumin, prealbumin or transferrin. Such preoperative nutritional assessment may detect patients in whom malnutrition is a major concern for their operative procedure, but the correction of this malnourished state, which in part reflects their underlying disease process, may be

impossible in the preoperative period. Highlighting the problem, however, will allow nutritional support to be commenced at an early stage and consideration given to the insertion of a feeding enterostomy or a designated central venous feeding line at the time of surgery. Correction of a low preoperative serum albumin level with human albumin solution is an ineffective and expensive method of providing nutritional support and should not be considered unless as an adjuvant to full parenteral or enteral nutrition. (For a full discussion on nutrition see Ch. 11.)

Management of obesity

In many respects, the overnourished or obese patient presents as great, if not greater, risks for surgery than the malnourished patient. The obese patient (greater than 30% above ideal weight) has a markedly increased risk (approximately 40%) of operative mortality from ischaemic heart disease and almost 50% increased risk of dying from a cerebrovascular accident. In addition, there is an increased risk of deep vein thrombosis and both wound and intra-abdominal sepsis. Operative risks may be reduced by a careful search for risk factors for ischaemic heart disease and their appropriate investigation and treatment. Prophylaxis against deep vein thrombosis is vital.

Management of the diabetic patient

Diabetic patients are high-risk candidates for any surgical procedure. In addition to their susceptibility to infection and impaired wound healing, they are at risk of vascular complications due to their accelerated atherosclerosis. Careful investigation for evidence of ischaemic heart disease, peripheral vascular disease or cerebrovascular disease is essential, and careful preoperative documentation of peripheral pulses is important. The risks of surgery can be minimized by keeping the blood sugar level carefully controlled. The overall management must be tailored to the severity of the diabetes as well as the operative procedure being performed. While tight glycaemic control is desirable, it is important to avoid hypoglycaemia, particularly when the patient is under or recovering from a general anaesthetic. For maturity-onset diabetics controlled by diet or oral hypoglycaemics who are undergoing minor surgery, it is sufficient to avoid the morning dose of oral hypoglycaemics with monitoring of blood sugar levels and the recommencement of oral hypoglycaemic therapy postoperatively. Start insulin-dependent diabetics undergoing major surgery on a 'sliding scale' of intravenous insulin doses depending on hourly blood sugar estimations. Alternatively, an intravenous infusion of insulin, glucose and potassium may provide adequate glycaemic control. All insulin-dependent diabetics undergoing major surgery should be discussed directly with the endocrinologist involved.

Treatment of preoperative anaemia or polycythaemia

Patients who have developed an iron-deficiency anaemia and are awaiting elective surgery may be treated by oral iron supplementation. Those requiring surgery more urgently with a haemoglobin less than 10 g dl⁻¹ should be transfused, but blood transfusion immediately prior to surgery (<48 hours) should be avoided as the oxygen-carrying capacity of stored blood is poor. Polycythaemia is less frequently encountered, but is a predisposing factor to postoperative deep vein thrombosis and should therefore be treated by repeated venesection until a satisfactory haemoglobin level is obtained.

Emergency surgery

The results of emergency surgery are less satisfactory than elective procedures, for a variety of reasons. The emergency nature of the surgery does not allow sufficient time for investigation and treatment of associated medical problems. Do not cut corners, and adhere to your elective preoperative protocols as far as possible. These patients are commonly dehydrated and hypovolaemic; if that is the case, their initial management must include insertion of wide-bore venous access and prompt rehydration. Consider putting in a central venous line and a urinary catheter to assess the adequacy of rehydration. Such patients are often septic as well, and require systemic antibiotic treatment. Place a nasogastric tube if there is insufficient time to allow for the usual period of fasting, or if you suspect bowel obstruction. Give careful consideration to the timing of the operation, and involve your senior colleagues in that decision-making process. The morbidity and mortality audit performed by the Royal College of Surgeons of England (Campling et al 1993) suggests that the majority of patients with acute surgical problems are better managed by active resuscitation prior to surgery being performed on a scheduled operating list by an experienced surgeon.

PREPARATION FOR SURGERY OF SPECIFIC PATIENT GROUPS

The preoperative preparation of patients for surgery is dependent on the procedures to be performed and the stage of the underlying pathology. However, some selected patient groups are worthy of particular mention.

Large bowel surgery

Most surgeons would consider that bowel preparation of some form is essential for the reduction of sepsis. Surprisingly, several recent controlled studies have failed to support the value of bowel preparation prior to colonic surgery and its value is therefore open to question. For elective surgery, bowel preparation is most commonly achieved by placing the patient on a liquid diet several days prior to surgery and administering oral purgatives on the day prior to surgery. The latter include sodium picosulphate (Picolax) 10 mg morning and night, or polyethylene glycol/sodium salts (Klean-Prep), 4 sachets in 4 litres of water taken 250 ml every 15 minutes. If this does not produce satisfactory cleansing of the bowel it may be combined with mechanical washouts via a rectal tube. Elderly patients may require intravenous hydration whilst undergoing bowel purgation due to associated fluid loss. In patients with an obstructing lesion, bowel preparation may not be possible. In this group of patients some have advocated on-table colonic lavage with the infusion of fluid via a caecostomy or appendicostomy with the effluent being drained by insertion of a wide-bore tube in the distal colon proximal to the obstruction. Warn all patients undergoing bowel surgery of the possibility of colostomy formation and mark the most practical site for a colostomy on the abdominal wall. The site should be carefully chosen preoperatively with the patient standing and with consideration for movement of the abdominal wall fat; input from the stoma therapist is often useful in this decision making.

Preparation of patients for upper gastrointestinal surgery

Patients presenting for upper GI surgery are often anorexic, resulting in a poor nutritional state which requires correction by enteral or parenteral nutrition both pre- and postoperatively. Vomiting results in dehydration, electrolyte depletion and possible acid–base imbalance, which again must be corrected preoperatively by adequate rehydration. If there is evidence of obstruction, insert a nasogastric tube and empty the stomach to prevent aspiration at the time of induction of anaesthesia. Vomiting may be associated with episodes of aspiration and an assessment of respiratory function from the patient's history along with a chest X-ray, respiratory function tests and blood gas analysis are helpful.

The oesophageal lumen becomes rapidly contaminated in the presence of disease or partial obstruction.

For 24 hours before operation give 10 ml of 0.2% chlorhexidine mouthwash and swallow, 6 hourly.

The jaundiced patient

The risks of surgery in patients with obstructive jaundice can be significantly reduced by careful preoperative management. Whether resolving the obstructive jaundice by preoperative insertion of a biliary endoprosthesis reduces the risk of surgery is controversial and is likely to relate to the age of the patient, the risk factors for surgery and the nature of the underlying disease. As a general rule, preoperative drainage should be considered in elderly patients who are deeply jaundiced and in all patients with biliary tract sepsis. Jaundiced patients may be deficient in the vitamin K-dependent clotting factors II, V, VII, IX and X, resulting in a bleeding tendency. Vitamin K should be given to all patients with obstructive jaundice prior to surgery (10 mg intramuscularly or intravenously). A coagulation profile should be checked, and those in whom a significant coagulopathy is present, but who require urgent surgery, should be given fresh frozen plasma at the time of surgery. Renal failure secondary to obstructive jaundice (hepatorenal syndrome) may be reduced by adequate preoperative hydration. It is essential that this patient group is not kept nil by mouth prior to surgery without intravenous fluid replacement. The value of the osmotic diuretic mannitol and the inotrope dopamine (in a low dose resulting in renal vasodilatation) in preventing hepatorenal failure is unproven, though they are frequently used. Infective complications are more common in patients with obstructive jaundice, and antibiotic prophylaxis is mandatory. Patients presenting with acute cholangitis require systemic administration of fluids and antibiotics and urgent biliary tract drainage either endoscopically or percutaneously.

Endocrine surgery

Patients undergoing surgery for thyrotoxicosis should have a period of treatment to reduce thyroid activity (e.g. carbimazole 10–15 mg three times daily) and β-blockers to prevent thyrotoxic crisis (e.g. propranolol 20–40 mg, 8 hourly for 10 days preoperatively). The movement of the vocal cords should be checked prior to surgery by indirect laryngoscopy to exclude an unsuspected idopathic unilateral palsy. The extent of a retrosternal goitre can be clearly demonstrated on computed tomography. Patients with phaeochromocytoma require preoperative medication to block the α and β adrenergic effects of catecholamines, and may require admission a week before surgery. Usually α blockade by phenoxybenzamine is commenced first,

followed 48 hours later by β blockade with atenolol or metoprolol.

The paediatric patient

The common surgical procedures in childhood are often performed by general surgeons with a training and interest in paediatric surgery. Complex congenital defects and surgery in neonates requires specialist surgical expertise and specific preoperative preparation. The management of all paediatric surgical cases should be carried out with the involvement of a paediatrician. Children should have surgery at the beginning of an operating list to minimize their period of fasting. If delayed, intravenous fluids should be commenced, venous cannulae should be inserted using topical anaesthetic cream to reduce discomfort and fluids administered according to body weight (40–60 ml kg^{-1} per 24 hours). Heparin and antibiotics are not required for routine clean surgical procedures.

Thoracic surgery

Assessment of respiratory function is the most important aspect of preoperative preparation (see above). Active preoperative physiotherapy, treatment of any respiratory infection with antibiotics and good postoperative analgesia should minimize the risk of postoperative respiratory failure. This patient group often has associated coronary and cerebral vascular disease due to atherosclerosis, and evidence of this should be sought and a cardiologist's opinion obtained if necessary. Pulmonary emboli are well recognized after thoracic surgery, and subcutaneous heparin is routine, as is antibiotic prophylaxis.

Vascular surgery

Atherosclerosis is a generalized disease and patients presenting with symptoms from vascular insufficiency (e.g. intermittent claudication) should have a careful search for cerebral, coronary and renal arterial disease. Ideally, severe ischaemic heart disease should be treated by drugs, angioplasty or coronary artery grafting prior to any surgery for peripheral vascular disease (see above). Diabetic patients with limb ischaemia should have careful diabetic control and treatment of infected skin lesions with appropriate antibiotics. Smoking is a common predisposing factor to atherosclerosis. It reduces small vessel blood flow and should therefore be stopped preoperatively. Smoking also predisposes to chronic obstructive airways disease and bronchial carcinoma. A careful history of respiratory problems should therefore be taken and a chest X-ray performed.

Sputum should be sent for culture and sensitivity plus cytology. Remember to check the serum lipid profile to rule out correctable hyperlipidaemia.

Orthopaedic surgery

The most common orthopaedic operations are for the treatment of joint abnormalities secondary to osteoarthritis. This patient group is elderly and their preparation for surgery must include a detailed search for medical problems prevalent in this age group such as ischaemic heart disease and chronic obstructive airways disease. These should be fully investigated and treated preoperatively. Joint replacement is major surgery associated with a significant blood loss, and cross-matching of blood is essential. The increased use of prostheses in orthopaedic surgery has allowed earlier mobilization of patients but carries the risk of infection around the foreign material. Antibiotic prophylaxis should be used which covers contamination from skin commensals such as staphylococci and streptococci. Thromboembolism is a major cause of mortality in orthopaedic patients, especially those undergoing pelvic surgery, and prophylaxis with standard or low-molecular-weight heparin is essential (see above).

Summary

1. Preoperative preparation requires close attention to detail.
2. Specific patients groups have specific needs.
3. High risk patients should be identified early and appropriate measures taken to reduce complications.

References

Campling E A, Devlin H B, Hoile R W, Lunn J N 1993 Report of the National Confidential Enquiry into Perioperative Deaths 1991/1992. London

Cogo A, Bernardi E, Prandoni P et al 1994 Acquired risk factors for deep vein thrombosis in symptomatic outpatients. Archives of Internal Medicine 154: 164–168

Goldman L, Caldera D L, Nussbaum S R 1977 Multifactorial index of cardiac risk in noncardiac procedures. New England Journal of Medicine 297: 845–850

Knaus W A, Draper E A, Wagner D P et al 1985 APACHE-II: a severity of disease classification system. Critical Care Medicine 13: 818–824

Knaus W A, Wagner D P, Draper E A et al 1991 The APACHE III prognostic system. Risk prediction of hospital mortality for critically ill hospitalised adults. Chest 100: 1619–1636

Paluzzi R G 1993 Antimicrobial prophylaxis for surgery. Medical Clinics of North America 77: 427–441

Thromboembolic Risk Factors (THRIFT) Consensus Group 1992 Risk of and prophylaxis for venous thromboembolism in hospital patients. British Medical Journal 305: 567–574

Velanovich V 1994 Preoperative laboratory screening based on age, gender and concomitant medical diseases. Surgery 115: 56–61

Wheatley T, Veitch P S 1997 Recent advances in prophylaxis against deep vein thrombosis. British Journal of Anaesthesia 78: 118–120

17

Premedication and anaesthesia

M. W. Platt

Objectives

- **To understand the role of preoperative medication in the work-up for surgery.**
- **To have a general understanding of the function of the anaesthetist, the effects of anaesthesia and the perioperative medical management of the patient.**
- **To realize the importance of analgesia in minimizing the stress response and its significance in reducing post-operative complications.**
- **To understand the basic pharmacology and toxicology of local anaesthetic agents and their use.**

PREMEDICATION

Premedication is the prescribing of drugs to be administered preoperatively. These are usually agents prescribed by the anaesthetist, at the preoperative visit, to allay anxiety, relieve pain, to dry saliva, and to maintain the dosage of intercurrent medication. After a brief discussion of intercurrent medication, the broad topic of anaesthetic premedication will be considered.

Intercurrent medication

Many patients coming to surgery have other medical problems which are treated by a variety of different drugs. Refer to the section on medical problems for detailed notes (see Ch. 7).

Some patients who need special consideration include: those on antihypertensive therapy; those on antiarrhythmic therapy; anticoagulated patients; patients on diabetic therapy (oral hypoglycaemics or insulin); those on endocrine replacement therapy (particularly thyroxine); those on adrenocortical replace-

ment or augmentation therapy; those patients undergoing treatment for asthma or chronic obstructive airways disease with bronchodilators and allied treatments; and those having cardiac failure therapy and diuretics.

Because of fasting, and sometimes the surgical problem itself, it is not always possible for this medication to be continued. However, many drugs need to be continued up to the time of surgery. Sometimes a parenteral form of the agent can be substituted.

Anaesthetic premedication

1. Anxiolysis
2. Drying secretions
3. Analgesia.

Anxiolysis (Table 17.1)

Patients attending for surgery are normally anxious about the outcome. They may have a fear of the unknown, of pain, of dying, of cancer, or non-specific fears. Although the preoperative visit by the anaes-

Table 17.1 Anxiolytic agents in common use

Agent	Dose	Approx. duration (h)
Benzodiazepines		
Diazepam	0.05–0.3 mg kg^{-1}	36–200
Temazepam	0.15–0.5 mg kg^{-1}	5–20
Lorazepam	0.015–0.06 µg kg^{-1}	10–20
Midazolam	0.07–0.08 mg kg^{-1}	0.5–2
Phenothiazines		
Promethazine	0.2–0.5 mg kg^{-1}	8–12
Prochlorperazine	0.1–0.2 mg kg^{-1}	

thetist does much to allay anxiety by reducing the unknown element, waiting for an operation may be unpleasant. Anxiolytics calm the patient and help to reduce time spent 'dwelling' on fears. Agents specifically used for anxiolysis are the benzodiazepines, particularly the shorter-acting agents such as temazepam, usually given orally 2 hours preoperatively. For major operations such as cardiopulmonary bypass, a long-acting drug such as lorazepam may be used. Opioid analgesics calm and sedate the patient and are often used, especially if analgesia is required (see below).

Phenothiazines may also be used, usually in combination with an opioid. Promethazine is frequently combined with pethidine. These agents are useful, especially in the elderly, since they calm the patient without too much sedation. Phenothiazines are also appropriate in atopic individuals (e.g. asthmatics), where their antihistaminic action may be useful. Prochlorperazine is used for its combined sedative and antiemetic properties.

Butyrophenones, such as droperidol, are now no longer used for sedation since they cause dysphoria and the so-called 'locked-in syndrome'. The latter is a state of fear elicited in the patient by a feeling of not being able to communicate with the outside world, although they appear very calm. In very low doses (e.g. 0.01 mg kg^{-1} of droperidol), however, these agents are very potent antiemetics.

Drying secretions (Table 17.2)

In the days of ether anaesthesia, it was particularly important to dry oral secretions, because ether stimulates salivary secretions on induction, potentiating the possibility of laryngospasm. With modern anaesthesia it is less of a requirement, although it may be useful to dry secretions prior to dental surgery, bronchoscopy or surgery on the lung and for paediatric patients in whom salivation can be a problem. In addition to drying secretions, muscarinic receptor antagonists also prevent bradycardia, a common side-effect of general anaesthesia, especially in very young children.

Hyoscine, in contrast to atropine, contributes to the sedative properties of premedication. Glycopyrrolate does not cross the blood–brain barrier, and is a more potent inhibitor of salivary secretions, with less effect on the vagus nerve and hence on the heart rate. Atropine has also been shown to have a small antiemetic effect, presumably through inhibition of the vagus nerve, as well as a slight bronchodilator effect.

Analgesia (Table 17.3)

There are two main reasons for using opioid analgesia as part of the anaesthetic premedication, apart from the excellent sedative properties. Patients with painful conditions such as fractured hips and other types of trauma need analgesia for a comfortable transfer to theatre. Opioid analgesics are also used preoperatively to provide a continuous background of analgesia to aid the anaesthetic and extend analgesia into the postoperative period. Recent evidence suggests that preoperative medication with analgesics such as opioids or possibly even non-steroidal analgesics, reduces postoperative analgesic requirements.

Premedication with an opioid is usually combined with anticholinergic agents, such as glycopyrrolate, to dry secretions and (in the case of hyoscine) to potentiate sedation.

Table 17.3 Analgesic agents in common use

Agent	Dose (mg kg^{-1})	Approx. duration, i.m. (h)
Morphine	0.1–0.2	4
Papaveretum	0.2–0.4	3
Pethidine	1.0–1.5	3–4

Notes:
1. Papaveretum is a mixture of alkaloids which contains morphine (45–55% dry weight), codeine, papaverine, thebaine and noscopine. It should not be used in women of child-bearing age, because noscopine has been shown to be a gene toxin.
Papaveretum is most commonly used as a premedication in combination with hyoscine, and comes in a premixed ampoule containing papaveretum 20 mg ml^{-1} and hyoscine 0.4 mg ml^{-1}.
2. Pethidine is often premixed with promethazine as pethidine 50 mg ml^{-1} and promethazine 25 mg ml^{-1}. Atropine is sometimes given in addition.
3. Morphine, often used alone for both its sedative and analgesic properties, is usually combined with a drying agent such as atropine (also useful to prevent bradycardia), or in combination with an antiemetic drug.

Table 17.2 Drying agents in common use

Agent	Dose (mg kg^{-1})	Approx. duration i.v.	i.m.
Atropine	0.02	15–30 min	2–4 h
Hyoscine	0.008	30–60 min	4–6 h
Glycopyrrolate	0.01	2–4 h	6–8 h

Generally speaking, the choice of premedication depends very much on the individual patient. For example, a moribund patient will not benefit, and may indeed suffer from such side-effects as respiratory or cardiovascular depression, whereas a young, fit, anxious patient could perhaps benefit from anxiolysis or sedation, besides possible analgesic requirements, especially in trauma.

GENERAL ANAESTHESIA

The anaesthetist is responsible for the perioperative medical management of the patient. This will include management of acute blood loss, maintenance of normal cardiorespiratory physiology and protection of organ function. This may include minimizing the stress response to surgery and the effects of the stress hormones on organ function (e.g. cardiac and renal function). General anaesthesia is a reversible, drug-induced state of unresponsiveness to outside stimuli, characterized by non-awareness, analgesia and relaxation of striated muscle. Older agents such as ether need to be given in large amounts to achieve these aims, and they take a long time for induction and recovery.

With the advent of newer, more specifically acting agents such as the muscle relaxants, modern general anaesthesia is a balance between the triad of 'relaxation', 'analgesia' and 'hypnosis' (lack of awareness).

A general anaesthetic may be considered in three phases, analogous to an aircraft flight:

- 'take-off' = 'induction'
- 'cruising' = 'maintenance'
- 'landing' = 'reversal and recovery'.

Each part of the triad of general anaesthesia will be considered separately, under the heading of each phase of the anaesthetic.

Induction of anaesthesia

Hypnosis at induction of anaesthesia

In the anaesthetic room, patients are induced using one or other of several intravenous anaesthetics. In approximate order of frequency, those shown in Table 17.4 are the most commonly used agents. When drugs are taken up in the bloodstream, initial distribution is to 'vessel-rich' tissues and those taking a large fraction of the cardiac output. Thus the brain, which is vessel rich and also taking a large fraction of the cardiac output, receives a considerable portion of intravenous anaesthetic given as a bolus. Subsequently, drugs diffuse out of the brain, down a concentration gradient formed by the falling blood concentration, and are redistributed to other vessel-poor tissues. This results in an initial short redistribution half-life. The longer elimination half-life of a drug represents its metabolism and elimination from the body. In some instances, this can appear to take a long time, due to the slow leaching out of drug from vessel-poor fat tissues.

Thiopentone, a very short-acting barbiturate, was the first widely used intravenous induction agent. It was first used to great effect on casualties from the bombing of Pearl Harbor in 1942. However, the ability of thiopentone to depress the myocardium was tragically evident in the deaths of young sailors already shocked from hypovolaemia. It was soon learned to reduce the dose and only give enough thiopentone to cause sleep (a 'sleep dose'), titrating carefully with each patient – especially those with a low cardiac reserve.

Propofol has a very short half-life, and tends to be used particularly in day-case surgery, where rapid recovery is indicated. It is also used to abate the effects of procedures which occasionally cause laryngospasm, such as laryngeal mask placement and anal stretching. Propofol is sometimes infused intravenously to maintain anaesthesia, because of its short half-life. The

Table 17.4	Anaesthetic agents		
Drug	Dose (mg kg^{-1})	Distribution half-life (min)	Elimination half-life (h)
Thiopentone	3–5	3–14	5–17
Propofol	1–3	2–4	4–5
Etomidate	0.3	2–6	1–5
Ketamine			
i.v.	1–2	10	2–3
i.m.	5–10	15	2–3
Methohexitone	1–3	3–8	26
Midazolam	0.03–0.3	6–20	1–4

initial bolus of propofol sometimes causes a profound fall in blood pressure and inhibits compensatory increases in heart rate. Preinduction administration of glycopyrrolate or atropine may attenuate this.

Etomidate is indicated only for induction of anaesthesia. As a side-effect, it causes a reversible suppression of an enzyme in the adrenal cortex, leading to inhibition of cortisol secretion – this is especially important if it is used as an infusion. Etomidate is indicated in patients with poor cardiac reserve, or other patients in whom a fall in cardiac output could prove catastrophic, because it tends to maintain cardiac output. It is relatively long acting, and is associated with a higher incidence of postoperative nausea and vomiting.

Ketamine is used in shocked patients, because it stimulates the sympathetic nervous system and prevents a fall in cardiac output. However, patients already on full sympathetic drive will still suffer a reduction in cardiac output and blood pressure. Ketamine produces a state known as 'dissociative anaesthesia' with profound analgesia. It is structurally related to LSD.

Benzodiazepines given intravenously, particularly midazolam (the most efficacious in this respect), are occasionally used to induce or assist induction of anaesthesia.

Opioids in very high doses are used to induce anaesthesia in some situations. The most commonly used agents for this are the highly potent synthetic derivatives fentanyl, alfentanil and sufentanil. Fentanyl is used in a dosage of up to 1.0 mg kg^{-1}, particularly in cardiac anaesthesia, since it avoids hypotension and maintains cardiac output. Without other agents, awareness may occur, however, and chest rigidity, preventing adequate ventilation, occasionally occurs (easily reversed with the use of muscle relaxants).

Generally, with the exceptions outlined above, all intravenous anaesthetic agents depress the myocardium.

Relaxation at induction

On induction, muscle relaxation is necessary to facilitate (tracheal) intubation. Relaxation during maintenance of anaesthesia is discussed below.

Suxamethonium is a depolarizing relaxant used primarily for difficult intubation and crash induction. It only lasts approximately 5 minutes, after a dose of 1.5 mg kg^{-1}. Suxamethonium is essentially two acetylcholine molecules joined together. Its great similarity to acetylcholine results in activation of the receptor and depolarization of the muscle membrane. However, this depolarization lasts some 5–10 minutes, and muscles become unresponsive to acetylcholine. As it lasts some 5–10 minutes, suxamethonium is useful, apart from intubation, for very short surgical procedures.

Side-effects of suxamethonium include:

1. *Histamine release.* 'Scoline rash' is very common following intravenous administration of suxamethonium. An erythematous rash is seen spreading over the upper trunk and lower neck anteriorly. Very occasionally, suxamethonium will cause bronchospasm and other more severe sequelae.

2. *Bradycardia.* This is seen particularly if a second or subsequent dose is given, especially in children. Atropine is given to prevent or reverse this effect.

3. *Generalized somatic pain.* The actual cause of this is unknown, but may be a result of widespread fleeting muscle contractions, termed 'fasciculations', caused by the depolarization of muscle fascicles.

4. *Hyperkalaemia.* Suxamethonium causes the release of potassium from muscle cells. This may be accentuated in acute denervating injuries such as spinal cord trauma or burns, and can lead to cardiac arrest.

5. *Persistent neuromuscular blockade.* Some patients may have deficient or abnormal plasma pseudocholinesterase, resulting in prolonged action of suxamethonium, sometimes called 'scoline apnoea'. This is genetically related. The completely silent gene is rare, occurring in approximately 1 : 7000 of the population.

6. *Malignant hyperthermia.* This is a condition occurring in some 1 : 100 000 of the population. It occurs as a reaction to certain anaesthetic drugs, of which suxamethonium and halothane are the commonest. Muscle metabolism becomes uncontrolled because of an abnormality of intracellular calcium flux. Body temperature rapidly rises at the rate of at least 2°C every 15 minutes, and $P_a\text{CO}_2$, reflecting the massively raised metabolic rate, also increases with alacrity. Treatment is with ventilation and surface cooling and intravenous Dantrium given promptly before death ensues.

'Crash induction'

This consists of a rapid-sequence intravenous induction, cricoid pressure and tracheal intubation, with the aim of preventing regurgitation and aspiration of stomach contents. The patient is given a precalculated dose of thiopentone (3–5 mg kg^{-1}), immediately followed by suxamethonium (1.5 mg kg^{-1}), currently the fastest-acting muscle relaxant, acting within one circulation time. A trained assistant applies pressure to the cricoid cartilage simultaneously compressing the oesophagus between cricoid ring and vertebral column. The trachea is intubated with a cuffed tracheal tube, and the cuff inflated. Only when the anaesthetic circuit is attached and cuff seal confirmed is cricoid pressure relaxed at the request of the anaesthetist.

The following patients are at risk of aspiration of stomach contents on induction of anaesthesia:

- All non-fasted patients
- Patients with a history suggestive of hiatus hernia
- Any emergency trauma patient (trauma slows stomach emptying)
- Intestinal or gastric obstruction or stasis
- Pregnancy (stomach emptying slowed and cardiac sphincter relaxed)
- Any other intra-abdominal tumours that may cause slowing of gastric emptying.

Maintenance of anaesthesia

Hypnosis during anaesthesia

Anaesthesia is usually maintained with volatile agents, which are hydrocarbons, liquid at room temperature, with high saturated vapour pressures and lipid solubility. Diethyl ether was the earliest agent used, and is still used commonly in other parts of the world. Ether is flammable and explosive. By adding fluoride and other halogens, however, the hydrocarbon molecule becomes much more stable. Modern agents are non-inflammable, non-explosive, and much more potent than ether. Being less soluble in blood (as indicated by the blood/gas partition coefficient), they also have a much faster uptake and elimination time than diethyl ether. Table 17.5 shows the most commonly used anaesthetic volatile agents (with ether as a comparison).

Halothane. A hydrocarbon with fluorine, chlorine and bromine atoms. This was the first modern volatile anaesthetic agent which was not explosive or flammable. Synthesized in 1951 and first used clinically in 1956, it was the most commonly used anaesthetic agent for 30 years. Halothane is a potent anaesthetic which allows a smooth induction (which is important especially for gaseous induction of children), and relatively rapid onset of anaesthesia. In the body, up to 20% is metabolized by the liver, the majority being eliminated unchanged via the lungs. The recovery time from halothane anaesthesia is also brisk and smooth. The most common side-effects of halothane are secondary to its effects on the heart. Halothane slows the sinoatrial node, slowing heart rate and causing variations in the p–q interval. It reduces myocardial workload. Like verapamil, halothane produces these effects by blocking calcium channels in the heart. However, it also sensitizes the heart to catecholamines and may precipitate arrhythmias (which is especially important in the presence of adrenaline-supplemented local anaesthesia and if the arterial carbon dioxide tension, P_aCO_2, is elevated). By reducing cardiac output, halothane attenuates splanchnic blood flow, diminishing hepatic blood

Table 17.5 Anaesthetic volatile agents

Agent	Structure	MAC	Blood/gas partition coefficient
Diethyl ether	$CH_3CH_2{-}O{-}CH_2CH_3$	1.92	12
Halothane	$CF_3CHClBr$	0.75	2.3
Enflurane	$CHF_2O{-}CF_2CHFCl$	1.68	1.9
Isoflurane	$CHF_2O{-}CHClCF_3$	1.05	1.4

Notes:
1. MAC: the minimum alveolar concentration of a gas or vapour in oxygen required to keep 50% of the population unresponsive to a standard surgical stimulus (opening of the abdomen). MAC is expressed as a percentage concentration.
2. Blood/gas partition coefficient: indicates how rapidly a gas or vapour is taken up from the lungs. The higher the blood solubility, the longer it takes for the brain to gain adequate anaesthetic concentrations.
3. Summary of effects of modern vapours on organ systems:
   (a) *Heart:* generally cause depressed contractility: halothane > enflurane > isoflurane (halothane causes more arrhythmias)
   (b) *Blood vessels:* generally cause vasodilation: isoflurane > enflurane > halothane
   (c) *Respiration:* depressed by all agents: enflurane > isoflurane > halothane
   (d) *Brain:* All may cause vasodilation and raised intracranial pressure: halothane > enflurane > isoflurane (isoflurane safe up to 1 MAC).

flow and possibly aggravating its effects on the liver. Using very fine indicators of hepatic performance, it has now been shown that even the briefest exposure to halothane will cause some degree of liver dysfunction. This is probably related to the large amount of halothane that is metabolized (up to 20%). There is also an idiosyncratic reaction which occurs after halothane exposure in some patients, known as 'halothane hepatitis'. The latter is a fulminant centrilobular necrosis of the liver which appears 2–5 days postoperatively. The incidence is 1 : 35 000 of the population (from the National Halothane Study, USA, 1966), with a mortality of over 50%. Halothane is now used in only 10% of anaesthetics given in the UK, the majority of these being for paediatric anaesthesia.

Enflurane. Enflurane is an ether synthesized in 1963 and first used in 1966. It is halogenated with fluorine and chlorine atoms to render it non-explosive and non-inflammable. Enflurane is more efficacious in reducing peripheral vascular resistance and is less likely to cause cardiac arrhythmias, nor does it sensitize the heart to catecholamines. However, its pungent odour makes it unsuitable for gaseous induction in children. Enflurane causes greater respiratory depression than halothane or isoflurane, and so it is less suitable for maintaining anaesthesia in the spontaneously breathing patient. Enflurane is only slightly metabolized by the liver (up to 2.5%) and appears not to cause hepatitis.

Isoflurane. Isoflurane is the most recent volatile agent in common use. It was synthesized in 1965 and first used in 1971. It is actually a structural isomer of enflurane, but with different properties. Isoflurane tends to act on the peripheral vasculature as a calcium antagonist, causing a reduction in peripheral vascular resistance. Although it has minimal effects on the heart, isoflurane may cause 'coronary steal', a phenomenon whereby blood is diverted from stenosed coronary arteries to dilated unblocked coronary arteries, possibly compromising ischaemic areas of myocardium. This is still a controversial area, however, and isoflurane generally causes minimal depression of contractility. In the brain, isoflurane has the least effect on cerebral blood flow, causing no significant increase up to 1 MAC. Isoflurane causes least respiratory depression and is suited to the spontaneously breathing patient. Only up to 0.2% of isoflurane is metabolized by the liver and no cases of hepatitis have been reported.

Desflurane is proving very popular for anaesthetizing day-care patients because of its rapid recovery, although it is very pungent and often causes patients to cough. It is unsuitable for gaseous induction for this reason.

Sevoflurane is very popular as a gaseous induction agent, especially in children, because of its rapid onset and non-pungent characteristics.

The last two are characterized by remarkable molecular stability, with very little hepatic metabolism. They also have a very low blood gas solubility coefficient, resulting in very rapid onset and recovery.

Xenon is currently undergoing trials as an anaesthetic agent. It is an extremely stable molecule and gives excellent cardiovascular stability with a rapid onset and offset and no metabolism. However, it is very expensive and has required the development of special anaesthetic machines which allow the gas to be recycled for further use.

Nitrous oxide. Nitrous oxide (N_2O), unlike the volatile agents, is a gas at atmospheric pressure and room temperature. It has a MAC of 103% at sea level. The requirements of keeping the patient well oxygenated mean that it can never be relied upon to provide anaesthesia in its own right. It is, however, a very potent analgesic agent. Fifty per cent N_2O is equivalent in efficacy to approximately 10 mg morphine sulphate. It continues to enjoy popularity as the main background anaesthetic gas, usually given as 70% in oxygen.

In concentrations greater than 50% it causes amnesia and contributes significantly to the overall anaesthetic.

Relaxation during anaesthesia

To allow the surgeon access to intra-abdominal contents, or to allow artificial ventilation of the patient, for example in chest surgery, muscle relaxation (paralysis) is required.

Agents used specifically to relax muscles are called *relaxants*. Relaxants are agents which block acetylcholine receptors on muscle end-plates. There are two types of relaxant: depolarizing and non-depolarizing.

Depolarizing muscle relaxants. Only one depolarizing relaxant is still in common use, *suxamethonium*, which is described above in relation to induction.

Non-depolarizing muscle relaxants. There are many different relaxants available today. Due to the side-effects of suxamethonium, research continues to find a non-depolarizing relaxant with a very rapid onset and very short half-life. Non-depolarizing relaxants have an onset time of the order of 2–3 minutes, and last from 20 minutes to 1 hour. They are competitive inhibitors of the acetylcholine receptors on muscle end-plates, preventing access of acetylcholine to receptor, resulting in non-transmission of nerve impulse to muscle. *Curare* was the first relaxant of this class, developed from an arrow poison used by the indigenous people of the Amazonian rainforests to kill animals for food. Only the dextrorotatory isomer is active; the term 'tubo-' refers to the bamboo tubes in which it is carried – 'D-tubocurare'. Modern relaxants tend to be shorter acting, with fewer side-effects (Table 17.6).

Analgesia during anaesthesia

The final part of the triad of general anaesthesia during its maintenance consists of analgesia. The anaesthetized patient derives analgesia from three potential sources: from the premedication, from anaesthesia supplementation with opioids, and from the analgesic properties of volatile and gaseous agents.

Premedication. Opioids used in premedication, as discussed earlier, will tend to last intraoperatively and into the postoperative period. In this way, premedication affects both the anaesthetic and postoperative analgesia.

Anaesthetic opioid supplementation. Intraoperatively, opioids are often administered to deepen the effect of the anaesthetic, or to reduce the amount of volatile agent used (often because of their side-effects such as hypotension). To limit the effects of opioids to the perioperative period, anaesthetists often use highly potent short-acting agents such as fentanyl, alfentanil

Table 17.6 Non-depolarizing muscle relaxants

Agents	Dose (mg kg⁻¹)	Duration of effect (min)	Side-effects
D-Tubocurare	0.5	30–60	Sympathetic ganglion blockade, histamine release, hypotension
Alcuronium	0.3	20–40	As above
Pancuronium	0.01	45–120	Vagolytic: tachycardia, increase blood pressure
Vecuronium	0.01	30–45	Bradycardia
Atracurium	0.06	15–40	Histamine release

Notes:
1. With the exception of atracurium, all these agents require renal and hepatic function for their clearance.
2. Atracurium is excreted by two mechanisms: Hoffman elimination (up to 40%) and hepatic metabolism. Hofmann elimination results in breakdown of the atracurium molecule as a result of pH and temperature. It is used in those patients with renal failure.
3. The histamine release associated with atracurium is only a quarter of that associated with tubocurare, and tends not to cause the hypotension seen with the latter agent.
4. The duration of effect with each agent varies slightly according to anaesthetic technique. The use of volatile agents, particularly enflurane and isoflurane, potentiates the effect of non-depolarizing muscle relaxants. Hypothermia also potentiates non-depolarizing relaxants.
5. The shorter-acting agents atracurium and vecuronium are often used as infusions for long cases and in intensive care.
6. Muscle relaxants have no intrinsic anaesthetic effect.

or sufentanil. These agents are all much more potent than morphine, and much shorter acting (of the order 20–30 minutes). They may need to be reversed at the end of the operation, to facilitate spontaneous respiration. However, this is at the expense of analgesia. Longer acting opioids such as morphine, papaveretum, or pethidine may also be used – especially if postoperative analgesia may be a problem.

Modern non-steroidal anti-inflammatory agents, such as diclofenac and ketorolac, are increasingly used for postoperative analgesia, either on their own for minor surgery or in combination with opioid techniques to give a much better quality of analgesia. Side-effects include renal failure (prostaglandin inhibition may lead to renal shutdown), gastric ulceration and bleeding (inhibition of platelet function). Different agents have different degrees of complications, but their careful use has revolutionized the aftercare of patients, particularly after day-care surgery.

Analgesic properties of volatile agents. Modern volatile anaesthetic agents have poor analgesic properties and contribute little to this part of the anaesthetic. However, N_2O is a very good analgesic (see above) and is also used for analgesia during labour (as a 50% mixture with oxygen, known as Entonox).

Recovery from anaesthesia

At the end of surgery, anaesthesia is terminated. Volatile agents and nitrous oxide are turned off on the anaesthetic machine and oxygen alone administered. Anaesthetic gases and vapours diffuse down concentration gradients from the tissues to alveoli of the lungs and out via the airway.

Reversal of muscle relaxation

Competitive muscle relaxants usually need to be reversed to ensure full return of muscle power. The degree of neuromuscular blockade can be monitored with a peripheral nerve stimulator.

Neostigmine (0.05 mg kg⁻¹) or *edrophonium* (0.5 mg kg⁻¹) is given intravenously. These agents block acetylcholinesterase in the neuromuscular junction, resulting in accumulation of acetylcholine. This overcomes the competitive blockade of the relaxant molecules in favour of acetylcholine. However, both neostigmine and edrophonium cause acetylcholine accumulation at both muscarinic and nicotinic sites. Muscarinic receptors are those cholinergic receptors in the heart, gut, sweat glands, etc. Therefore, to prevent bradycardia, profuse sweating, and gut overactivity, atropine (0.02 mg kg⁻¹) or glycopyrrolate (0.01 mg kg⁻¹) must be given with the anticholinesterase.

Full reversal of muscle relaxation is only apparent by appropriate neuromuscular monitoring, or when the patient is able to maintain head lifting. This aspect of recovery from anaesthesia is crucial, since full muscular control is necessary for coughing and for good control of the airway. Indeed it highlights the importance of adequate recovery facilities in the theatre suite.

REGIONAL ANAESTHESIA

Definition

Regional (local) anaesthesia is the reversible blockade of nerve conduction by regionally applied agents, for the purpose of sensory ablation, either of traumatized tissue, or to enable minor surgery. These agents are referred to as 'local anaesthetics'. Both motor and sensory nerves may be blocked, depending on the agent used and the anatomical region where the agent is applied.

Nerves may be blocked anywhere between the central nervous system and the site of required sensory loss. Local anaesthetics are used to block pain fibres as they enter the spinal cord: epidural, spinal and paravertebral techniques. They may also be blocked along their anatomical route in the neurovascular bundles: field blocks, or specific nerve blocks. Finally, local infiltration around the required site may be performed (for example, skin and subcutaneous infiltration), to block conduction at the nerve endings.

Types of nerve fibre

The speed with which local anaesthetic agents are taken up by nerve fibres depends on their size and whether they are myelinated. Nerve fibres are classified according to their size and speed of conduction (Table 17.7).

Sensitivity to local anaesthetics

The smaller fibres are more sensitive to local anaesthetic agents than the larger fibres. Hence, 'C' fibres conducting pain are more sensitive than motor fibres in the 'A' group. This is why patients may still be able to move limbs, even during regional anaesthesia.

The reason for the differential is most likely due to more rapid absorption and uptake of local anaesthetic into the smaller fibres within neurovascular bundles.

Local anaesthetic agents

Drugs used as local anaesthetics all tend to have 'membrane stabilizing' properties.

Local anaesthetic agents act by inducing a blockade of nerve transmission in peripheral nerve impulses. This occurs as a result of obstruction to sodium channels in the axon membrane, preventing ingress of sodium ions necessary for propagation of an action potential.

Local anaesthetic agents belong to one of two chemical classes according to their structure, which consists of an amide or ester linkage separating an aromatic group and an amine:

Aromatic group >–< Amine group
Amide or ester

Ester class

The only ester still in frequent use is *cocaine*, which is an ester of benzoic acid. It is used generally only for topical anaesthesia of mucous membranes in the nose and sinuses.

Amethocaine is still used occasionally as a topical agent, as is *benzocaine*.

Amide class (Table 17.8)

The first amide to be synthesized was *lignocaine*. This was shown to be safer than cocaine and has remained a mainstay for local anaesthetic practice. *Prilocaine* has the highest therapeutic index, and is considered the safest agent for intravenous blockade. Other amides in common usage include *bupivacaine*, *mepivacaine* and

Table 17.7	Types of nerve fibre			
Fibre	Type	Function	Conduction velocity (ms)	Diameter (μm)
A	α	Motor, proprioception	70–120	12–20
	β	Touch, pressure	30–70	5–12
	γ	Motor (spindles)	15–30	3–6
	δ	Pain, temperature, touch	12–30	2–5
B		Preganglionic autonomic	3–15	<3
C		Dorsal root: pain, reflexes	0.5–2	0.4–1.2
		Sympathetic: postganglionic	0.7–2.3	0.3–1.3

Table 17.8   Amide class

Drug	Maximum dose (mg)	Side-effects
Lignocaine	300 (500 + adr.)	No unusual features. CNS excitation with toxicity
Prilocaine	600	Least toxic. Methaemoglobinaemia >600 mg
Bupivacaine	175 (225 + adr.)	Sudden cardiovascular collapse. Not indicated for intravenous blockade
Cocaine	150	Cardiac arrhythmias. CNS excitation. Topical use only

Notes:
1. The table includes only those agents currently in common use and maximal doses relate to adult size (70 kg body weight). The bracketed dosages refer to maximal doses in the presence of adrenaline.
2. All local anaesthetic agents have membrane-stabilizing properties. Their toxic effects therefore relate to this property and involve mainly the cardiovascular and central nervous systems.

  Toxic effects on the central nervous system include fitting and coma, leading to death from hypoxia without adequate resuscitation. Cardiovascular effects from toxicity include hypotension, cardiac arrhythmias and acute cardiovascular collapse.

  Bupivacaine has a high affinity for cardiac muscle cells – a property which is thought to be responsible for the high incidence of cardiovascular collapse associated with its use for intravenous blockade (Bier's block), for which it is no longer recommended.
3. Toxic effects may also occur with the accidental intravascular injection of drug.
4. Concentration of local anaesthetic agents varies. Bupivacaine comes as 0.5% or 0.25%, with or without adrenaline. Lignocaine generally comes as 0.5, 1.0, 2.0% concentrations, again plus or minus adrenaline. The higher concentrations obviously have lower maximum safe volumes (1% = 10 mg ml^{-1}, 2% = 20 mg ml^{-1}).
5. Local anaesthesia techniques should always be performed where adequate resuscitation facilities are present.
6. Adrenaline and other vasoconstricting agents, such as felypressin, allow higher doses of local anaesthetic to be used, the vasoconstriction resulting in reduced absorption.

etidocaine. Bupivacaine is longer acting than lignocaine and is commonly used in epidural analgesia.

Clinical application

1. *Local infiltration* is used for surgery alone or in combination with general anaesthesia. Used with adrenaline, it reduces bleeding at the operative site. It also produces good postoperative analgesia. EMLA (eutectic mixture of local anaesthetics), a mixture of lignocaine and prilocaine produces good analgesia when applied topically to skin. It is useful for insertion of intravenous lines, arterial lines and removal of minor skin lesions. It needs to be applied some 2 hours before the procedure.

2. *'Field' blocks and nerve blocks* are useful for pro-ducing wider areas of anaesthesia and analgesia, for example in inguinal hernia repair, brachial plexus blockade for the upper limb and femoral and sciatic blocks of the lower limb.

3. *Spinal, epidural and paravertebral blockade* produce widespread anaesthesia and analgesia. The pain of labour and childbirth involves nerve roots of lower thoracic, lumbar and sacral regions of the spinal cord. Epidural techniques, involving the epidural placement of a catheter, allow continuous analgesia or anaesthesia, alleviating pain from all these groups of fibres. Regional anaesthesia such as this is frequently employed for urological and other surgery in the lower half of the body. It should be noted, however, that spinal and epidural techniques also block sympathetic ganglia at the appropriate levels. Hypotension will occur unless adequate precautions are taken.

Summary

1. Pre-emptive analgesia has gained popularity with the recent publication of data suggesting that the administration of analgesia preoperatively, either systemically as with an opioid, or regionally as in use of local anaesthetic techniques, reduces the patient's need for analgesia postoperatively. This has been reinforced by the finding that use of epidural analgesia for 3 days prior to leg amputation produces a marked reduction in the incidence of phantom limb pain. Thus the use of regional techniques combined with general anaesthesia is becoming more popular.

2. The widespread development of acute pain services is enabling the continuation of regional local analgesic techniques from the operating theatre into the general wards, improving the standards of postoperative pain control and perhaps reducing the incidence of postoperative nausea and vomiting secondary to opioids.

Further reading

Atkinson R S, Rushman G B, Lee A 1987 A synopsis of anaesthesia, 10th edn. Wright, London

Barash P G, Cuplen B F, Stoelting R K 1989 Clinical anaesthesia. Lippincott, Philadelphia

Gilman A G, Goodman L S, Rall T W, Murad F 1985 Goodman and Gilman's pharmacological basis of therapeutics, 7th edn. Macmillan, London

Miller R D 1990 Anesthesia, 3rd edn. Churchill Livingstone, Edinburgh, vols I–II

Nimmo W S, Smith G 1989 Anaesthesia. Blackwell Scientific, Oxford, vols I–II

Stoelting R K 1987 Pharmacology and physiology in anesthetic practice. Lippincott, Philadelphia

Vickers M D, Morgan M, Spencer P S J 1991 Drugs in anaesthetic practice, 7th edn. Butterworths, Oxford

18

Operating theatres and special equipment

M. K. H. Crumplin

> ### Objectives
>
> - **To understand the prevention of sepsis in theatre.**
> - **To learn the safe positioning of patients whilst they are unconscious.**
> - **To respect and understand the principles of diathermy, laser, cryosurgery and X-ray usage in a theatre environment.**
> - **To comprehend principles of the use of fibreoptics and microscopes.**
> - **Operating theatre design and environment**

INTRODUCTION

A large proportion of a surgeon's life is spent within the environment of an operating theatre. Here there are physical, chemical, and infective hazards to medical staff, nurses and patients, thus making the operating department the most hazardous part of the hospital. An understanding of this environment and the risks to both staff and patients must be clearly understood. In the operating theatre, the patient is totally helpless, and under full control of the theatre staff. A basic comprehension of management of patients under anaesthesia and of the equipment used will encourage surgeons to be responsible for the actions they undertake within that area.

THE OPERATING THEATRE

The operating theatre environment must provide a safe, efficient, user-friendly environment that is as free from bacterial contamination as possible. Operating theatre suites should be sited near to each other for efficient flexibility of staff movement. The theatres should preferably be situated on the first floor, away from the main hospital traffic. Ideally, operating rooms should be

on the same level and adjacent to intensive care units and surgical wards. The suite should incorporate the theatre sterile supply unit. There should be minimum distance between operating rooms and the accident and emergency (A&E) unit and X-ray facilities, which will both be sited on the ground floor. All district general hospitals should now have a multidisciplinary user committee to optimize efficiency and safety. This should be composed of surgeons, anaesthetists, operating theatre and anaesthetic nurses, microbiologists, a manager and a finance officer in line with recent Department of Health recommendations. This committee should meet on a regular basis. It is highly desirable to have an incident reporting system in place to audit adverse incidents in theatre.

Although there is no such entity as a standard operating theatre, an attempt was made by the Department of Health and Social Security in 1978 to introduce the nucleus concept, which at least provided hospitals with theatre suites appropriate to the average district general hospital requirements. Naturally, with orthopaedic, cardiac, neurosurgical, laser and other specialist requirements, there would have to be adjustments to the standard design, for example the Charnley tent, controlled areas for laser therapy and the provision of a pump preparation room off a cardiac bypass theatre.

The antiseptic environment

In any operating theatre suite an attempt should be made to minimize bacterial contamination, especially in the vicinity of the operating table; thus the concept of zones is useful:

- An outer, or general access zone – e.g. patient reception area and general office
- A clean, or limited access zone – e.g. the area between the reception bay and theatre suite, dispersal area, corridors and staff rest room
- a restricted access zone, for those properly clothed personnel engaged in operating theatre activities, anaesthetic room, and utility and scrub up rooms

- An aseptic or operating zone – the operating theatre.

To provide a minimally contaminated environment for surgeons and patients at the operating table, various principles must be employed.

Air flow

Directional air flow (laminar air flow) may be vertical or horizontal. Here, in addition to normal turbulent air flow through theatre which is necessary to maintain humidity, temperature and air circulation, an increased rate of air change is necessary to reduce the number of contaminated particles over the patient (i.e. aerobic counts of less than 35 micro-organism-carrying particles per cu mm). Air is pumped into the room through filters and passed out of vents in the periphery of the operating room and does not return into the operating suite. Most theatres have 20–40 air changes per hour, but this rate may increase to 400–600 per hour in the vertical laminar flow system of a Charnley tent.

Wearing of disposable, non-woven fabrics

This reduces dispersal of bacteria-laden particles which may emanate from the operating or nursing staff. Optimally, everybody would wear these gowns, but this might prove costly. Masks are not essential for the surgeon, but should be worn when the patient is particularly susceptible to infection, when a prothesis is being inserted, or when the surgeon or nurse has an upper respiratory tract infection.

Body exhaust suits

Here personal air circulation takes place within a specially designed operating suit and helmet so that exhaust air is removed from the suit by a pipe.

The operating tent environment

There is a high vertical laminar flow within the tent, and clean air from above the table is expelled down to floor level in a funnel shape, thereby reducing contamination. By using suitable exhaust suits and such tents, infection in hip replacement may be kept as low as 0.5%.

Behaviour in theatre

It is solely the surgeon's responsibility to ensure that:

- The correct patient is present
- Informed consent is obtained
- The operation site is marked

- The appropriate preoperative investigations have been performed
- Blood is cross-matched if relevant
- Ancillary investigations (frozen section, X-rays, etc.) are available.

It is desirable that the minimum number of people should be in the operating theatre, to provide safe and efficient management of the patient. The bacteriological count in theatre is related to the number of persons and their movement in the operating room.

Temperature and humidity control

A steady level of temperature and humidity during surgery is desirable for comfort and may be varied to suit individual preference. The temperature in the operating theatre will need to be higher for neonates, children, elderly patients and for prolonged surgery. The usual comfortable temperature range in the operating room would be 20–22°C (68–71.6°F). Temperature and humidity control should be integral to the air-conditioning system which, while maintaining a constant working milieu, will require approximately 20–40 air changes per hour. Patients will become hypothermic if the temperature is below 21°C (69.8°F) during prolonged procedures. Loss of heat may be reduced by using warming blankets placed on the sorbo-rubber table surface and by infusing warmed intravenous fluids. This is achieved by passing the blood, crystalloid or colloids through a coiled plastic infusion pipe in a heated waterbath. Postoperatively heat loss may also be minimized by wrapping the patient in aluminium foil.

OPERATING TABLES

Operating tables need to be heavy and stable, easily manoeuvrable, comfortable for the patient and highly adjustable in terms of positioning the patient correctly for a particular operative procedure. There are two basic types of operating table. First, and most common, are those which are completely mobile, thus allowing replacement if necessary. The second type of table is one which has a fixed and permanently installed column in the centre of the operating room with a variety of table tops which can be mounted on the column. These tables are usually expensive and have a remote control for their various movements. The problem is that if a fault develops with the table that theatre will be out of service. The advantage of the fixed-base system is that there is efficiency of patient handling and flexibility in operating-room scheduling using interchangeable table tops.

Essential characteristics of operating tables

It is important that the surface upon which the patient is placed is sympathetic to the contours of the patient. This is generally achieved by soft sorbo-rubber padding, which moulds to the patient to a certain degree. These pads are removable and easily cleaned. The sorbo padding will lift the patient above the metal table, for it is imperative that no part of the patient should come into contact with the metallic structure of the table. There should be easily accessible table controls, which may be motorized or hand operated. The table should be capable of two-way tilt, and breaking at its centre so that positions such as the lateral nephrectomy or jack-knife position may be used. The bottom half of the table must be easily removed so that various types of leg support and stirrups may be employed for gynaecological, urological, orthopaedic and pelvic surgery. With these leg supports it is important that joints are not overstressed and that undue pressure does not fall upon any point of the patient's lower limb. Tables for general surgery and urology should have a radiolucent section so that static X-ray films or an image intensifier may be used. A variety of arm rests, screen support bars, shoulder and pelvic supports should be available.

Safety and position on the operating table

In addition to the soft cushion support surfaces which line the hard surface of the operating table, it may be desirable to have built-in lumbar supports which are adjustable. Alternatively, partially filled intravenous fluid infusion bags can be placed under the patient's lumbar lordosis. When patient's arms are positioned either by their side, over their head or at right angles to the body, care must be taken that joints, ligaments and nerves are not overstressed. Various nerves are at risk from injury or pressure due to inappropriate positioning on the table. The brachial plexus may be stretched during arm movements, the ulnar nerve damaged at the elbow during pole insertion into the canvas sheet before transfer of a patient, and the lateral popliteal nerve may be damaged by pressure against a leg support bar. If the patient has osteoarthrosis this may be aggravated either by rough handling during transfer or excessive joint movement or distortion during the operative procedure. Should a patient have spinal or joint disorders it is perfectly reasonable to rehearse the position on the table with the patient prior to anaesthesia to make sure it is comfortable, e.g. cervical extension during thyroid surgery. Great care must be taken when moving patients on and off the operating table, and it should be ensured that no tubing attached to the patient is dislodged during transfer. Transfer of patients is best carried out using the Patslide, a tough plastic board, which acts as a bridge, on which the patient is carefully slid from trolley to table, or vice versa. At least three people should be involved in moving an unconscious patient.

Operating table fixtures for specialist procedures

Orthopaedic surgery

There are a great variety of limb attachments to an operating table to enable circumferential access to a limb and manoeuvrability, and also to allow the surgical team to use the image intensifier following fixation or reconstructive procedures.

Neurosurgical procedures

Access to the cranial cavity may be optimized by having the patient sitting up and an appropriate padded head support placed opposite the surgical field to keep the head in a comfortable and safe position.

SPECIAL EQUIPMENT IN THE OPERATING THEATRE

Tourniquets

Abuse of tourniquets may lead to vascular damage or thrombosis. Soft tissue and nerve injury may also occur. To avoid these problems follow these precautions:

- Exsanguinate the limb using an Esmarch bandage
- Apply the tourniquet cuff over soft padding at the appropriate site
- Inflate the tourniquet above the systolic blood pressure
- Record the time when the tourniquet is inflated and do not allow it to remain inflated for more than 2 hours.

Diathermy

Principles and effects

Surgical diathermy involves the passage of a high-frequency alternating current (AC) through body tissue: where the current is locally concentrated (a high current density), heat is produced, resulting in temperatures up to 1000°C. Low-frequency AC such as mains electricity (50 Hz) causes stimulation of neuromuscular tissue. The severity of the 'electrocution' depends on the current (amps) and its pathway through the body. Five to ten milliamps can cause painful muscle contractions, while 80–100 mA passing through the heart will cause ventricular fibrillation. However, if the current frequency is increased there is a reduction in the neuromuscular response; at current frequencies above 50 000 Hz (50 kHz) the response disappears. Surgical diathermy involves current frequencies in the range 400 kHz to 10 MHz. Currents up to 500 mA may then be safely passed through the patient. Heat will be produced wherever the current is locally concentrated.

Monopolar and bipolar diathermy

Monopolar diathermy is the most common configuration (Fig. 18.1). High-frequency current from the diathermy generator (or 'machine') is delivered to an active electrode held by the surgeon. Current density is high where this electrode touches body tissue and a pronounced local heating effect occurs. Current then spreads out through the body and returns to the diathermy generator via the patient plate electrode (often incorrectly called the 'earth plate'). This plate should be in good contact with the patient over at least 70 cm² (preferably twice this or more). This ensures that the current density at the plate is so low as to cause minimal heating. Misapplication of the patient plate is by far the most common cause of inadvertent diathermy burns.

Bipolar diathermy (Fig. 18.2) avoids the need for a plate and uses considerably less power. The surgeon holds a pair of forceps connected to the diathermy generator. Diathermy current passes down one limb of the forceps through a small piece of tissue to be coagulated, and then back to the generator via the other limb of the forceps. This inherently safer system has not gained wide use for two main reasons:

1. It cannot be used for 'cutting' (see below): cutting involves a continuous arc (spark) between the active electrode and the tissue involved. In bipolar diathermy an arc could only be struck between the limbs of the forceps.

2. It will not work with the common surgical practice of holding bleeding vessels with ordinary surgical forceps and 'buzzing' them with the active diathermy electrode. No current will pass through the tissue held by the surgical forceps. Bipolar current will only pass directly from one diathermy forceps limb to the other.

Cutting, coagulating and blend

Cutting diathermy involves the generator producing a continuous output, causing an arc to be struck between the active electrode and tissue. Temperatures up to 1000°C are produced. Cell water is instantly vapourized, causing tissue disruption with some coagulation of bleeding vessels. Coagulating diathermy involves a pulsed output. This results in desiccation and the sealing of blood vessels with the minimum of tissue disruption. Most diathermy generators have a 'blend' facility. This only functions when in cutting mode, and allows a combination of cutting and coagulation waveforms to increase the degree of haemostasis during cutting.

Earth referenced and isolated diathermy generators

Earth referenced generators. Older diathermy generators, many of which are still in everyday use, have valves and spark gaps to generate high-frequency current. These unsophisticated circuits produce a wide frequency range which includes frequencies above 1 MHz, and large earth leakage currents are unavoidable. The patient plate on these generators is earthed via a capacitor. The capacitor allows easy passage of high-frequency current such as in diathermy, but presents a large resistance to low-frequency currents such as mains electricity. (The patient is therefore not earthed for mains (50 Hz) current to reduce the risk of electrocution.)

As long as the patient plate is correctly applied, the patient is kept at earth (zero) potential for alternate sites such as electrocardiogram (ECG) electrodes or a drip stand accidentally touching the patient's skin. Unfortunately, if the patient plate is omitted, diathermy current will still flow (though a higher setting may be required) using the ECG electrodes or drip stand for

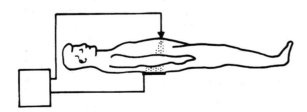

Fig 18.1   Monopolar diathermy.

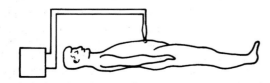

Fig 18.2   Bipolar diathermy.

the return pathway. An ECG electrode or drip stand presents skin contact of 1–5 cm², so a severe burn is inevitable.

Isolated generators. The more modern, often smaller, generators use transistors and 'solid-state' circuitry to produce the high-frequency current. Sophisticated electronics result in a much tighter frequency range (400–600 kHz) and a considerable reduction in earth leakage currents. Some of these solid-state generators (but by no means all) are designated 'isolated': the diathermy circuit is not earthed. This type of generator is inherently safer than an earth-referenced machine. Diathermy current can only pass back to the generator via the patient plate; there is no pathway back via earth. If the plate is omitted no current will flow.

Safety

General safety. Whenever electrical equipment is to be used on patients it is vital that the equipment meets the required safety standards and is properly maintained. Everyone using the equipment should be properly trained in its use. At the very least, read the user's manual: all diathermy machines are supplied with one.

Responsibility. The thorny problem of exactly who has overall responsibility for surgical diathermy is often not considered until a diathermy disaster occurs. In many operating theatres the diathermy is set up by nurses, or ODPs, and the anaesthetist is often the only doctor present when the patient plate is applied. Few surgeons check the diathermy prior to use. The surgeon using the diathermy must realize his overall responsibility, and check the alarm wiring and patient plate before use.

Alarms. Monopolar diathermy depends on the patient plate for its safety. All diathermy machines in use will alarm when switched on if the plate is not connected to the machine (plate continuity alarm), but only a few possess any alarm system that will ensure the plate is attached to the patient. Safe practice demands rigid adherence to correct procedures: first the patient plate is connected to the patient; the return lead is connected to the plate; the diathermy machine is switched on and the plate continuity alarm will sound; only then is the return lead connected to the diathermy machine, thus silencing the continuity alarm. Never do this in the reverse order. At the end of every case all these connections must be undone and the diathermy machine switched off. If the continuity alarm fails to silence, change the patient plate and lead first, not the machine. Some modern diathermy generators (e.g. Eschmann and Valleylab) possess systems that monitor the patient–plate interface. These systems will be explained

in the user's manual. Never disregard these alarms – check the patient plate contact carefully.

The patient plate. The most common cause of accidental diathermy burns is incorrect application of the patient plate. It may not be applied at all. More often there is a failure to follow guidelines. The plate should be sited close to the operation, while ensuring that diathermy current is moving away from ECG and other monitoring electrodes. The area under the plate should have a good blood supply to remove any heat generated: avoid bony prominences and scar tissue. All the plate must have good skin contact: shave hairy skin and ensure the plate is not kinked or crinkled. Do not let skin preparation fluids seep under the plate.

The patient. The second most common cause of diathermy burns is the patient touching earthed metal objects such as drip stands, uninsulated 'screens', and parts of the operating table. These small skin contacts can become alternative return pathways for the diathermy current, and the local current densities may be enough to cause a burn.

Sensible diathermy. The third most common cause of diathermy burns is careless technique. For safe diathermy:

- Check the dial settings before use
- If a spirit-based skin preparation fluid is used, ensure it has all evaporated or been wiped away before starting or the diathermy may set it alight
- Only the surgeon wielding the active electrode should activate the machine
- Always replace the electrode in an insulated quiver after use
- If diathermy performance is poor, carefully check the patient plate and lead rather than increase the dial settings
- Beware of using diathermy on or inside the gut (intestinal gas contains hydrogen and methane and the result is often inflammable and explosive)
- Beware of using diathermy on appendages (salpinx or penis) or isolated tissue (testis). In these circumstances a high current density can persist beyond the operative site.

If a burn occurs. Diathermy burns are often poorly investigated and remain unexplained. Other skin lesions such as chemical burns from preparation solutions or pressure sores may masquerade as diathermy burns. Definite electrothermal burns are rarely due to a fault in the diathermy machine, but usually to lapses in procedure. The operating-theatre record for all patients subjected to diathermy should include the site of the patient plate, and when the plate and monitoring electrodes are removed the underlying skin should be inspected. If a possible burn is discovered at the end of a surgical case, the patient and all attached equipment should remain in the operating theatre and the electromedical safety officer summoned. If the alleged burn is discovered after the patient has left theatre, all personnel involved in the case should be contacted: the precise arrangement of equipment and patient plate should be determined. Then all electrical equipment used should be tested, including the patient plate lead. Diathermy burns are usually full thickness and will require excision. The patient should be informed of the misadventure.

Diathermy and pacemakers.   There are two possible dangers:

• The high-frequency diathermy current may interact with pacemaker logic circuits to alter pacemaker function, resulting in serious arrhythmias, or even cardiac arrest.
• Diathermy close to the pacemaker box may result in current travelling down the pacemaker wire, causing a myocardial burn. The result will range from a rise in pacemaker threshold to cardiac arrest.

For safe use of diathermy with pacemakers:

• Contact a cardiologist. Information required includes the type of pacemaker, why and when it was put in, whether it is functioning properly, what is the patient's underlying rhythm (i.e. what happens if the pacemaker stops?).
• Avoid diathermy completely if possible. If not, consider bipolar diathermy.
• If monopolar diathermy has to be used, place the patient plate so that diathermy current flows away from the pacemaker system. Use only short bursts, and stop all diathermy if any arrhythmias occur.

 Key points

Remember you are in overall charge of the safe use of diathermy

Laparoscopic procedures. Sometimes the working space can be 'crowded', and inadvertent contact may be made between an instrument and the bowel. This may also occur when there is contact between the electrode and another metal instrument which is touching bowel. In a similar way, current can pass along an organ, which is resting against the gut, and pass out via the indifferent electrode. Insulation of instruments should be complete, and sparking between bowel wall and electrode avoided. An adequate view, CO_2 pneumoperitoneum, and using well-insulated instruments should be the aim. Careful technique, such as avoiding

excessive use of the diathermy and making an effort to 'tent' structures into space before current is applied, is important. Lower voltage currents, or bipolar diathermy can be used to minimize spread of current and sparking.

Lasers

The laser is a device for producing a highly directional beam of coherent (monochromatic and in phase) electromagnetic radiation, which may or may not be visible, over a wide range of power outputs.

Laser is an acronym for Light Amplification by the Stimulated Emission of Radiation. This describes the principle of operation of a laser. Energy is pumped into the lasing medium to excite the atoms into a higher energy state to achieve a population inversion in which most of the atoms are in the excited state. A photon emitted as a result of an electron spontaneously falling from the excited to the ground state, stimulates more photons to be emitted and lasing action starts. After reflection back and forth many times from a pair of mirrors at opposite ends of the resonant optical cavity containing the lasing medium, the number of photons is amplified, i.e. the light intensity or power is increased. One of the mirrors is only partially reflecting and allows a small part of the laser light to emerge as the laser beam. The lasing medium is commonly gaseous (e.g. argon or carbon dioxide), but may be crystalline (e.g. neodymium, yttrium, aluminium, garnet (NdYAG)). It is the lasing medium which determines the wavelength emitted. It is mainly the wavelength of the laser which determines the degree of absorption in tissue. However, the surgical applications also depend on the power density, the duration of exposure being just sufficient to produce the effect required. The delivery systems are designed to allow the laser beam to be transported, aimed and focused onto the treatment site. Argon and NdYAG lasers, for example, are transmitted down fibre optics to a slit lamp or into an endoscope. Carbon dioxide laser light is usually routed via a series of mirrors through an 'articulated arm', and thereafter through a micromanipulator attached to a microscope or colposcope.

Types of laser

1. Carbon dioxide infrared laser light has a wavelength of 10.6 μm. It is invisible and is rapidly absorbed by water in tissue and has very little penetration. It is therefore useful for vapourizing the surface of tissue, and water or wet drapes can be used as a safety barrier. There is a very small margin of damaged tissue and

healing is rapid, with minimal scarring. Treatment is relatively pain free.

2. The NdYAG laser penetrates more deeply, to 3–5 mm. The wavelength is 1.06 µm and is in the invisible infra-red light range. It is useful for coagulating larger tissue volumes and leaves behind an eschar of damaged tissue.

Both the above types require a visible guiding beam which is usually a red helium/neon beam.

3. Argon laser light is blue/green and hence absorbed by red pigment. The principal wavelengths are 0.49 and 0.51 µm. It is used principally in ophthalmology and dermatology.

Clinical applications

Gastrointestinal tract. The NdYAG laser is frequently used in the treatment of gastrointestinal problems. It can be employed for vapourizing and debulking recurrent or untreated advanced oesophageal carcinoma. Its use is predominantly in fairly short malignant strictures and may be superior to intubation. However, expanding covered metal stents may well prove an improved palliative alternative. Laser ablation is labour intensive and requires treatments every 6–8 weeks. This laser can be used for controlling gastrointestinal haemorrhage from the stomach, oesophagus and duodenum, destruction of small ampullary tumours in the duodenum and palliative resection of advanced rectal carcinomas. In the future, photosensitization may prove to be of value. The use of lasers in laparoscopic surgery is, perhaps, less frequent at present. There is a risk of carbon dioxide gas embolism.

Urology. The NdYAG laser can be used to treat low-grade, low-stage transitional cell lesions in the bladder and is suitable for treating outpatients under local anaesthetic. Here again, photosensitizing agents such as haematoporphyrin (Hpd) may be used in conjunction with a laser light wavelength of 630 nm. The beam is directed at sensitized tissues which are then more easily destroyed.

Ophthalmology. The NdYAG laser can be used to destroy an opaque posterior capsule during extracapsular cataract extraction. The argon laser may be employed for trabeculoplasty, to decrease intraocular pressure in patients with open-angled glaucoma. Laser photocoagulation has become standard treatment for patients with various retinal diseases such as diabetic retinopathy, and as a prophylactic measure in patients at risk from retinal detachment. Most ophthalmic photocoagulators are argon lasers.

Otolaryngology. A carbon dioxide laser may be used for haemostasis, removal of benign tumours and premalignant conditions. The argon laser has been used in middle ear surgery.

Vascular surgery. Laser angioplasty (carbon dioxide, NdYAG and argon) has been used to vapourize atheromatous plaques. Only approximately 50% of patients benefit, and significant complications are reported (e.g. perforation of vessel wall).

Plastic surgery. Pulsed ruby lasers may be used to remove tattoos, and port wine stains selectively absorb the argon laser beam. The carbon dioxide laser may be employed to resect atretic bony plates in congenital bony choanal atresia.

Gynaecology. There are several uses in gynaecology. Perhaps the most frequent is the treatment with a carbon dioxide laser of cervical and vulval precancerous lesions which are identified by colposcopy.

Classification

Lasers are classified according to the degree of hazard:

Class 1 (low risk). These are of low power and are safe. The maximum permissible exposure (MPE) cannot be exceeded.

Class 2 (low risk). These are of low power, emitting visible radiation. They have a maximum power level of 1 mW. Safety is normally afforded by natural aversion responses, e.g. the blink reflex.

Class 3a (low risk). These emit visible radiation, with an output of up to 5 mW. Eye protection is afforded by natural aversion. There may be a hazard if the beam is focused to a point, e.g. through an optical system.

Class 3b (medium risk). These emit in any part of the spectrum and have a maximum output of 0.5 W. Direct viewing may be dangerous.

Class 4 (high risk). These are high-power devices with output in any part of the spectrum. A diffusely reflected beam may be dangerous and there is also a potential fire hazard. Their use requires caution. Most medical lasers are in this class.

Hazards

The manufacturers are required to classify and label the product according to hazard level.

1. *Patient hazard*: inevitably, burning of normal tissue or perforation of a hollow viscus may occur with increasing depth of treatment (e.g. perforation of oesophagus) or damage to trachea or lungs during ear, nose and throat (ENT) procedures.

2. *Operator hazard*: usually the operator is not exposed to laser beams, but should accidental exposure occur it is frequently the eyes or skin that are damaged. Eye protection is important as some laser beams will penetrate and be focused on the retina. Also corneal

burns or cataract formation have occurred with less penetrating beams.

Safety measures

1. There should be a laser protection advisor (LPA) to consult on the use of the instruments throughout the hospital and to draft local rules.

2. A laser safety officer (LSO) should be appointed from the staff of the appropriate department using each laser. This person may well be, for example, a senior nurse and will have custody of the laser key.

3. All persons using the laser should be adequately trained in its use and be fully cognizant with all safety precautions.

4. There should be a list of nominated users.

5. A laser controlled area (LCA) should be established around the laser while it is in use. There should be control of personnel allowed to enter that area and the entrance should be marked with an appropriate warning sign, usually incorporating a light which illuminates while the laser is functioning.

6. While in the laser controlled area adequate eye protection should be worn. This must be appropriate to the type of laser used. The laser should not be fired until it is aimed at a target, and usually there will be an audible signal during laser firing.

7. The laser should be labelled according to its classification. Lasers in classes 3a, 3b and 4 should be fitted with a key switch and the key should be kept by a specified person. The panels which constitute the side of the laser unit should have an interlocking device so that the laser cannot be used if the panels are damaged.

There are various safety features which are required by way of shutter devices and emergency shut-off switches. Foot-operated pedals should be shrouded to prevent accidental activation. Medical lasers require a visible low-power aiming beam which may be an attenuated beam of the main laser, should this be visible, or a separate class 1 or 2 laser, e.g. helium/neon. The laser must be regularly maintained and calibrated.

8. Environment: reflective surfaces should be avoided in the laser controlled area. However, matt-black surfaces are not necessary. Adequate ventilation must be provided and should include an extraction system to vent the fumes produced. These fumes are known as the 'laser plume'.

Attention should be paid to the avoidance of fire as class 4 lasers will cause dry material (e.g. drapes or swabs) to ignite. Thus, damp drapes will provide an effective stop (e.g. for a carbon dioxide laser beam).

Fibre optics in theatre

Flexible instruments

The advent of fibre optics has undoubtedly made an immense impact on the management of patients. There is little evidence, however, that the use of instruments which incorporate fibre optics necessarily reduces mortality. Hollow viscera may be carefully inspected, and both diagnostic and therapeutic procedures can be performed under clear vision. Fibre-optic instruments are integral to the development of minimal access surgery (e.g. ureteric or bile duct stone retrieval).

In the 1950s, Professor Harold Hopkins of Reading University, UK, developed the earlier work of John Logie Baird (the inventor of television) to further the design of fibre-optic bundles which not only could transmit a powerful light beam but also, when suitably arranged, deliver an accurate image to the viewer. In the 1960s, urological instruments were developed incorporating multiple flexible glass-fibre rods. Each fine fibre rod is constructed of high-quality optical glass and transmits the image (or light beam) by the process of total internal reflection. This principle allows light to travel around bends in the fibre. Each fibre is small (8–10 μm in diameter), and to achieve the principle of total internal reflection must be covered by a coating of glass of low refractive index to prevent light dispersion. Many such coated fibres are bound together in bundles which can bend. For light transmission, fibres may be arranged in a haphazard manner (non-coherent) but for clear-image transmission the fibres must be arranged in a coaxial way (coherent) (Fig. 18.3). The following are examples of currently available flexible endoscopes utilizing fibre-optic light bundles:

- Oblique (for endoscopic, retrograde, cholangiopancreatography (ERCP) and end-viewing gastroscopes
- Laryngoscope
- Bronchoscope
- Fibre-optic sigmoidoscope and colonoscope
- Cystoscope (pyeloscope)
- Choledochoscope
- Arterioscope.

Each instrument has similar design principles incorporating the following:

- Coherent fibre bundles for high-quality visual image transmission
- Non-coherent fibre-optic bundles for light transmission
- A lens system at a tip and near the eyepiece of the instrument
- A proximal control system to manoeuvre the tip of the instrument and also to control suction and air/water flow

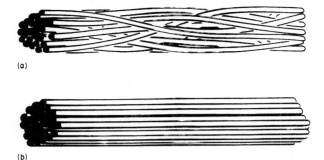

(a)

(b)

Fig 18.3 (a) Non-coherent fibre bundles for light transmission. (b) Coherent fibre bundles for viewing. Reproduced from Ravenscroft & Swan (1984) by permission of Chapman & Hall.

- Channels for blowing air or carbon dioxide and water down the instrument, and for suction – the latter doubles as a biopsy channel
- A wire guide incorporated to control tip movement, which takes place in four directions, each usually allowing a deformity of greater than 180° movement
- A cladding, consisting of a flexible, jointed construction, covered by a tough outer vinyl sheath.

Figures 18.4 and 18.5 show the basic structure of a typical endoscope, and Figure 18.6 shows the tip of an instrument, illustrating the lenses for light transmission and viewing, a suction channel (which should be large for use in the presence of gastrointestinal haemorrhage) and a small nipple directed over the lens, to enable the wash solution to clear the lens of debris.

Light sources should emit a powerful beam and the intensity is usually 150 W. Many light sources employ a halogen bulb, which needs to be fan cooled.

Rigid endoscopes

Optical systems in rigid endoscopes also employ the principle of total internal reflection, but there are several lens systems in addition. The objective lens systems are nearest the image and the relay lens systems nearer the eyepiece of the rigid instrument, through which the observer views a rectified and magnified image. A light cable (non-coherent fibres or liquid electrolyte solution) is employed and the fibres direct the light coaxially with the lens systems in the rigid tube. Some of the longer lenses are made of high-quality optical glass and act as a single large optical fibre for image transmission. Examples of rigid instruments are:

- Cystoscope, urethroscope, pyeloscope, ureteroscope
- Choledochoscope
- Laparoscopes.

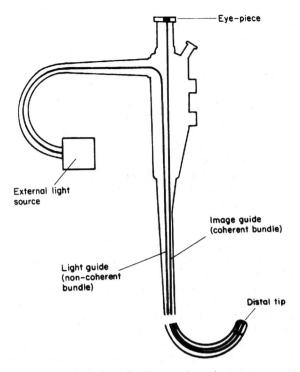

Fig 18.4 Basic design of a fibre-optic endoscope. Reproduced from Ravenscroft & Swan (1984) by permission of Chapman & Hall.

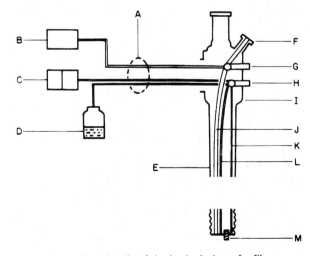

Fig 18.5 Further details of the basic design of a fibre-optic endoscope. A, endoscopic 'umbilicus'; B, suction pump; C, air pump; D, water reservoir; E, endoscopic insertion tube; F, biopsy port; G, suction button; H, air/wash button; I, endoscope control head; J, combined suction biopsy channel; K, water channel; L, air channel; M, combined air/water port. Reproduced from Ravenscroft & Swan (1984) by permission of Chapman & Hall.

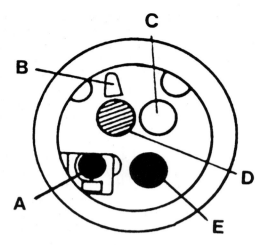

Fig 18.6 The top of an end-viewing fibre-optic instrument. A, forceps raiser; B, wash jet; C, image guide; D, light guide; E, biopsy/suction channel. Reproduced from Ravenscroft & Swan (1984) by permission of Chapman & Hall.

The lenses at the far end of the instruments will vary to allow differing fields of view and minimize peripheral field distortion.

Care of fibre-optic instruments

1. Instruments must be properly cleaned and disinfected before use. Debris may block channels and make suction and insufflation of air and liquid difficult. After use, the instruments should be cleaned internally by utilizing one of several automatic cleansing machines and externally with a suitable detergent solution. 'Q-tips' may be employed to clean lenses. Instruments should be soaked for at least 5–10 minutes between patients and a 2% gluteraldehyde solution is frequently used, though 70% alcohol and low-molecular-weight povidone–iodine are alternatives.

2. Avoidance of damage to the instrument: in most district hospitals endoscopies are performed in dedicated units where the care is certainly superior. When a variety of people handle and clean the instrument, damage is more likely to occur. Forcible distortion, dropping and, particularly, crushing of the instruments (e.g. by patients' teeth) must be prevented. In the latter instance, biting may be prevented by insertion of a suitable mouth gag. Individual fibres may break and become opaque, appearing as black dots down the instrument.

Key points

- **Take care to handle these delicate instruments carefully. They are very expensive**

Cryosurgery (syn. cryotherapy or cryocautery)

Cryosurgery is the freezing of tissue to destruction. Although cells are destroyed at $-20°C$ they may recover at higher temperatures than this. After freezing, the destroyed tissue sloughs off and reveals a clean, granulating base. The treatment is relatively pain free and minimizes blood loss. The object is to destroy abnormal tissue growth and preserve adjacent, healthy areas. This is achieved by the production of an ice ball at the tip of a cryoprobe (Fig. 18.7). To control the volume of tissue destroyed the size of the ice ball produced may be watched. The size of the lesion produced by cryosurgery depends on the temperature at the tip of the ice probe, the size of the tip and the number of freeze–thaw sequences. The size of the iceball will increase until the heat loss at the edge of the iceball is too small to permit further freezing of adjacent tissues. The size of an iceball and the extent of destruction can then be increased by a further freezing sequence. It is usually recommended to allow spread of the iceball 2–3 mm into healthy tissue to ensure adequate destruction of the diseased area. Inevitably, freezing a wart on

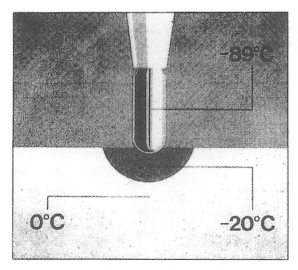

Fig 18.7 An ice ball at the tip of a cryoprobe. Reproduced by permission of Eugene A. Felmar, Santa Monica Hospital Medical Center, USA.

the sole of the foot is less critical than reattaching a retina, and for all the tasks demanded of cryosurgery there are various probe tips available.

Principles of therapy

The Joule – Thompson principle is that when gas expands heat is absorbed from the surrounding matter. The simplest example of this is spraying ethyl chloride on skin, which subsequently freezes. With a cryoprobe, however, the liquid gas (usually nitrogen or carbon dioxide) is sprayed against the inside of a hollow metal probe. The gas then expands in the tip and freezes the tissue on contact (Fig. 18.8).

Cell injury with cryotherapy

1. *Immediate phase*: rupture of the cell membrane caused by formation of ice crystals in the cell (most effective with rapid freezing (e.g. greater than $5°C\ s^{-1}$)).
2. *Intracellular dehydration*: this will result in increased and toxic levels of intracellular electrolytes.
3. *Protein denaturation*: this occurs to the lipoprotein structure of the cell membrane, nucleus and mitochondria.
4. *Cellular hypometabolism*: this results in enzyme inhibition.

Later in the course of injury there is also a loss of blood supply which causes tissue necrosis, and the resultant slough, before separation, will protect the tissues deeper to the injury so that when the slough separates it will leave a clean ulcer.

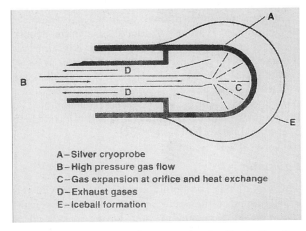

A – Silver cryoprobe
B – High pressure gas flow
C – Gas expansion at orifice and heat exchange
D – Exhaust gases
E – Iceball formation

Fig 18.8 Cross-section of a cryoprobe tip, illustrating the Joule-Thompson principle. Reproduced by permission of Eugene A. Felmar, Santa Monica Hospital Medical Center, USA.

As nerve endings are susceptible to cold injury, painful lesions can be rendered insensitive. Also, the treatment is not particularly painful to the patient, and local analgesia is usually unnecessary. Adjacent neurovascular structures are relatively safe as collagen and elastic tissue resist freezing. Thus, the advantages of cryotherapy are that it is a relatively pain-free and simple method of destroying tissue, usually leaving clean wounds, often with a reasonable scar.

The disadvantages of the technique are that frozen tissue cannot be analysed histologically, and thus this method of treatment is unsuitable for any lesion requiring microscopic examination. It may sometimes be difficult to gauge the exact penetration in the depth of the tissues treated. Thus, its use may be limited in curative treatment of malignancy, but obviously is of value in palliation. There may also occasionally be some bleeding and discharge after the slough separates (e.g. in the cryosurgical treatment of haemorrhoids).

Clinical applications

Given the various shapes of probe tips, a reasonable variety of therapeutic applications is available. When placing the probe tip, freezing must occur through a wet contact to ensure proper thermal conductivity. Two to three freeze–thaw cycles may be applied with overlap of areas treated if necessary.

Examples. Examples of the clinical application of cryosurgery include the following:

- Proctology: haemorrhoids and warts
- Gynaecology: cervical erosions and warts
- Dermatology: warts, low-grade skin cancers, herpetic lesions
- ENT: pharyngeal tonsillar remnants, carcinoma of the trachea, hypophysectomy
- Ophthalmology: cataract extraction, glaucoma, detached retina
- Neurosurgery: Parkinson's disease and cerebral tumours.

Ultrasound in the operating theatre

Ultrasound probes are employed during surgery to identify tumour deposits and anatomical landmarks such as blood vessels. In this way, clear guidance may be obtained as to the resectability of tumours or the presence of clinically undetected metastatic deposits. Not only may hand-held ultrasound probes be employed at open operations, but small laparoscopic instruments are also used for staging and anatomical purposes. At open surgery, for example, small islet cell tumours of the pancreas may be located accurately.

During laparoscopic cholecystectomy, a probe may not only identify structures, but also locate common bile duct stones.

Ultrasonic surgical aspirator

There are various ways in which the liver parenchyma may be dissected, with minimal blood loss. One of the most widely used, and efficient, is the CUSA (Cavitron UltraSonic Aspirator). The operating titanium tip of the instrument vibrates longitudinally at 23 000 oscillations per second (23 kHz). The way the instrument works is that electromagnetic energy is converted to mechanical movements. An electrical coil wrapped around metal laminations sets up a magnetic field, thus causing the metal to vibrate. The fine hollow tip of the instrument disrupts solid parenchyma by its fine vibrations and the heat generated. When debris is shed, it is mixed with fluid jetting from the instrument and the mixture is sucked away. More solid and fibrous structures, such as ducts and blood vessels, are not disrupted, and may then be clipped or ligated. Not only may this instrument be useful for open, solid parenchymal dissection, but it may also be used during laparoscopic dissection of the gallbladder or mobilization of the colon.

X-rays in theatre

Preoperative work-up

Normally completed prior to surgery, the preoperative work-up should address details of diagnosis and, where appropriate, anatomical or physiological factors which could affect the conduct or outcome of surgery. It should go without saying that appropriately labelled radiographs must be available in theatre at the time of operation.

The preoperative chest X-ray is generally unhelpful in the absence of cardiothoracic symptoms and should be reserved for older patients or those with specific indications.

Perioperative procedures performed in X-ray

Example: needle localization for impalpable breast lesions. Coordination between the surgeon and radiologist is vital, and each needs to understand what the other is doing. Premedication can make the procedure very difficult; for example, the patient may faint while sitting upright for mammography. It is imperative for the surgeon to inspect the postlocalization mammogram for the relationship between the wire and the suspected abnormality. Remember that mammograms are performed with the patient sitting and the breast subsequently compressed. The breast usually adopts a different configuration when supine. The excised specimen should be radiographed to confirm a satisfactory biopsy before the patient is wakened.

Example: retrograde pyelogram. This examination can be performed in theatre at the time of cystoscopy using fluoroscopy, or subsequently in the X-ray department where the radiologist has the advantage of being able to turn the patient and obtain films.

Intraoperative procedures

These fall into two categories. The first is purely diagnostic.

Example: on-table cholangiography. Use sufficiently dilute contrast medium to allow one to 'see through' the common bile duct on the film. The biliary tree should be adequately filled to show the main intrahepatic ducts as well as the common bile duct. Contrast medium is heavier than bile and tends to gravitate to dependent ducts. If the ampulla is patent, contrast medium flows into the duodenum, which is clearly recognizable by its mucosal pattern. Remember to put a 20° lateral tilt on the table to eliminate the overlap of contrast on the vertebral column.

Example: intraoperative angiography. Films may be exposed following a steady intra-arterial injection in theatre and adequate results obtained. Adverse reactions to modern contrast media while under general anaesthetic are very rare.

The second category consists of procedures where imaging is used to facilitate a therapeutic procedure. They require fluoroscopy and range from simple procedures such as reducing fractures to the sophisticated techniques of interventional uroradiology. Many of these techniques can be performed either in the operating room or in the X-ray department, but it is fair to say that facilities for fluoroscopy are usually better in X-ray while asepsis is better in theatre. X-ray machines are difficult to clean and a potential source of cross-infection. Specialist centres may have dedicated complex X-ray rooms which are organized in a fashion similar to operating theatres (or vice versa).

Equipment

This may be static or mobile, and it is the latter which is usually found in the operating theatre. Image intensification allows 'screening' without having to dark-adapt your eyes first! A mobile image intensifier for use in theatre will be mounted on a small 'C' arm. The table top must be radiolucent and there must be space under as well as over the table for the X-ray tube and the image intensifier. If films only are required, the table top will need a 'tunnel' to admit the X-ray cassette under the patient. Alternatively, the cassette may be draped in sterile towels. This would be necessary, for example, if intraoperative mesenteric angiography was to be performed on bowel lifted out of the abdomen at laparotomy. For a small field, the X-ray cassette can be placed on the image intensifier itself, and film obtained. Some modern machines can produce dry silver images directly from the TV monitor.

Biplane screening is a luxury not usually available in the operating theatre. The mobile 'C' arm is, nevertheless, quite versatile and the effect of 'parallax' can help to judge 'depth'.

Mobile X-ray sets operate from designated 13 A sockets which are on a separate ring main from other essential equipment. Modern mobile sets use 'sparkless' switching and should not therefore ignite inflammable gases. It is desirable to keep the mobile X-ray machine in the operating suite.

X-rays and the law

X-rays (and scalpels) can be weapons of assault if not used with care and a prospect of benefit to the patient. Medical staff clinically directing examinations employing ionizing radiation are required to have obtained a certificate demonstrating that they have received some training in radiation protection. It is hoped that eventually this will be included in the undergraduate curriculum. Staff physically directing exposure must be either a radiologist, radiographer, or hold an approved qualification.

Equipment must be regularly serviced and calibrated, and 'local rules' applied. The radiation protection supervisor in the hospital is the point of contact if in any doubt.

Safety

Look after yourself, other staff in the theatre and the patient. Use the lead aprons. Remember that the patient 'scatters' the X-ray beam. The inverse square law applies, so staff should not be unnecessarily close. Be aware of the screening time and record it.

The abdomen of pregnant patients should be X-rayed only if absolutely necessary. The last menstrual period should be established before the patient is anaesthetized.

Sundry points

1. Maintain a close relationship with the department of radiology.
2. Discuss problems before surgery. Radiologists (generally) will want to know the outcome. Remember that this includes anatomical details as well as the diagnosis.
3. Give the radiographer as much notice as possible.
4. Dim the theatre lights when using fluoroscopy and use viewing boxes to view films.
5. Take an interest in imaging, as 'a picture is worth a thousand words'.

Microscopes in the operating theatre

Microscopes have been introduced very gradually to the operating theatre; however, they have now become indispensable in a wide variety of surgical fields.

Advantages

The microscope offers an improved view of the surgical field, more precision, greater flexibility and less trauma to delicate tissues. It provides good stereoscopic appreciation of depth, through a narrow surgical approach, much smaller than the unaided surgeon's own interpupillary distance would allow.

Historical

Spectacles have been available for nearly 700 years and the compound microscope for about 300 years, but it was only 70 years ago that a microscope was used in theatre and only 30 years ago that its usage became more widespread.

A Swedish otolaryngologist, Nylen, introduced his monocular microscope in the surgical treatment of otosclerosis in 1921. A year later his chief, Professor Holmgren, used a binocular microscope for the same condition. In 1925, Hinselman used a microscope for colposcopy, but aside from this for 3 decades only otolaryngologists continued to use microscopes. In Chicago, Perritt used a microscope for ophthalmic surgery in 1950, and Zeiss started to mass-produce their MiI surgical microscope in 1953. Clinical applications then expanded: Jacobson in vascular surgery in 1960; Kurle in neurosurgery and Burke in plastic surgery in 1962.

Features of an operating microscope

Eyepieces. There is an adjustment for interpupillary distance and each eyepiece has a range of 5 dioptres.

Binocular tube. This can be straight or inclined.

Beam splitter. This is for connection of extra viewing tubes for observation and assistance. It also makes the use of still and video cameras possible as teaching aids.

Magnification system. Magnification is available as a Galilean system, variable in steps (e.g. × 6, × 10, × 25, × 40), or as a zoom system.

Objective lens. This affects working distance by changing lenses with variable focal lengths. For example:

$f = 150, 175, 200$	for ophthalmology and plastic surgery
$f = 250$	for otology and vascular surgery
$f = 250$ or 300	for tubal surgery (gynaecology)
$f = 300$ or 400	for neurosurgery
$f = 400$	for laryngoscopy.

Depth of field. The stereoscopic depth of field is less at higher magnification. It is best to focus at higher magnification first, then to reduce to working magnification so as to have the best focus at the centre of the depth of field.

Light. A powerful coaxial halogen light is incorporated in the body of the microscope. Oblique light is available for eye surgery.

Instruments used with microscopes

Each speciality has developed microsurgical instruments for its own needs. However, the following basic instruments are common to many specialities.

Spring-handled needle holder. Needle holders such as Borraquer or Castrovieso, ophthalmic, are available.

Spring-handled microscissors. These can be straight or curved. The straight are for cutting vessels and the curved for cutting tissue and thread.

Jewellers' or watchmakers' forceps. A wide variety of these are available.

Microsurgical clips. Scoville–Lewis microsurgical clips or fine Heifetzs neurosurgical clips can be used for vessel anastomosis.

Microelectrode. Monopolar or bipolar cautery is necessary.

Suture material. (a) Blood vessel anastomosis: 9.0 or 10.0 nylon on a 3–6 mm needle with a tapered end. (b) Nerve anastamosis: as above, but the needle needs a cutting point. (c) Fallopian tube work: no. 7.0 or 8.0 absorbable non-reactive suture with a 4 mm or 6 mm reverse cutting needle.

Sterilization. Sterile rubber cups or drapes are available to cover the controls.

Adjustment. Versatility in position needs several interlocking arms, counterbalanced vertical movement as well as a geared angled coupling between the microscope carriage arm and body. This will enable the microscope to swing from side to side while mounted in an oblique axis.

Mounting. This can be on a solid, well-balanced mobile floor stand, or a fixed ceiling mounting. Wall-mounted microscopes are also available.

Control of tremor

Counteracting surgical tremor is of vital importance. The key is that the instrument or the limb on which it is held must be firmly supported as close to the point of work as possible.

The future

The combination of the laser with a micromanipulator to the objective lens of the microscope will enhance the use of both instruments in the future.

Summary

1. Remember to optimize your behaviour and technique in the operating room to minimize infection.
2. Position and move patients carefully and gently while they are unconscious.
3. You are in charge of the tourniquet, diathermy, laser, cryoprobe and X-rays in theatre, so learn to respect all safety regulations.
4. Lead by example in the operating room by adopting careful and responsible attitudes to delicate and potentially dangerous equipment.

Acknowledgements

I am deeply grateful for help with writing this chapter to: Mr John Bancroft for the diathermy section; Dr David Parker for the section on X-rays in theatre; Mr Derry Coakley for the section on microscopes; and to my wife for her help in the section on lasers. I should also like to thank Miss Sharon Langford for typing the manuscript.

 Further reading

Brigden R J 1988 Operating theatre technique, 5th edn. Churchill Livingstone, Edinburgh

Douglas D M (ed) 1972 Surgical departments in hospitals: the surgeon's view. Butterworth, London

Johnston I D A, Hunter A R (eds) 1984 The design and utilization of operating theatres. Edward Arnold, London

Diathermy

Dobbie A K 1974 Accidental lesions in the operating theatre. NAT News December

Earnshaw J J, Keene T K 1989 Gastric explosion: a cautionary tale. British Medical Journal 293: 93–94

Editorial 1979 Surgical diathermy is still not foolproof. British Medical Journal 12: 755–758

Pearce J A 1986 Electrosurgery. Chapman & Hall, London

Lasers

1982 General guidance on lasers in hospitals. Medical physics and bioengineering working group. Welsh Scientific Advisory Committee (WSAC)

1983 Guidance on the safe use of lasers in medical practice. HMSO, London

Murray A, Mitchell D C, Wood R F M 1992 Lasers in surgery – a review. British Journal of Surgery 79: 21–26

Fibre optics

Ravenscroft M M, Swan C M J 1984 Gastrointestinal endoscopy and related procedures – a handbook for nurses and assistants. Chapman & Hall, London

X-rays

Ionizing Radiation Regulations 1985, 1988

Mound R F Radiation protection in hospitals (Medical Sciences Series), Adam Hilger, Bristol

Microscopes

Taylor S 1977 Microscopy. Recent advances in surgery. Churchill Livingstone, Edinburgh, ch 8

Adjuncts to surgery

A. L. G. Peel

    Objectives

- **Recognize the importance of good theatre management.**
- **Ensure basic understanding of usage and care of theatre instruments, accessories and special equipment.**
- **Appreciate the place of implants and tissue glues in modern surgical practice.**

INTRODUCTION

In health service economics an operating suite requires large capital and revenue budgets and this is favourably influenced by careful management of utilities. Good care of quality instruments ensures their long use, appropriate ordering and stocking means the shelf-life of equipment is not exceeded, wastage due to change in practice is reduced to a minimum and storage space is efficiently used. The avoidance of an unnecessarily wide range of equipment and materials allows better use of capital.

From the medicolegal aspect, the establishment of simple protocols aids efficient management within the theatre complex and helps to reduce errors, such as breakdowns in sterility or retention of swabs or instruments in patients.

A practical example of the rapidly changing scene in surgical practice is illustrated by orthopaedic surgery, where considerable expansion has occurred, particularly in prosthetic joint replacement, and in this field infection can result in very costly failure in terms of patient morbidity and financial implications to the health service.

In the attempt to 'abolish' infection to elective orthopaedic surgery the following factors are considered important.

    Patient screening for occult infection

Give particular attention to:
- **Possible urinary tract infection in females**
- **Carrier status – elective surgery should be postponed until pathogens are eliminated (e.g. *Staphylococcus aureus* in the nares)**

THEATRE MANAGEMENT

1. *Orthopaedic theatre.* A theatre should be dedicated to orthopaedics in which no dirty or contaminated orthopaedic surgery and no general surgery whatsoever is carried out.

2. *Clean air enclosures.* The routine use of clean air enclosures has resulted in the infection rate in prosthetic joint surgery (hip and knee) falling from 1.5% in the conventionally ventilated theatre to 0.6% (Lidwell et al 1982). Unidirectional air systems, especially with a downflow direction, reduces bacteria-carrying particles from 400–500 m^{-3} to 30–40 m^{-3}. Power tools produce additional problems since they produce an aerosol spray which effectively disseminates bacteria and viral particles.

3. *Theatre gowns.* Airborne bacterial dispersion can be further reduced by the use of appropriate fabric clothing. It is not widely appreciated that, in either conventional or unidirectional airflow theatres, the use of disposable fabric gowns alone in lieu of cotton gowns has not achieved a significant reduction in bacteria-carrying particles.

    Drawbacks to conventional sterile cotton pyjamas and gowns

- **Bacteria from surgeon tend to be pumped by air through or out of the clothing and into theatre air**

- Bacteria from surgeon being drawn through wet clothing by capillary action and hence contaminating the sterile operative area and wound
- Contamination of surgeon with patient's fluids

Alternatives to cotton gowns
- **Charnley total exhaust gown**
- **Disposable non-woven clothing**
- **Breathable plastic membrane fabrics**
- **Close-woven polyester or poly-cotton fabrics**

Of the alternatives to cotton gowns listed above, the use of the first is well established in clean orthopaedic surgery; the second, Sonta (manufactured by Du Pont Ltd), has been shown to be effective; the third requires seals at the neck and trouser opening, with the result that the wearer soon becomes hot and uncomfortable. The fourth option is expensive, but represents a significant improvement over conventional garments. Although the cost is high, this must be equated with the significant costs of morbidity due to infection. It has been stated that pharmaceutical manufacturing areas would be closed down if they used clothing currently worn in the majority of operating rooms (Whyte 1991).

Antibiotic prophylaxis: principles

- Single dose or three dose regimen
- High dose
- Appropriate microbiological spectrum
- Administer before or at induction of anaesthesia.

Theatre technique

- Disinfect hands in prescribed manner preoperatively
- *Use brushes for cleaning nails only*
- Use closed gloving technique to avoid contamination
- In orthopaedic implant surgery or with the use of power tools: *double glove.*

Dressings: desirable features

- Effective non-allergic adherence
- Non-bulky
- Transparent (allows *sterile* inspection).

INSTRUMENTS

Surgeons and instrument makers have combined to produce a wide range of instruments. Some, such as certain scissors, forceps and retractors, may be used in several different fields of surgery. Others are more specific; for instance, those used in anal surgery (Park's anal retractor and Lockhart–Mummery fistula probes). You should consider your requirements for instruments and appreciate the range and potential of different instruments. One advantage of a training rotation scheme is that it allows experience to be gained in a number of surgical disciplines and permits you to observe the use of instruments in different surgical disciplines. This knowledge can be reapplied to particular problems in whatever field you subsequently work.

Instruments are a sound investment and, whenever possible, use those of the highest quality. Of equal importance is the investment in maintenance care, not forgetting the basics of mechanical and chemical cleansing, particularly of hinge joints, adjustment of misalignment and regular sharpening of cutting instruments. In this context you have a very important role in avoiding damage to the instruments by not dropping them or using them inappropriately.

Sterilization

The majority of instruments are autoclaved (moist heat under pressure for a prescribed time) and this process needs constant monitoring, with care in the packing of the autoclave and verification that the temperature, pressure and time are correct.

Where steam autoclaving is impracticable and may cause damage, alternatives include (see Ch. 20):

- Formaldehyde autoclave
- Ethylene oxide
- Gluteraldehyde 2% solution (prolonged immersion)
  Note: – rendered ineffective by organic debris
  – toxic – causes skin irritation and requires a well ventilated room (alternatives are being developed)
- γ-Irradiation (wide commercial use for plastics).

Instrument sets

It is of considerable advantage to have the instruments required for a particular surgical procedure packed and sterilized in a single set. Within this set, as far as possible, each type of instrument should be in multiples of five. Thus each separate design or size of artery forceps may be grouped in separate fives or tens, whereas scissors of differing size and design are grouped in fives, etc. A standardized typed list of contents and numbers for each particular tray is routinely retained in the sterilized set. This reduces the number of single packed instruments that need to be opened and, more importantly, simplifies the instrument count at the beginning and end of each procedure.

Develop a close liaison between the central sterile supply department (CSSD) and theatre management to ensure adequate supplies of trays to meet the demand of a full schedule of operating lists, particularly when carrying out many minor procedures with a quick turnover.

LIGATURES, SUTURES, STAPLES AND CLIPS

When selecting a ligature or suture, consider several factors with regard to the material itself:

- Whether the material is to be absorbed
- The tensile strength
- The thickness
- The handling and knotting properties
- The intensity of the body's inflammatory reaction to the material.

A fine, absorbable suture is frequently selected for anastomoses in the gastrointestinal tract, and catgut is being replaced by the more reliable and less reactive synthetic monofilament polydioxanone (PDS or PDS II) or polyglactin 910 (coated Vicryl – the coating comprising glycolide, lactide and calcium stearate). When longer-lasting tensile strength is required, polymers, such as polyamide (Nylon), polypropylene (Prolene) or polytetrafluoroethylene (PTFE, Goretex) have proved to be of considerable value in, for example, abdominal wound closure and vascular anastomoses.

Metal clips are valuable alternatives to ligatures where access is difficult. They were originally made of stainless steel and were frequently used to demarcate an area for subsequent radiotherapy, or to assess by radiology the response of a neoplasm to treatment by radiotherapy or chemotherapy. They may produce a stellate shadow, obscuring detail in computed tomography (CT) scans, so they are now made from titanium.

 Key point

- **For skin, Steristrips or metal staples are useful alternatives but subcuticular sutures are less expensive.**

The majority of sutures are now atraumatic, which facilitates passage through the tissues and also relieves the scrub nurse of the arduous and tedious job of threading needles. The older practice of adding a half-hitch at the needle eye to prevent unthreading of the suture is especially traumatic to tissues.

When choosing a needle, consider the following:

- Shape:
  - (i) straight – infrequently used with the abandonment of hand needles
  - (ii) curved – becoming universal and held with a needle holder

- Tip
- Size and thickness: consider the tissue to be sewn, for example:
  - (i) skin or tough fibrous tissue, use a cutting needle
  - (ii) breast, use round bodied needle.

The introduction of a variety of staples for use in visceral tissues has also involved a number of changes in practice. You need to be aware of the range, the indications and contraindications for each type of instrument, including staple size, and the differences in design between manufacturers. Remember that surgical technique may need to be adapted as compared with the standard suture procedure. However, staple techniques are not as versatile as suturing and, as a trainee, you should concentrate on mastering the traditional method of uniting tissues.

I am of the opinion that staples should be used in preference to the sutures only when:

- The procedure can be carried out with greater safety (e.g. anastomotic leak)
- Operative time is significantly reduced and this is considered important
- The incidence of late complications (stenosis) is low (e.g. low anterior resection of the rectum or oesophagogastric anastomosis high in the chest).

SWABS AND PACKS

All cotton or fabric swabs and packs used during surgery must have radio-opaque marking. The size must be appropriate to the procedure and the purpose must be defined, e.g. small 'patty' swabs for neurosurgical procedures, narrow swabs for tonsillar surgery, large packs or gauze rolls for keeping abdominal viscera out of the operative field, for limiting gross contamination or for haemostatic control of raw surfaces.

Although haemostasis is usually achieved by electrocoagulation, ligation, undersewing or the use of clips, it is invaluable in certain situations to use certain manufactured haemostatic agents in the presence of a slow ooze. There is a choice between Surgicel, Oxycel or Sterispon, and again experience of the particular properties of each of the above is important. The application of Surgicel to the gallbladder bed with overlying pressure from a warm, moist swab controls a slow persistent ooze. When the overlying swab is removed, the haemostatic agent remains undisturbed. In neurosurgery the more delicate Sterispon may be preferred.

DISPOSABLE ACCESSORIES

Included in this category are accessories that remain on the surface of the body, skin or epithelial lining, or those that attain access to the interior of the body, usually for a limited period. Remember that they cause tissue irritation and create a break in the body's defence system.

Categories of disposable accessories

- Vascular cannulae, catheters and specialized equipment (e.g. Fogarty embolectomy catheters, Swan–Ganz catheters).
- Urological catheters and stents.
- Alimentary tract stents and catheters, for example:
  - (i) Straight, curved, cuffed or expansile stents for oesophageal and biliary malignant stricture
  - (ii) Balloon dilating catheters for strictures
  - (iii) Enteral feeding tubes.
- Stoma appliances.

 Key point

Remember the value of a skilled stomatherapist and the use of appropriate appliances in a patient with a high volume proximal intestinal fistula – very important adjuncts.

- Neurological valved shunts.
- Drains.

 Key point

Define the purpose and, therefore, duration of use. *Use closed systems.*

ENDOSCOPES

The development of endoscopes and their application in diagnosis and therapy continues. Instruments can be passed in the upper and lower respiratory tracts, the upper and lower alimentary tracts (including the biliary tree and pancreas), the upper and lower urinary tracts,

the female genital tract, and into joints, the peritoneal cavity and along blood vessels. Design modifications have resulted in a wide range of instruments with considerable therapeutic capabilities, often with the use of specialized accessories. They must be stored carefully, and maintained, cleaned, decontaminated and disinfected expertly, otherwise there is a risk of transmitting infection, particularly viral infection such as hepatitis B and C and human immunodeficiency virus (HIV).

Flexible instruments are usually disinfected by immersing them in a buffered 2% solution of gluteraldehyde for 20 minutes. Modern cystoscopes, for instance, may now be autoclaved.

> Do not neglect to master the use of the simple proctoscope, anal retractor, such as Park's or Eisenheimer's retractors, and sigmoidoscope.

IMPLANT MATERIALS

Prosthetic surgery continues to expand, and perhaps the greatest impact has been in orthopaedic surgery where successful joint replacement is well established in the hip, knee and interphalangeal joints and to a more limited extent in the shoulder and elbow joints. Prosthetic implants are also used widely in general, vascular, cardiac, urological, plastic and other branches of surgery, and there is wide variation in the materials used. Basic considerations and principles apply:

- Ease and reliability of manufacture and cost.
- Appropriate tensile strength and durability, e.g. some joint replacements need revision after a number of years, due to wear and tear causing fragmentation.
- Reaction between prosthetic materials themselves and the body tissues, e.g. the metal and plastic components of certain artificial hip replacements or between the joint prosthesis, cement and the bone.
- Platelet aggregation and plasma protein precipitation that occur around intravascular prostheses.
- The degree of incorporation into the body. Both metallic and silicone implants are surrounded by a collagen capsule but PTFE (Goretex) allows the ingrowth of fibroblasts.

Implant materials in orthopaedic surgery

1. Surgical-grade stainless steel is used for joint replacement bearing surfaces, plates, screws and wires.
2. Alloys, including Vitallium, are also used in joint replacement surfaces, wires and, less frequently now

owing to the preference for compression steel plating for internal fixation, in plates.

3. High-density polyethylene (ultra-high molecular weight) is used for joint replacement bearing surfaces to articulate with steel or Vitallium.

4. Silicone is used for hinge-type joint replacement, but not in bearing surfaces where debris produces a synovitis. It has been used very successfully in metacarpophalangeal and proximal interphalangeal joints.

5. Dacron and PTFE are materials that can be used under tension (e.g. synthetic ligament repair). Carbon fibre has been abandoned due to fragmentation and foreign body reaction.

The risk of infection

This is one of the most serious complications of prosthetic surgery:

Risk factors

- Immune compromised host
- Active infection present elsewhere in the host or in contacts
- Positive carrier state in patient or staff
- Cross-infection in hospital
- Failure of sterilization and/or packaging
- Inadequate air ventilation in the operating theatre and ineffectual operating theatre clothing
- Poor operative technique with contamination, poor haemostasis or ischaemic tissue
- Inadequate antimicrobial prophylaxis.

The time-scale of presentation is of significance, and this is one of the areas where *late infection up to a year or more after surgery may occur, particularly with the deep insertion of a prosthesis*. The implant itself can be of significance: whereas a smooth surface is bacteriostatic and non-wettable, a textured surface allows the entrapment of blood, serum, particles and bacteria in the crevices.

In deep infection occurring late around implants (e.g. hip) the bacteria may produce changes: *Staphylococcus aureus* produces a thickening of the capsule and *S. epidermidis* produces a polysaccharide slime. The prosthesis becomes loose, causes pain and may need removal.

Do not use an implant unless there is no natural alternative. Thus, in vascular surgery use vein grafts for lower limb arterial bypass surgery such as infra-inguinal bypass and especially for below-knee femoropopliteal bypass. Synthetic materials, Dacron (collagen-coated knitted Dacron) or Goretex (PTFE) may be used, particularly where large vessels need to be bypassed or replaced.

Tissue response to foreign material

Tissue reaction varies according to the material and the roughness of the surface. Marked inflammatory response, with microabscess formation, occurs around a buried silk or linen knot. By comparison, minimal response occurs around polypropylene, with not only a reduced likelihood of bacterial infection but also increased tensile strength, depending on the material used, and a lack of surrounding tissue inflammatory infiltrate.

Silicone forms a capsule. Fibroblasts orientate themselves to the surface of the foreign material and the collagen is formed in mirror image to the specific surface. As collagen matures it contracts. Fibroblasts cease to secrete collagen when they are in contact with other fibroblasts, but not when in contact with other cells. Thus over a smooth surface sheets of collagen are produced with increased contractile force of the capsule. Gradually, fibroblastic activity on the free surface subsides, collagen deposition is completed and moulding takes place, producing a mature capsule at approximately 3 months after surgery. Collagen production against the smooth inner capsular surface continues because the fibroblasts are not in contact with each other and, as a result, the cavity diameter decreases and the contractile force increases. By comparison, roughened surfaces allow fibroblasts to conform to the crevices; the fibres of collagen are then orientated at random with counteracting contractile forces and the fibroblasts lie in different planes and directions, allowing a greater chance of contact with each other, thus reducing the collagen deposition and resulting in a thinner capsule. Silicone particles are found in phagocytes in the capsule wall adjacent to lymphatic vessels, in the outer layer of capsules, and may reach the lumen of lymphatic vessels since they are found in regional lymph nodes.

Metal-on-metal joint replacement produces small particulate debris which is incorporated into the synovium, producing foreign-body giant cells.

Acrylic cement (polymethylmethacrylate), used in the fixation of prostheses, becomes encapsulated by fibrous tissue, the inner layer of which is sometimes hyaline and acellular and sometimes contains histiocytes and multinucleate giant cells. There is no evidence for malignant transformation or chronic inflammatory reaction with sinus formation (Charnley 1970). Revisional surgery of the cemented prosthesis is difficult. Alternatives under trial are based on isoelastic or mesh coating of the prosthesis to allow fibrous tissue to grow in.

The controversy over the safety of silicone mammary prostheses

In 1992 in the USA a moratorium was placed on the use of silicone gel breast implants because of the possible association with connective tissue disorders. In the UK, an independent expert advisory group reported to the Department of Health in 1993 that there was no evidence of an increased risk in implanted patients (Park et al 1993). In 1994, the Medical Devices Directory supported the Chief Medical Officer in stating that there was no evidence for a change in policy:

1. Selective reporting and bias was found in some articles.
2. There was confusion with the effects of the polyurethane coating of implants.
3. Difficulty was encountered in interpreting the psychological effects of breast implants.
4. Since the incidence of connective tissue disorders in the population is low and the latent period is long, large numbers and prolonged follow-up are needed.
5. Silicone, like any foreign body, may initiate an antibody and cell-mediated inflammatory response, but this is not in itself suggestive of an adverse effect on the immune system.

A further report is anticipated. There is currently no evidence that breast-implanted patients have an enhanced risk of developing either autoimmune connective tissue disease or mammary carcinoma. Silicone implants do, however, reduce the value of mammography. Newer tryglyceride-filled prostheses may be preferred; the shell is still textured silicone but mammography and ultrasonography are satisfactory (Trilucent, Lipomatrix).

TISSUE GLUES

Research into new methods of surgical tissue repair has yielded the prospect of using tissue glues. One such method is fibrin adhesion, based on the conversion of fibrinogen into fibrin on a tissue surface by the action of thrombin. The fibrin is then cross-linked by factor XIIIA to create a firm stable fibrin network with good adhesive properties.

The addition of aprotinin prevents premature dissolution of the fibrin clot by plasmin. In the presence of heavy bleeding the fibrin glue tends to be washed away before sufficient polymerization of the fibrin has occurred. The use of collagen mesh sheet with fibrin glue dispersed over the surface has been of considerable practical value. Note that the sheet should be kept in contact with the surface by gentle pressure for 3–5 minutes.

The indications are for tissue adhesion, haemostasis and suture support (see also Box 19.1).

There has been concern that the use of human fibrinogen and factor XIII might allow the transmission of

Box 19.1 Example of the use of tissue glues

General surgery
- Trauma to or surgery of liver, spleen, pancreas
- Haemostasis in gallbladder bed (cheaper agents currently available)
- Support anastomosis e.g. pancreaticojejunal anastomosis

Neurosurgery
- Repair of dural tear, sealing CSF leak
- Peripheral nerve anastomosis

Orthopaedic surgery
- Acetabuloplasty (cement-free prosthesis)
- Tendon repair
- Re-attaching osteochondral fragments

Cardiovascular and thoracic surgery
- Prosthetic implant in combination with collagen sheet to seal lung air leaks

Ophthalmic surgery
- Cataract operations

ENT surgery
- Tympanic membrane surgery
- Sealing CSF leaks

Urology
- Haemostasis, especially after TURP

Plastic surgery
- Attaching skin grafts

viral agents such as hepatitis B, hepatitis C or HIV. Commercial inactivation of a virus is achieved by pasteurization with purification of the proteins and then

Summary

1. Good theatre management is cost-effective and enhances safety for both patient and surgical team.
2. All surgeons need to know the basic principles of sterilization.
3. In the market place, the range of sutures and needles and staples is enormous – consider using a small selection to the dual advantage of reduced cost and storage space, and increased effectiveness.
4. Implants can transform a patient's quality of life but the surgery is costly and complications can be serious and prolonged.

heating the solution for 10 hours at 60°C. Laboratory studies have demonstrated that this process not only inactivates the hepatitis B and HIV viruses, but also herpes simplex virus and cytomegalovirus. Particular care is taken to use human fibrinogen from hepatitis B antigen negative, anti-HIV-negative and anti-hepatitis-C-negative plasma of healthy donors.

Marked arterial or venous bleeding renders the system ineffective. Hypersensitivity reactions have been described. The process is under evaluation in the UK.

 References

Charnley J 1970 Acrylic cement in orthopaedic surgery. E and S Livingstone, Edinburgh

Lidwell O H, Lowbury E J L, Whyte W et al 1982 Effect of ultraclean air in operating rooms in deep sepsis in the joint after total hip or knee replacement: a randomised study. British Medical Journal 285: 10–14

Park A J, Black R J, Watson A C H 1993. Silicone gel breast implants, breast cancer and connective tissue disorder. British Journal of Surgery 80: 1097–1100

Whyte W 1991 Operating theatre clothing: a review. Surgical Infection 3: 14–17

20

Prevention of infection in surgical practice

A. Davies, C. Kibbler

Objectives

- **Appreciate the importance of surgical sepsis as a significant cause of morbidity.**
- **Understand the principles of hospital infection control and its role in preventing infections.**
- **Be aware of methods by which asepsis and antisepsis are achieved, and when they are necessary.**
- **Know when antibiotic prophylaxis is desirable and when it is not.**
- **Recognize the benefit of infection audit with feedback to surgeons as a means of reducing the infection rate.**

INTRODUCTION

The Hungarian obstetrician Ignaz Semmelweiss was the first to demonstrate the importance of antisepsis, working in Vienna in the early 1850s. He found that on his obstetric ward attended by medical students almost one-fifth of all his patients died, usually of puerperal sepsis. On another ward, without medical students, the mortality was about 3 in 100.

He realized that the medical students came straight from the autopsy room and proceeded to examine his patients without so much as washing their hands. Having insisted that each student should do so with soap and water and then in chlorinated lime solution before entering the ward, he saw the mortality rate drop to less than 2 in 100.

Despite this dramatic result Semmelweiss was largely ignored and even ridiculed. It was not until Joseph Lister built on Pasteur's germ theory of disease in Glasgow in the late 1860s that antisepsis was looked at seriously.

Since then, the improved prevention and management of infections in surgical practice has been one of the most important factors allowing the development of surgery as we now know it. Even so, surgical wound infections remain an important cause of morbidity. Over 70% of hospital acquired infections occur in patients who have undergone a surgical procedure. Of these infections, wound infections are those which increase hospital costs and length of hospital stay the most. On average, wound infections prolong the hospital stay of the patient by 7 days.

Surgical wounds are traditionally classified as:

- Clean (Class I)
- Clean-contaminated (Class II)
- Contaminated (Class III)
- Dirty (Class IV).

Clean

These are wounds created during surgical procedures, in which the respiratory, genitourinary or gastrointestinal tracts have not been entered. The usual causes of infections in these wounds are airborne or exogenous bacteria that have entered the wound during surgery, or, in the case of prosthetic implants, the patient's own skin flora. The infection rate should not exceed 2%.

Clean-contaminated

This term describes wounds in elective surgery where the respiratory, gastrointestinal or genitourinary tracts have been entered. The primary cause of infection is the endogenous flora of the organ which has been surgically resected. The infection rate has been found to be approximately 5%.

Contaminated

These are wounds where at surgery acute inflammation was found (but not pus), or where there was spillage of gastrointestinal contents. They become infected with bowel/endogenous flora at a rate of about 20%.

Dirty

These are wounds where pus was found at operation, usually following organ perforation, although this category also includes contaminated traumatic wounds. The infection rate is up to 40%.

Not only are surgical infections extremely important to the outcome for individual patients and costly for hospitals, but they have also assumed medicolegal significance. All departments and surgeons should ensure that their infection rates compare favourably with those in other units, using methods which will be discussed later in this chapter.

 Strategies for minimising infection rates:

- Control of resistant organisms in all areas of the hospital
- Asepsis and antisepsis
- Surgical technique
- Use of prophylactic antibiotics
- Audit

1. CONTROL OF RESISTANT ORGANISMS

Antibiotics have been in use for more than 50 years and many organisms are now resistant to the older agents. For example, in many hospitals more than 50% of isolates of *E. coli* are resistant to ampicillin. The development of newer agents with increased activity and wider spectrum has allowed the benefits of antimicrobial therapy to be maintained and even improved. However, increasing use of these has led to the emergence of resistance in some important pathogen groups.

The most obvious example is methicillin resistant *Staphylococcus aureus*, known as MRSA. This is resistant to the commonly used anti-staphylococcal agent flucloxacillin and has to be treated with drugs such as glycopeptides (e.g. vancomycin, teicoplanin). The drawbacks are that as well as being more toxic, these agents also penetrate less well into soft tissues and wounds, can only be given parenterally and are more expensive. MRSA is of particular concern in fields such as burns, plastics and orthopaedics where tissue penetration of the antibiotic is of paramount importance and where an infection may result in removal of a prosthesis or failure of a graft. Even more worrying is the reported emergence of vancomycin resistant *S. aureus* (VRSA) in Japan and the USA. At the time of writing the extent of the problem was still being defined but there is a real danger that in the not too distant future we shall again be unable to treat *S. aureus* infection.

Enterococci are also posing major problems with resistance; vancomycin resistant enterococci (VRE) are now found in many UK hospitals and although they are less virulent than MRSA, they may cause life-threatening sepsis in patients whose immune defences are already impaired by trauma and poor nutrition.

Gram-negative organisms such as *Pseudomonas aeruginosa* may also be multi-resistant. The increasing use of third generation cephalosporins appears to be encouraging the emergence of Gram-negative bacilli such as *Klebsiella pneumoniae* and *Enterobacter cloacae* resistant to these and other beta-lactams.

Attempts must be made to keep the prevalence of resistant organisms within a unit to a minimum, and to prevent their spread between patients.

 Basic principles for the control of resistant organisms

- Handwashing and basic infection control practices
- Screening at-risk patients to identify those who are colonized
- Isolation of colonized or affected patients
- Control of movements of colonized patients between departments
- Judicious use of antibiotics

Handwashing and basic infection control practices

The importance of **handwashing** cannot be overemphasized. Studies have repeatedly shown that this is the single most important and successful method of controlling the spread of infection in hospital. Most hospital acquired infections are transmitted on the hands of staff. Hands should always be washed after any physical contact with any patient, either with soap/chlorhexidine/povidone–iodine solutions and water or with alcohol rubs or gels if the hands are not visibly soiled. Many lives could be saved by handwashing!

Screening of at-risk patients to identify those who are colonized

This is usually reserved for detecting MRSA. The aim of identifying colonized patients is to enable precautions to be taken to prevent spread of the organism to other patients, and also to reduce the risk of infection in those planned for high risk surgery such as vascular graft procedures and prosthetic orthopaedic surgery. Swabs of nose, throat and perineum are usually taken.

Colonized patients are asymptomatic and do not require systemic antibiotic treatment. Only if they show clinical evidence of infection should antibiotic treatment be undertaken. However, attempts should be made to eradicate MRSA (as opposed to clinical treatment) in colonized patients, although this will often fail in the presence of foreign bodies such as percutaneous feeding tubes, and persisting wounds. This is generally done with topical agents.

If there is evidence of an outbreak on a unit then staff may also be screened in case there are carriers, but this should only be done at the request of the infection control team.

In most UK hospitals the management of patients and staff in units affected by MRSA is based upon national guidelines. (Duckworth et al 1998).

Isolation of colonized or infected patients

Once patients have been found to be colonized with a significant multi-resistant organism they should enter 'wound and enteric' or 'source' isolation, which normally means that they should be nursed in a side-room. All staff should wear disposable gloves and aprons when in contact with the patient and medical staff should remove their white coats before entering the side-room. Ideally the patient should be nursed by the same nursing staff throughout the shift and all other staff such as porters, physiotherapists, phlebotomists, domestics, etc. should be aware of the significance of 'wound and enteric/source isolation' and the relevant precautions to be taken.

Control of movements of colonized patients between departments

Patients known to be carrying multi-resistant organisms should be operated upon at the end of the surgical list, so that the theatre can be cleaned thoroughly afterwards. Theatres should be made aware in advance of the patient's status. The same applies to visits to other departments such as radiology, physiotherapy, gym, etc. Movement of the patient within the hospital should be kept to a minimum and patients should only be transferred between wards when absolutely necessary.

Judicious use of antibiotics

Antibiotics should be used only when there is evidence of clinical infection or as part of a policy regarding perioperative prophylaxis. The choice of antibiotic should be rational and if there is any doubt the microbiologist should be consulted for advice earlier rather than later. Overuse of antibiotics not only encourages develop-

ment of resistance in exposed organisms, it also destroys patients' normal flora and makes them more susceptible to colonization with hospital organisms. Furthermore it predisposes to infection with *Clostridium difficile* which can lead to pseudomembranous colitis: third generation cephalosporins are notorious for this.

It is the responsibility of each unit, aided by the infection control team and microbiologist, to adhere strictly to their agreed policy at all times. Failure to do so on only a few occasions may wipe out the benefit reaped by following it obsessively the rest of the time.

2. ASEPSIS AND ANTISEPSIS

The term 'asepsis' is used to describe methods which prevent contamination of wounds and other sites, by ensuring that only sterile objects and fluids come into contact with them, and that the risks of airborne contamination are minimized. Antisepsis is the use of solutions (e.g. chlorhexidine, iodine or alcohol) for disinfection but does not necessarily imply sterility.

THEATRE CLOTHING

 Theatre clothing

Gowns
- **Woven cotton clothing is relatively ineffective at preventing the passage of bacteria**
- **Disposable non-woven fabric, Goretex or tightly woven polycottons are the ideal**
- **The Charnley exhaust gown is of some benefit in prosthetic implant surgery**

Masks
- **Controversial. Used to protect user's mucous membranes**

Eye protection/visors
- **Protect mucous membranes**

Hair and beards
- **Must be fully covered by synthetic caps/balaclavas**

Footwear
- **Little role in spread of infection**
- **Must protect from sharps injury**

Gloves
- **Sterile. Protect patient and user. Double-gloving provides increased protection against blood-borne viruses**

Gowns

Normal cotton clothing does little to prevent the passage of bacteria, especially those on skin scales, as the diameter of holes at the interstices of the cloth is usually greater than 80 microns. In addition, once cotton material is wet its barrier properties are much reduced, allowing bacteria to penetrate through from the wearer's skin. Therefore if clothes become wet they should be changed.

Materials which reduce the dispersion of skin scales and bacteria are restrictive to wear so a compromise has to be reached. Clothing made from disposable non-woven fabric, e.g. Sontara (Fabric 450), is suitable but expensive, as the whole team must wear it to obtain a benefit. Breathable membrane fabrics such as Goretex, or other materials such as tightly-woven washable poly-cottons are also suitable, but need careful laundering. Special attention has to be paid to the design of the clothing so that bacteria are not 'pumped out' at the neck or the ankles. Most effective of all is the Charnley exhaust gown, which for maximum benefit must be used in conjunction with a unidirectional high-efficiency particulate air (HEPA) filter system. It is also very restrictive and so rarely used by general surgeons. However it can be valuable in orthopaedic prosthetic surgery.

Masks

The use of masks is controversial. Few bacteria are discharged from the mouth and nose during normal breathing and quiet conversation, and it is argued that for general abdominal operations masks are not required for the protection of the patient. They are certainly not required for staff members in theatre who are not directly assisting. If masks are worn, e.g. in implant surgery, a fresh mask must be worn for each operation, as re-use and manipulation will simply contaminate the outside of the mask with skin commensals.

An efficient mask has to be capable of arresting low velocity droplets. Paper masks become wet within a few minutes and lose their barrier qualities, so should not be used. Disposable masks made of synthetic fibres are better and contain filters made of polyester (e.g. Bard Vigilon) or polypropylene (e.g. Filtron). Surgical anti-fog masks with flexible nosebands are available which follow facial contours and retain a high efficiency of filtration.

Masks continue to be worn to provide protective function for the wearer against blood-borne viruses, as part of a policy of universal (or standard) precautions (see Ch. 21), although full face visors will afford similar protection.

Eye protection

Protective eyewear with masks, or visors should be worn during any procedure which is likely to generate droplets of blood or other body fluids, in order to protect the mucous membranes of the wearer from blood-borne viruses. A variety of lightweight anti-fog goggles, glasses and visors are available which do not obstruct vision.

Hair/beard cover

Long hair must be tied up and all hair must be completely covered by a close-fitting cap made of synthetic material. Beards should also be fully covered by a securely tied mask and hood of the balaclava type.

Footwear

There is little evidence that the floor plays a significant role in the spread of infections in hospital. Staff should wear clean, comfortable, antislip and antistatic shoes. If there is a risk of fluid spillage, e.g. in genitourinary surgery, then ankle-length boots should be worn which can then be cleaned with warm soapy water.

Footwear should fit well and avoid producing a 'bellows' effect. Construction should be sufficiently robust to protect the foot from sharps injury.

Gloves

These are essential to protect both surgeon and patient from blood-borne viruses and to prevent the wound becoming contaminated with the surgeon's skin flora. Worryingly, many gloves have been found to have pre-existing holes prior to use as a result of inadequate quality control and poor manufacture, and furthermore during surgery around 20–30% develop holes of which the wearer is often unaware.

Double gloving affords extra protection but at the expense of reduced sensitivity and dexterity, and possible discomfort. It is important to use single-use surgical gloves from a reputable source. The gloves should have been sterilized by irradiation.

Surgical gloves made of natural rubber (latex) are increasingly reported to cause hypersensitivity reactions. Non-latex gloves without powder are available.

The use of armoured gloves, thimbles, protective clothing and safe surgical practice is considered in more detail in Chapter 21.

THEATRE AIR

Airborne bacteria are generally believed to be a source of postoperative sepsis, although this has only been unequivocally proved in the case of prosthetic orthopaedic implant infections. The number of circulating bacteria is directly related to the number of people in theatre, and their movements, which should both therefore be minimized. It is also important to remember that the type of theatre clothing worn affects the airborne bacterial load.

Plenum ventilation systems

General operating theatres are equipped with *positive pressure* or *plenum* ventilation systems, with the pressure decreasing from theatre to anaesthetic room to entrance lobby. Thus airborne microorganisms tend to be carried out rather than in. In a conventional plenum system there should be a minimum of 20 air changes per hour. Routine checks of bioload are not required. Guidelines regarding theatre air ventilation and theatre design can be found in the Department of Health documents Health Technical Memorandum 2025, *Ventilation in Health Care Premises* and Health Building Note number 26, *Operating Department*.

Ultra-clean air systems

These are advocated for prosthetic implant surgery. In these systems, instead of the turbulent airflow associated with plenum pressure systems, there is unidirectional or *laminar* airflow at about 300 air changes per hour. The air is recirculated through high efficiency particulate air (HEPA) filters. This produces a reduction in circulating microorganisms compared with a conventional system. In these theatres regular bacteriological assessment should be undertaken.

Charnley (1979) developed a ventilation system for total hip replacements in which the team operated within an enclosure ventilated with ultra-clean air as described above. Each member of the team also wore exhaust-ventilated bacteria-proof operating suits. In this way he reduced the number of postoperative joint infections from around 10% to less than 1%, although he also introduced other improvements at the same time which may have been partly responsible. However a Medical Research Council multi-hospital controlled trial showed a greater than fourfold reduction in joint sepsis rates using ultra-clean air compared with plenum ventilation, with the best rates of all when exhaust ventilated clothing was also used.

It should be borne in mind that if the level of asepsis is otherwise only moderate, then the impact of ultra-clean air systems may be lost. Their role in clean surgery other than prosthetic implant surgery is uncertain.

PREPARATION OF THE SURGEON

Most theatre-acquired infections are of endogenous origin, but the scrub team must ensure that they are not putting their patients at risk. Surgeons should not operate with infected skin conditions or in the prodromal period of a viral illness.

The term 'scrubbing up' is unlikely to disappear from surgical practice but repeated scrubbing is counter-productive as it results in skin abrasions and more bacteria being brought to the surface. An initial scrub of 3–5 minutes at the start of a list is sufficient, followed by effective handwashing using an antiseptic between cases. Skin antiseptics act rapidly and have a cumulative effect. Brushes should be sterile, single-use and made of polypropylene, not wooden with bristles. Showering prior to surgery increases the number of bacteria shed from the skin and is not recommended.

Antiseptics commonly used are:

- Chlorhexidine gluconate 4% (Hibiscrub): this is rapidly active, broad spectrum and persists with a cumulative effect, even under surgical gloves. It is easy to use but requires running water to wash off the detergent-like effect.

Surgeons allergic to chlorhexidine can use:

- Hexachlorophane (pHisoHex): this is only effective against Gram-positive bacteria and has a slow action but a cumulative effect.
- Povidone–iodine (Betadine): This acts more rapidly than hexachlorophane and has a broader spectrum but does not have a prolonged effect.

Hands should be thoroughly dried using single-use sterile towels; hot-air drying machines are not recommended.

PREPARATION OF THE PATIENT

The longer a patient stays in hospital before surgery the greater the likelihood of a subsequent wound infection. The hospital stay prior to the operation should be as short as possible and as many tests as possible should be carried out beforehand as an outpatient.

Cultures from postoperative wound infections often suggest that organisms are transferred from other areas of the patient to the operative site (endogenous transfer) despite the use of antiseptics. A preoperative shower using hexachlorophane or chlorhexidine has reduced wound infections.

All skin infections in the patient should be identified and pretreated or covered with waterproof dressings.

Shaving

Wound infection rates are higher when skin has been shaved at the operation site, because of injury to the skin. If hair removal is necessary, clippers or depilatory cream should be used. If shaving is considered essential it should be performed as near as possible to the time of operation, preferably by the surgeon prior to scrubbing up.

Transport to theatre

After the patient has been changed into a clean operating gown he or she can be transferred directly to the theatre in a bed. Ward blankets should be removed before entering theatre. There is no need for a special transfer area, changing trolleys, porters putting on plastic overshoes, or passing the trolley wheels over a sticky mat. Trolleys should be cleaned daily.

Preparing the patient's skin

The area around and including the operation site should be scrubbed first with a sponge or swab impregnated with detergent. After the skin has been cleaned and degreased in this way, antiseptic solutions should be used. Alcohol or an alcoholic solution of chlorhexidine or povidone–iodine is used. Disinfection is best when the antiseptic is rubbed on until the skin is dry.

Care must be taken when using alcohol solutions with diathermy; alcohol should not be allowed to pool in the umbilicus or under the perineum.

For vaginal or perineal disinfection a solution of chlorhexidine and cetrimide (Savlon) is advisable.

Drapes

Traditionally the periphery of the proposed incision site was protected with sterile cotton drapes. However these soon become wet, diminishing their protective properties, and so the use of incisional plastic drapes has been advocated. Work by Cruse and Foord (1980) showed that applying adhesive plastic drapes to the operation area itself did not decrease the wound infection rate, and this has since been confirmed in a study of caesarean section.

The following processes are necessary to achieve asepsis and antisepsis and will now be considered:

- Sterilization
- Cleaning and disinfection.

STERILIZATION

This is defined as the complete destruction of all viable microorganisms including spores, viruses and mycobacteria. It is in practice defined in terms of the probability of a single viable microorganism surviving on 1 million items.

The term sterilization can only be applied to equipment and not to the skin, where only antisepsis can be achieved.

 Sterilization may be achieved by:

- **Steam**
- **Hot air**
- **Ethylene oxide**
- **Low-temperature steam and formaldehyde (LTSF)**
- **Irradiation**

Sterilization by steam

Steam under pressure attains a higher temperature than boiling water and the final temperature is directly related to the pressure. Instruments can be reliably sterilized by steam under pressure using autoclaves. The instruments should have been cleaned first. This process can kill bacteria (including *Mycobacterium tuberculosis*), viruses and heat-resistant spores.

The preferred cycle is 134°C (at 2 atmospheres) for a hold time of 3 minutes, which entails a total cycle time of at least 30 minutes to reach the required temperature. Instruments used on patients with known or suspected transmissible spongiform encephalopathy for neurosurgical, ENT, orthopaedic or ophthalmic surgical procedures should be destroyed by incineration (ACDP 1998). For other procedures on these patients, disposable instruments should be used where possible. Non-disposable instruments may be autoclaved using a cycle of 18 minutes at 134°C or six cycles of 3 minutes.

Autoclaves should be centralized in specialized units, e.g. the sterile service department (SSD) or theatre sterile service unit (TSSU) and maintained by highly trained personnel. Maintenance and performance tests are very strictly controlled.

Small portable autoclaves are used in some theatres for convenience. They have the disadvantage that they are not being used by staff who are trained to scrutinize them and may not be adequately maintained.

There are also bottle autoclaves for sterilizing fluids but this is usually done by industry or specialized pharmacy production units.

Sterilization by hot air

All microorganisms are killed by dry heat at 160°C for a hold time of not less than 2 hours.

The process is inefficient compared with steam sterilization, but has the advantage of being able to treat non-aqueous liquids, ointments and airtight containers. It is also useful for avoiding corrosion of non-stainless metals and instruments with fine cutting edges (e.g. ophthalmic instruments).

It should not be used for aqueous fluids or for materials that are likely to be damaged at 160°C for 2 hours, such as rubber and plastics.

Again this equipment is subject to rigorous checks and maintenance.

Sterilization by ethylene oxide

Ethylene oxide is a highly penetrative, non-corrosive agent with a broad cidal action against bacteria, spores and viruses. However it is also flammable, toxic, irritant, mutagenic and potentially carcinogenic, and should not be used where heat sterilization of an object would be possible.

Its main uses are for wrapped and unwrapped heat-sensitive equipment: it is ideal for electrical equipment, flexible-fibre endoscopes and photographic equipment. It is not recommended for ventilatory equipment and is inappropriate for items with organic soiling.

EO sterilization is mainly an industrial process for single-use medical devices. There are a limited number of NHS regional units. It is expensive and potentially dangerous and must be carefully controlled and monitored.

Sterilization by low-temperature steam and formaldehyde (LTSF)

This method uses a combination of dry saturated steam and formaldehyde to kill bacteria, spores and most viruses. The advantage is that sterilization is achieved at a low temperature (73°C) and so it is suitable for heat-sensitive equipment and items with plastic components which might be damaged by other processes. It cannot be used on items contaminated with body fluids, since hardened fixed protein deposits will be produced, or on narrow bore tubing which may contain condensed water with trapped formaldehyde which will be hazardous to patients, so endoscopes are excluded.

Sterilization by irradiation

This process employs gamma rays or accelerated electrons. It is an industrial process suitable for sterilizing large batches of similar products, such as catheters, syringes, etc.

CLEANING AND DISINFECTION

Cleaning is a process which removes visible contamination but does not necessarily destroy microorganisms. It is a necessary prerequisite of effective disinfection or sterilization.

Disinfection is a process which reduces the number of viable microorganisms to an acceptable level but may not inactivate some viruses and bacterial spores.

 Methods of disinfection include:

- **Low temperature steam (LTS)**
- **Boiling water**
- **Formaldehyde**
- **Other chemical disinfection**

Disinfection by low-temperature steam

This kills most vegetative microorganisms and viruses by exposure to moist heat. Typical conditions are exposure to steam at a temperature of 73°C for a period of 20 minutes at below atmospheric pressure. Following LTS disinfection, items can be easily cleaned as the coagulated protein residues are readily removable, unlike the baked-on residues produced following autoclaving. This makes it a useful process to render dirty instruments from theatre and clinics safe to handle prior to sterilization.

The process is carried out in a disinfector, usually in the TSSU.

Disinfection by boiling water

This kills bacteria, some viruses (including HIV and HBV) and some spores. It does not sterilize.

Soft water at 100°C at normal pressure for 5 minutes is satisfactory. Suitable instruments include speculae, proctoscopes and sigmoidoscopes.

Disinfection with formaldehyde

Formaldehyde gas is a broad-spectrum antimicrobial agent which can be used for disinfection. It is a hazardous substance, being flammable, explosive and irritant to the eye, skin and respiratory tract. The process has therefore to be monitored and controlled carefully. The gas is used at up to 50°C and has limited sporicidal activity.

It is used for large heat-sensitive equipment such as ventilators, suction pumps and incubators. Paper, rubber and some plastics are excluded.

Chemical disinfection

This is used where heat cannot be used. A good example is the use of glutaraldehyde 2% (Cidex) to decontaminate flexible endoscopes. It is rapidly active against most vegetative bacteria and viruses (including HIV and HBV), and slowly effective against TB and spores. It is toxic, irritant and allergenic.

It is important that those involved in the purchase and development of new instrumentation for surgery or investigation consider how it may be sterilized at the end of the procedure. Recent years have seen the introduction of increasing numbers of instruments which cannot be sterilized and can only be disinfected with difficulty.

DEALING WITH SPILLAGES

Body fluid spillages must be removed as soon as possible. They should be covered first with an appropriate disinfectant such as hypochlorite granules (Presept), then absorbent paper towels. Gloves and plastic apron should be worn.

WASTE DISPOSAL

Careful separation of clinical waste must occur as it is disposed of in different ways. Yellow sharps bins and yellow plastic bags are incinerated and this is the correct method of disposal for all combustible material of an infectious nature, such as needles, plastic syringes, disposable linen and contaminated protective clothing.

3. SURGICAL TECHNIQUE

The postoperative infection rate is influenced by the following factors:

• Length of time in theatre. The longer the operation the more likely the wound is to become infected. Operations should be performed as expediently as safety will allow.
• Operative trauma should be kept to a minimum and tissues gently handled.
• Incisions by sharp instruments are less likely to become infected than those produced, for example, by cautery. On the other hand, use of cautery means sutures can be avoided; sutures themselves can act as a nidus for infection. The thinnest ligature which is suitable should be used.

• Haematomas are at risk of becoming infected.
• Areas left necrotic or with poor blood supply are also vulnerable.
• Avoid leaving a dead space.
• Prophylactic drains are unwarranted and increase the risk of infection. If a drain is necessary it should not enter through the wound but at some distance from it. It should drain into an entirely closed system to decrease the chance of ascending infection, and it should be removed as soon as possible.

4. USE OF PROPHYLACTIC ANTIBIOTICS

It has been shown that for many contaminated and clean-contaminated procedures the postoperative infection rate can be decreased by use of appropriate prophylactic antibiotics given prior to surgery. The general principles of antibiotic prophylaxis are as follows:

1. Antibiotic prophylaxis should be used only when contamination of a wound is expected or when operations of a contaminated site may lead to bacteraemia. It is not required for clean-wound procedures except:
 – when an implant or vascular graft is inserted
 – in valvular heart disease to prevent infective endocarditis
 – during emergency surgery in a patient with pre-existing or recently active infection
 – if an infection would be very severe or have life-threatening consequences.
2. There is no evidence that prolonged prophylaxis has any advantage over short courses (24 hours). Prolonged administration may lead to superinfection. Normally in clean surgery one dose is considered sufficient. In contaminated surgery three doses are often given.
3. The antibiotic should be given parenterally and immediately prior to surgery to ensure effective tissue levels. Antibiotics given soon afterwards are unable to prevent infection. If surgery continues for more than 3–4 hours then a further dose should be given in theatre as tissue levels of the drug may no longer be satisfactory. In joint replacement surgery, acrylic cement containing gentamicin has been used with success.
4. Antibiotics should be chosen to cover relevant organisms. The agent to be used should be decided upon after discussion with the microbiologist regarding likely contaminants and local resistance patterns. For example, in orthopaedic surgery the main pathogens are staphylococci, but in bowel surgery cover is required for anaerobic and Gram-negative aerobic bowel flora.

The surgeon and microbiologist should work together to develop standard policies for the unit, and once in place these should be strictly adhered to.

5. FEEDBACK TO SURGEON AND UNIT

Using these four strategies, then, surgeons aim to keep their postoperative infection rate to a minimum. However, it is important that both the surgeon and the unit are aware of their infection rates and that they compare favourably with rates in other similar units. This may be achieved by:

- Surveillance programmes
- Infection audit.

Surveillance

The Study on the Efficacy of Nosocomial Infection Control (SENIC) was carried out in the USA over 10 years in the 1970s. A random sample of 1000 patients from each of 338 hospitals was studied and details about each patient were recorded and analysed. It was found that infections of the urinary tract were the most common nosocomial infections but, as already mentioned, wound infections were the most costly, both financially and in terms of delayed discharge from hospital.

SENIC data measured intensity of surveillance, control efforts, policy development and teaching and whether or not infection rates were fed back confidentially to individual surgeons. In hospitals with optimal performance in all these categories the wound infection rate was 38% lower. The key factor in this reduction appears to be confidential feedback to individual surgeons. This is known as the Hawthorne effect.

Surveillance is an expensive and very time-consuming process and the optimal surveillance system is not known. Different studies have tried various methods of recording the number of infections, for instance use of the nursing Kardex or daily wound examination by the surveillance team. Despite the drawbacks it is useful not only for feedback but also for rapidly identifying changes in epidemiology or a rise in infection rates, or for assessing the effect of implementing new preventive strategies.

Infection audit

Although a record of overall infection rates by surveillance is the ideal this is not generally practical, as discussed above. Clinical audit is a way of reviewing clinical practice and outcomes and has also been shown to be useful in surgical practice. All UK NHS units are required to carry out audit of their practices. Infection rates are important to audit. An acceptable standard exists and steps can be taken to improve rates in the process of closing the audit loop.

Summary

Postoperative wound infections are a cause of serious morbidity to patients and expense to hospitals. They can be minimized by attention to:

1. Infection control. **Handwashing** is the single most important measure in controlling the spread of infection between patients.
2. Asepsis and sterile technique. Surgeons should be aware of the rationale behind precautions taken in theatre and when to employ them, the methods available for sterilization and disinfection, and the acceptability of each technique for different instruments and procedures.
3. Antibiotic prophylaxis should be targeted and rational, and guided by agreed local policies.
4. Confidential feedback of infection rates to surgeons has been shown to lower the infection rate, and so the importance of infection audit or surveillance is stressed.

References

Advisory Committee on Dangerous Pathogens Spongiform Encephalopathy Advisory Committee 1998 Transmissable spongiform encephalopathy agents: safe working and the prevention of infection. HMSO, London

Cruse P J E, Foord R 1980 The epidemiology of wound infection: a 10-year prospective study of 62,939 wounds. Surgical Clinics of North America 60: 1

Duckworth G et al 1998 Revised guidelines for the control of methicillin-resistant *Staphylococcus aureus* infection in hospitals. Report of a combined working party of the British Society for Antimicrobial Chemotherapy, the Hospital Infection Society and the Infection Control Nurses Association. Journal of Hospital Infection 39: 253–290

Further reading

Ayliffe G A J, Lowbury E J L, Geddes A M, Williams J D (eds) 1992 Control of hospital infection, 3rd edn. Chapman and Hall Medical, London

Philpot-Howard J, Casewell M 1995 Hospital infection
    control. Saunders, London
Morgan D (ed) 1995 A code of practice for sterilisation of
    instruments and control of cross infection (amended).
    British Medical Association, London

21

The risks to surgeons of nosocomial virus transmission

D. J. Jeffries

Objectives

- **Understand the main surgically important viruses.**
- **Appreciate the sources and methods of viral transmission.**
- **Recognize how to reduce the risks of transmission during surgical treatment.**
- **Know what action to take if exposure to infection has occurred.**

Many different viruses have been associated with nosocomial spread and health care workers frequently become infected as part of a hospital outbreak. It may be difficult to define the extent of an outbreak of a nosocomial virus infection due to a virus such as influenza or respiratory syncytial virus, as there is usually evidence of a parallel oubreak in the community and new infections are likely to be introduced repeatedly by patients, visitors and staff. Some viruses (e.g. herpes simplex, varicella-zoster virus and viral haemorrhagic fevers) may be spread to health care workers by close patient contact, while others may be widely disseminated in a ward or outpatient unit, e.g. winter vomiting due to small round structured viruses (SRSV). The risk of acquiring a nosocomial virus infection is reduced by the following measures:

1. Education and awareness of the risks
2. Isolation or cohorting of patients when appropriate
3. Good hygiene and adherence to infection control procedures
4. Immunization, if vaccines are available
5. Post-exposure measures if available.

Close collaboration between microbiologists, virologists and other health care workers will ensure that staff are aware of the risks from individual infected patients and of the appropriate procedures necessary to control these risks. All health care workers in contact with patients or their samples are exposed to nosocomial virus infections and, provided that adequate protective clothing and other facilities are available, the risk of occupationally-acquired infection is accepted as part of the job. The surgeon is at no greater risk of acquiring most of the recognized nosocomial virus infections than any other health care worker (for detailed reviews of specific infections and their control see Breuer & Jeffries (1990) and Jeffries (1995a)). The nature of the work of surgeons exposes them to the risk of infection from three blood-borne viruses, human immunodeficiency virus (HIV), hepatitis B virus (HBV) and hepatitis C virus (HCV). All of these viruses may lead to a prolonged infectious carrier state and demonstration of persistent infection in a surgeon may lead to the need to change his/her practice to avoid exposure-prone invasive procedures or, if this is not possible, it may be necessary to change to another speciality. There are potentially serious outcomes from virus infections that may be acquired nosocomially; this chapter is therefore focused on these agents.

THE BLOOD-BORNE VIRUSES

The main features of human immunodeficiency virus and the hepatitis viruses are presented in the 1995 publication from the Advisory Committee on Dangerous Pathogens (ACDP), entitled *Protection against blood-borne infections in the workplace*, and in a review by Jeffries (1997).

Human immunodeficiency viruses (HIV-1, HIV-2)

The first cases of the acquired immune deficiency syndrome (AIDS) were recognized in 1981 and in 1983 a retrovirus (HIV-1) was identified which was subsequently shown to be the causative agent. In 1985, a second human immunodeficiency virus (HIV-2) was isolated from individuals from West Africa and this has now spread to other parts of Africa, India and Europe. The two viruses are very similar and their modes of spread and clinical effects are identical although there is some evidence that disease progression is slower in HIV-2 infection. In this chapter the two viruses are referred to collectively as HIV. HIV contains RNA and during the course of its replication the genetic material of the viral particle is reverse-transcribed by an enzyme, reverse transcriptase, into a DNA copy which is inserted into the chromosomes of an infected cell. This integrated package of viral genetic material (or provirus) produces new viral particles which are available to infect other cells. Thus, following primary infection with HIV, the virus persists within cells for the life of the cells and, because of continual transfer to other cells in the immune system and central nervous system, the infection persists for the life of the individual. Recent work indicates that an HIV-infected individual produces very high levels of virus, 10^9–10^{10} virus particles per day, and is consequently potentially infectious to others for life. In health care the nature of the viral particle, which is surrounded by a lipid-containing envelope, means that it is easily destroyed by heat, disinfectants and detergents. At ambient temperatures, however, the virus is protected from desiccation and may persist in dried blood or secretions for several days.

The major cellular receptor for HIV is the CD4 antigen which is present on helper T lymphocytes and cells of the antigen-presenting series. These are the main target cells for the virus and gradual depletion of these cells over a period of years leads to the opportunistic infections and tumours that are characteristic of AIDS.

Hepatitis B virus (HBV)

Hepatitis B virus (HBV) is a DNA virus which causes acute hepatitis; because of its long incubation period (45–180 days, mean 75 days) it was previously known as long-incubation hepatitis (or serum hepatitis). During the acute infection, and in carriers of HBV, viral particles released from the liver are present in circulation. The surface coating of the particles is present in excess and this material, hepatitis B surface antigen (HBsAg), is identified by serological tests as the main indicator of active infection. A second antigen, HBeAg, which is derived from core particles of the virus present in the liver, indicates continuing activity of the virus in the liver and the presence of HBeAg in the blood correlates with high levels of infectivity. As with all types of viral hepatitis, the degree of illness produced is variable and ranges in different individuals from asymptomatic infection to acute hepatic failure. The immune response is a major factor in determining the severity of disease. In the immunologically immature or immuno-compromised, asymptomatic infections are common, but the risks of proceeding to long-term carriage of the virus are high. The long-term carrier rate following neonatal infection is >90%, in children aged 1–10 years it is 23%, and in adults 5% or less become carriers. This high rate of persistence following infection in early life largely explains the estimated 250–300 million carriers in the world, the majority of whom are in resource-deprived countries where 15–20% of the population may be infected.

The carrier of HBV presents a potential risk of horizontal transmission to others, predominantly via sexual intercourse and blood transfer. The HBeAg positive mother is also very likely to infect her baby during delivery.

Persistent replication of HBV in the liver of HBeAg positive carriers carries a risk of progressive liver damage, leading to chronic active hepatitis, cirrhosis and an increased risk of hepatocellular carcinoma.

Hepatitis C virus (HCV)

Following the identification of HBV, the continued occurrence of post-transfusion hepatitis led to the realization that there were other blood-borne hepatitis viruses (termed non-A, non-B hepatitis). The RNA virus, HCV, is now recognized as the major cause of non-A, non-B hepatitis. Hepatitis C is predominantly blood borne and infection is common in injecting drug users and recipients of unscreened blood and/or blood products. The acute phase of HCV infection is usually asymptomatic and only approximately 10% of individuals have overt hepatitis. Following primary infection, however, the majority (about 80%) proceed to become persistent carriers of the virus and, as with HBV infection, there is a long-term risk of chronic liver disease with cirrhosis and hepatocellular carcinoma.

SOURCES OF INFECTION

As the term implies, the major blood-borne viruses, HIV, HBV and HCV, are found predominantly in the circulation and most occupational infections occur as a result of exposure to blood. Other body fluids may contain infectious virus, however, and these are listed in Box 21.1. Percutaneous inoculation is the major route of infection in health care and there is no evidence of transmission of any of the common blood-borne viruses by the airborne route or from occupational or social contact that does not involve body fluid exposure.

Box 21.1 Body fluids, etc. which should be handled with the same precautions as blood

1. CSF
   Semen
   Vaginal secretions
   Breast milk
   Amniotic fluid
   Peritoneal fluid
   Pleural fluid
   Pericardial fluid
   Synovial fluid
2. Any other body fluid containing visible blood
3. Unfixed tissues and organs

Table 21.1 Factors affecting percutaneous transmission of HIV during occupational exposure*

Factor	Odds ratio†	95% C.I.
Deep injury (intramuscular)	16.1	6.1–44.6
Visible blood on device	5.2	1.8–17.7
Needle used in a blood vessel	5.1	1.9–14.8
Source patient with AIDS	6.4	2.2–18.9
AZT prophylaxis used	0.2	0.1–0.6

*Adapted from Centers for Disease Control (1995)
†Significant at $p < 0.01$.

RISKS OF INFECTION

Hepatitis B immunization has dramatically altered the level of risk to surgeons and other health care workers. Prior to the introduction of safe and potent HBV vaccines and subsequent checks of immune status, the risk of infection could be as high as 30% after percutaneous injury involving the blood of a HBeAg positive patient. Transmission of HBV has also been associated with mucous membrane exposure to blood and with bites from HBV infected patients but the risk of infection from these routes has not been quantified.

The overall risk of acquiring HIV following a single percutaneous inoculation with HIV-infected blood is approximately 0.36% (1 in 275). The results of a case-control study of 31 healthcare workers infected occupationally, compared to 679 control subjects, identified several factors which affected the risks of percutaneous transmission of HIV (Centers for Disease Control 1988). These are listed in Table 21.1. It will be noted from the table that, in this case-control study, the use of the antiviral drug AZT reduced the transmission rate by 80%. This will be returned to later.

The risk of acquiring HIV from mucous membrane or conjunctival exposure to blood from infected individuals is lower than from percutaneous inoculation. One seroconversion was reported on follow up of 1107 exposures (Jeffries 1995b). The risk of percutaneous transmission of hepatitis C virus has not been clearly defined and rates of 0–10% have been reported. In a small study of 68 health care workers in Japan, who sustained percutaneous exposure to the blood of HCV RNA-positive patients with chronic renal failure or HCV-related liver disease, seven (10%) developed markers of infection. In a survey of 3267 orthopaedic surgeons in the USA, HCV antibodies were present in 0.8%. The antibody prevalence increased from 0% in the 20–29 years age group to 1.4% in those over 60 years. For comparison, 12% had evidence of past or current HBV infection (ranging from 2.9% in the 20–29 year age group to 26% in those 60+) and two surgeons were HIV positive (both had other risk factors apart from surgery).

REDUCING THE RISKS OF INFECTION

General measures

It is neither cost-effective nor reliable to embark on routine screening of patients for blood-borne viruses. The marker tests for infectivity, HIV and HCV antibodies and HBsAg, become positive up to 12 weeks, 26 weeks and 26 weeks respectively after infection and a patient may be highly infectious before positivity is demonstrated. Similarly, it is unreliable to attempt to identify carriers of the viruses by designation of 'risk groups'. Although the blood-borne viruses HIV and HCV were originally associated with homosexuality and drug use, the spread of infection outside of perceived risk groups and control of infection in those previously perceived to be in risk groups by education, needle exchange schemes, etc. means that 'risky activity' by anyone should raise the suspicion of possible infection. Faced with the ever present risk of occupational infection, the surgeon is advised to adopt a policy of 'universal precautions' with regard to carrying out procedures with a risk of contact with high risk body fluids and tissues (see Box 21.1). The basis and procedure of using universal precautions was presented by the Centers for

Disease Control (1987, 1988, 1991) and by the UK Health Departments (1990, 1998). As percutaneous inoculation is the major route of infection, care should be taken when handling sharp instruments and any passing of sharp instruments to others should never be direct but through the vehicle of a rigid container such as a kidney dish. In some studies, approximately 40% of inoculation injuries of staff have occurred during attempts to re-sheathe needles. This should never be attempted unless a suitable safe re-sheathing device is available. In the absence of such a device, needles (and other disposable sharps) should be discarded directly into approved sharps containers. Suture needles and scalpels should never be left on trays for others to clear away. Cuts and abrasions should be covered with waterproof dressings and disposable gloves should be worn if there is a risk of contamination of the hands with blood. Protective eye-wear and a mask should be worn if splashing with blood or other body fluids is likely.

It is possible to produce guidelines for the use of protective clothing on the basis of an assessment of likely exposure to blood (Table 21.2).

Blood spillages on surfaces should be removed by first applying a suitable disinfectant, such as sodium hypochlorite (10 000 parts per million available chlorine) and then washing thoroughly with detergent and water.

Hepatitis B virus infection is preventable by immunization with the current, safe, genetically-engineered vaccines. All staff likely to be exposed to blood, tissues or other body fluids in the course of their work should be immunized and their antibody levels should then be checked to ensure that protective immunity is present. Those who fail to respond to the vaccine should be made aware of the fact that they are non-responders and, in the event of exposure to known or suspected HBV-positive blood, they should be offered passive protection with HBV immunoglobulin (HBIG).

Reducing blood exposure of the surgeon and patient during surgery

In an observational study by Tokars et al (1992), the rate of inoculation injury was recorded during the course of different types of surgical operation. Percutaneous injury rates to the main operator per 100 procedures were 4 for orthopaedics, 8 for general surgery, 9 for coronary artery bypass grafting, 17 for gastrectomy and 21 for vaginal hysterectomy. Inspection of gloves after operation has revealed a perforation rate for single glove use of 11–54% (Maffuli et al 1989, Church & Sanderson 1980, Brough et al 1988, Palmer & Rickett 1992, Smith & Grant 1990). The wearing of two pairs of surgical gloves has been reported to result in perforation of the inner glove in 2% of operations (Matta et al 1988). Penetration of the glove material by a sharp instrument or needle has a significant wiping effect and this reduces the volume of blood and amount of virus transferred. Studies using a paper pre-filter model in vitro and an ex vivo porcine tissue model

Table 21.2 Categorization of procedures according to risk of exposure to blood*

Category	Examples of procedures	Protective measures
A(i) Contact likely: risk of uncontrolled bleeding	Major surgery Gynaecology Obstetrics	Full range of protective clothing (gloves, water–repellent gown and apron, protective headware, mask, protective eyewear, protective footwear)
A(ii) Contact probable – splattering unlikely	Intra-arterial puncture Insertion/removal of intravenous/intra-arterial lines Dentistry	Gloves to be worn Masks/protective eyewear to be available
A(iii) Low likelihood of blood contact	i.m., i.d., s.c. injections	Gloves available
B No risk of blood contact	Most ward/clinic work	None necessary

*Adapted from UK Health Departments (1990)

demonstrated a reduction of blood transfer of 46–86% depending on whether a solid or hollow needle was used and on the gauge of the latter (Mast et al 1993). Thus, although standard disposable latex gloves offer no protection against needle penetration, this evidence of reduction of exposure to blood provides strong support for the use of gloves, even in simple procedures such as venepuncture, if there is a risk of injury to the operator, for example in the case of an uncooperative patient.

A number of aspects of surgical technique are worthy of appraisal in the interests of reducing the risk of percutaneous injury. Care in ensuring that no more than one person is working in an open wound or body cavity at any one time and the use of a 'hands-free' technique, where the same sharp instrument is not touched by more than one person at the same time, should be considered unless the nature of the operation renders it impossible. The need for care in passing instruments to others has already been stressed. Needles, scalpels and other sharp instruments should not be left in the operating field. These should be removed promptly by the scrub nurse after they have been deposited in a neutral zone such as a tray or kidney dish. Instruments, rather than fingers should be used for retraction and for holding tissues during suturing. Instruments should be used to remove scalpel blades from handles and all needles and sharp instruments should be directed away from the non-dominant, or assistant's hand. Suture needles should be removed before tying sutures, and instruments, rather than fingers, should be used for tying.

In addition to attention to the discipline of carrying out surgical techniques, it may be worth considering alternative equipment. The use of electrocautery, blunt-tipped needles and stapling devices may reduce the need for sharp instruments and needles. The use of sharp clips for surgical drapes should be avoided. Blunt clips are available as are disposable drapes incorporating self-adhesive film. The use of scalpels which are disposable, have a blade release device or retractable blades, will remove the risk of injuries associated with assembly or disassembly of these instruments.

The risks of contact with infected blood will vary depending on the local prevalence of infections and the nature of the patient population. With the current distribution of blood-borne viruses, however, all operating theatre staff will be exposed from time to time. The decision to introduce double-gloving for all surgical procedures may depend on a local risk assessment, but other measures to reduce exposure to blood and other body fluids can be applied to all operative procedures.

Post-exposure measures

Key point

- **As soon as possible after percutaneous inoculation or, in the case of operative surgery, as soon as the patient is stable and can be left to the care of others, wash the site of injury liberally with soap and water.**

Avoid scrubbing, encourage bleeding. Do not use antiseptic preparations as the effect of these on local defences is unknown. Wash out splashes into the eye or mouth by irrigating with copious volumes of water. Complete an incident form and contact the Occupational Health Department or another doctor designated with the responsibility of caring for staff, as specified in the local guidelines.

Key point

- **Seek advice at once; if post-exposure prophylactic drugs for HIV are to be considered, they should be commenced without delay, and ideally within 1 hour of exposure.**

It is normal practice to take a blood sample from the staff member at this time as the stored serum can then be used as a baseline for further testing. Laboratory testing of the source patient, after pre-test discussion and obtaining fully informed consent, will aid further management by clarifying the risks, if any, of exposure to blood-borne viruses.

If the source patient is known or suspected to be a HBV carrier, the prophylactic regimen will depend on the immune status of the health care worker. Those who have never had vaccine should receive hepatitis B immunoglobulin (HBIG) within 48 hours of exposure and a course of hepatitis B vaccination should be started as soon as possible. In those who have been vaccinated, the recommendation of the occupational health adviser is likely to depend on the record of the person's antibody response. If there is a recorded antibody response of more than 100 miu ml^{-1} within the previous year, no further action is necessary. If the person's blood has not been tested within the year, or if a lower titre was recorded, a booster dose of vaccine followed by retesting of antibody status may be necessary. Health care workers who have failed in the past to respond to the vaccine should be offered protection with HBIG.

There is currently no prophylaxis for HCV and follow up consists of monitoring liver function and testing for anti-HCV antibodies. There is some anecdotal evidence to suggest that health care workers who become infected with HCV may respond favourably by treating, at the earliest sign of infection, with interferon-α.

Guidelines for the use of post-exposure chemoprophylaxis to prevent HIV infection of health care workers were issued in the UK in June 1997 (UK Health Departments 1997). Post-exposure prophylaxis is recommended when there has been significant exposure to material known, or strongly suspected, to be infected with HIV. Significant routes of exposure are percutaneous inoculation, exposure of broken skin or contact with mucous membranes including the eye, and high risk material (listed in Box 21.1). As in equivalent guidelines issued in the USA, the first line drugs for post-exposure prophylaxis are zidovudine (AZT) 200 mg t.d.s. or 250 mg b.d., lamivudine (3TC) 150 mg b.d., and indinavir 800 mg t.d.s. Treatment should commence as soon as possible, ideally within 1 hour of exposure, and should be continued for 1 month. A negative test for HIV antibody 6 months after the exposure confirms the absence of occupationally acquired infection.

INFECTED HEALTH CARE WORKERS

Guidelines issued by the General Medical Council, General Dental Council and the United Kingdom Central Coordinating Committee for Nurses, Midwives and Health Visitors (UKCCC) stress the importance of health care workers who consider that they have been at risk of infection with HBV or HIV seeking appropriate pre-test discussion and testing. If found to be infected they have a responsibility to be under regular medical supervision. Guidelines issued in the UK recommend that those who are infected with HIV or who are 'high infectivity' (HBeAg) carriers of HBV should not perform exposure-prone invasive procedures (UK Health Departments 1993, 1994). Exposure-prone procedures are defined as:

Those where there is a risk that injury to the worker may result in the exposure of the patient's open tissues to the blood of the worker. These procedures include those where the worker's gloved hands may be in contact with sharp instruments, needle tips or sharp tissues (spicules of bone or teeth) inside a patient's body cavity, wound or confined anatomical space where the hands or fingertips may not be visible at all times.

For some surgeons and other health care workers, confidential discussion between the person concerned and his/her health adviser may lead to minor changes in practice which would allow work to continue with the avoidance of exposure-prone procedures. If there is any doubt, advice should be sought from a specialist occupational health physician who may, in turn, wish to present the situation anonymously to the UK Advisory Panel for Health Care Workers Infected with Bloodborne Viruses (UKAP).

Some specialities, e.g. dentistry, are concerned almost totally with activities that are, by definition, exposure-prone. For HIV and HBeAg positive carriers working in such specialities, the only option in the UK is for retraining in another speciality.

No recommendations have been issued in the UK for health care workers found to be carriers of HCV unless they have been demonstrated to have transmitted their virus to a patient, in which case exclusion from exposure prone procedures has been advised. Recent reports of transmission of HBV from carrier surgeons who are HBsAg positive but HBeAg negative has led to a need to review the guidelines on staff who were previously thought to be at low risk of transmitting to their patients. It is now known that some carriers who are HBeAg negative have mutant forms of the virus and the virus is unable to generate HBeAg. Pending further guidelines, health care workers who are HBeAg negative and who have been shown to have transmitted HBV to patients are excluded from exposure-prone procedures.

CONCLUSIONS

Surgeons will continue to be at risk, albeit small, of acquiring blood-borne viruses from their patients. The level of risk will vary depending on the prevalence of viruses in the local population. Adoption of universal precautions and careful attention to operative technique will reduce the risks to the operator and other staff to a minimum. There is considerable cause for concern if surgeons are expected to operate in situations where, for lack of resources, there is inadequate provision of protective clothing, such as impermeable gowns and disposable gloves, and hepatitis B vaccine. A significant exposure to the blood of a patient causes considerable anxiety for a period of up to 6 months and until laboratory tests confirm negativity. There is no reason for a surgeon to avoid exposure-prone procedures during this period providing he/she is aware that there is a possibility of infection developing and a high standard of infection control is practised. It may be necessary, however, for the individual's medical adviser to recommend lifestyle changes such as condom usage for sexual intercourse and avoidance of donating blood, semen, etc. to prevent transmission to others by non-occupational routes. In the UK, as described earlier, guidelines for HIV and HBV (HBeAg) infected health care workers advise strongly against participation in exposure-prone procedures. This approach is not adopted in many other countries where either no restriction is placed on clinical practice or exposure-prone procedures can continue providing the patient is informed of the situation.

Summary

1. Recognize the procedures that raise the risks of viral transmission.
2. Take precautions on behalf of yourself, your patients and your colleagues.
3. Do not abandon universal precautions in emergency circumstances.
4. Learn what to do if an incident has exposed you or anyone else to the risk of contamination.

References

Advisory Committee on Dangerous Pathogens (ACDP) 1995 Protection against bloodborne viruses in the workplace: HIV and hepatitis. HMSO, London

Breuer J, Jeffries D J 1990 Control of viral infections in hospital. Journal of Hospital Infection 16: 191–221

Brough S J, Hunt T M, Barrie W M 1988 Surgical glove perforation. British Journal of Surgery 75: 317

Centers for Disease Control 1987 Recommendations for prevention of HIV transmission in health care settings. Morbidity and Mortality Weekly Record 36(2S): 1S–18S

Centers for Disease Control 1988 Update: universal precautions for prevention of transmission of human immunodeficiency virus, hepatitis B virus, and other bloodborne pathogens in health care settings. Morbidity and Mortality Weekly Record 37: 377–388

Centers for Disease Control 1991. Recommendations for preventing transmission of human immunodeficiency virus and hepatitis B virus to patients during exposure prone invasive procedures. Morbidity and Mortality Weekly Record 40(RR–8): 1–9

Church J, Sanderson P 1980 Surgical glove punctures. Journal of Hospital Infection 1: 84

Jeffries D J 1995a Viral hazards to and from health care workers. Journal of Hospital Infection. 30(Supp): 140–155

Jeffries D J 1995b Surgery and bloodborne viruses. PHLS Microbiology Digest 12: 150–154

Jeffries D J 1997 Viral agents of bloodborne infections. In: Collins C H Kennedy D A (eds) Occupational bloodborne infections. C.A.B. International, pp 1–16

Maffulli N, Capasso G, Testa V 1989 Glove perforation in elective orthopaedic surgery. Acta. Orthop. Scand. 60: 565–566

Mast S T, Woolwine J D, Gerberding J L 1993 Efficacy of gloves in reducing blood volumes transferred during simulated needlestick injury. J Infect Dis 168: 1589–1592

Matta H, Thompson A M, Rainey J B 1988 Does wearing two pairs of gloves protect operating theatre staff from skin contamination? British Medical Journal 297: 597–598

Palmer J D, Rickett J W S 1992 The mechanisms and risks of surgical glove perforation. Journal of Hospital Infection 22: 279–286

Smith J R, Grant J M 1990 The incidence of glove puncture during caesarean section. Journal of Obstetrics and Gynaecology 10: 317–318

Tokars J L, Bell D M, Culver D H et al 1992 Percutaneous injuries during surgical procedures. Journal of the American Medical Association 267: 2899–2904

UK Health Departments 1990 Guidance for clinical health care workers. Protection against infection with HIV and hepatitis viruses. Recommendations of the Expert Advisory Group on AIDS. HMSO, London

UK Health Departments 1993 Protecting health care workers and patients from hepatitis B. Department of Health, London

UK Health Departments 1994 AIDS/HIV-infected health care workers: guidance on the management of infected health care workers. Department of Health, London

UK Health Departments 1997 Guidelines on post-exposure prophylaxis for health care workers exposed to HIV. Department of Health, London

UK Health Departments 1998 Guidance for clinical health care workers. Protection against infection with bloodborne viruses. Department of Health, London

Operation

22

Good surgical practice

J. L. Dawson

Objectives

- **Understand your responsibilities.**
- **Ensure you have obtained informed consent.**
- **Work within your capabilities.**
- **Keep good notes.**

Good surgical practice will provide effective control of clinical practice as well as protecting you from legal pitfalls which await the unwary. Good surgical practice is a hard taskmaster. It demands self-discipline at all times in order to organize yourself and your commitments and combine this with honesty to your patients, your colleagues and, not least, yourself.

It is important to develop the right surgical working habits from the very beginning of training, especially:

- Time keeping
- Note keeping.

Your day should be organized so that all inpatients have been seen and assessed before the first fixed commitment. Always be on time for ward rounds, outpatients, operating lists and clinical meetings.

The essential discipline of writing concise clear contemporaneous notes cannot be overemphasized. They should contain an objective account of the history and clinical findings. Avoid judgemental or flippant comments. The notes may, for a few patients, be used as a legal record of the patient's care and progress.

The organization of modern hospital practice has led to a serious erosion of the continuity of care by one doctor for an individual patient. The notes now provide the written record of what was previously carried in the mind of the attending resident. A duty doctor is now regularly called to see patients who are under the care of a different firm. Accurate and comprehensive notes are essential for a proper assessment to be made in the event of such an emergency call. There is no doubt that the number of complaints about clinical management and clinical care is increasing: accurate clinical records are an essential safeguard to rebut any inappropriate or vexatious complaints.

Emotional neutrality

It is essential that all surgeons, of whatever grade, maintain a completely neutral stance and do not get into any sort of emotional conflict with patients, relatives or indeed professional colleagues who are responsible for patient care. Emotional conflict clouds judgement and should be avoided at all costs. Always resist responding to provocation, however tempting it may be.

Surgical team

The organization of the delivery of surgical care and training is centred around a unit or firm, usually consisting of two to three consultants plus junior staff. With the shortening of the period of surgical training, firm timetables are being adjusted to allow space for continuing surgical education. The basis of this includes a regular audit meeting at which the patient's notes are scrutinized. The basic surgical trainees are usually responsible for producing the clinical information for these audit meetings. One consultant member of the team is usually designated as the trainer responsible for a particular trainee's education. Loyalty to the firm and good rapport with your trainer are the hallmarks of a successful training programme.

Many surgical patients require imaging of one sort or another to make or confirm the diagnosis or to monitor progress after surgical treatment. Regular meetings with the radiology department are now the norm in most hospitals, but you should develop the habit of calling in to the X-ray department to arrange urgent investigations personally; in this way you will find you enjoy maximum cooperation which contributes enormously to the smooth running of the treatment of patients under your care.

Patient's understanding

Before proceeding to operate you must ensure that both the patient and relatives understand the aim of the operation and that their expectations of the outcome are realistic (see Ch. 15). The fact that the patient signs a consent form will not be accepted as evidence that he or she has received an adequate explanation of the operative procedure. In principle, the explanation of the operative procedure should be given by the person undertaking the operation. With more complicated procedures resulting in serious permanent changes, such as mastectomy or establishing a stoma, more than one consultation is necessary with the patient, and preferably with a spouse or relative present as well as a nurse counsellor. This is important so that the patient does not feel rushed into making a decision which later may be regretted. There is now widespread use of printed leaflets explaining the common procedures.

Emergency admissions

History and physical examination remain the basis for diagnosis in the majority of surgical patients. However, clinical assessment of emergency referrals may be much more difficult. The patient and relatives are more anxious and there is a degree of urgency to make a diagnosis and decide upon action. It will be rapidly apparent to you that the florid abdominal signs elicited in the casualty department may later, after a period of warmth and security in a hospital bed, have largely disappeared. Reassessment and re-examination is an essential part of the process of evaluating a patient referred as an emergency. It follows that the signs and symptoms of each examination should be carefully recorded in the notes, together with the time and also the results of any emergency investigations undertaken.

For emergency patients difficulties do arise when the patient is too ill or too young to understand the implications of what is proposed. In these circumstances it is highly desirable to speak to close relatives or other responsible persons to explain what is proposed. However, the guiding principle is that you should always act in the best interests of the child or adult, and very occasionally this may require recourse to making an application to the court.

Avoidance of errors

The surgeon responsible for the operation should also mark the lesion to be operated upon before any premedication is given. Once an operating list has been agreed and published, any change to the order is best avoided. If it is necessary, alert the theatre staff and the anaesthetist so that no error can occur.

Prophylactic measures

Ensure that the patient is in the best possible mental and physical condition and all appropriate prophylactic measures have been taken to minimize complications. These are easily overlooked in an emergency, especially prophylaxis against venous thrombosis, which is especially important in those patients who are taking a contraceptive pill.

Operation notes

At the completion of any operation, write up the notes personally. These should include a clear and accurate account of the pathology found and also a description of precisely what procedure was done and what was the state of affairs on completion. Record any intraoperative testing (e.g. anastomoses or blood flow following revascularization procedures). The importance of these notes cannot be overemphasized.

Delegation

The surgeon in training is the responsibility of the trainer. The delegation of any operative procedure must take place only when there is adequate supervision either by assisting, watching or being readily available for advice. Avoid embarking on any procedure which you regard as beyond your capability. Increasing specialization and expertise together with the introduction of new techniques (e.g. minimal access surgery) has focused patients' (and lawyers') attention on the matter of professional competence. The rapid expansion of workshops devoted to instructing the trainee in new techniques using simulation material are an essential part of surgical training and experience.

Day surgery

Day surgery presents special problems. Make sure you see all patients before undertaking the list to confirm what is to be done and carry out any necessary marking. At the end of the day, before the patient is discharged home, check that the patient is fully recovered and that there are no untoward symptoms or signs. Make proper arrangements for the patient's further care. Given an adequate and legible discharge note for the GP's information, and an emergency call number for the patient, so that advice is available should anxieties arise in the hours after returning home.

Postoperative course

You learn the variations which may occur from patient to patient during normal recovery, only from assiduously looking after large numbers of patients. Experience at the bedside is of paramount importance. It is almost impossible to learn these things from a textbook. Over time the expected pattern of recovery becomes second nature, and deviation from this pattern instinctively prompts appropriate and expeditious action. The decision to re-explore a patient is always difficult, but early evacuation of blood clot or arrest of continued bleeding may prevent serious complications later on (e.g. infection of a haematoma within the peritoneum leading to prolonged and life-threatening sepsis).

Daily note-making in the postoperative period helps to imprint on your mind the variation in recovery patterns.

Surgical audit and continuing medical education

Carefully audit and self-review outcomes throughout your professional career as an essential part of maintaining surgical standards (see Ch. 42). For individual surgical teams this is ideally done on a weekly basis. Only in this way can the head of the team maintain an overall view of precisely what is happening.

Delegation of audit to a hospital audit department does not remove responsibility from individual surgeons for producing accurate data about the service provided. If an accurate weekly record is kept it is no great burden to produce monthly and annual figures on the activities of the firm. Although most surgical teams do this for inpatients, the activities in the day surgery unit and outpatient department may receive less careful scrutiny. Control of what happens in the outpatient department is particularly difficult, especially when locums are employed. Unless there is some form of audit a patient attending an outpatient clinic can often be subjected to various procedures and investigations and even be put on the waiting list for operative treatment without the consultant having any knowledge. Regular audit meetings also provide a forum to discuss policy change and encourage a cohesive team approach. They are an excellent and essential basis for the continuing surgical education of all grades of surgeon.

Summary

1. Organize your time.
2. Inform your patient.
3. Ensure that the patient is well prepared.
4. Operate within your capabilities.
5. Keep good notes.
6. Maintain a personal audit.

23

Surgical access, incisions and the management of wounds

D. J. Leaper

Objectives

- **Be aware of technical factors which contribute to wound infection.**
- **Understand the general principles of access to the abdomen and chest.**
- **Understand the principles of wound care.**
- **Be aware of responsibilities of care of instrument and swabs during operations.**

INTRODUCTION

There are records which describe successful wound management from as long ago as the time of the Assyrians and the ancient Egyptian empire. Techniques using sutures and threads, linen adhesive strips and skin 'clips' of soldier ant heads have all been described historically. Dressings have been equally diverse, their value often being based on erroneous principles, but in the last 30 years there has been increasing interest resulting in many tailor-made and improved types of dressing.

The scourge of successful wound healing is infection, which was well recognized by Hippocrates and Galen, although some of their remedies were far from adequate. Microscopic confirmation of Celsian hypotheses and observations (the calor, rubor, tumor et dolor of acute inflammation) was slow in coming, but the understanding of the physiology of wound healing has advanced greatly over the last 2–3 decades and is continuing to do so. The correct concepts and control of infection became established with the introduction of antisepsis through Semmelweis and Lister, associated with the work of Pasteur. Aseptic techniques were adopted at the turn of this century. Antibiotics are now an integral part of surgical management, particularly in prophylaxis, and again we have seen continuing advances since the days of Ehrlich, Fleming, and Florey and Chain.

In retrospect, our surgical repertoire seems to have met no bounds or restrictions. Operative surgery and anaesthesia allow procedures such as heart–lung transplantation to be undertaken safely. Our forebears would not believe what is now possible, but the natural processes of wound healing must not be forgotten. The aphorism of 'cut well, sew well, get well' depends on a knowledge of wound-healing mechanisms and the adverse effects which may influence them.

SURGICAL ACCESS AND INCISIONS

Hair removal

Body hair is conventionally removed from a proposed operative field the day before surgery. This is done for aesthetic reasons and also to allow painless removal of dressings, particularly the currently popular polymeric transparent sheet dressings (such as Opsite or Bioclusive) which were introduced as incise drapes. It has been shown, however, that the time of shaving is critical: when performed over 12 hours before surgery clean wound sepsis rates increase from 1–2% up to more than 5%. Inexpert or unsupervised shaving by patients worsens these rates. Minor skin abrasions and cuts which are exuding by the time of surgery allow emergence of skin commensals to the surface and colonization by pathogens.

Clipping of hair or the use of depilatory creams, which are messy, reduces infection rates to a tenth of those following shaving. Shaving, if it is necessary, should be undertaken shortly prior to surgery. Avoidance of shaving altogether does not increase wound infection rates.

Operative drapes

Following skin preparation, usually with 0.5% chlorhexidine or 10% povidone–iodine (1% available iodine) in 70% alcohol, the operative field needs to be delineated with operative drapes. Conventionally these are resterilized double-thickness linen sheets which are held with towel clips. These need substantial care for further use: as well as the need for steam sterilization, they have the drawback of allowing permeation related to the weave.

Disposable fabrics do not allow penetration by body fluids and their waterproofing is a benefit when operating in the face of contamination or when there is a risk of human immunodeficiency virus (HIV) or hepatitis infections. They are expensive. Incise drapes of adhesive polyurethane film were introduced over 30 years ago. They are widely used in prosthetic or vascular surgery when there is an increased risk of opportunist infection by skin organisms such as *Staphylococcus epidermidis*. There is no definite indication that they reduce infection, and in fact the wound bacterial count at the skin surface increases during their use.

Antiseptic impregnation has little added protective effect. However, in general surgical operations incise drapes avoid the need for towel clips and can isolate stomas or an infected nearby focus (such as an infected separate wound). Wound guards can be placed into the wound but do not reduce the risk of wound infection, although they reduce bacterial contamination during open viscus surgery.

Principles of access incisions

Incisions are usually made for exploration or to reach particular structures. In 'open', or conventional surgery the incision enables the operator to view the target area directly. There has been a revolution, the extent of which is difficult to prophesy, for operations to be performed within cavities through minimal incisions; the target is viewed indirectly through a telescope. For open surgery there are several considerations that may be in conflict:

- **Access.** In order to perform any procedure competently, you must have good access. This is not just for viewing but to offer the ability to manipulate the tissues, if necessary view the rear aspect, perhaps control other structures that may not lie within the minimal exposure. A linear incision can be temporarily converted into an ellipse by retracting the sides. In some cases it may not give sufficient access and an angled incision then offers better exposure, the side within the angle being widely retractable.
- **Avoiding incidental damage.** Important structures often lie along the line of the most direct incision. Nerves or tendons are sometimes at risk. The vascular supply to important structures may be damaged and prejudice healing. Injury to some tissues prejudices future function – for example, damage to muscles and

ligaments around a joint and longitudinal scar contraction along a limb may cause later restriction of movements.

- **Tissue planes.** An intimate knowledge of tissue planes is vital in gaining correct exposure. This is particularly important in the presence of disease, which often distorts the tissues. Dissection in the wrong plane can risk causing damage or risk not completely encompassing disease such as a neoplasm.
- **Cosmetic aspects.** The resulting skin scar is the only part of the operation visible to the patient. This is particularly important following facial surgery but in modern society there are few areas of the body that are now permanently covered. A young woman is permanently embarrassed by an ill-planned and distorting breast scar.
- **Vascular supply and wound healing.** Linear incisions infrequently fail to heal because of injury to the vascular supply, but angled incisions may do so. However, when an incision is made parallel to a previous one, the intervening tissue is rendered ischaemic and healing will be prejudiced.
- **Bleeding.** There are few incisions that can be made without causing some bleeding. If this is not carefully controlled, there is a high risk that blood will collect within the wound, separating the tissues; this will prevent healing and, at worst, become infected and complicate recovery.
- **Infection.** An initially clean area should not become infected as a result of operation. However, on many occasions the operation is performed to deal with infection, or it may be encountered unexpectedly. As exposure is increased there is a risk of contaminating previously sterile tissues.

Closure

- **Apposition.** To obtain perfect healing, the various tissues on each side of the incision should be brought together, and prevented from separating until the cells have bridged between them. If differing tissues are apposed, or if other structures are interposed, then healing cannot take place.
- **Tension.** When tissues are excised, there is a possibility that the margins of excision will be brought together under tension unless special measures are carried out. At the simplest this may be a 'relieving' incision or a more complicated flap may be created to fill the defect. There are circumstances in which tension is inevitable and must be accepted and allowed for.
- **Layers.** As a general rule each layer of tissue is repaired separately in order to restore the tissue planes. This may be very important if structures that move such as tendons could adhere to firm tissues and

become fixed if they are not resheathed in flexible areolar tissue.

• **Materials.** The opposing edges are most frequently united using sutures. The materials are chosen to provide the maximum security and minimum tissue reaction. In the past, natural substances were usually employed but these have now largely been replaced by synthetics that behave in a reliable fashion, whether they are intended to be reabsorbed or to remain relatively unchanged. Again, as a result of much work by our predecessors, the choice has become increasingly standardized.

Laparotomy incisions

Opening the abdomen has some special aspects. The choice of incision depends on the purpose of the intended operation. When operation is performed for carrying out a specific procedure, the incision is placed so that it gives the maximum exposure (Fig. 23.1). Exploration is often carried out through midline vertical incisions in adults, and a time-honoured approach is paramedian through the rectus sheath but pulling aside the medial part of the intact rectus muscle which will act as a shutter subsequently (Fig. 23.2). In infants, who have different proportions, transverse incisions may be more appropriate.

Closure of the abdomen inevitably carries the difficulty that intra-abdominal pressure cannot be prevented and therefore tension is inevitable. Indeed, if there is distension of the abdominal contents it will increase tension.

A layered closure may be used for a traditional paramedian incision. However, this general principle that usually applies elsewhere is not usually adhered to in the abdomen. This is as a result of the work of Jenkins (1976), a surgeon at Guildford in Surrey. He showed that using a non-absorbable, continuous mass suture at

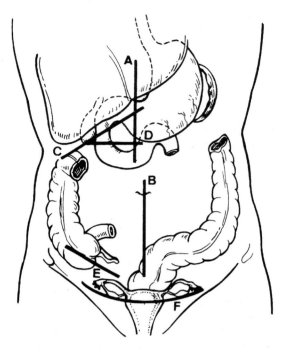

Fig 23.1 Favoured laparotomy incisions: **A**, paramedian; **B**, midline; **C**, Kocher; **D**, transverse; **E**, Lanz; **F**, Pfannenstiel.

least four times the length of the incision, wound dehiscence is virtually eliminated. The needle 'bites' are about 1 cm from the edge and the suture tension is just sufficient to appose the edges.

Chest incisions

There are three principal routes into the chest. The lateral thoracotomy follows the line of the upper edge of a

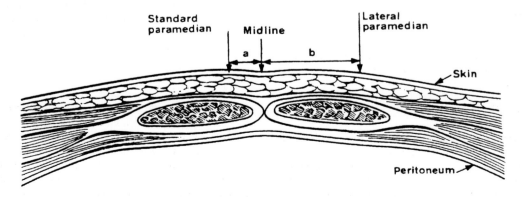

Fig 23.2 Lateral and standard paramedian incisions *a* = 2 cm; *b* = two-thirds from midline to lateral rectus sheath.

rib. In some cases a combined thoracoabdominal incision is used. This usually continues the line of an incision along one of the lower ribs and is carried through the costal margin into the abdomen. Access to the pericardium, heart and great vessels is achieved through a median sternotomy.

PRECAUTIONS AGAINST LOSS OF INSTRUMENTS OR SWABS

The following precautionary measures are essential:

Precautionary measures

- **Correctly organize instrument trays, limiting the number of individually packed instruments as far as possible.**
- **Arrange swabs and packs in 'fives' bound together with red cotton or, if small, carefully packaged (e.g. on a safety pin).**
- **Check the number of instruments on trays against printed lists incorporated in each pack.**
- **Record all sutures, swabs, packs, needles and extras clearly and legibly on a board in the theatre.**
- **Use of special swab racks, including the modern disposable wallets, which facilitate counting at the end of a long complex operation during which many swabs are used.**
- **Mark radio-opaque, non-implantable, non-metallic equipment such as drains and the laparomat.**
- **The theatre record book must be signed by the scrubbed and assistant nurses.**
- **Record and sign that the count was correct at the end of the operation note in the patient's records.**

The way to reduce errors is to establish a simple, well-disciplined routine of accountability, including a permanent and accurately maintained record.

SKIN CLOSURE

Skin closure should be cosmetically acceptable, with avoidance of inversion of the edges, and should avoid infection, hypertrophic scars or keloid formation. Several techniques are available: continuous or interrupted, simple or mattress and subcuticular. All are acceptable, but the last gives the best results.

Tape closure and clip sutures are associated with a low infection rate and also give good cosmetic results. The use of a polyurethane adhesive sheet dressing (Bioclusive, Opsite) over a sutured wound acts as a large tape closure, allowing easy inspection.

Cyanoacrylate skin adhesives are expensive and demand near-perfect haemostasis. There is no definite evidence that reducing dead space with subcuticular sutures or drains is effective, nor that it prevents wound infection.

Undue tension must be avoided to allow postoperative swelling.

Sutures require removal at, as a working rule, 3–5 days (head and neck), 7 days (inguinal and upper limb), 10 days (other abdominal incisions, lower limb) and up to 14 days for dorsal incisions. Knots placed well to the side of the incision facilitate removal. Special instruments allow painless removal of clips (rapidly if necessary after thyroidectomy).

Langer's lines

These are low-tension lines in the skin and correspond to natural skin creases. If an incision crosses them at right angles then there is a risk that resultant scars become hypertrophic and cosmetically unacceptable. Whenever possible, therefore, Langer's lines should be followed for incisions. When these lines have to be crossed for surgical access, particularly in operations on small joints for example, then skin crease lines should be crossed obliquely or incisions employing Z-plasties or an S-shape should be planned.

Hypertrophic skin scars

These show a proliferation of scar tissue, but this stays within the boundaries of the wound and not beyond it as keloids do. They tend to occur in scars around joints and in areas of skin tension. With the passage of time they become avascular and may regress to form a white, stretched, widened scar.

Contractures

These should not be confused with the normal process of wound contraction. Contractures follow delayed wound healing and occur after infection, and inadequate treatment of burns in particular. Deep burns which are not excised are prone to contracture. Established contractures can be released by plasty incisions, excised and covered with split-thickness grafts or with transposition flaps.

Keloids

These are formed by abnormal collagen metabolism and result in a proliferation of scar tissue beyond the boundaries of the original wound. They occur in dorsal areas of the body and over the face and deltopectoral region. Keloids occur in dark-skinned people and may be encouraged to form as a cultural body decoration.

Excision of keloids is almost always followed by a more exuberant recurrence. X-rays have been used but topical steroid creams or steroid injections are more definitely effective. Pressure on an excised keloid can prevent recurrence, a useful example being the use of a clip or peg on an earlobe that has developed a keloid after piercing for earrings.

SURGICAL DRESSINGS

The last 30 years have seen an increased depth of understanding of wound-healing processes and many dressings are being manufactured to provide the requirements of the ideal wound environment. There is no clear-cut evidence, however, that wounds should be left open with a dry surface and a fibrinous coagulum, which seals the wound, or whether they should be covered (and hidden from view). Exuding wounds are at risk of secondary infection and may not be protected by a dressing. If covered by an absorptive dressing, pathogenic organisms can track through a soiled wet dressing from its surface (strike-through). The requirements of an ideal surgical dressing are listed in Box 23.1. Some of their requirements are theoretical, but many are based on sound experimental evidence. The armamentarium of modern surgical dressings is mainly directed at management of chronic open wounds such as venous leg ulcers.

Polyurethane incise drapes have become popularized as a primary wound dressing for sutured wounds and skin donor sites. They maintain moisture which enhances epithelial closure, and allow easy inspection and aspiration of excessive excudate. On donor sites they are claimed to relieve pain. They are gas and water-vapour permeable but excessive maceration risks secondary infection, although the dressings are impermeable to organisms. More traditional wound dressings include Melolin or non-adherent sheet dressings which require a secondary pad dressing if there is excessive exudate.

For open wounds such as a healing pilonidal sinus cavity or a superficially dehisced, infected abdominal wound we are spoilt for choice. The moulded polymeric Silastic form dressing is ideal, allowing pain-free wound care, by the patient if necessary. Other bead and

> **Box 23.1 The ideal surgical dressing (which does not exist)**
>
> - Absorbent and able to remove excess exudate
> - Maintain moist environment and aid own tissues to debride necrotic material and promote healing
> - Prevent trauma to underlying healing granulation tissue or to prevent shed of foreign particles into the wound
> - Be leakproof and prevent strike-through and secondary infection
> - Maintain temperature and gaseous change
> - Allow simple dressing changes, easy, less frequent application and removal, and be pain free
> - Be odourless, cosmetically acceptable and comfortable
> - Not be expensive

powder dressings may be equally useful; they absorb exudate and maintain the moist environment (examples are Debrisan, Iodosorb and Intrasite). Sheet polymeric dressings are reserved for more superficial open wounds. They may be fully occlusive (Comfeel Ulcer Dressing or Granuflex) or semiocclusive (Geliperm) or with a biological source (the alginates Kaltostat or Sorbsan). The list of dressings increases, and satisfactory trials are required to show their merit and comparative relative worth. Biologically active dressings and living skin equivalents are examples of these.

PRINCIPLES OF WOUND MANAGEMENT

An operation is a responsibility to be undertaken with informed consent of the patient and should be performed in optimal circumstances. This should be tailored with management of the intercurrent illness, nutrition, the need for resuscitation and prophylaxis against infection and phlebothrombosis. Surgery is based on ritual and it is difficult to measure the quality of operative surgery, although we achieve much through audit, and morbidity and mortality meetings.

Lord Moynihan taught that an operation should start with a clean sweep of the knife. Techniques of aseptic procedures and swab and instrument counts are easy to teach. Gentle handling of tissues is more difficult to learn – some surgeons in training find it comes naturally, whereas others take time to be able to oppose cut tissues perfectly without undue suture tension. It is logical to secure haemostasis in surgical wounds; it is poor technique that leads to a wound needing resuture or evacuation of a haematoma. Excessive use of diathermy or the failure to avoid dead space are signs of poor surgery, but evidence to show impaired healing or increased infection risk is hard to prove. The use of drains to evacuate dead space, to 'protect' against the consequences of an anastomotic leak or to remove fluid collections or body fluids effectively is a classical example of an ingrained surgical technique which again still needs clear scientific evidence that it works.

Summary

1. Decide on several adjuncts to surgical practice which may influence wound healing or infection, such as shaving and incise drapes.
2. Be sure to use the most appropriate incision for the operation you are about to undertake.
3. Know your anatomy for making and closing the incision and choose the most appropriate suture material.
4. Ensure you have optimal retraction, lighting and infallible rules to avoid loss of swabs or instruments.
5. Choose the dressing which is most appropriate in postoperative management of your wound.

References

Jenkins T P N 1976 The burst abdominal wound: a mechanical approach. British Journal of Surgery 63: 873–876

Further reading

Anonymous 1986 Dressings for ulcers. Drug and Therapeutics Bulletin 24: 9–12

Cox P J, Ausobsky J R, Ellis H, Pollock A V 1986 Towards no incisional hernias: lateral paramedian versus midline incisions. Journal of the Royal Society of Medicine 79: 711–712

Harland R N L, Irving M H 1988 Surgical drains. Surgery 1: 1360–1362

Leaper D J 1985 Laparotomy closure. British Journal of Hospital Medicine 33: 317–322

Leaper D J 1985 Local effects of trauma and wound healing. In: Burnand K G, Young A E (eds) Ian Aird's companion to surgical studies. Churchill Livingstone, Edinburgh, ch 2, p 27–35

Leaper D J 1992 Surgical factors influencing infection. In: Taylor E W (ed) Infection in surgical practice. Oxford University Press, Oxford, ch 3, p 18–27

Leaper D J, Foster M E 1990 Wound healing and abdominal wound closure. In: Taylor I (ed) Progress in surgery. Churchill Livingstone, Edinburgh, vol 3, ch 2, p 19–31

Lucarotti M E, Billings P J, Leaper D J 1991 Laparotomy, wound closure and repair of incisional hernia. Surgery. 10: 1–6

Wadstrom J, Gerdin B 1990 Closure of the abdominal wall: how and why. Acta Chirurgica Scandinavica 156: 75–82

24

Minimal access surgery

A. Darzi

Objectives

- **Understand the nomenclature and boundaries of minimal access surgery.**
- **Recognize that minimal access surgery aims to accomplish surgical therapeutic goals with minimal somatic and psychological trauma.**
- **Recognize the limitations of minimal access surgery in its current state considering future improvement in training and technology.**

Diseases that harm call for treatments that harm less.

William Osler

Minimal access surgery is a marriage of modern technology and surgical innovation which aims to accomplish surgical therapeutic goals with minimal somatic and psychological trauma. Technology is often blamed by those who claim to detect a deterioration in the doctor–patient relationship and is frequently cited as a major cause of the upward spiral of health-care costs. Although these are valid concerns, the properly controlled development of minimal access surgery with well-considered pre- and postoperative management offers benefits, including cost benefits, without sacrificing the quality of care of the patient as a whole individual. Minimal access techniques are less invasive, less disabling and less disfiguring. With increasing experience they offer cost-effectiveness to both health services and employers by shortening operating times, shortening hospital stays and allowing faster recuperation. State-of-the-art video recording can help communication, bring the patient and family closer to the process, improve clinical decision-making and enhance rapport.

NOMENCLATURE

The urologists Wickham & Fitzpatrick (1990), who were instrumental in highlighting the need for techniques which reduced therapeutic and surgical trauma, advocated the term 'minimally invasive therapy', but there remains much debate about the most accurate title for this new discipline (Box 24.1). Cuschieri (1992), argues that this terminology is inappropriate because it inaccurately implies increased safety, a connotation which is fallacious because there is no correlation between invasiveness and risk. The most important argument against the use of this terminology is that it fails to emphasize the essential attribute of the approach which is the reduction of surgical trauma. The alternative terminology, minimal access surgery (MAS), is more accurate and descriptive (Cuschieri 1992).

Technology has effectively miniaturized our eyes and extended our hands to perform microscopic and macroscopic operations in places which formerly could be reached only with large incisions. It has also provided new ways to look at tissues, using light, sound waves and magnetic fields which can detect disease and guide therapy (Darzi et al 1993). These same technologies, more highly focused and used at much higher power, can also be used to give highly controlled resection and tissue destruction. It is vital that surgeons understand the principles of these devices so that they

---

Box 24.1 Minimal access surgery: nomenclature

- Endoscopic surgery
- Keyhole surgery
- Laparoscopic surgery
- Minimally invasive surgery
- Minimal access surgery

can help to shape the future development of minimal access surgery and not become the servants of the machines they use.

BOUNDARIES OF
MINIMAL ACCESS SURGERY

Techniques

- Laparoscopy
- Thoracoscopy
- Endoluminal endoscopy
- Perivisceral endoscopy
- Arthroscopy and intra-articular joint surgery
- Combined approach.

Minimal access surgery has crossed all traditional boundaries of specialities and disciplines. Shared, borrowed and overlapping technologies and information are encouraging a multidisciplinary approach which serves the whole patient rather than a specific organ system. Broadly speaking, minimal access techniques can be categorized as follows:

Laparoscopy. A rigid endoscope is introduced through a metal sleeve into the peritoneal cavity which has been inflated with a carbon dioxide pneumoperitoneum. There is little doubt that laparoscopic cholecystectomy has revolutionized the surgical management of cholelithiasis and has become the mainstay of management of uncomplicated gallstone disease. With improved instruments and more experience, it is likely that other advanced procedures, currently regarded as controversial, will also become fully accepted.

Thoracoscopy. A rigid endoscope is introduced through an incision in the chest to gain access to the thoracic contents. Many feel that the benefits of thoracoscopy will prove to be even greater than those of laparoscopy.

Endoluminal endoscopy. Flexible or rigid endoscopes are introduced into hollow organs or systems, such as the urinary tract, upper or lower gastrointestinal tract, respiratory and vascular systems.

Perivisceral endoscopy. Body planes can be accessed even in the absence of a natural cavity. Examples are mediastinoscopy, retroperitoneoscopy and retroperitoneal approaches to the kidney, aorta and lumbar sympathetic chain. Other more recent examples include subfascial ligation of incompetent perforators in varicose vein surgery.

Arthroscopy and intra-articular joint surgery. Orthopaedic surgeons have long used arthroscopic access to the knee and have now moved their attention to other joints, including the shoulder, wrist, elbow and hip.

Combined approach. The diseased organ is visualized and treated using an assortment of endoluminal and extraluminal endoscopes and other imaging devices.

SURGICAL TRAUMA IN OPEN AND
LAPAROSCOPIC SURGERY

Morbidity of open surgical wounds

- **Pain leads to reduced mobility, leading to increased pulmonary collapse, chest infection and deep venous thrombosis**
- **Infection**
- **Dehiscence**
- **Bleeding**
- **Herniation**
- **Nerve entrapment**

Most of the trauma of an open procedure is inflicted because the surgeon must have a wound large enough to give adequate exposure for safe dissection at the target site. The wound is often the cause of morbidity, including infection, dehiscence, bleeding, herniation and nerve entrapment. The pain of the wound prolongs recovery time and, by reducing mobility, contributes to an increased incidence of pulmonary collapse, chest infection and deep venous thrombosis.

Mechanical and human retractors cause additional trauma. Body wall retractors tend to inflict localized damage which may be as painful as the wound itself. By contrast, during laparoscopy the body wall is retracted by the low pressure pneumoperitoneum, giving a diffuse force applied gently and evenly over the whole body wall, causing minimal trauma.

Exposure of any body cavity to the atmosphere also causes morbidity through cooling and fluid loss by the evaporation of body fluid. There is also evidence from the literature to suggest that the incidence of postsurgical adhesions have been reduced by the use of the laparoscope because there is less damage to delicate serosal coverings. In handling intestinal loops the surgeon and assistant disturb the peristaltic activity of the gut and provoke adynamic ileus.

In minimal access surgery the trauma of access and exposure are reduced, while visualization is magnified and improved.

DISADVANTAGES OF MINIMAL ACCESS SURGERY

Limitations of minimal access surgery

- **Difficulties in hand–eye coordination due to:**
  - **2 dimensional imaging**
  - **Lack of navigational cues to judge depth**
- **Lack of tactile feedback**
- **Difficulties in dissection and haemostasis in more advanced procedures**
- **The need to make incision to deliver specimens in excisional surgery**
- **Possible local biological factors leading to increased incidence of wound recurrence**

To perform minimal access surgery with safety, the surgeon must operate remote from the surgical field using an imaging system which provides a 2 dimensional representation of the operative site. The endoscope offers a whole new anatomical landscape which the surgeon must learn to navigate without the usual cues which make it easy to judge depth. The instruments are longer and sometimes more complex to use than those common in open surgery. The result of all this is that the beginner in minimal access surgery is faced with significant problems of hand–eye coordination. Stereoscopic imaging for laparoscopy is still in its infancy. Future improvements in these systems will greatly enhance manipulative ability in critical procedures such as knot tying and dissection of closely underlying tissues. There are, however, some drawbacks, such as reduced display brightness and interference with normal vision due to the need to wear glasses. It is probable that brighter projection displays will be developed, at increased cost. However, the need to wear glasses will not be easily overcome. Looking further to the future, it is evident that the continuing reduction in costs of elaborate image-processing techniques will make a wide range of transformed presentations available. It will ultimately be possible for a surgeon to call up any view of the operative region that is accessible to a camera and present it stereoscopically in any size or orientation, superimposed on past images taken in other modalities. It is for the medical community to decide which of these many imaginative possibilities will contribute most to effective surgical procedures.

Another problem occurs when there is intraoperative arterial bleeding. Haemostasis may be very difficult to achieve endoscopically because blood obscures the field of vision and there is a significant reduction of the image quality due to light absorption.

Some of the procedures performed by this new approach are more technically demanding and are slower to perform. Indeed, on occasions a minimally invasive operation is so technically demanding that both patient and surgeon are better served by conversion to an open procedure. Unfortunately, there seems to be a sense of embarrassment or humiliation associated with conversion, which is quite unjustified. It is vital for surgeons and patients to appreciate that the decision to go for an open operation is not a complication, but rather usually implies sound surgical judgement.

Another disadvantage of laparoscopic surgery is the loss of tactile feedback. Laparoscopic ultrasonography might substitute the need to 'feel' in intraoperative decision-making. Although ultrasonography has progressed significantly in the past several years, laparoscopic ultrasound remains in its infancy. The rapid progress in advanced laparoscopic techniques, including biliary tract exploration and surgery for malignancies, has provided a strong impetus for the development of laparoscopic ultrasound. Although incompletely developed, laparoscopic ultrasound already offers advantages that far outweigh its disadvantages

Advantages of laparoscopic ultrasound

- **Substitutes for the sense of touch**
- **Allows visualization through tubular fluid-filled and solid organs as well as vascular structures**
- **Permits differentiation of solid and cystic masses**
- **Allows evaluation of the wall layers of hollow viscera**
- **Allows evaluation of the dimensions, infiltration and dissemination of tumours for better staging**
- **Helps formulate an optimal surgical plan**
- **Avoids unnecessary tissue dissection**
- **Allows guided biopsies**
- **Easily performed, safe, and economic**
- **Does not use ionizing radiation or contrast media**
- **Can be employed at any time during surgery**
- **Can be used during pregnancy**
- **Has no contraindications**

In more advanced techniques the large piece of resected tissue, such as the lung or colon, has to be extracted from the body cavity (Monson et al 1992). Occasionally, the extirpated tissue may be removed through a nearby natural orifice, such as the rectum or the mouth. At other times a novel route may be employed. For instance, a benign colonic specimen may be extracted through an incision in the vault of the vagina. Although tissue 'morcellators, mincers and liquidizers' could be used in some circumstances, this has the disadvantage of reducing the amount of information available to the pathologist. Recent reports of tumour implantation in the sites of portholes has raised important questions about the future of the laparoscopic treatment of malignancy.

There is growing need for improvement in dissection techniques in laparoscopic surgery, and specifically of improving the safe use of electrocautery and lasers. Ultrasonic dissection and tissue removal has been utilized by a growing number of specialities for several years. The adaptation of the technology to laparoscopic surgery grew out of the search for alternative, possibly safer, methods of dissection. The current units combine the functions of three or four separate instruments, reducing the need for instrument exchanges during a procedure. This flexibility, combined with the ability to provide a clean, smoke-free field, improves safety while shortening operating times.

Although dramatic cost savings are possible with laparoscopic cholecystectomy the position is less clear-cut with other procedures. There is another factor which may complicate the computation of cost versus benefit. A significant rise in the rate of cholecystectomy followed the introduction of the laparoscopic approach as the threshold for referring patients for surgery lowered. The increase in the number of procedures performed has led to an overall increase in the cost of treating symptomatic gallstones.

TRAINING FOR MINIMAL ACCESS SURGERY

It is probably true to say that no previous surgical innovation has aroused so much public questioning of how surgeons are trained. While the pioneers of a new technique are inevitably self-trained, there comes a time when patients rightly demand that all those who offer a new technique have had proper training to perform it safely and effectively. This is particularly so in laparoscopic surgery, which employs skills that are not commonly used in everyday life.

The importance of training in minimal access surgery has been recognized with the establishment of several training centres dedicated to teaching the fundamentals of safe minimal access surgery. These centres, including the Minimal Access Therapy Training Unit (MATTU) at the Royal College of Surgeons of England, are working to develop training methods using various forms of simulation which will allow surgeons to complete a significant part of their skills training before they begin to operate on patients. The sophistication of these simulation techniques seems likely to increase with the development of virtual-reality machines, which will generate an artificial environment in which the surgeon can practise with complete safety.

THE FUTURE

Although there is no doubt that minimal access surgery has changed the practice of surgeons, it has not changed the nature of disease. The basic principles of good surgery still apply, including appropriate case selection, excellent exposure, adequate retraction and a high level of technical expertise. If a procedure makes no sense with conventional access, it will make no sense with a minimal access approach.

Improvements in instrumentation and the development of structured training programmes are the key to the future of minimal access surgery. It is certain that there is much that is new in minimal access surgery. Time will tell how much of what is new is truly better.

The cleaner and gentler the act of operation, the less the patient suffers, the smoother and quicker his convalescence, the more exquisite his healed wound.

Lord Moynihan of Leeds

Summary

Minimal access techniques:
1. Less disabling and less disfiguring.
2. Cross all traditional surgical boundaries.
3. Encourage multidisciplinary approach which serves the whole patient rather than a specific organ.
4. Have some limitations.
5. Training in the techniques cannot be overemphasized.

 References

Cuschieri A 1992 A rose by any other name: minimal access or minimally invasive surgery. Surgical Endoscopy 6: 214

Darzi A, Goldin R, Guillou P J, Monson J R T 1993
Extracorporeal shock wave thermotherapy: new
antitumour option. Surgical Oncology 2: 197–204
Monson J R T, Darzi A, Carey P D, Guillou P J 1992
Prospective evaluation of laparoscopic assisted colectomy
in an unselected group of patients. Lancet 340: 831–833

Nduka C, Super P, Monson J R T, Darzi A 1994b Cause and
prevention of electrosurgical injury in laparoscopic
surgery. Journal of the American College of Surgeons 179:
161–179
Wickham J, Fitzpatrick J M 1990 Minimally invasive surgery
[editorial]. British Journal of Surgery 77: 721

 Further reading

Nduka C, Monson J R T, Darzi A 1994a Abdominal wall
metastases following laparoscopic surgery. British Journal
of Surgery 81: 648–652

25

Principles of skin cover

D. M. Davies, L. E. Ion

Objectives

- **Understand the principles of wound assessment.**
- **Understand the reasons for failure of skin cover.**
- **Develop a plan for wound management.**
- **Develop a ladder of skin cover reconstruction.**

INTRODUCTION

Skin cover and wound healing should be understood as two aspects of the same goal: the restoration of the functional envelope of the human body. You should understand the basic science and physiology of wound healing. The cellular sequences of repair and their controlling factors are not discussed in this chapter.

When faced with closure of a wound, regardless of its aetiology, make sure that you have covered in your mind a checklist of the most relevant aspects:

- Are there patient factors affecting the wound healing?
- Are there local factors likely to influence healing?
- Do I have experience of the surgical techniques that I plan to use?

Never forget that basic surgical principles are basic because they are usually simple but fundamental to the care of each and every patient that you treat.

Take a history from the patient, or eyewitnesses, regarding the mechanism of injury. This will give you precious information about the quality of the tissues surrounding and underlying the wound. Do not forget to inquire about the patient's general state; your management plans will need to make adjustments for patients with diabetes, cachexia, cytotoxic medication, or anticoagulants.

Examine the patient carefully. In particular, in the face area detect whether there is a fracture of the underlying facial bones, or damage to structures such as the eye, facial nerve and also the parotid duct. Injuries with functional consequences can often only be diagnosed preoperatively and not at the time of surgical exploration. Remember that what is not recorded prior to surgery may be ascribed to the surgical act.

Assess the wound itself and ask yourself if its appearance is consistent with the history (e.g. degloving injury or a heavy crush).

Lastly, carry out investigations, including wound swabs where indicated, X-rays for bony fractures, proceeding occasionally to ultrasound, CT, or MRI.

PRINCIPLES OF WOUND MANAGEMENT

1. *Assess the patient.* If there are correctable medical factors like poor nutrition, diabetes, anaemia etc., try to improve these before attempting wound cover.

2. *Assess the area.* An ulcer on an ischaemic leg may heal with dressings if the ischaemia is corrected. A pressure sore on an insensate foot may be better treated by a change of shoe. A small sinus over osteomyelitis will need debridement of bone.

3. *Assess the wound.* Evaluate any wound considered for closure for the level of necrotic tissue, debris and bacterial contamination. Necrotic tissue requires sharp debridement. Irrigation will aid in the removal of foreign bodies, and pulsating jet lavage is an improved modification. Bacterial contamination can be measured by taking a wound biopsy. When quantitative bacteriology shows in excess of 100 000 organisms per gram of tissue in general the take of skin grafts and primary wound healing is poor. Manage such contamination by excision/debridement, with or without topical antiseptic agents. Systemic antibiotics have little local effect when dead tissue persists or if there is excessive thick granulation.

Surgical debridement is the poorest performed operation by junior hospital doctors, but it is the key to reaching bacterial balance. If there is any doubt about the viability of tissue then a second-look policy should be undertaken 24–48 hours later. This can be repeated several times until there is absolutely no doubt that what is left in the wound is alive and viable and not seriously contaminated by bacteria. Only when this is achieved can effective wound closure be obtained.

 ## Closure of acute wounds

- **Primary/delayed primary closure**
- **Secondary closure**
- **Tertiary closure**

Closure of acute wounds may be divided into *primary*, *delayed primary*, *secondary* and *tertiary*. This bears a relationship to the classically described healing by *primary* and *secondary intention*. You could view this as a case of synchronous healing of the wound at all depth levels as opposed to asynchronous healing of the deeper layers and epithelium.

In *primary closure* the wound is usually closed by direct approximation of the wound edges without tension. Larger defects may be closed by skin grafts or flaps. In general, traumatic injuries and surgical wounds should be closed primarily, if appropriate. In *delayed primary closure*, an interval of several days between injury and closure is used to ensure wound decontamination. In both cases, however, there is a synchronicity of the wound healing processes through the wound depth.

In *secondary closure* the wound is left open and the processes of wound contraction and epithelialization occur from the edges. There is obviously a time difference between the healing of the deeper tissues and epithelial recovery, which can lead to the formation of granulation tissue and delay in healing. This sometimes requires active tertiary intervention.

Tertiary closure can be defined as the active intervention to provide skin cover to a wound that either has a delay in healing or is stagnant. As in all other cases, bacterial balance is mandatory before attempting closure of the wound, but perhaps more difficult to achieve with chronic wounds.

In general, a dressing should maintain a moist wound environment to facilitate re-epithelialization. Topical agents, whether antibacterial or debriding, need to be justified by the characteristics of the specific wound. Attempts are made continuously to change the characteristics of the dressings and improve their ability to protect the wounds while providing more pain relief

and comfort for the patient. Remember though that they are only the finishing touch to your wound management, not a substitute for it. The cheapest, quickest and still the best debrider of a wound is the scalpel.

The reconstructive surgeon's approach to providing skin cover is algorithmically structured as a reconstructive ladder. Going up the ladder is justified either by the impossibility of using a simpler approach or by functional or cosmetic requirements.

 ## Reconstructive ladder

- **Conservative management**
- **Direct closure**
- **Skin grafts**
- **Tissue expansion**
- **Flaps**

CONSERVATIVE MANAGEMENT

Conservative management is commonly bypassed for functional and cosmetic requirements. It can however, be an excellent option for some fingertip injuries in children, for some facial abrasions and for acute pressure sores. It is inevitably used in some ulcers when the medical state of the patient precludes surgery, or when uncorrectable local factors would condemn any method of reconstruction. In such cases, the choice of the dressing as well as the nursing care play an important role in achieving improvement or cure.

DIRECT CLOSURE

Wound edges should be accurately opposed to permit healing. There should be no skin edge step off and sutures should not be so tightly approximated that ensuing oedema causes further ischaemia to the edges of the wound. The major strength in the skin is in the dermis; the collagen fibres in the dermis will give the wound its tensile strength. Good approximation of the dermis is therefore vital. Sutures placed in fat generally give little strength, cause necrosis and serve as a foreign body and a nidus for infection. The fascia has sufficient collagen to permit approximation with sutures, but underlying muscle will not support sutures. Thus the best closure of a wound extending through muscle includes good approximation of the fascia and dermis. A buried dermal closure with an inverted suture will place the knot in the depth of the wound and minimize the likelihood of its erosion to the surface and the formation of a stitch abscess. Except in the face, where accurate epidermal skin edge approximation is required, interrupted cutaneous sutures are very rarely indicated.

The epidermis in the face can be approximated with a non-adsorbable suture such as nylon which will best approximate the wound edges accurately. These sutures should be removed prior to invasion by epithelium into the suture holes. The density of the dermal appendages in the area will determine the timing of the suture removal.

In areas such as the face, which has a high density of dermal appendages, suture track marks may occur when the stitches are left in place for as little as 4 days. Areas such as the palmar and plantar surfaces have such a low density of dermal appendages that the sutures may be left in place for as long as 3 weeks.

SKIN GRAFTS

A skin graft is the transfer of a segment of skin which has been totally separated from its blood supply. All skin grafts initially adhere to the recipient bed by fibrin, which must be vascular enough to support the metabolism of the graft. The thinner the graft the less nutrition it requires and the more likely it is to take. Within 48 hours capillaries will grow from the underlying bed into the graft, a process known as *inosculation*, and the graft becomes vascularized.

Skin grafts are of two types. The workhorses of reconstruction are split thickness skin grafts, but on the face in particular, where a more cosmetic reconstruction is required, full thickness skin grafts are often employed. Remember that a donor site for a partial thickness skin graft will always leave a cosmetic abnormality and thus, particularly in a young patient, skin should be taken from the buttock whenever practical rather than the thigh.

Since a graft must derive its new vascularity from the recipient bed, some general observations may be made.

1. Skin grafts should do well on well vascularized non-infected wounds, clean granulation tissue or wounds created following the excision of tissue. Irregular or less well vascularized surfaces such as fat are less predictable.

2. Grafts do not require pressure, but they do require immobilization and thus patient cooperation is necessary.

3. The best results are accomplished when the donor tissue matches the recipient bed in texture and colour.

4. Avascular wounds, such as bone without periosteal cover, tendon without peritenon, denuded cartilage and irradiated wounds, are incapable of nourishing a graft.

5. Heavy contamination by microorganisms is an important cause of graft loss. Usually this is because the fibrin is degraded by the fibrinolytic cascade initiated by the presence of large amount of bacteria; quantities exceeding 100 000 organisms per gram of tissue frequently results in the non-take of grafts.

6. Grafts cannot survive on a blood clot. Pressure may help prevent seroma/haematoma formation and will also help immobilize the graft. Immobilizing some areas of the body (e.g. the back) can be notoriously difficult, and in such areas graft failure is common.

If the patient is cooperative, if the wound is appropriate for a graft, if the wound has been properly prepared, if the graft is applied accurately and if the postoperative management is conducted well, then a skin graft will always take. Every surgeon should be capable of harvesting a partial thickness skin graft, either by a dermatome or using a protected skin graft blade (e.g. a Humby knife or later modifications by Watson and Cobett). Acquire this skill by practising on a cadaver. Also be aware of the fact that in many instances meshing the skin graft will allow both expansion of the graft and also an increased chance of take by allowing seroma to escape between the perforations.

Be aware of the long-term management of a skin graft. Provide external support to a graft on the lower limb by using Tubigrip and apply moisturizing creams to dry pruritic donor sites and grafts. Later, prevent or treat hypertrophic scarring by the use of Jobst pressure garments.

Full thickness skin grafts are used commonly on the head and neck area, particularly the eyelids and nose. The principles that apply for the successful take of a partial thickness skin graft apply even more to a full thickness skin graft, as the initial metabolic requirements of a full thickness skin graft are relatively greater. Postoperatively, a full thickness skin graft usually provides a better cosmetic match and is less likely to contract.

FLAPS

If a wound bed is avascular, such that it is unlikely to be able to support a skin graft, then skin that retains its blood supply has to be used to cover a wound. This is the definition of a skin flap.

Random pattern flaps

One of the several functions of skin is temperature regulation and thus skin has a blood supply many times in excess of its metabolic requirements. Skin can be moved as a flap and survives being nourished through its base or pedicle. In a random pattern flap there is no specific blood vessel in the pedicle, the flap being nourished by the dermal plexus. Experience shows that, provided the length of the flap is not greater than 1.5–2 times the width of its base, then it should survive. Random flaps are not new – Sushruta in the Samhita in India used such flaps for nasal reconstruction in about 600 BC. Random flaps can be based on the geometry of 2:1 and can be used to fill a local defect, either by rotation or transposition.

This geometric design obviously presented limitations in covering larger skin defects.

Axial flap

Towards the end of the 1960s, McGregor and his colleagues in Glasgow questioned why flaps in the groin area and forehead could be safely designed 4–5 times as long as the base and commonly survive. They found that the skin in the groin area is supplied by a specific blood vessel (the superficial circumflex iliac artery) and, provided this artery with its accompanying venae commitans is included in the base of the flap and not damaged, then a skin flap can be raised on a very narrow pedicle right out over the most lateral part of the iliac crest. The groin flap was introduced into reconstructive surgery in the early 1970s and was a major breakthrough.

It was soon recognized, however, that there were only a few other axial pattern flaps in the body, e.g. the deltopectoral flap (on the chest) based on the perforating vessels of the internal mammary artery, and the forehead flap based on the anterior branch of the superficial temporal artery.

Myocutaneous flaps

Following further investigations in the postmortem room, it became apparent that skin in large areas of the body is supplied by blood vessels which come through from the underlying muscles. The rediscovery of the latissimus dorsi myocutaneous flap by Olivari in Germany and the further discovery of other myocutaneous and muscle flaps (the important ones being the latissimus dorsi, pectoralis major, rectus abdominus, tensor fascia lata, gluteus maximus, and gastrocnemius) allowed a vast expansion in reconstruction.

The principle of a myocutaneous flap is that the skin overlying a muscle will survive provided the pedicle to the muscle, which is usually a dominant vessel at one end, is not divided. Thus a paddle of muscle with overlying skin can be rotated over an arc of 360° to cover a local skin defect.

Fascial flaps

Further investigations into the blood supply of skin, particularly in the limbs where the muscles tend to be long and narrow, show that perforating vessels come between the muscles and supply a vascular plexus just superficial to the deep fascia. Thus, if the fascia is included together with the perforating vessel in the skin flap, then long flaps, much greater than the original random patterned 2:1, can safely be raised. These are fasciocutaneous flaps, and are of particular importance in repairing skin defects on the lower limb, where they can be based either proximally or even distally.

Free flaps

Despite the wealth of flaps available, two problem areas remain for the closure of large wounds. These are the top of the head and the lower third of the leg. In the late 1970s, microvascular surgery (i.e. the repair of small blood vessels below 1–2 mm in diameter) became a practical proposition, although Carrel had been able to undertake successful anastomoses of small blood vessels experimentally in the early part of this century. This ability to join blood vessels, however, allows the pedicle of axial and myocutaneous flaps to be divided and the vessels reanastomosed to local blood vessels, adjacent to the wound on the head or lower leg. This is the basis of so-called 'free flaps' and is the top rung of our ladder of reconstruction.

TISSUE EXPANSION

Tissue expansion, introduced by Neuman and refined by Radovan and Austad, is a method of introducing skin and hypodermis to cover a wound. It relies on the tissue's ability to stretch and proliferate under continuous moderate tension, similar to the abdominal expansion during pregnancy. The procedure involves the subdermal insertion of a tissue expander – essentially a soft silicone bag – that is gradually inflated through an injection port placed subcutaneous or external. Once the tissue expansion is achieved – usually 6–8 weeks – the expander is removed and the excess tissue is designed as a flap for closure of the defect.

Summary

1. Assess the wound and the patient.
2. Correct (if possible) negative factors.
3. Debridement is the best wound preparation.

Summary (contd.)

4. Manage bacterial contamination.
5. Plan the reconstruction.
6. Discuss your plan with the patient.
7. The simplest solution is usually the best solution.
8. Convert a dirty open wound to a clean open wound.
9. Convert a clean open wound to a closed wound.

 Further reading

Ashton SJ, Beasley RW, Thorne C N M (eds) 1997 Grab and Smith's plastic surgery, 5th edn. Lipincott-Raven

McGregor I A, McGregor A D, 1995 Fundamental techniques in plastic surgery and their surgical applications. Churchill Livingstone, Edinburgh

26

Transplantation

P. McMaster, L. J. Buist

Objectives

- Appreciate the causes of organ rejection.
- Understand the principles of transplantation and immunosuppression.
- Be aware of the source of transplanted organs, and the associated ethical and legal considerations.

Box 26.1   Forms of tissue transfer

Transfer of tissue
- Blood
- Bone marrow

Transfer of solid organ
- Skin
- Cornea
- Kidney
- Heart
- Liver
- Pancreas

BASIC PRINCIPLES

Early Christian legends attest to the attempts by man to replace diseased or destroyed organs or tissues by the transfer from another individual. The father of modern surgery, John Hunter, carried out extensive experiments on the transposition of tissues and concluded what he thought were successful experiments on the transposition of teeth! However, it was not until the dawn of the 20th century that the practical technical realities of organ transfer were combined with sufficient understanding of the immunological mechanisms involved to allow transplantation to become a practical reality.

While it had long been recognized that successful blood transfusion was in large measure dependent on matching donor and recipient cells, it was only in the 1950s that Mitchison (1953) demonstrated that, while cell-mediated immunity was responsible for early destruction and rejection, it was the humoral mechanism with cytotoxic antibodies that was primarily involved in the host response to foreign tissue. It became increasingly recognized that all tissue and fluid transfer was governed by basic immunomechanisms (Box 26.1).

The need in the Second World War to find improved ways of treating badly burned pilots led Gibson & Medawar (1943) to carry out a series of classic experiments on skin transplantation. They were able to conclude that the transfer of skin from one part of the body to another in the same individual (an *autograft*), survived indefinitely, whereas the transfer of skin from another individual (an *allograft*) was in due course destroyed and that the recipient retained memory of the donor tissue and further transfers or allografts were destroyed in an accelerated mechanism. Thus the wider recognition of the universal acceptance of autografts became realized, whereas the failure of an allograft was recognized as part of an immune response. An alternative source of organs is, of course, the animal world, and the transfer from another species is known as a *xenograft*.

FIRST CLINICAL PROGRAMMES

The recognition that an autograft would be universally acceptable led to the first successful attempts at organ grafting in man. In the early 1950s, Murray et al (1955) at the Peter Bent Brigham Hospital in Boston, were able to demonstrate the successful transfer of a kidney graft from an identical twin with acceptance and successful function, and to develop a programme of renal transplantation between monozygotic twins. Living related organ transfer continues to be the most successful form of grafting without the need to alter the recipient's immune mechanism, as it fails to recognize the donor tissue as foreign.

Some of the recipients of kidney transplants from identical twins remained well more than 30 years after grafting. However, grafts between unrelated living individuals performed by this same group invariably failed, although not as quickly as experimental studies might have suggested.

RESPONSE

The other major human source of organs, other than from living relatives, is from individuals who have died as a result of road traffic accidents or cerebral injuries. Cadaveric organ grafting from non-related individuals is now the major source of organs. Within Europe, more than 90% of all organs transplanted are from brain-dead donors.

Thus, although technical considerations presented the initial formidable barrier to organ transfer, it was increasingly the understanding of the immune response causing organ destruction by rejection which led to clinical schedules permitting practical transplantation services to be established. The body's immune response to destroy the invading organ we now recognize as *rejection*.

REJECTION

Early experimental studies involving tissue transfer suggested genetic regulation of the rejection process. It was suggested in the 1930s that rejection was a response to specific foreign antigens (alloantigens) and that they were similar to blood groups of other species. The development of inbred lines of experimental animal models allowed the demonstration of antigens present on red blood cells and the concept of histocompatability. This suggestion of an immunological theory of tissue transplantation stimulated Medawar's (1944) work in rabbits and later in mice, and led to similar studies in man with the discovery of the human leucocyte antigen (HLA) system.

Further experimental studies defined the concept of rejection into three primary categories: *hyperacute rejection*, which can occur in a matter of hours due to preformed antibodies in a sensitized recipient; *acute rejection*, which takes place in a few days or weeks and is usually caused by cellular mechanisms; and *chronic rejection*, which occurs over months or years and remains largely undefined, but involves primarily humoral antibodies. A detailed review of experimental and modern transplantation biology is quite beyond the scope of this chapter, but increasing understanding of

this area will allow more refined changes in rejection management and increasingly successful organ grafting.

AVOIDING REJECTION

The degree of disparity between donor and recipient is an important key element in the severity of the immune rejection response. In xenografting (transfer between species) the presence of preformed antibodies leads to rapid endothelial damage, causing vascular thrombosis, gross interstitial swelling and necrosis of the graft, all within a matter, usually, of hours.

Similarly, when transfer occurs between human beings, the degree of compatibility between donor and recipient is important to the success, or otherwise, of the graft.

As indicated earlier, transfer between identical twins is associated with universal success, without the need to modulate the immune mechanism. However, transfer between non-identical relatives or using cadaveric organs produces the recognition of non-self by the recipient and the mounting of an immune response. It is the avoidance or modification of this immune response which has been the main target over the last 25 years and the avoidance of overwhelming rejection has been a prime goal.

Two approaches have been taken to the problem: tissue typing, and reduction of immune response.

Tissue typing

In the attempt to match the donor and recipient more closely, the concept of typing has become widely developed. Early work demonstrating that blood transfusion was dependent on matching between donor and recipient was extended into experimental and then clinical transplantation studies in the 1960s and 1970s.

The human chromosome 6 contains the genetically determined major histocompatability complex (MHC), i.e. the HLA-A, HLA-B, HLA-C (class 1) and HLA-DR (D-related; class 2) loci. A whole series of additional genetic regions have been linked to the HLA complex, although in clinical terms these are probably less significant.

Thus it has become increasingly possible, using serological studies, to genetically map an individual on the basis of the HLA region of this chromosome. Since one chromosome is inherited from each parent and each individual has two HLA haplotypes, there is a 25% chance that two siblings will share both haplotypes (i.e. identical) and, by standard and Mendelian inheritance, a 50% chance that they will share one haplotype. Thus in first-degree relatives when the donor and recipient are matched for HLA-A and B antigens there is an excellent likelihood of graft success, whereas because of the complexity of the MHC allele, the wide divergence of antigens and random cadaveric donors, even if matched for one or two antigens, there may still be very substantial disparity.

Thus, in order to avoid rejection, the concept of tissue typing trying to match more accurately the donor and the recipient has gained wide acceptance. Serological methods allow class 1 HLA antigens to be defined using typed serum obtained from nulliparous women. Using a microcytotoxicity assay, multiple antisera against HLA-A, B, C and DR antigens are provided on Terasaki trays and then frozen until needed. When needed, the trays are thawed and the donor lymphocyte cells are added to the wells containing complement and the antisera against specific HLA types. If the antibody causes the cells to lyse, acridine orange (a dye) enters the damaged cell and appears orange under fluorescence microscopy. Thus by using microcytotoxicity tests it is possible to identify quite rapidly the HLA class 1 antigens present in a donor.

Until recently, class 2 antigen typing required a mixed leukocyte reaction to determine individual constituents, but more recent techniques have avoided this laborious investigation. From the clinical standpoint the practical importance of identification of the degree of compatibility between donor and recipient is clearly defined in many organ-grafting systems. Cadaveric grafting can only achieve this level when beneficially matched donor and recipient pairs, in which all major class 1 and class 2 antigens are identical, are grafted. This so-called 'full house' HLA match can give 1 year cadaveric graft survival approaching 90%. However, this is only when combined with chemical non-specific immunosuppression.

When grafts are transferred between donor and recipient with a complete mismatch an additional 20–25% of grafts will be lost over the ensuing 5 years. Thus, in cadaveric grafting the degree of matching has an important role in determining the severity of the immune response and the ultimate success, or otherwise, of the graft.

Nevertheless, no matter how good the matching is in cadaveric situations, modulation of the immune response continues to be necessary to ensure graft survival.

Reduction of immune response

Reduction in the immune response occurs frequently in clinical practice in such situations as uraemia, profound jaundice and in patients with advanced malignancy and acquired immunodeficiency syndrome (AIDS). The controlled reduction of an immune response to foreign antigen on the graft requires careful clinical judgement. Initial attempts using widespread radiation produced severe depletion of not just lymphocytes but also a pancytopenia, and although skin grafts and other organs were readily accepted immunologically by the recipients, the majority of patients quickly died from overwhelming infection.

A refinement of this technique in which partial lymphocyte irradiation was used has been successful both experimentally and in clinical practice, depleting the immune response so that grafts can be accepted.

Chemical immunosuppression

Since the mid-1950s the primary mode of immunomodulation has been the administration of chemical agents. A demonstration by Hitchings & Elion (1959) over 40 years ago that 6-mercaptopurine had immunosuppressive potential allowed Schwartz & Dameschek (1959) to treat rabbits stimulated by foreign antigen. The treated animals did not produce antibodies to the antigen stimulation, and work by Calne in 1960 showed that 6-mercaptopurine could also inhibit the immune response in dogs. A number of other agents were studied at that time and those found to be of clear benefit were steroids, reducing the cellular response, and eventually azathioprine, which showed improved results when compared to 6-mercaptopurine.

For more than 20 years chemical immunomodulation with the combination of steroids (prednisolone) and azathioprine was to be the main non-specific immunosuppressant used. They inhibited the immune response largely by depressing circulating T cells.

The production of antilymphocytic globulin by sensitization in animals was also demonstrated to inhibit the immune response, although variability and efficacy limited its clinical use.

Cyclosporin. Clearly the ultimate goal of selectively inhibiting the recipient's immune response remains a long way off, and in clinical practice non-specific agents continue to be used. In 1976, Borel and colleagues working in Sandoz laboratories assessed the potent immunosuppressive properties of cyclosporin A, a cyclical peptide with 11 amino acids. The demonstration of both the in vitro and in vivo immunosuppressive activity was quickly followed by extended clinical studies. It was clearly demonstrated that cyclosporin could suppress both antibody production and cell-mediated immunity, exhibiting a selective inhibitory effect on T-cell-dependent responses. Of critical importance was the observation that the drug was neither profoundly lympho- nor myelotoxic and had no influence on the viability of the mature T cells or the antibody-producing B cells. Further agents have recently been introduced to clinical practice, perhaps resulting in less rejection still (FK506 or tacrolimus).

CURRENT CLINICAL IMMUNOSUPPRESSIVE USE

For nearly 25 years the mainstay of clinical immunosuppression was the combined use of steroids and azathioprine. With increasing clinical experience it became possible to adjust the dosage of these agents so that in many individuals it was possible to maintain immunosuppression and thus prevent rejection, while minimizing the risk to the recipient of overimmunomodulation, a delicate balance which requires considerable clinical skill.

Patients receiving steroids and azathioprine required careful, meticulous monitoring for signs of early infection and the presence of organ rejection. Progressive reduction in haemopoietic production leads to thrombocytopenia and leucopenia, with the attendant risk of infection (bacterial, fungal and viral). The major complications of long-term steroid and azathioprine immunosuppression are outlined in Box 26.2.

Thus considerable clinical skill was needed to avoid the risks of infection, and in cadaveric grafting, when the degree of matching between donor and recipient was often less than optimal, death from infection was the commonest cause of death in the first 3 months after grafting. In addition, the need to administer steroids continually became a major limiting factor, particularly in children where the complications of steroids can be so crippling (Box 26.3).

Box 26.2   Side-effects of steroids and azathioprine

Steroids
- Avascular necrosis of bones
- Diabetes
- Obesity
- Cushing's syndrome
- Pancreatitis
- Cataract
- Skin problems
- Psychosis

Azathioprine
- Bone marrow suppression
- Polycythaemia
- Hepatotoxicity

Box 26.3   Side-effects of steroids in children
- Growth retardation
- Cushingoid appearance
- Diabetes
- Obesity

The results of organ grafting using prednisolone and azathioprine left much to be desired, and so the introduction of cyclosporin into clinical trials in the early 1980s was an important step forward in the more selective use of immunomodulation. Not only could steroids be minimized or avoided in some individuals, but pancytopaenia was rarely encountered. Nevertheless, cyclosporin was rapidly found to have its own attendant problems and difficulties and nephrotoxicity remains a persistent problem (Box 26.4).

With increasing clinical experience, however, many of these toxic effects can now be minimized such that excellent rehabilitation can be achieved and organs can now be grafted which previously would have been unsuccessful in the prednisolone and azathioprine era. The overall results of cyclosporin will be outlined in the individual sections, but there have been no clinical series in which the results of cyclosporin have been inferior to the treatment with azathioprine and prednisolone, and for the most part an improved benefit of between 15% and 20% of graft survival at 1 year has been reported.

Postoperative monitoring of all patients with transplanted organs involves regulation of the immunosuppressive regimen, detection of the development of organ rejection and constant vigilance for signs of infection.

Box 26.4   Side-effects of cyclosporin
- Nephrotoxicity
- Hepatotoxicity
- Tremors, convulsions
- Skin problems
- Gingival hypertrophy
- Haemolytic anaemia
- Hypertension
- Malignant change

CADAVERIC ORGAN DONATION

The concept of the diagnosis of brain death and increased awareness by both the public and doctors alike of the need for organ donation have improved the supply of cadaveric organs for grafting. In the UK, about a third of patients who become organ donors have died from spontaneous intracranial haemorrhage, although head injuries and road traffic accidents also provide a significant number.

SPECIFIC ORGAN TRANSPLANTATION

KIDNEY

Kidney transplantation is now well established as the most effective way of helping patients with end-stage renal failure. Despite a significant expansion in the number of kidney transplants, long waiting lists exist for those on dialysis awaiting treatment. In the UK an integrated approach has shown a steady increase in the proportion of patients treated by transplantation, such that nearly 50% of patients now have a functioning transplant.

Patient selection

With kidney transplantation affording the optimal quality of rehabilitation, few patients will be denied the prospect, although the patient's age and underlying renal condition may need to be taken into account.

Age

In general, children do very well after transplantation, although infants below the age of 5 years present a more controversial issue because of the difficulty of management of immunosuppressive agents. The newer immunosuppressive regimens, however, allow adequate growth and physical development. The goal for children must be the establishment of normal renal function before maturity and to take full advantage of the growth spurt that occurs at puberty.

While in the early days patients over the age of 55 years were frequently denied transplantation, many centres now offer renal transplantation to patients over 65 or 70 years. Patient and graft survival has been very satisfactory in this group, but immunosuppressive schedules frequently need to be reduced in the elderly to ensure that overwhelming infection does not occur.

Renal disease

Renal transplantation is now offered for many primary and secondary renal conditions resulting in chronic renal failure, including glomerulonephritis, pyelonephritis and polycystic disease. Some types of autoimmune glomerulonephritis antibodies have been demonstrated to cause damage to the transplanted kidney, but this is not a contraindication to transplantation since probably less than 10% of grafts will be seriously injured.

Assessment of potential recipient

Careful review of both the physical and psychological status of the patient is needed prior to transplantation and factors which may increase the hazards of surgery or immunosuppressive management require evaluation. Patients in renal failure frequently suffer from cardiovascular problems (hypertension with left ventricular hypertrophy, and coronary artery disease) and the symptoms are increased by anaemia. There is a high incidence of peptic ulceration in uraemic patients and of metabolic bone disease, causing renal osteodystrophy. All these associated conditions must be optimally treated or controlled prior to transplantation surgery. Sources of underlying or potential infection such as an infected urinary tract or peritoneal cavity from peritoneal dialysis must be eradicated or treated and the patient's status for viruses such as hepatitis B, HIV and cytomegalovirus must be known to minimize activation following immunosuppression. Careful surgical review related to previous abdominal operations, peripheral vascular ischaemia, or the presence of ileal conduits following previous urogenital surgery needs also to be carefully taken into account and a surgical plan initiated.

Careful counselling and support are also needed to ensure that the patient understands and is prepared for transplantation.

Surgical technique

The technique of renal implantation has remained unchanged now for nearly 40 years, with the donor kidney being implanted extraperitoneally in one of the iliac fossae. The renal artery is anastomosed to either the internal or the external iliac artery, and the renal vein to the recipient's external iliac vein. The donor ureter is then implanted into the recipient's bladder. Over 100 000 kidney grafts have been performed around the world, but total transplantation rates vary significantly from one country to another.

Postoperative problems

Monitoring of the kidney allograft is required to detect signs of rejection, suggested by a reduction in urinary output and an elevation in serum creatinine, and then confirmed by biopsy or aspiration cytology. This allows the prompt recognition of acute rejection crisis and its treatment by steroids.

With increased clinical experience the hurdles of acute rejection and infectious complications can usually be overcome, and patient survival at 1 year is in excess of 95% in many programmes, with over 85% of kidney grafts functioning well. However, a steady attrition of renal grafts will occur over the next 10 years, so that only just half of all renal transplants will be functioning well at 10 years, with many having been lost from the slow process of chronic rejection.

Rehabilitation can be spectacular, allowing patients the freedom to eat without restriction on salt, protein or potassium, the resolution of anaemia and infertility and an improvement in their overall sense of well-being.

Renal transplantation in the diabetic patient can be combined with pancreas transplantation, with implantation of the whole organ and drainage of the pancreatic duct into the gastrointestinal tract or the urinary bladder. Transplantation of isolated pancreatic islets is in its infancy.

HEART

While the patient afflicted by renal disease has the benefit of chronic haemodialysis, the individual with progressive cardiac problems has no life-support system and death invariably ensues unless cardiac transplantation is undertaken. Initial efforts in the late 1960s by Barnard (1967) led to a progressive expansion of increasingly successful programmes. The majority of patients will suffer from cardiomyopathy, terminal ischaemic cardiac disease or, more rarely, some congenital form of cardiac disease. Donor selection must be rigorous because immediate life-sustaining function is required of the graft.

Orthotopic replacement of the diseased heart has been the most frequently undertaken procedure, although the heterotopic placement of auxiliary cardiac implants has been undertaken. The donor atria are anastomosed to the posterior walls of the corresponding chambers of the recipient prior to joining the pulmonary artery and the aorta.

Postoperative cardiac function is monitored and endomyocardial biopsy allows histological examination of heart muscle for ventricular cellular infiltration indicative of acute rejection. While the early attempts at cardiac grafting resulted in poor overall survival, the situation has improved remarkably. A 1-year survival of over 85% and a 5-year survival of 60% of patients with excellent quality of rehabilitation is most encouraging.

This solid foundation of cardiac grafting inevitably led to an extension to combined heart and lung transplantation, primarily for those suffering from pulmonary hypertension, or for some terminal lung diseases, such as cystic fibrosis or emphysema. If the recipient has lung disease but a good functioning heart on receipt of a combined heart–lung graft, the heart from the first recipient can be implanted into a second cardiac patient – the domino procedure. As a result of technical advances, transplantation of single lung is now possible. Because of the risk of infection in the implanted lungs, immunosuppressive management is critical. Sputum cytology and even lung biopsy may be needed to differentiate infection from rejection. In spite of this, the Stanford University Series now reports 2-year survival of over 60% in heart–lung recipients.

LIVER

Although the first attempts at liver transplantation were made in the early 1960s, the formidable technical, preservation, immunological and organ availability difficulties meant that it was only in the early 1980s that successful programmes were established. The majority of adult patients coming to liver grafting have extensive cirrhosis (primary biliary cirrhosis, chronic active hepatitis and hepatitis B) or, less frequently, primary liver cancer. In the paediatric group the most common indication for liver transplantation is biliary atresia.

The liver is particularly susceptible to ischaemic injury and the ability to harvest and store livers for only a few hours led to an extremely complex surgical procedure, undertaken often in the most difficult emergency situations.

The liver is placed orthotopically after removal of the diseased organ, and to reduce the physiological changes during the anhepatic phase venovenous bypass is employed. Improvements in organ preservation (principally the introduction of the University of Wisconsin solution) mean that livers can now be stored for 12–14 hours and transferred from one country to another. The evidence that tissue matching is important in liver grafting has yet to be fully established, but as in other forms of transplantation this may prove to be the case.

Patients coming to liver grafting are frequently critically ill with multi-system failure, and the complexity of the operation inevitably has meant that technical failures have been frequent. In spite of this, results have continued to improve, and with nearly 7000 liver transplants performed in Europe alone and 1-year survival of over 75%, liver transplantation is increasingly being established as one of the most effective modalities of treatment for liver disease. In some groups the results have shown even more impressive improvement. Infants and children with biliary atresia undergoing grafting stand a greater than 90% chance of 1-year survival, with the majority going on for many years. The longest survivor is now over 20 years after transplantation.

The major limiting factor in liver grafting now is donor availability and, while in the UK some 550 grafts were performed in 1994, the need is probably double that. The most acute shortage is of paediatric organs, and often a larger liver has to be divided and only part transplanted into a child.

ETHICAL ISSUES

The development of transplantation in the 1950s and 1960s caught not just the imagination of the medical profession but the public as well, and led to the reappraisal of fundamental beliefs in many areas. The concept of death was challenged from the traditional one of the cessation of the heart beat to that of the concept of brain-stem death, and wide public and professional debates ensued. Death, the great taboo of the 20th century, was addressed in a new fundamental way. The majority of countries enacted legislation or medical guidelines identifying new criteria which would allow more effective recognition of an individual's incapacity to regain essential and vital functions. Some of these issues were challenged in courts of law and were often widely reported in the media.

Thus ethical and moral issues were raised from the very outset of organ grafting. With the increasing success of organ transplantation these pressures have grown. The rights of the individual to dispose of his or her own organs as they wish has been a matter of debate, and the profession has loudly condemned the commercialism which is in danger of entering clinical practice. The purchase or sale or organs is now condemned by almost all international transplantation organizations.

Should a living individual during his lifetime voluntarily donate an organ to another? The first successful grafts between identical twins from within a family were clearly perceived to be an act of great charity and compassion. Living-kidney grafting in the USA accounts for more than a third of all grafts, but should such altruism be permitted between non-family members, or those in whom a loving and caring bond does not exist? These new issues continue to be addressed by society.

One other issue has particularly focused on cardiac and liver transplantation and this relates to the consumption of economic resources for an individual. In the UK the cost of renal transplantation in total is approximately £8000–10 000, whereas the cost of dialysis per year per patient approaches £15 000. While renal transplantation is clearly the most cost-effective way of dealing with renal failure compared with some other forms of medical and surgical treatment and perhaps health-care initiative, it is seen as being expensive. Cardiac and liver transplantation can equally be seen to consume an inappropriate amount of the health resources available in some areas, and indeed the state of Oregon has now withdrawn financial support from liver transplantation programmes, giving them a very low priority compared with their other health schedules.

Each new development in science and clinical medicine raises its own issues which need to be addressed, and as these modalities of treatment spread to other countries different cultural approaches may be required. It will be for the individual community to decide whether such treatments are appropriate for its members and what extent of resources can be made available.

Clinical organ transplantation has evolved rapidly over the last 25 years, affording treatment to many thousands of patients who would otherwise be dead or enduring an existence of chronic illness. Further advances are sought in the fight against the recipient immune response and to procure donor organs of the highest quality, thus enabling even more patients to experience the increasing benefits of transplantation.

Summary

1. Successful whole organ transplantation has depended on a number of advances in understanding of infection and immunosuppression.
2. Awareness of the public and of doctors has increased the supply of cadaveric organs.
3. Results have improved because of better monitoring and management, rather than from any technical changes.

References

Barnard C N 1967 The operation. A human cardiac transplant: an interim report of a successful operation performed at Groote Schuur Hospital, Cape Town. South African Medical Journal 41: 1271–1274

Borel J F, Feurer C, Gubler H U, Stahelin A 1976 Biological effects of cyclosporin A: a new antilymphocytic agent. Agents and Actions 6: 468–475

Calne R Y 1960 The rejection of renal homografts: inhibition in dogs by 6-mercaptopurine. Lancet i: 417–418

Gibson T, Medawar P B 1943 The fate of skin homografts in man. Journal of Anatomy 77: 299–309

Hitchings G H, Elion G B 1959 Activity of heterocyclic derivatives of 6-mercaptopurine and 6-thioguanine in adenocarcinoma 755. Proceedings of the American Association for Cancer Research 3:27

Medawar P B 1944 Behaviour and fate of skin autografts and skin homografts in rabbits. Journal of Anatomy 78: 176–199

Mitchison N A 1953 Passive transfer of transplantation immunity. Nature 171: 267–268

Murray J E, Merrill J P, Harrison J H 1955 Renal homotransplantation in identical twins. Surgery Forum 6: 423–426

Schwartz R, Dameschek W 1959 Drug induced immunological tolerance. Nature 183: 1682–1683

Malignant disease

27

Pathogenesis of cancer

K. Eagle, D. Hochhauser

Objectives

- **Recognize that cancer cells exhibit defects in cell cycle control.**
- **Explain that molecular biology has revealed some of the genetic events which occur in tumours.**
- **Understanding these events will lead to new treatment strategies.**

Table 27.1 The commonest sites of malignancy comparing UK with Japan

UK	Japan
Lung	Stomach
Breast	Lung
Colorectal	Liver
Prostate	Colorectal
Stomach	Breast

INTRODUCTION

Cancer is a process in which uncontrolled cell proliferation occurs with invasion and metastasis. About one quarter of all deaths in the UK are due to cancer which is the second leading cause of mortality behind cardiovascular diseases. There is a striking geographical variation in the incidence of different cancer types. In the Western world the commonest are lung, large bowel, breast and prostate cancer, whereas in Asia the incidence of carcinoma of the stomach and hepatocellular carcinoma is higher (Table 27.1).

PATHOGENESIS

Key points

- **The normal cell cycle is controlled by a series of intracellular and extracellular signals.**

The interval between each cell division is termed the cell cycle (Fig. 27.1). Quiescent cells that are not actively growing remain in a resting state or G_0. During the cell cycle duplication of genetic material occurs, followed by division of the replicated chromosomes to daughter cells. There are checkpoints which occur dur-

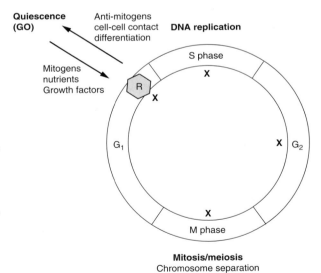

Fig 27.1 Schematic representation of the cell cycle. Resting or quiescent cells in G_0 can be driven into cycle by the action of mitogens. Once the cell passes through the restriction point (R) it is committed to progress through S phase where DNA replication occurs. Chromosomes are segregated in mitosis. The black crosses indicate cell cycle checkpoints which allow the fidelity of the DNA duplication and accuracy of chromosome separation to be monitored.

ing different stages of the cell cycle allowing the fidelity of DNA replication and the accuracy of chromosome segregation to be monitored. The restriction point (START) in G_1 is the critical point at which a cell becomes committed to enter S phase (DNA synthesis). Before the cell passes this point it requires specific mitogenic growth factors and nutrients, e.g. epidermal growth factor (EGF), but after this point progression through the rest of the cell cycle is independent of these factors.

Cancer cells exhibit a number of different features from normal cells

The cardinal features of cancerous growth are invasion and metastasis. These occur because tumour cells are not governed by the same growth constraints as normal tissues. One example is contact inhibition found in normal cells which cease proliferating once they achieve confluence; this phenomenon is abolished in tumour cells. There are also frequent alterations in cell surface glycoproteins and lack of differentiation (anaplasia) with accompanying loss of function.

Abnormal cell cycle checkpoints are a feature of cancer cell growth

Disruption of cell cycle checkpoints is a common feature of cancer cells (Fig. 27.1). The critical G_1/S transition (restriction point) is governed by the availability to the cell of nutrients and growth factors. There may also be important inhibitory influences at this point such as transforming growth factor beta (TGFβ). Cancer cells usually have an aberration in the restriction point enabling proliferation of cells to occur despite the lack of necessary growth factors. These abnormalities may occur through deletion or mutation of genes which govern the orderly transition of cells into S phase, e.g. the retinoblastoma gene. In addition, many growth factors or their receptors may be inappropriately expressed or overexpressed (e.g. mutations in TGFβ which override the lack of mitogenic signals and cause the cell to pass through G_1 in the absence of growth factors).

Many cancers result from environmental carcinogens

There are many factors which are carcinogenic (i.e. can cause cancer). These include, most significantly, tobacco smoke as well as occupational sources (asbestos), chemicals (aromatic amines), toxins (aflatoxin), ionizing radiation and viruses (Table 27.2). The mechanism of damage for some of these agents has been identified and, in the case of cigarette smoke, may

Table 27.2 Carcinogenic agents

Agent	Tumour type
Viral	
Hepatitis B and C viruses	Hepatocellular cancer
Epstein–Barr virus	Burkitt's lymphoma, nasopharyngeal carcinoma, Hodgkin's disease
Human papilloma virus	Anogenital cancer
Human T-lymphocyte virus-I	Adult T cell lymphoma, leukaemia
Chemical factors	
Cigarette smoking	Lung, laryngeal, bladder cancer
Polycyclic hydrocarbons	Lung
Asbestos	Mesothelioma
Nickel, chromates, arsenic	Lung
Aromatic amines	Bladder
Polyvinyl chloride	Angiosarcoma of the liver
Aflatoxin	Hepatocellular
Physical factors	
Ionizing radiation	Leukaemia, breast cancer
Ultraviolet radiation	Melanoma, basal and squamous cell carcinoma of the skin

involve DNA mutation (mutagenesis). However, there are clearly other undefined environmental factors involved in cancer development as shown by data from migrant populations where the incidence of colorectal cancer in Japanese immigrants to the USA is similar to that of native Americans but five times higher than that in Japan (Haenszel & Kurihera 1968).

Cancers may occur as a result of activation of cellular genes termed oncogenes

Proto-oncogenes are normal cellular genes that function as a positive regulators of growth and can be converted to oncogenes by mutation, deletion or overexpression. Therefore an oncogene encodes a dominantly activated protein that promotes the process of cellular transformation. Activation may be triggered by viruses. The association between viruses and cancer was first shown in 1911 by Peyton Rous, who demonstrated that a virus could produce sarcomas in chickens (Rous 1911). These viral DNA sequences were subsequently found to be similar to sequences in human DNA and their protein products involved at all stages of cell growth, including growth factors, growth factor receptors together with cytoplasmic and nuclear proteins. The function of these genes can be altered by mutation or overexpression which may result in uncontrolled cell division or invasive growth. These genes were termed dominant oncogenes because only a single copy of the gene (allele – any one of the alternative forms of a specified gene) needs to be mutated to produce a dominant alteration in function. Examples include the *ras* family (Kirsten *ras*, Harvey *ras*, N-*ras*) which were first identified as the oncogene of acutely transforming RNA tumour viruses. The *ras* family is frequently mutated in human cancers (e.g. K-*ras* in pancreatic cancer and H-*ras* in bladder cancer). The *ras* gene product binds guanine nucleotides and normally functions as part of the cell-signalling cascade which can be initiated by activation of certain growth factors (e.g. binding of EGF to its receptor). In its physiological state *ras* is bound to guanine diphosphate (GDP) and on activation this is exchanged for guanine triphosphate (GTP) which activates downstream signalling until the molecule is hydrolysed and de-activated by intrinsic GTPase activity. Mutation of the *ras* gene can cause loss of this GTPase activity causing it to remain in an active state which promotes continued signal transduction and, consequently, DNA synthesis and cell growth.

Cancers may occur by inactivation of cellular genes

Some genes may exert a negative influence on cell growth and inhibit cell proliferation. Mutation or deletion of these genes, termed tumour suppressor genes (recessive oncogenes), results in loss of normal growth constraints. Unlike proto-oncogenes, both copies of a tumour suppressor gene must be defective to result in loss of function.

The Knudson (two hit) hypothesis

The best example of this is the retinoblastoma gene (Rb gene) which, when mutated, gives rise to a tendency to form retinoblastomas. There are two groups of patients who develop these tumours. In the first group the tumours are commonly bilateral and occur in young infants (mean age 14 months); the mean age of the second group is older and the tumours are always unilateral but the overall incidence is low. Knudson postulated that there was a single genetic locus responsible which has subsequently been identified as the Rb gene. In the first group the patients inherit one defec-

tive copy of the gene and one normal allele. Mutations in the normal allele subsequently lead to a complete loss of function of the Rb gene and tumour formation early in life (the 'two hit' hypothesis). In the second group, patients inherit two normal Rb alleles and very rarely (1 in 30 000) two independent mutations occur to inactivate the gene and lead to tumour formation (Fig. 27.2) (Knudson 1971).

p53 gene and protein

The p53 gene (so named due to its molecular weight) is a tumour suppressor gene whose protein product causes cells to arrest at G_1 in the cell cycle following DNA damage, allowing time for repair or, if there is significant damage, cell death pathways may be activated (apoptosis). Mutations of this gene are common in cancer (up to 60%) and the majority cause production of a faulty p53 protein (mutant p53). Cells with the mutant

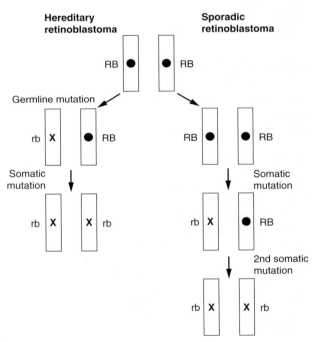

Fig 27.2 Knudson's two-hit hypothesis. RB: normal retinoblastoma gene; rb: mutated retinoblastoma gene. Patients who inherit one defective copy of the gene and one normal allele have a high risk of acquiring a somatic mutation at an early age leading to loss of function of the RB gene, hence the incidence in young infants and tumours are commonly bilateral. Patients who inherit two normal copies of the gene require two somatic mutations (1 in 30 000) and therefore the mean age of onset is older and the tumours are unilateral.

p53 do not arrest in G_1 which can result in accumulations of mutations and genomic instability which may be critical for the formation of tumours. Germline mutations of the p53 gene can also occur (Li–Fraumeni syndrome) predisposing the individual to develop sarcomas and other tumours at an early age (Malkin et al 1990).

Cancer arises by accumulation of mutations in oncogenes and tumour suppressor genes

One of the best models of tumour progression, associated with stepwise genetic alterations, is colorectal cancer. There is a clear progression of events that may occur over a period of time. Approximately 10% are associated with inherited genetic defects such as familial adenomatous polyposis – an autosomal dominant disease in which there is a mutation in the adenomatous polyposis coli (APC) gene. Mutations in the APC gene also occur in approximately 40% of patients without an inherited tendency and this is therefore thought to be a key mutation which allows the development of colorectal adenomas and has been termed a 'gatekeeper' gene. Thus the earliest lesions which are thought to be pre-cancerous, known as aberrant crypt foci, have been found to possess APC mutations. Following this, a further series of mutations in important cellular genes must then occur (including K-*ras* and p53) which results in progression of a small benign adenoma to a carcinoma displaying invasive and metastatic properties (Fig. 27.3). Other tumours may also arise following a similar progression, including Barrett's oesophagus and oesophageal carcinoma.

Pathogenesis

- **The cardinal features of a cancerous growth are invasion and metastasis.**
- **The function of normal cellular genes can be deranged by mutation or overexpression which results in loss of the normal growth constraints and tumour cell proliferation (oncogenes).**
- **Some genes exert a negative effect on cell growth. Mutation of such tumour suppressor genes results in loss of normal growth constraints.**
- **Cancer arises by accumulation of mutations in oncogenes and tumour suppressor genes.**

Cancer metastasis is a complex event involving an alteration in cell adhesion and new blood vessel formation

Most patients die due to the presence of metastatic disease. This is a complex mechanism beginning with the neoplastic transformation of a normal cell. The tumour cells proliferate with support of nutrients present in their microenvironment, but, in order to grow beyond 1 to 2 millimetres, new vessel formation (angiogenesis) must occur. The development of new blood vessels is mediated by factors released by both the tumour and host cells which include vascular endothelial growth factor (VEGF) and transforming growth factors (TGF) α and β. These new vessels have a number of different features from normal vessels, including differences in cellular composition, permeability, stability and regulation of their growth. This expansion in vascularity may increase the probability of tumour cells entering the circulation and metastasizing.

In order for metastasis to occur there may be a downregulation of adhesion molecules allowing an increase in cell motility and detachment from the primary tumour. For example, in epithelial tumours there is down regulation in expression of E-cadherin which is an adhesion molecule responsible for the organization, maintenance and morphogenesis of epithelial tissues. Reduced levels of E-cadherin are associated with a decrease in cellular/tissue differentiation and increased grade in different epithelial neoplasms. Detachment of tumour cells may also be aided by a number of enzymatic factors released by the tumour, including the metalloproteinases, which disrupt normal tissue architecture, allowing penetration of the basement membrane and cellular dissemination into capillaries and small lymphatics. Circulating single cells are usually destroyed by the host's immune system but aggregates of cells may survive and arrest in capillary beds of distant organs. These may then proliferate within the lumen of vessels or extravascate. Locally produced growth factors can stimulate growth of the tumour cells to produce a new tumour mass which then develops its own microvasculature.

The pattern of metastases may be regulated by the organ environment

The pattern of metastasis depends upon the cell of origin. Paget's hypothesis was based on the post-mortem examination of patients who died of breast cancer and other neoplasms. In 1889 he proposed that metastasis was not due to chance but that certain tumour cells ('seed') had a special affinity for the growth milieu provided by specific tissues or organs ('soil'); this would seem to be compatible with the site-specific pattern of distant organ metastases (e.g. bony metastasis in patients with prostate cancer). In regional metastatic involvement the process may be due to anatomical or mechanical considerations such as lymphatic drainage of the primary tumour, e.g. axillary lymph nodes in patients with breast cancer.

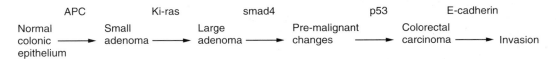

Fig 27.3 The multi-step pathway to colorectal cancer. The accumulation of 5–10 mutations in several tumour suppressor genes or oncogenes over a lifetime results in cancer.

Invasion and metastasis

- **Most patients die because of metastatic disease.**
- **Neoplastic transformation of a normal cell results from an imbalance and dysregulation of stimulatory and inhibitory cellular events.**
- **Angiogenesis is mediated by factors released by both the tumour and host cells.**
- **Invasion is mediated by release of enzymatic factors from the tumour cells.**
- **Prior to invasion, a downregulation of adhesion molecules occurs, allowing an increase in cell motility and their detachment.**

Future developments

The overall survival for most patients with solid tumours remains poor. Recent expansion in molecular biology has allowed identification of key genetic events involved in the pathogenesis of certain malignancies. These genetic abnormalities may be used to select a group of prognostic factors and, in some cases, these may predict the probability of a patient to responding to therapy. c-erbB$_2$ is a growth factor receptor overexpressed in 20–30% of patients with breast cancer and is associated with resistance to chemotherapy and radiotherapy and a poor prognosis. Identification of such patients may therefore allow modification of treatment to suit the individual such as antibodies to c-erbB$_2$ (Hayes 1996, Slamon et al 1987).

The goal of any cancer treatment is to specifically kill tumour cells whilst sparing normal cells and most conventional agents achieve this by inducing apoptosis (programmed cell death). p53 mutations, which occur commonly in cancer, are associated with resistance of cells to apoptosis and may explain in part why many tumours with mutant p53 are resistant to therapy. The production of p53 mimetics (agents that restore normal p53 function) which induce apoptosis is being investigated and their use may allow tumours with mutant p53 to become more susceptible to treatment.

Alternatively, by identifying critical mutations in the production of the malignant phenotype (i.e. the result-ing structural or functional characteristics of a tumour), it may be possible in the future to target these lesions (e.g. by gene therapy) and prevent tumour formation.

Summary

1. The cardinal features of a cancerous growth are invasion and metastasis.
2. Cancer is a disease caused by aberrant growth due to loss of the normal growth constraints.
3. Oncogenes are normal cellular genes that promote cell growth which can be activated by point mutation, amplification or dysregulation leading to abnormal cell growth. Such genes are dominant because mutation of a single allele will lead to an alteration in function.
4. Tumour suppressor genes are normal cellular genes which exert a negative effect on cell growth. Mutation results in loss of normal growth constraints. Both alleles must be mutated to result in a loss of function.
5. Cancer arises by accumulation of a number of mutations in oncogenes and tumour suppressor genes.
6. Most patients die due to the presence of metastatic disease.
7. Cancer metastasis is a complex event involving an alteration in cell adhesion and new blood vessel formation.

References

Haenszel W, Kurihera M 1968 Studies of Japanese migrants: mortality from cancer and other diseases among Japanese in the United States. Journal of the National Cancer Institute 40: 43–68

Hayes D F 1996 Should we treat HER, too? Journal of Clinical Oncology 14: 697–699

Knudson A G Jr 1971 Mutation and cancer: statistical study of retinoblastoma. Proceedings of the National Academy of Science USA 68: 820

Malkin M D, Li F, Strong L C 1990 Germ line p53 mutations in a familial syndrome of breast cancer, sarcoma and other neoplasms. Science 250: 1233–1238

Paget S 1889 The distribution of secondary growths in cancer of the breast. Lancet 1: 571

Rous P 1911 A sarcoma of the fowl transmissible by an agent separable from the tumour cells. Journal of Experimental Medicine 13: 397

Slamon D J, Clark G M, Wong S G, Levin W J, Ullrich A, McGuire W L 1987 Human breast cancer: correlation of relapse and survival with amplification of the HER-2/neu oncogene. Science 235: 177–181

Kohn E C, Liotta L A 1998 Invasion and metastasis. In: Fauci A S, Braunwauld E (eds) Harrison's principles of internal medicine. McGraw-Hill, USA, pp 520–523

Perkins A S, Stern D 1997 Oncogenes. In: DeVita V T, Hillman S, Rosenberg S A (eds) Molecular biology of cancer, 5th edn. Lippincott-Raven, Philadelphia, vol. 1, pp 79–102

Weinstein I B, Carothers A M, Santella R M, Perera F P 1995 Molecular mechanisms of mutagenesis and multistage carcinogenesis. In: Mendelsohn J, Howley P M, Israel M A, Liotta L A (eds) The molecular basis of cancer. W B Saunders, London pp 59–85

Further reading

Fidler I J 1997 Invasion and metastasis. In: DeVita V T, Hillman S, Rosenberg S A (eds) Molecular biology of cancer, 5th edn. Lippincott-Raven, Philadelphia, vol. 1, pp 135–152

28

Principles of surgery for malignant disease

P. J. Guillou

Objectives

- **Appreciate the importance of histological diagnosis.**
- **Realize the multidisciplinary implications of management.**
- **Accept that surgery may be valuable even when cure is no longer possible.**

INTRODUCTION

In 1996, malignant disease accounted for just under a quarter of all deaths in the UK, being second only to cardiovascular disease, including strokes (42.4% of all deaths), in the league of individual causes of death (Office of Population Statistics and Census Monitor 1997). In England and Wales, total cancer registrations rose from 209 431 in 1990 to 249 681 in 1992; this represented a real rise in true incidence per 10 000 population. Table 28.1 indicates the contribution of different types of malignant disease to the total figure. Lung cancer constitutes the greatest overall number of cancer deaths, although amongst women carcinoma of the breast is more common. Cancer arising in the gastrointestinal tract constitutes 27% of all cancer deaths (Table 28.2). Over the past 2 decades there have been major improvements in the results of treatment of some solid organ malignancies such as testicular cancer, whereas in others progress has been much slower. For example, the overall survival rate from colorectal cancer has improved little over the past 20 years and, as can be seen from Tables 28.1 and 28.2, remains over 50%. However, even here there is promise of some improvement with newer surgical techniques for rectal cancer, radiotherapy and chemotherapy.

Surgery has a diagnostic and staging role in the management of most common cancers but in addition is therapeutic for a number of solid organ malignancies

Table 28.1 The most common cancers in 1996 (figures in parentheses represent percentages of total malignancies registered)

	Males	Females
Lung	24 746 (24%)	11 749 (11%)
Prostate	14 140 (14%)	
Breast		30 787 (28%)
Colorectal	13 835 (13%)	13 879 (13%)

Table 28.2 Gastrointestinal cancer deaths, 1996

	Males	Females
Oesophagus	3580	2280
Stomach	4252	2526
Colon	5021	5524
Rectum	2826	2144
Pancreas	2829	3044

such as cancer of the breast, lung, urogenital tract and gastrointestinal tract. In all instances the design of therapeutic and staging surgery follows identical principles based on knowledge of the modes of spread of the tumour in question.

Spread of malignant tumours

Malignant tumours are spread by:

- Direct involvement of adjacent tissues and organs.
- Lymphatic drainage to regional glands and via major ducts into the blood stream.
- Venous drainage to the right heart, to the lungs and then to the left heart and the systemic circulation.

Alternatively via the portal vein to the liver, then to the right heart
- Within body cavities – transcoelomic (Latin: *trans* = across + Greek: *koilos* = hollow).

Presenting features

Presenting features are very varied, including:

- Palpable swelling
- Obstructive symptoms in tubular structures such as the digestive, biliary and urological tracts.
- Haemorrhage – anaemia, haematuria, rectal bleeding, or bleeding from cutaneous lesions
- Local compression or invasion such as nerve roots
- Metastatic effects such as ascites, pleural effusion, lymphadenopathy, hepatomegaly or effects of cerebral metastases
- Asymptomatic incidental findings.

ASSESSMENT

The physical findings, endoscopy, and the demonstration of tumour markers may assist in assessing the disease. The extent of the disease may be assessed using imaging techniques (see Ch. 5). The localization of metastases of some tumours may be determined by conjugating a radioisotope to a monoclonal antibody which specifically identifies an epitope; this is a small part of the antigen with a structure complementary to its corresponding antibody expressed on the surface of the tumour cell. The marked cells are identified using an isotope scanner.

In almost every patient, histological or cytological examination is essential (see Ch. 6). The tissue may be obtained using fine needle aspiration cytology (FNAC), needle biopsy, wedge biopsy, and excision biopsy. This usually confirms or excludes the diagnosis, and offers information on cell type, differentiation and, in some cases, extent of invasion.

Always confirm the histological diagnosis of malignant disease before planning management.

SURGICAL MANAGEMENT

This is usually determined by a multidisciplinary team of clinicians including radiotherapists and medical oncologists. Selection is determined by assessment of the extent of the disease, its aggression, the availability and effectiveness of alternative and adjunctive therapy. Added to this is the general health of the patient and the patient's understanding, and acceptance of the need to undergo surgery. For example, the patient must be aware of the likely benefits and possible disabilities, such as loss of important functions, the need for a colostomy following a bowel resection, or the cosmetic loss of a breast following mastectomy (see Ch. 15).

Coexisting disease must be detected (see Ch. 7). Nutritional support may be valuable (see Ch. 11). Meta-analysis of trials of preoperative parenteral nutrition in appropriate cases suggests that overall morbidity may be reduced by one fifth and mortality by almost one third. There are also advantages in postoperative enteral (via jejunostomy), or parenteral nutrition if there is likely to be delayed oral feeding. The patient must be carefully prepared for any likely procedures (see Ch. 16), and if necessary given prophylactic antibiotic cover (see Ch. 20).

In spite of many diagnostic advances, it may be impossible to make a final decision until the operation is performed:

- The tumour may be fixed. Frequently, it can still be successfully resected in continuity with the attached – but potentially infiltrated – tissue. Safe circumnavigation of the growth without encroaching on it demands an intimate knowledge of the anatomy and of the results of distortion brought about by the disease process.
- The tumour may prove to be unresectable.
- It may be resectable but there are unsuspected metastatic deposits that throw into doubt the value of resecting it. In some cases, however, this may not preclude resection; for example, secondary deposits of colorectal cancer in the liver may be subsequently investigated and found to be resectable.
- There may be synchronous, previously undetected primary tumours – or incidental disease.
- If resection is unadvisable, palliative (Latin: *palliare* = to cloak), procedures may be appropriate in order to mitigate the effects of the disease.

Emergency presentation of tumours portends a poorer prognosis. For example, intestinal obstruction or perforation of a bowel tumour may make radical resection inappropriate, so that palliation alone is possible; in the case of colonic obstruction, this may need to be limited to the construction of a colostomy.

Curative surgery for primary malignant disease

Curative surgery implies removing the whole tissue containing the tumour together with an intact covering of normal tissue to avoid shedding viable tumour cells, and leaving the margins of resection free of malignant tissue. This demands an aggressive approach, carrying a higher risk of postoperative sequelae, both short and long term. It is useless to submit a patient to such a procedure yet leave viable malignant cells that will cause recurrence.

In order to achieve success you must know the directions of tumour spread. In tubular organs longitudinal and lateral spread are both important. For example, in the oesophagus, cancer cells spread longitudinally submucosally beyond the visible limits, so the longitudinal resection must be extensive in order to avoid the future development of anastomotic recurrence. In rectal carcinoma it is recognized that tumour cells spread a relatively short distance longitudinally but at least as importantly, it has a propensity to spread laterally in the lymphatic vessels into the pelvic mesorectum.

The great American surgeon William Halsted identified a further principle of effective cancer surgery – you must not transgress the lymphatic connections between the primary tumour and the regional lymph nodes draining the area. He elucidated this in relation to breast carcinoma at a time when no alternatives to ablative radical surgery were available. To achieve it he developed radical (Latin: *radix* = root; hence, 'by the roots') mastectomy in which the breast, the lymph nodes and the intervening tissue were removed in one piece ('en bloc'). The same logic is applied to organs secondarily invaded from the primarily affected organ; for example, if gastric carcinoma invades contiguous organs such as the body and tail of the pancreas, the transverse colon, or the retroperitoneal nodes and spleen, they are resected en bloc with the stomach.

Curative surgery for secondary malignant disease

The development of local or locoregional recurrences of malignant disease should not necessarily occasion surgical despair. In some cases further surgical treatment is valuable, for example:

- Regional nodal metastases from malignant melanoma, following earlier excision from a limb or trunk, in the absence of detectable distant secondaries, should be treated by block dissection. Survival rates for 5 years of 20–25% can be expected.
- Recurrent colorectal cancer suspected clinically, or through regular monitoring of plasma carcinoembryonic antigen (CEA; see Ch. 31) and liver ultrasound, may be indications for 'second look' surgery. Locally recurrent colorectal cancer is rarely cured by further resection but valuable palliation can often be provided. In contrast, consider resection of detected liver metastases, provided extrahepatic disease can be excluded. Approximately 10% of such patients prove to have

disease suitable for resection; there must be fewer than four metastases confined to no more than two anatomical segments. A 5 year survival of 35% can be achieved.

Reconstructive surgery for malignant disease

Ablative radical surgery for malignant disease often demands subsequent reconstruction (rebuilding or remodelling), restitution (restoration), or substitution (replacement). The essential requirement is a sound blood supply for the tissues to be used. Examples are:

- Stomach mobilized and supplied only by the right gastric and gastroepiploic arteries can be drawn up to the neck to replace the pharynx or oesophagus resected for carcinoma. The left gastric and short gastric arteries are divided and the duodenum is mobilized to allow the pylorus to reach up to the oesophageal hiatus.
- Following mastectomy, myocutaneous reconstruction can be achieved using a rectus abdominis flap. The flap can remain attached because of the anastomosis between the superior and inferior epigastric arteries. Similarly, a latissimus dorsi flap can remain attached, being supplied by the thoracodorsal vessels.
- Reconstruction can be achieved in other regions using myocutaneous flaps. In some cases free tissue transfer may be employed, anastomosing the divided supplying vessels to local vessels, using microvascular surgical techniques.
- Where skin and tissue has been lost, as following mastectomy, it may be replaced by first achieving healing of the skin and then inserting an inflatable tissue expander to develop a space. The expander is then removed and replaced by a silicone implant or other substitute for the breast.

Palliative surgery for malignant disease

Although curative surgery may not always be possible, the symptoms can often be alleviated (Latin *ad* = to + *levis* = light; lightened or mitigated) by surgical means. For example:

- Obstruction of the oesophagus, stomach, small bowel or colon can often be relieved. Palliative resection, bypass or external stoma can usually be achieved. Open surgery may be avoided in some cases. Malignant obstruction of the oesophagus is usually amenable to endoscopic insertion of a stenting tube, or a self-expanding stent introduced under radiological control. The intraluminal incursion of the tumour can be temporarily burned off using a laser beam controlled endoscopically.
- In biliary obstruction, in spite of modern imaging techniques, it is often difficult to be certain whether or

not a malignant obstruction is amenable to curative surgery without operative assessment. Potentially, 25% of pancreatic cancer patients and 35% of those with ampullary carcinoma may survive 5 years following resection. Alternatively, a stent may be inserted percutaneously or endoscopically, but it tends to block and then needs to be replaced. Consequently, there is considerable controversy about the management of malignant biliary obstruction.

• In some cases surgery may alleviate symptoms or reduce the need for treatment, even though it does not affect the outcome. For example, patients with incurable carcinoma of the stomach or colon may bleed chronically and require regular blood transfusions. Resection of the affected part stops the chronic bleeding and mitigates the symptoms of anaemia.

• Apart from relieving colic from obstruction, resecting locally invasive bowel tumours rarely reduces pain. Neurectomy occasionally helps but often results in motor loss. Coeliac axis block is usually more effective than systemic analgesia in relieving the deep infiltrating pain of, for example, unresectable pancreatic cancer.

ADJUVANT THERAPY

Adjuvant treatment (Latin: *ad* = to + *juvare* = to help), is an extra remedy added to the treatment to increase its effectiveness (see Chs 29, 30). When applied prior to surgery it is called neoadjuvant (Greek: *neos* = new – perhaps revived in a new form) therapy. Examples are preoperative radiotherapy for rectal cancer, chemoradiotherapy for oesophageal cancer and some stages of breast cancer. In these cases the intention is to 'downstage' the primary tumour.

Adjuvant therapy may be administered following surgery, when the histological staging is available. Patients at high risk of postoperative recurrence can now be identified and given additional therapy. An example of this is the administration of 5-FU and folinic acid to patients undergoing resection of Duke's stage 'C' colonic cancer (Cuthbert Dukes, pathologist at the famous St Mark's Hospital in London classified rectal cancers as 'A' if the tumour was limited to the rectal wall, 'B' if it extended through the wall but not

Summary

1. In the assessment of patients with suspected malignant disease, the clinical aspects are still paramount, in spite of the availability of valuable diagnostic aids.
2. Early diagnosis improves the prognosis. Emergency intervention carries a poorer outlook than elective surgery.
3. The management of malignant disease by surgery cannot be prescribed in isolation from other modalities.
4. Do not embark on dangerous or mutilating treatments, such as resectional surgery or chemotherapy, without first making exhaustive efforts to make a tissue diagnosis.
5. Although curative resection is ideal, operative intervention can be valuable even when the disease has extended beyond the scope of total excision.
6. The patient must be aware of the possibilities, and of the consequences of each course of action, before being asked to consent to treatment.
7. If cancer recurs after operative treatment do not necessarily exclude the possibility of further surgical intervention – usually only palliative, but occasionally curative.

involving adjacent lymph nodes, and 'C' when regional nodes were invaded). This adjuvant therapy provides a 30% improvement in 5 year survival compared with surgery alone.

 Further reading

Guillou P J 1990 Biological response modifiers in the treatment of cancer. Clinical Oncology 2: 347–353
Taylor I, Cooke T G, Guillou P J 1996 Essential general surgical oncology. Harcourt Brace Churchill Livingstone, Edinburgh

29

The principles or radiotherapy

R. A. Huddart

Objectives

- **Understand the physics and biology of radiation determining how radiotherapy is used.**
- **Understand the process of delivering a course of radiation.**
- **Recognize the role of radiotherapy treatment in modern oncology with emphasis on its interaction with surgical oncology.**
- **Understand the basis of radiation side effects and how they may interact with surgical treatment.**

SOURCES OF IONIZING RADIATION

Radiotherapy is the therapeutic use of ionizing radiation for the treatment of malignant disorders. Natural sources of radiation include radioactive isotopes which decay with the production of β-particles (electrons) and γ-rays (a form of electromagnetic radiation). Originally radium was used, but over the last 20 years this has been replaced by safer artificial isotopes such as cobalt-60, caesium-137 and iridium-192, which are generated in nuclear reactors. Isotopes are used mainly as sources implanted directly into tissues (e.g. iridium needles in the treatment of carcinoma of the tongue) or inserted into a cavity (e.g. caesium sources inserted into the uterus and vagina for the treatment of carcinoma of the cervix). Radioactive isotopes may also be given systemically (e.g. iodine-131 in the treatment of thyroid cancer).

External beam radiotherapy was revolutionized in the 1950s by the advent of megavoltage treatment machines; initially cobalt machines and later linear accelerators. The linear accelerator generates a stream of electrons which is accelerated to high speed by microwave energy before hitting a tungsten target. This interaction results in the emission of high-energy X-rays. The high-energy X-ray beam produced by a linear accelerator has several properties which make it well suited for present day radiotherapy:

1. The greater penetration of the γ-rays means that a high proportion of the dose applied to the body surface reaches the tumour.

2. All X-ray beams have a fuzzy edge (the *penumbra*) due to the reflection and scattering of the beam by tissues. High-energy X-rays suffer relatively little sideways scatter as they pass through tissues, and this helps to keep the edge of the beam sharp.

3. The forward scattering effect is also indirectly responsible for the point of maximum dose being 1–2 cm below the skin surface (Fig. 29.1). The skin therefore receives a low dose and is spared from radiation reactions. It was the high skin doses associated with low-energy X-ray machines that in the past caused the uncomfortable skin reactions and limited treatments of deep-seated tumours.

In addition, cyclotrons can be used to produce ionizing beams of heavier particles such as neutrons or protons. However, these machines are yet to find a place in routine clinical practice.

ACTIONS OF IONIZING RADIATION

X-rays (from linear accelerators) and γ-rays (from isotopes) are both forms of electromagnetic radiation and are biologically indistinguishable. High-energy X-rays consist of packets of energy (photons) which interact with the molecules of body tissues to cause ionization and release electrons of high kinetic energy. These electrons cause secondary damage to adjacent molecules, including DNA via an oxygen-dependent mechanism. The resultant DNA damage is mostly repaired by enzymes in a matter of hours, but certain DNA lesions

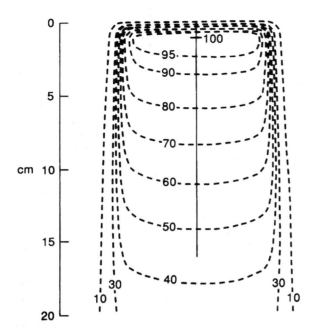

Fig 29.1 Dose distribution of a linear accelerator. Note the maximum dose is below the skin surface and 65% of the applied dose is present at 10 cm.

are irreparable. In some normal cell lineages (e.g. lymphoid, myeloid, germ cells) the DNA damage triggers immediate programmed cell death (apoptosis). Non-repairable DNA damage causes a variety of chromosomal abnormalities. This DNA damage does not stop most cells from performing their normal physiological functions effectively, but when the cell tries to divide it dies in the attempt. Thus damage is expressed when the cell undergoes mitosis, and in fully differentiated cells incapable of further division (e.g. muscle cells) this damage may never be expressed. Hence:

- Tissues may be severely damaged by irradiation but appear essentially normal; damage may be expressed only if they are stimulated to divide.
- Response to radiotherapy by tumours may be delayed, especially in tumours with slow rates of growth (e.g. pituitary tumours).

There are many data on the respective effects of radiotherapy on normal tissues and tumours. It appears that tumour cells may not differ greatly from the cell of origin in response to single doses of radiotherapy, although there may be differences in the ability of tumours and normal tissues to recover from the effects of cell damage. For example, normal tissues have a greater ability to respond to radiation-induced cell

depletion by accelerated repopulation, an ability which seems to be less developed in tumours. To eradicate a tumour within the limits of tolerance of surrounding normal tissues, radiotherapy must exploit these and other subtle differences in DNA repair and regrowth of normal tissues.

In external beam treatments, therapeutic advantage is generally achieved by dividing the total dose of radiotherapy into small parts over several weeks, a practice called *fractionation*. A full discussion of the effects of fractionation is not possible in this chapter but generally:

1. Reducing the dose per fraction allows certain critical normal tissues such as the nervous system, the lungs and other slowly proliferating tissues to repair damage more effectively than tumours.

2. Fractionation over a period of several days or weeks gives rapidly proliferating normal tissues such as skin and gut a chance to repopulate and hence recover from radiotherapy-induced damage faster than tumours.

3. Many tumours contain hypoxic areas. As the major effect of radiotherapy is by an oxygen-dependent mechanism, these areas are relatively resistant to radiotherapy. Each fraction of radiotherapy reduces the number of tumour cells and allows some hypoxic areas to become better oxygenated. Fractionation allows this process of reoxygenation which may take hours or days to occur and is thought to make tumours more radiocurable.

The above comments help to explain the empirical finding that radiotherapy is most effective when given daily over several weeks. A comparable effect to fractionation is seen with interstitial and intracavity treatments where a continuous low exposure over several days is biologically equivalent to multiple small fractions.

The ability to a cure a tumour probably depends on being able to eliminate every clonogenic tumour cell from the target volume. This is influenced by a variety of factors:

Size of tumour

A number of factors means that the larger the tumour the less successful radiotherapy tends to be:

- The larger the tumour the greater the number of cells present and hence a larger number of fractions will be necessary to have a high probability of eliminating the last clonogenic tumour cell. For example, the majority of 2 cm carcinomas can be controlled by 60 Gy, whereas a 4 cm carcinoma needs 80 Gy for similar control rates.

• Large tumours may contain large hypoxic areas which are relatively radioresistant and thus reduce the chance of cure.

• Large tumours usually need a larger treatment volume than small tumours. This usually increases the volume of normal tissue irradiated; the greater the volume of normal tissue the higher the chance that a part of that tissue is damaged by the radiotherapy and hence the normal tissue complication rate rises. To reduce this complication rate a dose reduction is often necessary, with a corresponding reduction in the chance of cure.

Radiosensitivity of tumour cells

The commonest histological types of tumour have cells of similar radiosensitivities (e.g. squamous carcinoma cells and adenocarcinoma cells). Differences in tumour cure between these common histological types probably relate more to differences in tumour bulk, oxygenation and proliferation. There are exceptions, with the cells of some tumours being more radiosensitive (e.g. seminoma and lymphoma) and others being more radioresistant (e.g. melanoma, glioma and sarcomas). The reasons for these differences are not clear. Radiosensitive tumours may be more sensitive due to a greater tendency to undergo apoptosis in response to DNA damage, but there is evidence, at least in vitro, that a variety of other mechanisms may have a role (e.g. melanoma seems to be more resistant to radiotherapy due to an increased ability to repair DNA damage).

Tolerance of normal tissues

The total dose which can be applied to a tumour is limited by the tolerance of the surrounding normal tissue. This varies greatly between tissues. If the tumour lies close to a sensitive organ (e.g. the spinal cord), then the total dose that can be safely delivered is much less than if the tumour lies within muscle or bone, for example. Hence the chance of cure may be reduced. The dose that can be applied will also depend on the volume needed to be irradiated. A good example of this is the lung. The tolerance dose for whole lung to be able to function after treatment is in the region of 20 Gy in 10 fractions of 2 Gy. Therefore, if the whole lung or large sections need to be treated (e.g. selected cases of Hodgkin's disease) this is the maximal fractionated tolerated dose. However, doses as high as 60 Gy can be given to portions of a lung, such as the lobe, because small areas of permanent damage are acceptable and have little overall effect on lung function.

RADIOTHERAPY PLANNING

The major principle of radiotherapy is to give the maximum possible dose to the smallest volume which will encompass all the tumour. This volume, termed the *treatment volume*, consists of:

1. The macroscopic tumour volume determined from clinical findings, imaging (X-rays, computed tomography (CT) scans, radioisotope scans, etc.) and operative findings termed the *gross tumour volume* (GTV).
2. A biological margin (often 0.5–1 cm) which allows for microscopic tumour; spread beyond the visible tumour: the *clinical target volume* (CTV).
3. A technical margin, usually 0.5 cm to allow for errors and variability in daily set-up (e.g. due to respiratory movements of the patient): the *planning target volume* (PTV).

Minimizing these errors and improving quality assurance is an area of active research. Techniques such as megavoltage imaging (in which an X-ray image of the patient is produced as the treatment beam passes through the tumour, showing how well the area actually treated corresponds to the treatment plan), may enter clinical practice in the future.

Accurately localizing the tumour in the patient is essential to the success of radiotherapy. In most cases the tumour cannot be visualized directly and localization depends on physical examination, imaging and operative notes. The importance of accurate and detailed operative records cannot be overemphasized. An operation is a unique opportunity to visualize the tumour directly, and full advantage of this opportunity must be taken to describe the extent of disease and acquire as much additional information as possible about local pathology. Limited information invariably leads to larger target volumes, increased radiotherapy morbidity and reduced cure rates.

Once the radiotherapist has determined the exact size, shape and location of the target volume the aim is to encompass the target volume with a radiation dose distributed as homogeneously as possible. A variation of under 10% is aimed for and achieved. Single fields are usually inadequate in this respect, except for superficial tumours. Opposing two fields at 180° to each other treats intervening tissue homogeneously. This arrangement is very simple to plan and is suitable for most low-dose palliative and a few radical treatments. Two opposed fields usually include more normal tissue in the high-dose volume than is strictly necessary (Fig. 29.2). Therefore, more complex multifield arrangements are normal for curative treatments to confine the high dose volume more closely to the target.

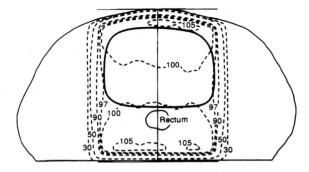

a.

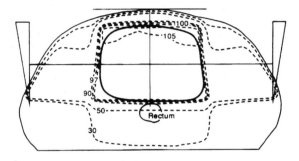

b.

Fig 29.2 Comparison of the dose distribution of different field arrangements. The parallel opposed field arrangement (a) adequately treats the target volume (the bladder) but gives a high rectal dose. A three-field arrangement (b) covers the target volume with a much reduced rectal dose and is therefore preferable.

These arrangements are usually planned by the cross-sectional target volume from CT scans of the patient in the treatment position.

Conventional therapy uses rectangular fields to encompass the target volume. As tumours are not cubes, an unnecessary amount of normal tissue is included in the treated volume. This causes increased morbidity and limits the doses that can be given (e.g. for pelvic tumours the dose given is limited by the amount of small bowel included in the target volume). Conformal therapy uses new engineering and computer technology to generate irregularly shaped fields so that tumours can be encompassed by high dose volumes which correspond more precisely to the tumour's shape. A recent randomized trial in prostate cancer at the Royal Marsden NHS Trust has demonstrated a reduction in the risk of late side-effects and has allowed dose escalation which should improve cure rates (Dearnaley et al, in press).

Directing several beams of radiation accurately to intersect across the target volume does not necessarily guarantee an even dose distribution because the X-rays have to pass through different amounts of tissue on the way from the entry point on the skin to the target volume. In addition, lung absorbs less energy than other tissues because of the air it contains. These potential sources of dose inhomogeneity throughout the target volume must be calculated and compensated for using a number of measures that alter the beam shape and profile (e.g. different weightings on each X-ray beam and the introduction of wedge-shaped filters which absorb different amounts of energy across the beam) (Fig. 29.3). Production of homogeneous dose distributions has been greatly facilitated by the introduction of planning computers and CT planning which can visualize and allow for tissue inhomogeneities directly. This area continues to develop rapidly, and in the future more sophisticated means of compensating for potential sources of uneven dose distribution will come into routine practice, as will more advanced beam-defining devices.

Once satisfactory dose distribution and treatment plans have been produced and checked, treatment of the patient can begin. It is important that treatment is applied in a reproducible fashion. The patient must be positioned, lying in a recorded position, with appropriate supports to maintain stability. Lasers are frequently used to help establish and monitor patient alignment. If extra accuracy is desirable (especially in the head and neck region) a light plastic shell may be used to immobilize the patient. The machine is then positioned according to skin markings and recorded settings determined during planning, and treatment is commenced.

 Planning radiotherapy

The radiotherapist:
- **Defines the volume to be treated.**
- **Designs radiation fields to encompass the volume to be treated. Complex 3 or 4 beam field arrangements are used for radical treatment to minimize the volume of normal tissue irradiated. Irregularly shaped ('conformal') fields are now being used to further reduce the volume of normal tissue treatment.**
- **Produces a radiotherapy plan which allows for dose imhomogeneity to produce a uniform dose distribution across the volume to be treated.**

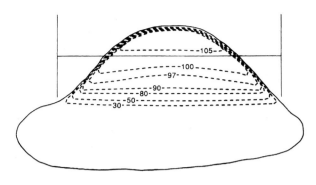

a.

b.

Fig 29.3 Treating the breast without compensation for breast curvature produces an inhomogeneous dose distribution (a). When this is compensated for by a wedge filter (b) the dose distribution is improved.

RADIOTHERAPY: THE FUTURE

In recent years several new techniques have improved the therapeutic ratio in selected circumstances.

Accelerated radiotherapy

This involves giving multiple daily treatments of the same size as used in conventional fractionation but given to shorten the overall treatment time from 6 weeks to less than 3 weeks. Recent research suggests that clonogenic tumour cells can proliferate significantly during a treatment course of 6 weeks and this could, theoretically, reduce the chance of tumour control. Reducing the overall treatment time could make an important difference, allowing less time for proliferation and leaving fewer tumour cells to kill. However, reducing treatment time also gives normal tissues less time to recover. Enhanced early skin and mucosal reactions may limit this approach.

Hyperfractionation

This delivers two or three smaller fractions a day over the conventional treatment period (i.e. the number of treatment days remains the same but the number of fractions is increased). Reducing fraction size reduces late tissue damage, with relatively less effect on tumour control. This has allowed dose escalation, with an increased chance of cure, especially in head and neck cancer (Horiot et al 1992).

CHART (continuous hyperfractionated accelerated radiotherapy)

This new regimen aims to combine the advantages of accelerated and hyperfractionated radiotherapy by giving three treatments a day over a 12-day period with no gaps (including no breaks for weekends and bank holidays). Results from a multicentre trial have shown that CHART improved survival in patients with localized lung cancer and, to a lesser extent, local control and survival in patients with head and neck cancer (Dische et al 1997).

Stereotactic radiosurgery

This technique utilizes fixation devices adopted for neurosurgical practice to localize tumours precisely in 3 dimensions, using fiducial markers. By using arcing radiation beams, conformally shaped fixed fields or multiheaded Cobalt units (Gamma knives), radiation beams can be delivered to a concentrated area with a high degree of precision.

Particularly applicable to cranial radiotherapy, this allows a high dose to be delivered to the target but very low dose to surrounding tissue. This technique can be used as a boost after conventional treatment course, retreatment of recurrences, or as a sole ablative treatment, e.g. in AV malformations not suitable for surgery (Brada & Ross 1995).

Conformal radiotherapy

Conformal radiotherapy (see above) is now entering routine clinical practice. Further technical advances, including the use of multileaf collimators (beam defining devices which allow irregular shaping of fields), which can vary during treatment administration, and 'inverse planning' where the radiotherapist determines what he/she wishes to achieve and the computer determines optimum field size, shape, direction and weighting, are likely to lead to further sophistication in treatment administration (including treatment of concave or annular shapes). This should further reduce radiation morbidity, particularly near sensitive structures (e.g. spinal cord, optic chasm, eye).

ROLE OF RADIOTHERAPY

Radiotherapy may be used in the management of malignant disorders in the following ways:

- As primary treatment.
- As adjuvant treatment prior to or following primary surgery (or chemotherapy).
- For palliation of symptoms.
- As a systemic treatment, either in the form of external beam total body irradiation or of systemic administration of a radioactive isotope.

Radiotherapy as primary treatment

When radiotherapy is used as the primary treatment the aim is to effect cure with the minimum of side-effects. It is an alternative modality of local control to surgery (Table 29.1). Radiotherapy, like surgery, is most effective at controlling small, well-localized and defined tumours, but has the advantage of preserving normal function. For many cancers, surgery and radiotherapy are equally effective modes of treatment and close liaison between surgeons and radiotherapists is essential if the appropriate modality of treatment is to be chosen for any given patient. This choice may vary between patients and depends on a variety of tumour (including site, stage and histology) and patient (including age and performance status) factors. Choice of modality of treatment is not restricted to either surgery alone or radiotherapy alone; a policy of initial radiotherapy followed by planned salvage surgery if this fails (as in many head and neck tumours) or initial combination therapy may best serve the patient.

Radiotherapy may be indicated as the initial treatment by a variety of circumstances, including:

1. Sites where surgery and radiotherapy are equally effective but radiotherapy gives better functional or cosmetic results (e.g. in bladder cancer where radical radiotherapy gives good results and avoids the necessity of cystectomy and ileal conduit, or laryngeal cancer where radiotherapy gives equal results to surgery but allows preservation of the voice).

2. Very radiosensitive tumours such as lymph node metastases from testicular cancers or early Hodgkin's disease.

Table 29.1 Results of curative radiotherapy

Site	Stage	Survival (5 years)	Comments
Skin	All	90–95%	Equivalent to surgery. Choice depends on site
Head and neck			
Tongue	T1	91%	50–60% for all stages
Glottis	T1	90%	
Other sites	All	30–80%	Local control rates with salvage surgery used for local relapse
Lung			
Conventional	T1	30%	40% 2 year survival
Gastrointestinal tract			
Oesophagus	All	9%	Equivalent to surgery
Anal canal	All	66%	Better results than anoperineal resection
Urology			
Bladder	T2/3	34%	Salvage cystectomy for local relapse. Surgery only 28% 5-year survival
Prostate	T1/2	80%	Equivalent to surgery
	T3	60%	
Penile	All	75%	Over 90% cure for stage 1 tumours
Gynaecology			
Cervix	1B	85–90%	Equivalent to surgery in randomized studies
	2A/B	61–85%	
Endometrium	All	60–65%	For patients unfit for surgery only
Vagina	Stage 1	75%	

3. Inoperable tumours. Occasionally radiotherapy can be used for attempted cure (e.g. brain-stem gliomas or pelvic sarcomas).

4. At sites where operations carry a high morbidity/mortality and equivalent results are gained by radiotherapy (e.g. carcinoma of upper or mid-oesophagus).

5. In patients unfit for radical surgery when surgery is otherwise the treatment of choice (e.g. patients with bronchial cancer and chronic airways disease).

All cases, however, need to be carefully assessed to decide the appropriate treatment option. In some cases where radiotherapy would normally be indicated other factors may make surgery preferable in that patient. For instance, it may not be possible to apply a radical dose because of an adjacent sensitive structure (e.g. if small bowel is adherent to the bladder, giving a full radical dose may be impossible without a risk of severe morbidity and cystectomy may be indicated). Alternatively, bone or cartilage involvement by tumour may have occurred (especially in head and neck cancer). In such cases the risk of osteoradionecrosis following radical radiotherapy is greatly increased, making surgery the preferred option.

Key points

- **Radiotherapy is an effective alternative modality to surgery to obtain local control**
- **The choice of radiotherapy versus surgery often depends on tumour and patient related factors**
- **Close liaison between surgeon and radiotherapist should lead to optimum treatment strategy being determined for each patient**

Adjuvant radiotherapy

For some tumours, preoperative or postoperative radiotherapy may improve local control. Adjuvant radiotherapy (Table 29.2) achieves this by controlling microscopic spread beyond resection margins, tumour spilled at operation or lymph node metastases. The low tumour burden means that lower doses than those normally used in radical treatments can be employed with a resultant reduced morbidity while obtaining a high rate of local control. If local control is an important determinant of survival, then this may equate with an improvement in overall survival. Even if metastases limit survival, adjuvant radiotherapy often has a valuable role in improving loco-regional control and quality of life. This may be especially important if symptoms of relapse cannot be easily controlled (e.g. rectal cancer).

Adjuvant treatment may be given to (a) the site of primary disease to reduce local recurrence or (b) sites of potential metastatic spread.

Postoperative radiotherapy has the advantages of the radiotherapist having details of surgical and pathological findings available in addition to clinical and radiological assessment. This allows for accurate staging and selection of those cases which would most benefit from radiotherapy.

However, the planning of postoperative radiotherapy can be more difficult, as the radiotherapist can no longer directly image the tumour. Accurate operation notes greatly aid localization of treatment, as does marking the tumour bed with clips. If the need for postoperative radiotherapy is anticipated prior to operation it is often helpful for the radiotherapist to see the patient preoperatively (e.g. prior to wide local excision of a small breast cancer). Postoperative radiotherapy is of proven value in reducing local recurrence at many sites, some of which are discussed below. At most sites postoperative radiotherapy is of no proven benefit in prolonging survival after complete resection of the primary tumour.

In selected circumstances, *preoperative radiotherapy* may be of value. Preoperative radiotherapy has the potential advantage of a downstaging effect which may allow an easier or less extensive operation to be performed (e.g. in rectal cancer or limb sarcomas). It may also reduce the risk of seeding at the time of operation and control microscopic disease at the edges of the tumour. Certain problems have limited the usefulness of this approach; foremost is the fear that radiotherapy increases the surgical morbidity. However, it is now thought that, as long as the operation is performed within 4 weeks of radiotherapy, this increase is minimal with doses of radiotherapy up to 40 Gy. A further problem is that the downstaging effect of the radiotherapy makes interpretation of the subsequent surgical specimen and pathological staging difficult. This also causes difficulties in comparing different series of patients, assessing prognosis and giving advice on further treatment. It is therefore a less established form of treatment, but has been used in bladder cancer, rectal cancer and sarcomas and, less often, in the treatment of oesophageal and endometrial cancers (Pollack & Zagars 1996, Graf et al 1997).

Radiotherapy to sites of lymph node spread has been used in the treatment of many cancers, especially when it was thought that blood-borne spread followed lymph node invasion. Increasingly, studies suggest that lymph node metastasis may be a marker of synchronous blood-borne metastasis and at several sites prophylactic lymph node irradiation has been shown to be of little

Table 29.2 Effect of adjuvant radiotherapy (RT) on local control and/or survival

Site	Stage	Criteria	Results		Comment
			No RT	RT	
Breast	T1/2 N0	LC	63%	88%	NSABP randomized trial of conservative surgery radiotherapy
	T1/2 N+	LC	57%	94%	
Central nervous system					
Astrocytomas	Gd1	S	25%	58%	
Oligodendrogliomas	All	10 year S	27%	50%	
Pituitary	All	10 year LC	10%	90%	RMNHST data
Craniopharyngioma	Incomplete excision	S	35%	90%	70% survival for complete excision
Lung small cell					
Thoracic	Limited stage	2 year LC	23%	48%	Overview of 9 randomized trials*
		2 year S	16%	22%	
Cranial RT	Limited stage	2 year LC	45%	84%	Danish trial†
		2 year S	16%	25%	
Gastrointestinal tract					
Pancreas	Operable tumour	2 year S	15%	42%	GITSG trial (NO RT V RT with 5-fluorouracil)
Rectum	Dukes' C	LC	65%	90%	MRC 3rd trial survival advantage in some series
Gynaecology					
Endometrium	Stage 1	LC	88%	99%	
	Stage 1	S	64%	81%	
	Stage 2	S	20%	56%	
Parotid					
Carcinomas	All	LC	62%	87%	
Plemorphic adenomas	Incomplete excision	LC	76%	98%	
Bladder	T2/T3B	S	28%	45%	Non-randomized data
Soft tissue sarcoma	Limited stage	LC	60%	75%	Review of French experience‡

*Warde & Payne (1992)
† Work et al (1996)
‡ Coindre et al (1996)

value in survival terms (e.g. bladder and prostate cancer) (Asbell et al 1988). Despite this, in a variety of cancers, lymph node irradiation is of value when initial spread is to lymph nodes and is an important determinant of survival (e.g. head and neck cancers) or relapse-free survival (e.g. seminoma). Prophylactic lymph node irradiation is also justified in reducing the risk of macroscopic nodal disease when symptomatic relapse is difficult to salvage. An example of this is supraclavicular fossa irradiation in axillary lymph-node-positive breast cancer. Node relapse at this site is difficult to salvage and has a high morbidity in terms of lymphoedema and brachial plexus neuropathy. The risk of such relapse is markedly reduced by applying adjuvant radiotherapy.

In a similar fashion, craniospinal irradiation improves prognosis when central nervous system (CNS) spread is common (e.g. medulloblastoma and ependymomas). Chemotherapy only poorly penetrates the CNS, and for some otherwise chemosensitive tumours the CNS may act as a sanctuary site (e.g. acute lymphoblastic leukaemia (ALL) and small cell lung cancer). If cerebrospinal fluid (CSF) metastases are common, cranial or craniospinal irradiation is a highly successful form of prophylaxis. For example, following the introduction of irradiation the incidence of CNS relapse in patients with acute lymphoblastic leukaemia has dramatically reduced and it has had a major impact on the chances of cure in this illness.

Key points

- **Adjuvant radiotherapy may significantly reduce the risk of loco-regional recurrence especially if the tumour is larger or excision is marginal**
- **Accurate pre-operative staging and operation records improve the effectiveness of radiotherapy**

Palliation

Of all modalities used to treat advanced cancer, radiotherapy is the most useful for the palliation of symptoms either from advanced primary or metastatic disease. The criteria of success must be in terms of quality of life rather than survival. The aim is therefore to give sufficient treatment to relieve symptoms without short-term side-effects for as long as the patient is expected to survive. The trend is towards short courses delivering a few large fractions of radiotherapy, thereby achieving maximum symptom relief with minimal interference in the patient's life. Frequently, a single large fraction of radiotherapy is all that is necessary to palliate symptoms. For example, most patients with lung cancer present with disease too advanced for any radical treatment. Such patients are frequently symptomatic with, for example, haemoptysis, dyspnoea, pain or cough. These are usually well controlled with one or two fractions of radiotherapy (Bleehen et al 1991). In certain circumstances in pelvic tumours, or recurrent chest wall breast cancer, longer fractionated courses to higher doses are necessary to offer a good chance of sustained symptom relief. In addition, palliative radiotherapy may be used for relief of symptoms due to metastases. The treatments of different types of metastasis are considered below.

Bone metastasis

Symptomatic bone metastases affect approximately 20% of patients at some stage during their illness. Radiotherapy is a highly effective means of controlling local pain due to such bone involvement. Recent work has shown that a single 8 Gy fraction of radiotherapy will relieve pain partially or completely in 80% of patients 4 weeks after treatment (Price et al 1986). Lesions with substantial cortical bone erosion should, however, be considered for orthopaedic fixation followed by radiotherapy to prevent fracture. Patients with extensive bone metastases (as frequently see in prostate cancer) obtain good palliation from wide-field hemibody irradiation given as a single treatment. The other

half-body can be treated 4–6 weeks later Approximately two-thirds of patients will obtain good pain relief from such treatments. An alternative approach is to use a radioactive isotope (strontium-89) which is taken up by bone metastases. It is given as a simple intravenous injection and may be repeated. In randomized studies (in prostate cancer) strontium-89 produced pain relief equivalent to local or hemibody irradiation, with the advantage of lower toxicity and the appearance of fewer new sites of pain on subsequent follow-up (Quilty et al 1994).

Spinal cord compression

This is an emergency which can cause devastating motor, sensory and sphincter disturbances. Metastatic disease can cause cord compression by direct extension from vertebral disease, epidural deposits or, rarely, intramedullary disease. There has been no large trial of radiotherapy versus surgery in the treatment of this disorder, but most series suggest radiotherapy alone, in most instances, is as effective as surgical decompression followed by radiotherapy. Surgical treatment should be considered when there is no diagnosis, in radioresistant tumours (melanoma, sarcomas), were evidence of spinal instability or progression through radiotherapy. Over 70% of patients will achieve good pain relief and 50% a useful response if treated before a major neurological deficit develops. Some patients will regain the ability to walk, but only 10% of total paraplegics regain useful function (Huddart et al 1997).

Brain metastases

This is a frequent complication of advanced cancer and is associated with a high morbidity. They are especially common in lung cancer, breast cancer (10% of all patients at some stage), melanoma, kidney and colon carcinomas. They are usually multiple and the prognosis is poor, with the median survival if untreated being 6 weeks. A 50% symptomatic response rate to radiotherapy and dexamethasone is expected, the radiosensitive tumours such as small cell lung, breast and colon cancers responding better than average. A good response to dexamethasone and good performance status also predict for good outcome. Frail patients with poor performance status tend to gain little and treatment may not be indicated in such patients. Short courses of treatment seem to be as effective as longer courses (Priestman et al 1996). Patients with a single metastasis have a better outlook, with a median survival of 4–6 months, and 30% of patients with breast cancer survive over 1 year. There is some evidence that surgical resection followed by whole-brain irradiation is better than whole-brain irradiation only (in selected patients fit for surgery). Recent work with stereotactic boost (see above) suggest that similar results may be obtained with radiosurgery (Wurm et al 1994).

Superior venal caval obstruction (SVCO)

SVCO is caused by enlarged right-sided mediastinal lymph nodes or tumours (especially lung cancers). It causes engorgement of veins to the neck, cyanosis, facial oedema and dyspnoea. Following mediastinal radiotherapy, 70% of patients gain relief within 14 days.

Other indications

Some other indications for palliative radiotherapy are retinal metastases, skin metastases and lymph node metastases.

Key points

- **Radiotherapy is effective at relieving symptoms of advanced local or metastatic disease**
- **Short courses of treatment are usually sufficient to palliate symptoms**
- **Longer courses of treatment are sometimes justified, especially to obtain loco-regional control**

Radiotherapy for the treatment of systemic disease

Radiotherapy is generally used to treat local disease. There are, however, two areas where radiotherapy is used to treat systemic disease: total body irradiation and radioactive isotopes.

Total body irradiation

A total body dose of >4 Gy will result in bone marrow failure. This has limited the usefulness of the technique for the treatment of malignant disease until the onset of bone marrow transplantation. Total body irradiation using a dose of 8–10 Gy as a single dose or a higher fractionated dose is a highly effective conditioning regimen for the treatment of leukaemias. It is also being examined in trials in the treatment of other radiosensitive tumours such as lymphomas.

Radioactive isotopes

This technique uses radioactive isotopes which emit short-range β-particles and/or γ-rays. If the tumour concentrates the isotope compared to the surrounding tissues it will be preferentially irradiated. The best example is the use of iodine-131 in the treatment of follicular and papillary thyroid cancer. The malignant tissue takes up and concentrates iodine, and hence residual tumour is irradiated to a high dose. Using this technique, lung and sometimes bone metastases can be eliminated. Other examples are the use of phosphorus-32 in polycythaemia rubra vera, strontium-89 in metastatic prostate cancer (see above) and m-iodo-benzylguanidine (MIBG) in neuroblastoma.

COMPLICATIONS

Normal tissue side-effects are due to cellular damage inflicted at the time of irradiation. This damage is largely expressed at the time of mitosis, so the sensitivity to and the expression of this damage depend on the proliferative characteristics of each tissue.

Acute effects

In some tissues, such as the epidermal layers of the skin, the small intestine and bone marrow stem cells, turnover is rapid and damage is expressed early. Skin is the classic example of such a tissue. Stem cells in the basal layers of the skin divide; the daughter cells differentiate and move to the surface over a 2-week period to replace shed cells. After irradiation, production of replacement cells is reduced or halted. The epidermis gradually thins and, if sufficient damage has occurred, epidermal integrity is lost and desquamation occurs. Recovery will occur over a period of days or weeks after the end of treatment by surviving stem cells producing enough daughter cells to cover the deficient area. It can be seen that:

- The time to onset of side-effects is determined by the skin turnover time, (i.e. 2 weeks for skin but 5 days for small intestine)
- The severity and length of time to recovery depend on the amount of damage to the stem cells and hence on radiation dose
- Provided there is a certain number of clonogenic cells surviving, recovery is likely to be complete.

Although this mechanism is responsible for most acute reactions the clinical effect will vary from site to site. For example, in the upper gastrointestinal tract acute reactions cause inflammation and discomfort (mucositis and oesophagitis, while small or large bowel damage by similar mechanisms causes vomiting, diarrhoea or, more rarely, ulceration and bleeding.

Other acute reactions, however, may operate by

different mechanisms and are less well understood (e.g. somnolence after cranial irradiation).

Late irradiation effects

Though acute effects are important for the tolerance of radiotherapy; the dose of radiotherapy applied is usually limited by long-term, late radiation effects.

Stem cell effects

Stem cell damage usually recovers completely but if it is severe, long-lasting effects can occur. The most important example of this is gonadal damage. Oocytes are particularly radiosensitive and even moderate doses of a few grays of radiation precipitate premature menopause. Spermatogenesis is also sensitive to radiotherapy. Doses in the region of 3 Gy cause oligospermia or azoospermia which may last 6 months to 1 year, but higher doses (>6 Gy) cause permanent sterility.

Depletion of parenchymal or connective tissues

In many tissues the parenchymal cells turn over very slowly. As radiation damage is expressed at mitosis, lethal damage will not be expressed until cells divide weeks, months or even years later. Irradiation of the thyroid gland, for example, leads to gradual depletion of thyroid follicular cells and can cause hypothyroidism over a period of many years.

Vascular damage

Damage to the vasculature is a common mechanism of damage, especially in tissues which never replicate (e.g. neurons or cardiac muscle) or which replicate only very slowly (e.g. fibroblasts). Radiation has a wide range of pathological effects on the vasculature due to damage to both endothelial cells and connective tissue. This leads to impairment of the fine vasculature, often in a patchy fashion. The damage can result in poor wound healing, tissue atrophy, ulceration, strictures and formation of telangectasia.

The precise clinical effect depends on the organ involved. For example, in the bladder the telangectasia can cause haematuria, while fibrosis, ulceration and tissue atrophy can cause a constricted fibrotic bladder which causes frequency and nocturia. Similar changes in the gastrointestinal tract may cause bowel obstruction by stricturing of the viscous or by peritoneal adhesions.

At other sites vascular damage is manifest differently. In the CNS glial tissues are depleted as a direct effect of radiation and via vascular effects, causing secondary demyelination and neuronal loss. Damage to the cardiac vasculature may result in early ischaemic heart disease if the dose is high enough, with myocardial infarction being an increasingly recognized cause of late morbidity and mortality in a minority of patients 15 years after internal mammary irradiation for breast cancer.

Lymphatic damage

High-dose radiotherapy can also damage lymphatic vessels, leading to reduced drainage and limb lymphoedema. The risk is increased if there has been previous or successive surgery. For example, radiotherapy to the axilla after complete axillary dissection for early-stage breast cancer carries a much higher risk of arm lymphoedema than either modality alone.

Late effects are usually irrecoverable and show a dose response. Low doses are less likely to cause damage, while progressively higher doses have a greater chance of causing complications and this damage becomes clinically relevant at an earlier stage. The radiation dose therefore has to be chosen carefully, taking into account normal tissue tolerance as well as predicted tumour cure dose and, as long as this is done, organs will function normally for the remainder of the patient's life. The actual dose chosen depends on a variety of factors. For each site an acceptable level of damage must first be decided and balanced against the chance of tumour control (Fig. 29.4). Damage to the

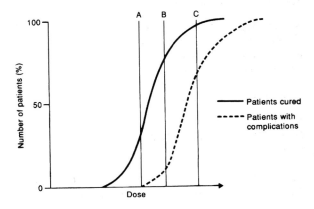

Fig 29.4 The relationship between cure and complications. A dose may be chosen with a very low risk of observable side-effects, but this may mean a very low chance of tumour cure as well (A). On the other hand, a high tumour cure rate may be associated with an unacceptable rate of complications (C) – forcing an intermediate dose to be chosen as optimal under a particular set of clinical circumstances (B).

spinal cord has such disastrous consequences that no morbidity can be accepted. A lower dose than that used at many other sites has to be accepted, even at the expense of tumour cure probability. Damage to other soft tissues (e.g. muscle and fat) is undesirable but of lesser importance and a higher dose and higher risk are accepted. As mentioned previously, the volume treated is important; the larger the volume, the greater the risk of damage and the lower the tolerable dose (e.g. for the spinal cord a short length of cord can be treated to 50 Gy, but long segments (i.e. over 10 cm) will not tolerate over 40 Gy). Other factors affecting tolerance include age (children and the elderly being less tolerant), pre-existing vascular disease and previous surgery.

Second malignancy

In addition to specific organ complications the problem of secondary malignancies is being increasingly recognized. This has been best studied in Hodgkin's disease, where an increased incidence of acute leukaemias are seen 3–10 years after irradiation, with a smaller increased risk of solid tumours following (Swerdlow et al 1992). The precise risk is difficult to quantify, but data give an overall risk of leukaemia of approximately 1–2% at 15 years. The risk is greatest if radiotherapy is given in conjunction with, or is followed by chemotherapy (especially chemotherapy with alkylating agents, e.g. cyclophosphamide or mustine), in one series being 0.2% if no chemotherapy is used and 8.1% if the patient receives multiple courses. Similar increased incidence of leukaemia has been seen in other cohorts of patients, including those with ankylosing spondylitis who have received spinal irradiation (Weiss et al 1994). Of perhaps more concern is the risk of solid malignancy which is increasingly recognized, estimates rising to 10% of patients surviving Hodgkin's disease 15–20 years following radiotherapy, though a disease-related phenomenon could also be responsible (Swerdlow et al 1992). This risk of secondary malignancy has to be balanced against the risks of dying from the primary disease in most cancer sufferers.

In conclusion, radiotherapy is set to remain the chief curative modality in patients with non-surgical cancer. As screening and other early detection methods diagnose an increasing percentage of individuals with truly localized disease its importance is likely to increase. This continued role in the curative treatment of cancer patients continues to stimulate research into the technical and biological basis of radiotherapy. In future years, further improvements in the efficacy and safety of radiotherapy should be expected to result from this research.

Summary

1. The physical and biological attributes of radiotherapy mean that the optimum application of radiotherapy means using multiple beams of high energy X-rays in treatment given daily over several weeks.
2. Radiotherapy is an effective alternative to surgery to obtain local control of many cancers.
3. Addition of adjuvant radiotherapy to surgery frequently improves local control.
4. Short course radiotherapy is useful in the palliation of symptoms due to advanced cancer.
5. Radiation dose is limited by the risk of late effects which may develop months or years after treatment.

References

Asbell S O, Krall J M, Pilepich M V et al 1988 Elective pelvic irradiation in Stage A-2, B carcinoma of the prostate: analysis of RTOG 77–06. International Journal of Radiation Oncology Biology Physics 15(6): 1307–1316

Bleehen N M, Girling D J, Fayers P M, Aber V R, Stephens R J 1991 Inoperable non-small-cell lung cancer (NSCLC): a Medical Research Council randomised trial of palliative radiotherapy with two fractions or ten fractions. British Journal of Cancer 63(2): 265–270

Brada M, Ross G 1995 Radiotherapy for primary and secondary brain tumors. Current Opinion in Oncology 7(3): 214–219

Coindre J M, Terrier P, Nguyen-Binh B et al 1996 Prognostic factors in adult patients with locally controlled soft tissue sarcoma: a study of 546 patients from the French Federation of Cancer Centers sarcoma group. Journal of Clinical Oncology 14(3): 869–877

Dearnaley D P, Khoo V S, Norman A et al (in press) Reduction of radiation proctitis by conformal radiotherapy techniques in prostate cancer: a randomised trial. Lancet (in press)

Dische S, Saunders M, Barrett A, Harvey A, Gibson D, Parmar M 1997 A randomised multicentre trial of CHART versus conventional radiotherapy in head and neck cancer. Radiotherapy and Oncology 44(2): 123–136

Graf W, Dahlberg M, Osman M M, Holmberg L, Pahlman L, Glimelius B 1997 Short-term preoperative radiotherapy results in down-staging of rectal cancer: a study of 1316 patients. Radiotherapy and Oncology 43(2): 133–137

Horiot J C, Le Fur R, N'Guyen T et al 1992 Hyperfractionation versus conventional fractionation in oropharyngeal carcinoma: final analysis of a randomized trial of the EORTC cooperative group of radiotherapy. Radiotherapy and Oncology 25(4): 231–241

Huddart R A, Rajan B, Law M, Meyer L, Dearnaley D P 1997 Spinal cord compression in prostate cancer: treatment outcome and prognostic factors. Radiotherapy and Oncology 44(3): 229–236

Pollack A, Zagars G Z 1996 Radiotherapy for stage T3b transitional cell carcinoma of the bladder. Seminars in Urology and Oncology 14(2): 86–95

Price P, Hoskin P J, Easton D, Austin D, Palmer S G, Yarnold J R 1986 Prospective randomised trial of single and multifraction radiotherapy schedules in the treatment of painful bony metastases. Radiotherapy and Oncology 6(4): 247–255

Priestman T J, Dunn J, Brada M, Rampling R, Baker P G 1996 Final results of the Royal College of Radiologists' trial comparing two different radiotherapy schedules in the treatment of cerebral metastases. Clinical Oncology 8(5): 308–315

Quilty P M, Kirk D, Bolger J J, Dearnaley D P et al 1994 A comparison of the palliative effects of strontium-89 and external beam radiotherapy in metastatic prostate cancer. Radiotherapy and Oncology 31(1): 33–40

Swerdlow A J, Douglas A J, Vaughan Hudson G, Bennett M H, MacLennan K A 1992 Risk of second primary cancers after Hodgkin's disease by type of treatment: analysis of 2846 patients in the British National Lymphoma Investigation. British Medical Journal 304(6835): 1137–1143

Warde P, Payne D 1992 Does thoracic irradiation improve survival and local control in limited-stage small cell carcinoma of the lung? A meta-analysis. Journal of Clinical Oncology 10(6): 890–895

Weiss H A, Darby S C, Doll R 1994 Cancer mortality following x-ray treatment for ankylosing spondylitis. International Journal of Cancer 59(3): 327–338

Work E, Bentzen S M, Nielsen O S et al 1996 Prophylactic cranial irradiation in limited stage small cell lung cancer: survival benefit in patients with favourable characteristics. European Journal of Cancer 32A(5): 772–778

Wurm R, Warrington A P, Laing R W et al 1994 Stereotactic radiotherapy for solitary brain metastases as alternative to surgery (Meeting abstract 050). British Journal of Cancer 70(Suppl 22): 21

Further reading

Dobbs J, Barrett A 1985 Practical radiotherapy planning. Edward Arnold, London

Horwich A 1995 Oncology: a multidisciplinary textbook. Chapman & Hall, London

Steel G G 1993 Basic clinical radiobiology for radiation oncologists. Edward Arnold, London

30

Chemotherapy — hormone therapy and cytokines

C. A. E. Coulter

Objectives

- **Appreciate the indications for chemotherapy.**
- **Recognize the importance of establishing a clinical response.**

INTRODUCTION

Localized tumours may be treated successfully by surgery or radiotherapy but metastases can only be cured by systemic therapy. Unfortunately, chemotherapy remains curative for a relatively small percentage of patients with cancer and in most situations palliation of symptoms with only modest improvements of survival will be the most that can be expected of treatment.

The combination of chemotherapy with surgery and/or radiotherapy may also increase local tumour control. Chemotherapy given after surgery or radiotherapy has been used to treat the primary disease is called *adjuvant chemotherapy*.

Neoadjuvant chemotherapy or *primary medical treatment* are terms which describe the use of chemotherapy as an initial treatment for patients who present with localized but extensive cancer (such as large primary breast tumours) where the local control may be improved by combining two modalities of treatment.

The word 'chemotherapy' was first used by Paul Ehrlich. He used rodent models to develop antibiotics and this led George Clowes in the early 1900s to work on rodents which could carry transplanted tumours. The modern chemotherapeutic agents were alkylating agents and their use followed the observation that seamen who were exposed to mustard gas had marrow and lymphoid hypoplasia. This led in the 1940s to the use of nitrogen mustard in humans with Hodgkin's disease and other lymphomas. The demonstration of successful regression of advanced cancer with these chemicals caused much excitement. Subsequent to this work at Yale, Sidney Farber's observations on the treatment of children with leukaemia and the successful treatment of children with Wilm's tumour led to a rapid increase in the number of cytotoxic drugs available and a rapid increase in the number of tumours in which they were used.

BASIC PRINCIPLES

The aim of chemotherapy is to selectively destroy tumour cells while sparing normal tissues. Growth characteristics of tumour cells allow selective tumour cell destruction and relative sparing of normal cells (Fig. 30.1).

Kinetic classification of anticancer drugs

Non-phase-dependent drugs kill cells exponentially with increasing dose and are equally toxic for cells in cycle and in G_0.

Phase-dependent drugs kill cells at lower doses but reach a plateau kill if given at higher doses because they can only kill cells in a specific part of the cell cycle.

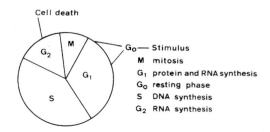

Cell death

G_0 — Stimulus
M mitosis
G_1 protein and RNA synthesis
G_0 resting phase
S DNA synthesis
G_2 RNA synthesis

Fig 30.1 Growth characteristics of tumour cells.

Predominantly phase-dependent:

- Etoposide
- Methotrexate
- Procarbazine
- Vinca alkaloids.

Non-phase dependent

- Alkylating agents
- Actinomycin D
- 5-Fluorouracil
- Anthracyclines.

Growth characteristics of tumours

The rate of proliferation during the lifetime of a tumour is not constant. In the early stages of tumour growth the growth fraction is high, but as the tumour enlarges the growth fraction is lower. The growth fraction peaks when the tumour is about 37% of its maximum size.

As the tumour enlarges, the growth fraction falls and the growth rate slows. Chemotherapy will be less effective in larger tumours because the growth fraction is smaller and the number of cells killed by a therapeutic dose of chemotherapy will be smaller.

Skipper et al (1964) formulated principles of tumour cell kill by drugs by using L1210 leukaemia in mice. He showed that the survival of the animal is inversely related to the tumour burden and that for most drugs there was a clear relationship between the dose of drug and the eradication of tumour cells. A given dose of drugs kills a constant fraction of cells not a constant number. This means that cell destruction by drugs follows first-order kinetics and a treatment reducing a population from one million to 10 cells should reduce a population of 100 000 to one cell. The implication of the fractional cell killing is that to eradicate a tumour population effectively it is necessary either to increase the dose of the drug or drugs within limits tolerated by the host, or to start treatment when the number of cells is small enough to allow tumour destruction at reasonably tolerated doses. The implication is not, as has sometimes been stated, that eradication of the last neoplastic cell is not possible with chemotherapy, but that the toxic effects on normal cells may be a limiting factor.

Development of new cytotoxic drugs

Phase I:

- Maximum tolerated dose
- Toxic effects
- Pharmacology.

Phase II:

- Evaluation of anticancer action.

If the drug has an objective response rate in a specific tumour type of 25% or more, it may then proceed to phase III testing.

Phase III:

- Controlled clinical trials.

Pharmacology of cytotoxic drugs

Alkylating agents. These compounds produce their effects by linking an alkyl group (R–CH–) covalently to chemical moieties in protein and nucleic acids.

Antimetabolites. Antimetabolites are agents that by virtue of their structural similarity with physiological intermediates are accepted as substrates for vital biochemical reactions and thus interfere with the required cell process.

Antitumour antibiotics. These drugs produce their effect by binding to DNA and intercalating between the base pair.

Plant derived agents. These are mitotic spindle poisons that bind to tubulin, which is a protein of the cellular microtubules.

Biological agents. Biological therapy is treatment that produces antitumour effects through the action of natural host defence mechanisms or the administration of natural mammalian substances.

Hormonal therapy. Hormonal agents are used in the management of patients with metastatic or locally advanced hormonally responsive cancers.

USE OF CYTOTOXIC AGENTS (Table 30.1)

Alkylating agents

Cyclophosphamide. Breast cancer, small cell lung cancer, Hodgkin's disease, non-Hodgkin's lymphoma, leukaemia and sarcomas.

Chlorambucil. Low-grade non-Hodgkin's lymphoma, ovarian and breast cancer.

Gemcitabine. Pancreatic and non-small cell lung cancer.

Dacarbazine. Melanoma, lymphoma and soft tissue sarcoma.

Cisplatin. Testicular teratoma and seminoma, ovarian cancer, bladder cancer, small cell cancer of the lung, head and neck cancer.

Procarbazine. Hodgkin's disease.

Table 30.1   Major cytotoxic agents

Class	Route	Dose (guidelines only) mg m^{-2}	Acute toxicity Plasma WBC	Platelets	Nausea/ vomiting	Other toxicity
Alkylating agents						
Cyclophosphamide	i.v./p.o.	50 mg to 1.5 g	Marked	Mild	Moderate	Cystitis/alopecia
Chlorambucil	p.o.	10 mg	Moderate	Moderate	Mild	Leukaemia
Melphalan	p.o.	10 mg	Moderate	Moderate	Mild	Leukaemia
Dacarbazine	i.v.	500 mg	Mild	Mild	Marked	Flu-like syndrome, painful arm
Cisplatinum	i.v.	100 mg	Moderate	Moderate	Severe	Neuropathy Otoxicity Nephropathy
Carboplatin	i.v.	400 mg	Mild	Moderate	Mild	
Procarbazine	p.o.	100 mg	Moderate	Moderate	Mild	Incompatible with cheese and alcohol
Gemcitabine	i.v.	1000 mg	Mild	Mild	Mild	Flu-like syndrome, skin rash
Antimetabolites						
Methotrexate	i.v./p.o/i.t.	50 mg to several grams (folinic acid given if dose greater than 50 mg m^{-2})	Mild	Mild	Moderate	Renal and liver dysfunction Mucositis
5-Fluorouracil	i.v.	400 mg	Mild	Mild	Minimal	Diarrhoea Conjunctivitis Hand–foot syndrome Cerebellar syndrome
Antitumour antibiotics						
Doxorubicin	i.v.	40 mg	Marked	Marked	Marked	Alopecia Cardiomyopathy
Mitozantrone	i.v.	10 mg	Moderate	Moderate	Moderate	Mild alopecia
Bleomycin	i.v./i.m./i.t.	15 000 i.u. (international units)	Minimal	Minimal	Minimal	Flu-like illnesses Discoloration and thickening of skin over joints Pulmonary fibrosis
Actinomycin D	i.v.	1 mg	Marked	Marked	Minimal	Alopecia Mucositis
Plant derived agents						
Vincristine	i.v.	2 mg (total dose)	Mild	Mild	Mild	Peripheral neuropathy, constipation
Vinblastine	i.v.	7 mg	Marked	Marked	Mild	Mucositis
Vindesine	i.v.	5 mg	Marked	Marked	Mild	Neuropathy
Vinorelbine	i.v.	15 mg	Marked	Mild	Mild	Neuropathy, constipation
Etoposide	i.v./p.o.	100 mg	Moderate	Moderate	Mild/ moderate	Neuropathy

Table 30.1 (Contd.)

Class	Route	Dose (guidelines only mg m^{-2})	Acute toxicity		Nausea/ vomiting	Other toxicity
			Plasma WBC	Platelets		
Plant derived agents (Contd.)						
Paclitaxel	i.v.	175 mg	Marked	Mild	Mild	Alopecia skin rash, neuropathy
Docetaxel	i.v.	100 mg	Marked	Mild	Mild	Alopecia Skin rash neuropathy

Antimetabolites

Methotrexate. Acute leukaemia, non-Hodgkin's lymphoma, breast cancer and sarcomas.

5-Fluorouracil. Breast and gastrointestinal cancer.

Antitumour antibiotics

Doxorubicin. Breast cancer, lymphomas, small cell lung cancer, ovarian cancer and bladder cancer.

Mitozantrone. Leukaemia, lymphomas and breast cancer.

Bleomycin. Testicular tumours, head and neck cancers and lymphoma.

Plant-derived agents

Vincristine. Lymphomas, leukaemia, small cell lung cancer and breast cancer.

Vinblastine. Testicular tumours, lymphomas and breast cancer.

Vindesine. Melanoma.

Vinorelbine. Non-small cell lung cancer, breast and ovarian cancer.

Paclitaxel. Ovarian and breast cancer.

Docetaxel. Breast and ovarian cancer.

Etoposide. Testicular tumours, extra-gonadal germ cell tumours, leukaemia and lung cancer.

Biological therapy

The pharmacopoeia includes recombinant cytokines which have immunomodulator activity and antitumour activity. These include interleukin-2 and α-interferon.

Interleukin-2 (IL-2) is a T-cell growth factor that is central to T-cell mediated immune responses. IL-2 has been approved for treatment of metastatic renal cell carcinoma. Response rates of 20% have been observed, and 50% of responding patients remain progression free 4–7 years following therapy. IL-2 has also demonstrated activity against malignant melanoma and the response rate approaches 20%.

Other recombinant cytokines, termed *colony stimulating factors (CSF)* exert effects on haematopoiesis and immune functions. They do not have antitumour effect but reduce chemotherapy-induced haematological toxicity and are useful adjuvants in high dose chemotherapy and bone marrow transplants. They are *erythropoietin* and *granulocyte CSF (filograstin)*.

Additional anticancer biologic reagents, including IL-2, IL-4, IL-6, IL-7 and IL-12, are currently being evaluated.

α-interferon (IFN-α) has demonstrated activity against many solid and haematogenous malignancies. A response rate of 80–90% has been observed among patients with hairy cell leukaemia. Survival appears to be prolonged compared with historical controls. Patients with chronic myeloid leukaemia respond to α-interferon but no survival benefit has been demonstrated. α-Interferon has been approved for use in Kaposi's sarcoma. There is a 30% response rate.

IFN-α-2B can be offered to high risk malignant melanoma patients (stage 3) after resection of primary tumour.

Hormonal therapy

Hormonal manipulation was the first form of system treatment offered to patients with cancer. In 1896 Beetson performed oophorectomy for metastatic breast cancer and observed objective responses. Endocrine responsive tumours constitute approximately 15% of all malignant disease. Hormonal treatment is used for patients with breast cancer, prostate cancer and endometrial cancer.

Breast cancer

Oestrogen receptors (ER) and progestogen receptors (PgR) should be assayed in primary breast tumours. If a tumour is ER positive, 60% of patients will respond to hormone manipulation. Progestogen receptors are made as a result of oestrogen action through functional oestrogen receptors. If the tumour is PgR negative the probability of response to hormone therapy is reduced. If ER and PgR are both positive there is 75% response rate. If it is ER positive and PgR negative there is a 35% response rate.

Agents used for treatment are as follows:

- Pre-menopausal patients
  - Oophorectomy
  - Lutenizing hormone-releasing hormone (LHRH) agonist
  - ?Tamoxifen.

- Post-menopausal patients
  - Tamoxifen
  - Anastrozole
  - Megestrol acetate.

Prostate cancer

Agents used for treatment are as follows:

- LHRH agonists
- Orchidectomy
- Non-steroidal anti-androgen e.g. flutamide and bicalutamide
- Diethylstilboestrol.

PHARMACOLOGY

The susceptibility of a tumour cell to a drug depends on the sensitivity of the cell to the action of the drug, to the cycling of the tumour cell and to the concentration delivered to the tumour.

There is evidence of a dose–response relationship for some cytotoxic drugs and in breast cancer doxorubicin has been shown to confer greater therapeutic benefit at high dose. Very high dose chemotherapy, with autologous bone marrow or stem cell support, is a technique used for treatment in acute leukaemia or as second-line therapy in lymphomas. The same technique is under trial as treatment for women with high risk breast cancer.

The dose of an anticancer drug is limited by its toxic effect on normal tissues. The cells which normally are turning over rapidly are the usual sites of dose-limiting toxicity. The bone marrow and intestinal epithelium are therefore problem sites. The dose given is usually calculated on the basis of milligrams or grams per metre of the surface area. Dose schedules are also affected by the function of major organs such as the liver and kidneys.

Liver

The liver is the principal site for metabolism and excretion of some drugs, and when the serum bilirubin is elevated doxorubicin, mitozantrone and the vinca alkaloids should be used with caution and the dose of the drugs reduced.

Kidneys

Drugs which are cleared by the kidney may cause increased toxicity if the patient has impaired renal function. Renal function must be checked carefully before each course of chemotherapy when certain drugs are given. The important drugs to note are cisplatin, cyclophosphamide, methotrexate, ifosfamide and procarbazine. When these drugs are given the patient should be well hydrated.

Carboplatin, which is similar in use to cisplatin, may be given with a low creatinine clearance.

COMBINATION CHEMOTHERAPY

The potential circumvention of resistance to treatment has historically been the most important factor prompting studies of drug combinations. Human tumours present with a greatly reduced percentage of cells in the proliferation pool. Effective chemotherapy has, in most cases, to be repeated over long intervals; under these circumstances exposure of tumour cells to chemicals can lead to chemical resistance. Because of this, combinations of drugs have been used to reduce resistance.

The major principles of combination chemotherapy are that all drugs included in the combination would be active against the tumour when used alone, that they should have different mechanisms of action and that they should have minimally overlapping toxicities.

METHODS OF ADMINISTRATION

Drugs may be given orally, intramuscularly, intravenously, or intrathecally. Venous access devices may be required for convenience, or because of poor veins or for infusional chemotherapy. Long-term catheters may be inserted into the right atrium; double lumen catheters (Hickman or Groshong) are normally used. Implanted venous access ports may be placed subcutaneously against the chest wall.

An implanted pump may be placed into the common hepatic artery to infuse chemotherapy continuously into the liver. This technique is being evaluated in patients with liver metastases from the colon and rectum.

COMPLICATIONS

Acute toxicity

Local toxicity

Doxorubicin and vinca alkaloids cause tissue destruction when extravasated. This devastating toxicity can be avoided by ensuring that the needle is within the vein and that the vein is tested by a non-vesicant substance before the injection of the vesicant drugs is started.

Bone marrow toxicity

For most drugs bone marrow toxicity is a dose limiting factor. It is mandatory that a full blood count is taken on the day of the treatment so that dose modifications or postponement of treatment can be considered.

Patients must be warned to alert the oncology department if they have a fever. If a fever develops and the patient has a granulocyte count of less than 0.5×10^9 they should be fully investigated to establish the exact nature of the infection and intravenous antibiotic therapy and treatment with G-CSF should be initiated as an emergency.

Bleeding does not usually occur until the platelet count falls to 20×10^9, but patients with low counts should be checked for signs of haemorrhage. Platelet support should be given if the count falls below 20×10^9 per litre.

Gastrointestinal toxicity

Nausea and vomiting are caused by cisplatin, cyclophosphamide, doxorubicin and actinomycin C. This is probably due to a combination of stimuli from the chemoreceptor trigger zone, the gut and cerebral cortex.

Patients receiving less toxic combinations of chemotherapy will respond to metoclopramide or domperidone and dexamethasone. For patients receiving highly emetogenic drugs such as cisplatin, treatment with a 5-hydroxytryptamine antagonist such as ondansetron or granisetron should be given prophylactically together with dexamethasone. Oral premedica-

tion with lorazepam will help the patient to relax before treatment.

Methotrexate may cause mucositis and oral hygiene should be given particular attention.

Vincristine may cause constipation and paralytic ileus. Treatment with laxatives is sometimes required.

5-Fluorouracil and cyclophosphamide may cause diarrhoea and prophylactic codeine may be given.

Alopecia

Doxorubicin, cyclophosphamide, etoposide, vincristine and paclitaxel cause alopecia. Hair loss due to doxorubicin may be much reduced by scalp cooling. All hair loss is temporary and patients can be reassured that there will be hair regrowth after treatment has been completed. Wigs are available and should be provided for patients before hair loss occurs. Hair loss will start at 18–21 days after the first injection of these drugs.

Long-term toxicity

Carcinogenesis

Long-term treatment with alkylating agents such as chlorambucil and melphalan is associated with the development of acute leukaemia. The risk is directly related to the total dose of the drugs given. This is an important reason for reducing the length of treatment and, therefore, the cumulative dose of these agents. The risk of developing a second solid tumour due to chemotherapy appears very low.

Gonadal damage

Alkylating agents are the drugs most commonly implicated in causing sterility. After combination chemotherapy for Hodgkin's disease, the majority of men are azoospermic. This is due to the combination of alkylating agents. All male patients should be offered sperm banking before chemotherapy is started. With modern assisted reproductive techniques it is possible to achieve ovum fertilization with a very low sperm count and the ICSI (intracytoplasmic sperm injection technique. Men do not need hormone replacement therapy.

For women over 30 years there is a very high risk of permanent amenorrhoea when they have received combination chemotherapy for Hodgkin's disease. It is now possible, but time consuming and expensive, to hyperstimulate the ovaries before chemotherapy to obtain ova which can be fertilized and frozen. Female patients will need hormone replacement therapy.

Patients receiving chemotherapy must receive counselling about the risk of long-term infertility and the inadvisability of pregnancy during chemotherapy. Men who receive treatment with cisplatin for germ cell tumours usually retain fertility as do women who have received chemotherapy for choriocarcinoma.

VALUE

Chemotherapy can cure some patients with advanced tumours. Cure is possible in the following tumours, which constitute about 12% of cancers.

Advanced tumours which are potentially curable

- Acute lymphoblastic leukaemia
- Germ cell tumours
- Choriocarcinoma
- Ewing's sarcoma
- Wilm's tumour
- Diffuse large cell lymphoma.

Tumours which are potentially curable by local treatment and adjuvant chemotherapy

- Breast cancer
- Lymphoma
- Ovarian cancer.

Tumours which have a response rate which leads to pro-longed survival

- Ovarian cancer
- Lymphoma
- Metastatic breast cancer
- Acute myeloid leukaemia
- Small cell lung cancer.

Tumours which have an overall response rate of 50% but no definite survival benefit

- Head and neck cancer
- Bladder cancer
- Stomach cancer
- Colorectal cancer.

Tumours which are poorly responsive to chemotherapy

- Pancreatic cancer
- Melanoma
- Soft tissue sarcoma
- Renal cancer
- Thyroid cancer
- Cervical cancer.

Summary

1. Chemotherapy can cure some patients but is used for palliative treatment for the majority of patients with metastatic disease.
2. Chemotherapy must be used only when a diagnosis of malignancy has been established histologically.
3. Objective evidence of clinical response must be established.
4. Biological therapy and hormone therapy may also prolong patients' lives.

References

Skipper H E, Schabel F M, Wilcox W S 1964 Experimental evaluation of potential anticancer agents. Cancer Chemotherapy Reports 35: 1–11

Further reading

Carmo-Pereira J, Costa F O, Henriques E et al 1987 A comparison of two doses of adriamycin in the primary chemotherapy of advanced breast cancer. British Journal of Cancer 56: 471–475

Chabner B A, Longo D (eds) 1995 Colon cancer chemotherapy; principles and practices, 2nd edn. Lippincott, Philadelphia. *A comprehensive review of chemotherapy.*

DeVita V T 1978 The evolution of therapeutic research in cancer. New England Journal of Medicine 298: 907–910

Fischer D S, Tish Knobf M, Durivage H J 1993 The cancer chemotherapy handbook, 4th edn. Mosby, St Louis, pp 5–7

Kaye S B, Cumming J, Kerr D 1985 How much does liver disease affect the pharmacokinetics of adriamycin? European Journal of Cancer 21: 893–895

Marshall E K 1964 Historical perspectives in chemotherapy. In: Goldin A, Hawking I F (eds) Advances in chemotherapy. Academic Press, New York, Vol. 1, pp 1–8

31

Tumour markers

G. J. S. Rustin

Objectives

- **Appreciate the potential uses of circulating tumour markers.**
- **Recognize which tumour markers are most commonly elevated in particular tumours.**
- **Understand how tumour markers can be used to affect management of certain tumours.**
- **Lead to more appropriate requesting of tumour marker measurements.**

INTRODUCTION

Tumour markers are substances present in the body in a concentration which is related to the presence of a tumour. A tumour marker does not have to be tumour specific. It may be secreted or shed into blood and other body fluids or expressed at the cell surface in larger quantities by malignant cells than by non-malignant cells. Tumour markers can be detected either by measuring the concentration of the marker in body fluids (usually by immunoassay) or by detecting the presence of the marker on the cell surface in paraffin sections or fresh biopsies (by immunohistochemistry). This chapter examines critically those situations where estimation of circulating tumour marker levels may be of clinical value.

DEFINITIONS

The terms most commonly used to describe the usefulness of a tumour marker are defined in Table 31.1. Sensitivity is a measure of how commonly a tumour marker level is elevated in the presence of that particular tumour. Specificity measures the proportion of patients without tumour who have normal marker levels, and

Table 31.1 Terms used to describe tumour markers

	Tumour Present	Absent
Assay positive	TP	FP
Assay negative	FN	TN
Sensitivity	$= \dfrac{TP}{TP + FN} \times 100$	
Specificity	$= \dfrac{TN}{FP + FN} \times 100$	
Positive predictive value	$= \dfrac{TP}{TP + FP} \times 100$	
Negative predictive value	$= \dfrac{TN}{FN + TN} \times 100$	

TP, true positive; FP, false positive; FN, false negative; TN, true negative

are therefore the true negatives. The positive predictive value is the percentage of positive results (i.e. elevated marker levels) which are true positives. An ideal tumour marker would have 100% sensitivity, thus detecting all cases of a particular tumour, and 100% specificity, being elevated only in the presence of that tumour and not in any other situations.

POTENTIAL USES OF TUMOUR MARKERS

The potential clinical uses of tumour marker estimation are:

- Screening
- Diagnosis

- Prognostic indicator
- Monitoring therapy
- Early diagnosis of relapse.

Examples of these uses will be given for the cancers where tumour markers are currently of greatest value. Although they will not be discussed in any further detail in this chapter, the existence of cell surface tumour markers is being exploited to localize a tumour either for imaging purposes, using a radiolabelled antibody, or as a treatment modality, using antibodies to carry radioactivity or toxins selectively to the tumour.

REVIEW OF THE USE OF TUMOUR MARKER ESTIMATION IN THE MANAGEMENT OF PARTICULAR TUMOURS

Gestational trophoblastic tumours (GTT)

The role of human chorionic gonadotrophin (HCG) in the management of GTT comes closest to the ideal use of a tumour marker. HCG is a glycoprotein produced by trophoblast cells. The α-subunit is identical to that of follicle-stimulating hormone (FSH), luteinizing hormone (LH) and thyroid-stimulating hormone (TSH), but the C-terminal end of the β-subunit is unique to hCG and provides the basis of the specific immunoassay. There are many different assays for HCG available. It is essential to know whether the assay in use locally recognizes just the β-subunit or the intact complete HCG molecule, as they can give quite different results.

Diagnosis and screening

Elevated levels of hCG are found with as few as 10^5 trophoblast cells, but elevated serum hCG levels are also found in normal pregnancy, in ectopic pregnancy, in patients with germ cell tumours and, occasionally, in patients with non-germ-cell tumours. Pelvic ultrasound examination therefore remains the best method for diagnosing hydatidiform mole. The great sensitivity of hCG, however, allows it to be used to screen a high-risk population. The first national screening programme for any cancer was set up in 1972 so that, following a diagnosis of hydatidiform mole, all patients are centrally registered. Patients are then followed using serial hCG measurements in blood or urine. This screening allows those patients with persistent trophoblastic disease after evacuation of hydatidiform mole to be detected on the basis of plateauing or rising tumour markers before any clinical evidence of disease develops (Bagshawe et al 1986).

Prognosis/monitoring response to treatment

Since hCG levels in patients with GTT reflect the total body burden of viable tumour, the level is a major factor in deciding whether a patient fits into a good or poor prognostic group. In patients with GTT, serial hCG estimation is used to monitor response to chemotherapy and to detect the development of drug resistance. The hCG value may initially increase after starting treatment, possibly due to tumour lysis or to increased syncytial differentiation induced by the therapy. The hCG level then falls at a rate which is a function of metabolic clearance and the rate of synthesis. Plateauing of hCG values or rising values during the course of chemotherapy indicate the development of drug resistance, and need to change chemotherapy.

Detection of recurrence

Serial measurement of hCG will detect any recurrence of GTT with 100% sensitivity. The accurate measurement of HCG in urine, which is stable in the post, increases the ease of monitoring and obviates the need for frequent hospital visits. A rise in hCG is not, however, diagnostic of recurrent disease, and a new pregnancy must always be considered and ruled out by ultrasound examination. Patients who have had a hydatidiform mole have a slightly increased risk of choriocarcinoma after any subsequent pregnancy and should have further hCG estimations at 4 and 12 weeks postpartum.

Germ cell tumours

α-Fetoprotein (AFP) and hCG are elevated, either singly or in combination, in more than 80% of patients with disseminated non-seminomatous germ cell tumours (NSGCT) and in approximately 60% of patients with localized, stage I disease (Bower & Rustin 1996). Other markers of use in patients with germ cell tumours include lactate dehydrogenase (LDH), but many laboratories only measure hydroxybutyrate dehydrogenase (HBD) which is mostly isoenzyme 1 and 2 of LDH. Placental alkaline phosphatase (PLAP), although elevated in about 50% of patients with seminomas and in smokers, adds little to clinical management as it is rarely greatly elevated and usually falls to normal so quickly on therapy that it adds little to monitoring (Nielsen et al 1990).

Diagnosis and staging

All patients who are suspected of having a germ cell tumour should have serum sent for tumour marker estimation before excision of the primary tumour. Patients whose clinical status could be compromised by a biopsy (e.g. a patient with severe dyspnoea due to extensive lung metastases) should be considered to have an NSGCT if the distribution of the disease is compatible with such a tumour and there is gross elevation of either hCG or AFP. Elevated hCG is associated with the presence of trophoblastic elements in an NSGCT, and can be produced by syncytial giant cells in a pure seminoma. AFP, a glycoprotein with a molecular weight of 63–70 kDa, is secreted by the yolk sac element of an NSGCT, and a patient with an elevated AFP should never be considered to have a pure seminoma, regardless of the histological findings.

Failure of tumour marker levels to fall to normal postoperatively indicates the presence of occult metastatic disease, even if all other staging investigations are normal. One further situation in which hCG estimation may be of diagnostic value is in the detection of brain metastases. A pretreatment cerebrospinal fluid hCG level that is more than one-sixtieth the serum hCG level indicates the presence of brain metastases; the normal ratio, however, does not exclude brain metastases (Bagshawe & Harland 1976).

Prognosis and staging

Initial tumour marker levels are now recognized as the single best predictor of failure to achieve complete response following chemotherapy. An international collaborative group has recently proposed a prognostic classification (Table 31.2) based on an analysis of 5202 patients which found tumour marker levels and the presence or absence of mediastinal and non-pulmonary, non-nodal visceral metastases as the important risk factors (International Germ Cell Collaborative Group 1997).

Monitoring response to treatment

In patients with elevated hCG or AFP, these markers are the most sensitive method for assessing response to treatment. Although, in general, successful chemotherapy is invariably accompanied by a fall in serial hCG and AFP levels, there are two situations in which this may not occur. Firstly, an initial rise in tumour marker levels may occur soon after starting the first course of chemotherapy due to tumour lysis. The second situation is a plateau or even a rise in AFP levels, despite evidence of response from all other investigations. This is thought to be due to AFP production by the liver in response to toxicity and appears to be more common in those patients receiving hepatotoxic drugs such as methotrexate and ifosfamide. The only situation where falling marker levels are not associated with a decreasing germ cell tumour mass is when there is enlargement of cystic differentiated teratoma. These masses require resection before they become inoperable.

Early detection of recurrence

All patients with germ cell tumours should continue to have serial tumour marker estimation after completion of chemotherapy to detect relapse early. The other situation in which serial marker estimation is invaluable, is in surveillance of patients with stage I disease following orchidectomy. Close follow-up by clinical examination, tumour markers, chest X-rays and CT scans will detect relapse early in the 25–30% of those in whom the disease is destined to recur and, with adequate treatment, virtually all patients will be cured. In view of the potential for tumour markers to double rapidly, it is important that markers are measured at least monthly, and more frequently if raised.

Table 31.2 Tumour markers in prognostic classification of germ cell tumours

	Marker		
	AFP (ng ml^{-1})	HCG* (ng ml^{-1})	LDH† (× N)
Good	<1000	and <1000	and <1.5 N
Intermediate	1000–10 000	or 1000–10 000	or 1.5 N–10 N
Poor	>10 000	or >10 000	or >10 N

*For HCG, 1 ng ml^{-1} is approximately equal to 5 iu l^{-1}
†N, upper limit of normal

Gastrointestinal tumours

There are a number of antibodies currently available which detect antigens expressed by gastrointestinal tumours. The most widely used are the antibodies which react with carcinoembryonic antigen (CEA), a 200 kDa glycoprotein. Assays dependent on monoclonal antibodies include CA 19.9, an antigen derived from a human colon adenocarcinoma cell line with an epitope structurally identical to the sialylated Lewis A antigen, and CA 50, which is similar but not identical to CA 19.9. Elevated levels of several other markers such as CA 72-4 have also been found.

Diagnosis and screening

Serum CEA is elevated in fewer than 5% of patients with Dukes' grade A colorectal cancer, about 25% of Dukes' grade B, 44% of Dukes' grade C and about 65% of patients with distant metastases (Begent & Rustin 1989). CEA can be elevated not only in cancers of the gastrointestinal tract but also in a variety of other conditions including: severe benign liver disease; inflammatory lesions, especially of the gastrointestinal tract; trauma; infection; collagen disease; renal impairment; and smoking. The low incidence of high serum CEA levels in early disease and its poor specificity explain its lack of value in screening normal populations for colorectal cancer. The low sensitivity precludes its being useful even for screening patients with ulcerative colitis or familial polyposis coli; although these patients are at high risk of developing colorectal cancer, both conditions may cause raised serum CEA in the absence of malignancy.

Prognosis/monitoring treatment

A raised preoperative CEA level has been shown to be associated with a poorer prognosis, but the value of preoperative CEA as an independent prognostic factor is unclear. Serum CEA levels should fall to normal within 4–6 weeks of complete resection of a colorectal carcinoma, the mean half-life being about 10 days. Levels usually rise with disease and fall with response to chemotherapy or radiotherapy. Failure of CEA to fall during radiotherapy usually indicates the presence of tumour outside the radiation field. Several studies have shown that survival is longer in patients who have a fall in serum CEA level during chemotherapy than in those in whom there is no change or an increased level (Allen-Mersh et al 1987). CA 19.9 is elevated in 75–90% of patients with pancreatic carcinomas and is increasingly used to monitor palliative chemotherapy.

Follow-up and detection of relapse

In approximately two-thirds of patients with recurrent colorectal cancer, a rise in serial serum CEA values predicts recurrence on average 11 months before it becomes clinically apparent (Begent & Rustin 1989). Surgical resection of isolated metastases of colorectal cancer has been advocated. Unfortunately, a randomized, multicentre trial under the auspices of the Cancer Research Campaign has failed to show any survival benefit from surgery after early detection of recurrence by rising CEA levels (Lennon et al 1994. However, further work is required to determine whether such patients would benefit from chemotherapy.

Ovarian cancer

The site and pattern of spread of ovarian cancer make it very difficult to detect and monitor using conventional clinical and radiological techniques, so a circulating tumour marker is potentially very valuable. CA 125 is the most commonly used tumour marker for ovarian cancer. CA 125 is found in derivatives of coelomic epithelium, including pleura, pericardium and peritoneum, but is not detected in normal ovarian tissue.

Diagnosis

CA 125 is elevated in over 95% of patients with advanced (stage III or IV) ovarian cancer, but in less than 50% of patients with stage I disease (Bast et al 1983). However, an elevated CA 125 is not diagnostic of ovarian cancer. Levels above 30 iu ml^{-1} are frequently seen during the first trimester of pregnancy, in patients with endometriosis or with cirrhosis, especially if ascites is present, and in 1% of healthy controls. In addition, over 40% of patients with advanced non-ovarian intra-abdominal malignancies have elevated CA 125 levels. None the less, in a patient suspected of having ovarian cancer, the presence of an elevated CA 125 should prompt the surgeon either to refer the patient to a gynaecological oncologist or to perform the surgery through a more extensive midline incision to allow adequate debulking of tumour.

Screening

Despite the low sensitivity of CA 125 for potentially curable stage I tumours, large screening studies have been performed. One study at the Royal London Hospital measured serum CA 125 in 22 000 postmenopausal well women. Those women who had CA 125 levels above 30 U ml^{-1} underwent pelvic ultrasound, and if that was positive a laparotomy was performed. In all there were 11 confirmed cases of epithelial ovarian cancer (true positives) and 11 cases in whom laparotomy did not reveal an ovarian tumour (false positives). Of note, however, is the fact that only 3 of the 11 patients with screen-detected ovarian cancers had stage I disease (Jacobs et al 1993). A large randomized trial is currently investigating whether serial CA 125 screening plus measurement of OVX1 can lead to improved survival. Apart form women at high risk of familial ovarian cancer, screening for ovarian cancer should not yet be offered to women outside a clinical trial.

Assessing completeness of excision

In order to decide optimum postoperative management, it is important to know whether one is dealing with a patient with completely excised, stage I disease, or whether the patient has residual tumour after surgery. A persistently elevated CA 125 after oophorectomy for suspected stage I disease is definite evidence of residual tumour.

Prognosis and response to treatment

Very high CA 125 levels prior to surgery are associated with a worse prognosis, but knowledge of this is unlikely to lead to any alteration in management. The exception is in women with stage 1 disease where a preoperative level > 65 U/ml has been shown to be a powerful adverse prognostic indicator (Nagele et al 1995). Such patients are candidates for chemotherapy rather than surveillance. Several groups have shown that the CA 125 level after one, two or three courses of chemotherapy, a long half-life or greater than sevenfold fall are the most important prognostic factors for survival. Prognostic information based on CA 125 should not be used to decide therapy, as in nearly 20% of cases where CA 125 predicts a poor prognosis the patient has no cancer progression in the next 12 months (Fayers et al 1993).

Recently, definitions for response based on serial CA 125 estimations have been proposed (Rustin et al 1995) and appear more accurate than scans for monitoring therapy. For use in clinical trials they have to be very precise and use mathematical logic in a computer programme. Put simply, response according to CA 125 has occurred if either of the following criteria are applicable:

- *Either* 50% response has occurred if there is a 50% decrease in serum CA 125 levels. There must be two initial elevated samples. The sample showing a 50% fall must be confirmed by a fourth sample (requires four CA 125 levels).

- *Or* 75% response has occurred if there has been a serial decrease in serum CA 125 levels of more than 75% over three samples (requires three CA 125 levels)

(In each the final sample has to be at least 28 days after the previous sample.) These definitions are particularly useful for clinical trials where they indicate which new treatments are active more easily and cheaply than by the use of standard response criteria.

Detection of progression or relapse

A serial rise of CA 125 of more than 25% appears the most accurate method of predicting progression of ovarian cancer during therapy and could lead to ineffective, toxic and expensive therapy being withheld. A confirmed doubling from the upper limit of normal during follow-up predicts relapse with almost 100% specificity. There is controversy about the role of serial CA 125 measurements during follow-up with the anxiety from knowing CA 125 levels inducing CA 125 *psychosis* in some patients. Although the use of CA 125 estimation to define progression may reduce the number of radiological investigations performed, there is no evidence at present that early reintroduction of chemotherapy or searching for a resectable site of relapse produces any survival benefit. A large MRC and EORTC trial is currently witholding all serial CA 125 results from clinicians and patients during follow-up until the levels double. Patients are then randomized between immediate therapy or the clinician not being informed of the result so the patient continues on observation. Until the results of this trial are available, monitoring by CA 125 during follow-up should be discouraged.

Prostate cancer

Prostate specific antigen (PSA) is the most useful tumour marker in patients with prostate cancer. PSA is a serine protease produced by prostate epithelium with the function of liquefying the gel which surrounds spermatazoa to enable them to become fully mobile. In serum, PSA is found either free or complexed to proteins. PSA has superseded prostatic acid phosphatase as it is elevated in a higher proportion of men with prostate cancer.

Diagnosis, screening and staging

Elevated levels of PSA (>4 ng ml^{-1}) occur in about 53% of men with intracapsular microscopic, and 77% of men with intracapsular macroscopic prostatic cancer, but can also occur in 30–50% of men with benign prostatic hypertrophy (BPH), a condition common in men of similar age group to those who develop prostate cancer (Dorr et al 1993). The combination of PSA and digital rectal examination, followed by prostatic ultrasound in patients with abnormal findings, is commonly used for screening in the USA but is not recommended in the UK as there is so far no evidence of survival benefit from early detection of prostate cancer. There is a vocal debate raging, with those who advocate screening stating that an individual with early prostate cancer may be cured by radical surgery or radiotherapy. Those against screening point out that despite a 9% chance of developing clinical prostate cancer there is only a 1% chance of dying from it and we cannot predict which cancers will be aggressive, so most patients will suffer the side-effects of therapy without any benefit. Furthermore, about 40% of those patients with PSA levels of 4.0–9.9 ng ml^{-1} at screening will already have tumour spread outside the prostate (Catalona et al 1991).

Several methods are being used to improve diagnostic specificity. The best appears to be the measurement of the ratio of free to total PSA as more of the PSA is protein bound in patients with prostate cancer than those with BPH. The ratio of free to total PSA is low (about 10%) in prostate cancer compared to >16% in BPH and prostatitis. Using this ratio increases the specificity for diagnosing prostate cancer from 30% to 61% (Froschermaier et al 1996). PSA density and PSA density of the transition zone rely on ultrasound size estimations leading to lack of precision, but some centres have shown this measurement to improve specificity. Another method is based on the observation that PSA levels generally rise by more than 20% per annum in cases of malignancy. The PSA velocity calculated from serial levels can improve specificity but at the expense of delaying diagnosis.

PSA is inferior to transurethral ultrasound in the detection of capsular invasion. A recently studied research tool is to use the ultrasensitive reverse transcriptase polymerase chain reaction to detect PSA gene expression on circulating prostate cells. This technique might improve staging by detecting preoperatively those patients with extracapsular extension who do not benefit from radical surgery. Patients with PSA levels of <20 ng ml^{-1} can be assumed to have no bone metastases and do not necessarily need bone scans. However, not all patients with a PSA of >20 ng ml^{-1} will have distant metastases. Lymph node metastases are usually associated with elevated PSA.

Prognosis/monitoring response/detection of recurrence

As the PSA level correlates with prostatic volume and tumour differentiation, it is not surprising that a high pretreatment PSA is associated with a poor prognosis. PSA levels fall rapidly to normal after complete removal of tumour by radical prostatectomy, although the rate of fall is slower after successful radiotherapy or endocrine therapy. A serial rise in PSA frequently precedes other evidence of disease progression in the patient with a past history of prostate cancer. The development of back pain in the presence of an elevated PSA level suggests the development of bone metastases.

Hepatocellular carcinoma

Serum AFP is elevated at presentation in 50–80% of UK patients with hepatocellular carcinoma (HCC). Although HCC is one of the most common malignant tumours in the world today, the relatively low incidence in the UK does not justify general population screening, although such screening may be justified in areas such as China with high-incidence populations. In the UK, serial AFP estimation and ultrasound examination can be justified, however, for selective screening of high-risk populations (i.e. patients with cirrhosis, chronic hepatitis B or haemochromatosis) because patients who have successful resection of a solitary, screen-detected tumour have a higher chance of long-term survival. Modest elevations of AFP occur in about 20% of patients with hepatitis, cirrhosis, biliary tract obstruction and alcoholic liver disease and in up to 10% of patients with hepatic metastases. Despite these caveats, a massively elevated AFP in a patient with known cirrhosis is virtually diagnostic of HCC.

Breast cancer

A variety of tumour markers have been studied in patients with breast cancer, including CEA and tissue polypeptide antigen (TPA) and several polymorphic epithelial mucin markers (HMFG1, HMFG2, MSA, MCA, CAM-26, CAM-29 and CA 15-3). The most widely investigated mucin marker in breast cancer is CA 15-3. The commercially available CA 15-3 kit utilizes a sandwich technique which employs two monoclonal antibodies: the 115D8 antibody as the capture antibody and the DF3 antibody as the tracer antibody.

Diagnosis and screening

Although elevated levels of CA 15-3 are found in 55–100% of patients with advanced breast cancer, serum CA 15-3 is raised in only 10–46% of patients with primary breast cancer and in about 10% of patients with early (T1-2 NOMO) operable disease. As 2–20% of patients with benign breast disease have elevated levels, it is clear that mucin assays such as

CA 15-3 are lacking in both specificity and sensitivity as a screening tool. No other tumour marker or combination of markers contribute to the diagnosis of breast cancer (Nicolini et al 1991).

Prognosis/monitoring response to treatment

Elevated preoperative levels of CA 15-3 have been shown to be associated with a poorer prognosis (Kallioniemi et al 1988). However, this may well be due to the association between CA 15-3 and tumour burden, and there is no convincing evidence to date that measurement of CA 15-3, or any other tumour marker, provides significant independent prognostic information. Although tumour marker levels can fall with reduction in tumour burden following systemic therapy, the variation between patients make tumour markers unreliable for assessing response.

Early detection of relapse

The observation that over 60% of patients who develop recurrent breast cancer have raised levels of CA 15-3 suggests a potential value in early detection of recurrence. The use of a panel of tumour markers might further increase the pick-up of recurrent disease. However, it is questionable whether such early detection of relapse will alter survival and thus whether the patient will benefit.

Other cancers

• Neuron-specific enolase is elevated in many patients with advanced small cell lung cancers and in children with neuroblastoma, where it is used for screening.
• Paraprotein levels are very important in the management of patients with myeloma where β_2-microglobulin may be of prognostic value.
• Carcinoid tumours can be monitored by urine levels of 5-hydroxyindole acetic acid (5HIAA), and polypeptides such as gastrin or glucagon are useful in the management of rare gastrointestinal tumours.
• Squamous cell carcinomas are associated with elevated levels of squamous cell carcinoma antigen (SCC) as well as cytokeratin fragments. SCC and CA 125 give valuable prognostic information in patients with cervical carcinoma, and may indicate relapse before scans.
• Calcitonin and calcitonin-gene-related peptide are used in the diagnosis and screening for medullary thyroid carcinoma.
• Serum S-100 and reverse transcriptase polymerase chain reaction to detect mRNA of tyrosinase on circulating melanoma cells are being studied for staging and following patients with melanoma.

There are many other markers not mentioned, either because they are not considered to be of clinical value or because information related to value is inadequate. Many cytokines, growth factors, shed receptors, oncogenes and oncogene products are being investigated as tumour markers, and some may well prove to be useful. Despite many claims, there are no markers that are of use as general cancer screens.

Summary

1. Tumour markers may have a high sensitivity in patients with advanced cancer but most have a low sensitivity in patients with early stage cancer.
2. When using a tumour marker to help in diagnosis it is essential to know its specificity.
3. The potential uses of tumour markers are best demonstrated by HCG, where it is used for screening, diagnosis, determining prognosis, monitoring therapy and in follow up of patients with gestational trophoblastic disease.
4. The most commonly used tumour markers are PSA for prostate cancer, CA 125 for ovarian cancer, CEA for colorectal cancer, and HCG and AFP for germ cell tumours.
5. Before requesting a tumour marker always consider whether the result would alter your management.

References

Allen-Mersh T G, Kemeny N, Niedzwiecki D et al 1987 Significance of a fall in serum CEA concentration in patients treated with cytotoxic chemotherapy for disseminated colorectal cancer. Gut 12: 1625–1629

Bagshawe K D, Harland S 1976 Immunodiagnosis and monitoring of gonadotrophin producing metastases in the central nervous system. Cancer 38: 112–118

Bagshawe K D, Dent J, Webb J 1986 Hydatidiform mole in England and Wales, 1973–1983. Lancet ii: 673–677

Bast R C, Klug T L, St John E et al 1983 A radioimmunoassay using a monoclonal antibody to monitor the course of epithelial ovarian cancer. New England Journal of Medicine 308: 883–887

Begent R J, Rustin G J S 1989 Tumour markers: from carcinoembryonic antigen to products of hybridoma technology. Cancer Surveys 8: 107–121

Bower M, Rustin G J S 1996 Serum tumor markers and their role in monitoring germ cell cancers of the testis. In: Vogelzang N J et al (ed) Comprehensive textbook of genitourinary oncology. Williams & Wilkins, Baltimore, pp 968–980

Catalona W J, Smith D S, Ratliff T L et al 1991 Measurement of prostate specific antigen in serum as a screening test for prostate cancer. New England Journal of Medicine 324: 1156–1161

Dorr V J, Williamson S K, Stephens R L 1993 An evaluation of prostate-specific antigen as a screening test for prostate cancer. Arch Intern Med 153: 2529–2537

Fayers P M, Rustin G J S, Wood R et al 1993 The prognostic value of serum CA 125 in patients with advanced ovarian cancer: an analysis of 573 patients by the Medical Research Council Working Party on Gynaecological Cancer. International Journal of Gynaecological Cancer 3: 285–292

Froschermaier S E, Pilarsky C P, Wirth M P 1996 Clinical significance of the determination of noncomplexed prostate-specific antigen as a marker for prostate carcinoma. Urology 47: 525–528

International Germ Cell Collaborative Group 1997 International germ cell consensus classification: a prognostic factor-based staging system for metastatic germ cell cancers. Journal of Clinical Oncology 15: 594–603

Jacobs I, Prys Davies A, Bridges J et al 1993 Prevalence for screening for ovarian cancer in postmenopausal women by CA 125 measurement and ultrasonography. British Medical Journal 306: 1030–1034

Kallioniemi O P, Oksa H, Aaran R et al 1988 Serum CA 15-3 assay in the diagnosis and follow up of breast cancer. British Journal of Cancer 58: 213–215

Lennon T, Houghton J, Northover J on behalf of the CRC/NIH CEA Trial Working Party 1994 Post-operative CEA monitoring and second-look surgery in colorectal cancer: trial results. British Journal of Cancer 70: 16

Nagele F, Petru E, Medl M et al 1995 Preoperative CA 125: an independent prognostic factor in patients with stage 1 epithelial ovarian cancer. Obstet Gynecol 86: 259–264

Nicolini A, Colombini C, Luciani L et al 1991 Evaluation of serum CA 15-3 determination with CEA and TPA in the postoperative follow up of breast cancer patients. British Journal of Cancer 64: 154–158

Nielsen O S, Munro A J, Duncan W et al 1990 Is placental alkaline phosphatase (PLAP) a useful marker for seminoma? European Journal of Cancer 26: 1049–1054

Rustin G J S, Nelstrop A E, McClean P et al 1995 Defining response of ovarian carcinoma to initial chemotherapy according to serum CA 125 Journal of Clinical Oncology 14: 1545–1551

Postoperative

32

The body's response to surgery

J. P. S. Cochrane

Objectives

- **Understand the wide range of reactions to surgical operations.**
- **Recognize the clinical features resulting from the body's response.**
- **Appraise the importance of reducing the effects of surgical trauma.**

The body responds to trauma with local and systemic reactions that attempt to contain and heal the tissue damage, and to protect the body while it is injured. The response is remarkably similar whether the trauma is a fracture, burn, sepsis or a planned surgical operation, and the extent of the response is usually proportional to the severity of the trauma.

The systemic response, produced by many different mediators, increases the metabolic rate, mobilizes carbohydrate, protein and fat stores, conserves salt and water, and diverts blood preferentially to vital organs. It also stimulates important protective mechanisms such as the immunological and blood clotting systems.

The response aids survival if no other help is available but some of its features are not ideal in a hospital setting. Moreover, severe trauma can lead to a harmful overreaction of the response in which systemic changes cause progressive organ dysfunction, with lethal consequences.

Key points

- **Surgical operation is a controlled form of trauma in which many aggravating factors can be controlled.**

INITIATION OF THE RESPONSE

Various noxious stimuli produce the response but they rarely occur alone, and multiple stimuli often produce greater effects than the sum of single responses. The response is modified by the severity of the stimulus, the patient's age, nutritional status, coexisting medical conditions, medication and if the trauma or operation has affected the function of any particular organ. Recent trauma or sepsis will also modify the response to a subsequent surgical operation.

Pain. Stimuli from the skin, the musculoskeletal system, the visceral stretch receptors and, especially, pulling on the mesentery stimulate the sympathetic nervous system, ACTH and vasopressin (AVP).

Tissue injury. Cell death leads to cytokine release. If sufficient cytokines are produced in the wound they will enter the systemic circulation and the acute-phase response occurs.

Infection. Endotoxin from the cell walls of Gram-negative bacteria is the most powerful stimulus for release of one of the cytokines, tumour necrosis factor (TNF), from macrophages. Infection can also enter the circulation from the bowel if the mucosal barrier is impaired.

Hypovolaemia. Most injuries lead to hypovolaemia, either from haemorrhage, plasma loss in burns or third-space losses. This stimulates baroreceptors, releasing AVP, catecholamines, renin–angiotensin and aldosterone, and leads to impaired excretion of sodium and water. If there is hypoperfusion, toxins and metabolites may be released into the circulation.

Starvation. If starvation accompanies trauma it causes the body to use muscle bulk as a source of protein and the immune response is impaired.

Hypoxia, hypercarbia or pH changes. Chemoreceptors in the carotid and aortic bodies react to these changes and stimulate the sympathetic nervous systems, ACTH and AVP.

Energy substrates. Hypoglycaemia stimulates ACTH, growth hormone, β-endorphin, AVP and catecholamines. Certain amino acids also have particular effects.

Fear and emotion. Stimulate the sympathetic nervous system, AVP and ACTH.

Temperature. Hypothermia, whether due to decreased heat production in prolonged hypovolaemia or starvation, increased heat loss in burns, or induced for cardiac surgery, stimulates the hypothalamus and leads to increased secretion of AVP, ACTH, growth hormone, thyroxine and catecholamines.

SYSTEMS CONTROLLING THE RESPONSE

Four principal systems produce the response:

1. *Sympathetic nervous system.* The immediate fight and flight reaction may help the injured person avoid further injury, but it has short-lasting effects on metabolism.

2. *Acute phase response.* The wound becomes a 'cytokine organ' whose metabolism and local healing responses are controlled by cytokines and other mediators that are produced by different cells in the wound. In severe trauma cytokines produce a systemic 'acute phase' response, with profound changes in protein metabolism, and immunological stimulation; these effects are mostly beneficial but in severe trauma can be lethal.

3. *Endocrine response.* This includes not only the hypothalamic–pituitary–adrenal (HPA) axis but also growth hormone, arginine AVP, thyroxine, insulin and glucagon, causing some metabolic effects, particularly changes in carbohydrate and fat metabolism. This response appears to protect not so much against the stress, but more against the body's acute phase response from overreacting.

4. *Vascular endothelial cell system response.* This affects vasomotor tone and vessel permeability, so it affects perfusion, circulating volume and blood pressure and can lead to septic shock.

Sympathetic nervous system

The central and peripheral sympathetic systems are stimulated particularly by pain and hypovolaemia, and this has direct actions, and indirect effects by releasing adrenaline from the adrenal medulla and noradrenaline predominately from peripheral ganglia. These catecholamines have both α and β effects on sympathetic receptors that prepare the body rapidly for fight or flight by cardiovascular, visceral and metabolic actions.

Cardiovascular effects

Blood is redistributed from the viscera and skin (α effects) to the heart, brain, and skeletal muscles (β_2 effects) and there is an increase in heart rate and contractility (β_1 effects).

Visceral effects

Non-essential visceral functions such as intestinal motility are inhibited and bladder sphincter tone is increased; other actions are: bronchodilatation (β_2); mydriasis (α_1); uterine contraction (α_1); and relaxation (β_2); visual field increases.

Metabolic and hormonal effects

Blood glucose rises due to increased breakdown of liver and muscle glycogen and by gluconeogenesis (α_1), and indirectly by suppression of insulin secretion (α_2) and stimulation of glucagon secretion (β). Other hormonal actions are stimulation of growth hormone (α) and renin (β_1). Lipolysis is stimulated in adipose cells, and ketogenesis is stimulated in the liver.

Acute-phase response

Local effects

Noxious stimuli such as infection, trauma, toxins, haemorrhage or malignancy attract granulocytes and mononuclear cells to the site of injury, and these cells, together with local fibroblasts and endothelial cells, release cytokines. *Cytokines* are peptides produced by a variety of cells (unlike true hormones) and produce mainly paracrine (direct cell-to-cell) effects. Interleukins (IL) 1, 2 and 6, tumour necrosis factor (TNF) and the interferons are the main cytokines. Their actions help to contain tissue damage by contributing to the inflammatory reaction through vasodilatation, increased permeability of vessels, migration of neutrophils and monocytes to the wound, activation of the coagulation and complement cascades, and proliferation of endothelial cells and fibroblasts.

Systemic effects

If cytokine production is large enough, systemic effects occur such as fever, malaise, headache and musculoskeletal pains that encourage energy conservation. They may also produce a leucocytosis, activation of immune function, release of ACTH and glucocorticoids, activation of clotting cascades, an increase in ESR, a decrease in circulating levels of zinc and iron (inhibiting the growth of micro-organisms requiring iron). They also affect the serum levels of *acute phase reactants* (APRs) which are host-defence proteins synthesized in the liver; most increase (such as C-reactive protein, fibrinogen, complement C3, α-antichymo-trypsin, caeruloplasmin, and haptoglobin), but the levels of albumin and transferrin decrease.

- *IL-6* is the main mediator of this altered hepatic protein synthesis.
- *TNF* (cachectin) released primarily from macrophages by bacterial endotoxin, causes anorexia, tachypnoea, fever and tachycardia, with proliferation of fibroblasts and widespread effects on neutrophils; it stimulates production of other cytokines, ACTH, APRs, and amino acids from skeletal muscle, hepatic amino acid uptake, and elevation of plasma triglycerides and free fatty-acids. High concentrations cause multiple-organ dysfunction syndrome (MODS).
- *IL-2* enhances immune function by T-lymphocyte proliferation and by enhancing the activity of natural killer cells.
- *IL-1* in low dosage causes fever, neutrophilia, low serum zinc levels, increased APR synthesis, anorexia, malaise, release of ACTH, glucocorticoid and insulin, and, in high dose, the features of MODS.
- *Interferons*, such as γ-interferon are glycoproteins produced by T lymphocytes which activate macrophages, enhancing both antigen presenting and processing as well as cytocidal activity; γ-interferon is synergistic with TNF, inhibits viral replication, and inhibits prostaglandin release.
- *Prostaglandins* are important components of the inflammatory response. They can be produced by all nucleated cells except lymphocytes, and they increase vascular permeability, cause vasodilatation and leucocyte migration.
- *Leucotrienes* are 1000 times as effective as histamine at increasing postcapillary leakage and they cause increased leucocyte adhesion, vasoconstriction and bronchoconstriction.
- *Kallikreins and kinins.* Bradykinin release is stimulated by hypoxia and it is a potent vasodilator that increases capillary permeability, producing oedema, pain and bronchoconstriction and affecting glucose metabolism.

Interactions between APRs and the endocrine response

IL-1 and IL-6 can activate the HPA axis by increasing ACTH secretion and also directly stimulate glucocorticoid (GC) release from the adrenal gland. GCs initially help cytokines to regulate APRs, but if GC levels remain elevated they inhibit cytokine production.

Endocrine response

The HPA axis is stimulated mainly by the injury itself, but probably its most important function is to control the effects of systemically released cytokines.

ACTH. This is released from the anterior pituitary by neurological stimuli reaching the hypothalamus, or by hormones such as AVP, angiotensin-II or catecholamines. The ACTH response to stress is not inhibited by administered steroids. ACTH stimulates the adrenal cortex to release glucocorticoids and also potentiates the action of catecholamines on cardiac contractility.

Glucocorticoids. These usually have only a 'permissive' action (allowing other hormones to function) but the increased levels after trauma have important metabolic, cardiovascular and immunological actions proportional to the severity of the trauma. *Cortisol* is the main glucocorticoid and its serum level usually returns to normal 24 hours after uncomplicated major surgery but may remain elevated for many days in extensive burns or if infection supervenes. It stimulates the conversion of protein to glucose (catabolic action); it stimulates the storage of glucose as glycogen; it is an antagonist of insulin and this assists gluconeogenesis to increase plasma glucose (diabetogenic action); it helps to maintain blood volume by decreasing the permeability of the vascular endothelium and enhancing vasoconstriction by catecholamines and suppressing synthesis of prostaglandins and leucotrienes (anti-inflammatory action); it also inhibits secretion of IL-1 and IL-2 antibody production and mobilization of lymphocytes (immunosuppressant action).

If the glucocorticoid response is absent (due to previous long administration of steroids or adrenalectomy) the injured person may die from hypoglycaemia, hyponatraemia or circulatory failure.

Aldosterone. The inevitable release of ACTH after trauma stimulates a short term release of aldosterone from the adrenal cortex, but the rise may be prolonged if other stimuli such as hypovolaemia or vasomotor changes (which activate the renin–angiotensin system in the kidney) occur. A rise in plasma potassium concentration can also stimulate aldosterone release. Aldosterone causes increased reabsorption of sodium and potassium secretion in the distal convoluted tubules and collecting ducts, and hence a reduced urine volume.

Arginine vasopressin (AVP). This is released from the posterior pituitary by pain, a rise in plasma osmolality (via osmoreceptors in the hypothalamus), hypovolaemia (via baroreceptors and left atrial stretch receptors), anaesthetic agents or a rise in plasma glucose. Its actions on the distal tubules and collecting ducts in the kidney lead to increased reabsorption of solute-free water; it causes peripheral vasoconstriction especially in the splanchnic bed and it stimulates hepatic glycogenolysis and gluconeogenesis. Its secretion increases for about 24 hours after operation, and during this time the kidney cannot excrete 'free' water (water that is not solute led) so the urine osmolality remains higher than plasma. After head injury, burns or prolonged hypoxia there may be continued secretion of AVP resulting in oliguria and hyponatraemia.

Insulin. In the ebb phase after injury plasma insulin concentration falls because catecholamines and cortisol make the β-islet cells of the pancreas less sensitive to glucose. Glucagon also inhibits insulin release and cortisol reduces the peripheral action of insulin; less carbohydrate is transported into cells and blood sugar rises. In the flow phase plasma insulin rises but blood sugar remains elevated because various intracellular changes make the tissues resistant to insulin.

Glucagon. Glucagon secretion from the α-islet cells of the pancreas increases after injury and this plays a small part in increasing blood sugar by stimulating hepatic glycogenolysis and gluconeogenesis. It also stimulates hepatic ketogenesis and lipolysis in adipose tissue. Cortisol prolongs its actions.

Thyroxine. Total T4 (but not usually free T4) and total and free T3 (the more active hormone) decrease after injury, because cortisol impairs conversion of T4 to T3.

Heat shock proteins (HSPs). These are produced by virtually all cells in response to many stresses (not just heat), mainly via the stimulus of the HPA axis, and they are also elevated in certain tissues in chronic diseases. The ability to produce them declines with age and they appear to protect cells from the deleterious effects of stress and to inhibit synthesis of APRs.

5-hydroxytryplamine. This is a neurotransmitter produced from tryptophan and found in enterochromaffin cells of the intestine and platelets. It is released when tissue is injured and it causes vasoconstriction and bronchoconstriction, increases platelet aggregation and increases heart rate and contractility.

Histamine. Histamine is released from mast cells, platelets, neurones, and the epidermis by trauma, sepsis and hypotension. Its main action is to cause local vasodilatation and increased vascular permeability, so large concentrations may lead to hypotension. It acts on H_1 cell surface receptors to increase histamine precursor uptake and cause bronchoconstriction, and increased intestinal motility and cardiac contractility; it also acts on H_2 receptors that inhibit histamine release and produce changes in gastric secretion, heart rate and immunological function.

Growth hormone. Growth hormone is released from the anterior pituitary as a result of neurological stimulation of the hypothalamus or by a rise in circulating levels of catecholamines, ACTH, AVP, thyroxine, or glucagon. Its plasma levels increase after trauma, hypovolaemia, hypoglycaemia, or a decrease in plasma fatty acids or increase in serum arginine. Its main effects are to promote protein synthesis and enhance breakdown of lipid and carbohydrate stores. It increases plasma fatty acids and ketone bodies through direct stimulation of lipolysis and potentiation of catecholamine effects on adipose tissue and by stimulation of hepatic ketogenesis. It is also associated with a fall in insulin levels that allows plasma glucose to rise.

Endogenous opioids. Endogenous opioids such as β-endorphin increase after trauma and produce analgesia, a rise in blood sugar, a lowering of blood pressure and effects on immune function.

The vascular endothelial cell system response

The scattered 'endothelial organ' weighs about 1.5 kg and after trauma produces short-lived substances that have primarily local actions affecting local vasomotor tone and coagulation, but which can also produce systemic effects on the immune function by affecting platelet and lymphocyte binding. Endothelial cells such as granulocytes can produce oxygen-free radicals (OFR) in response to ischaemia and shock; this leads to cell damage by peroxidation of cell membrane unsaturated fatty acids.

Nitric oxide (NO). This is a powerful vasodilator produced mainly by endothelial cells but also by macrophages, neutrophils, Kuppfer cells and renal cells. It is inactivated by haemoglobin and opposed by endothelins. Its other action is to increase production of APRs.

Endothelins (ET). These are a family of potent vasoconstricting peptides with mainly paracrine actions. They are released by thrombin, catecholamines, hypoxia, cytokines and endotoxins. They counteract NO and prostacyclins to maintain vasomotor tone.

Platelet-activating factor (PAF). This is released from endothelial cells by the action of TNF, IL-1, AVP and angiotensin II. When platelets come into contact with PAF they release thromboxane that causes platelet aggregation and vasoconstriction. PAF also reduces the permeability of endothelial cells to albumin and may also affect glucose metabolism.

Prostaglandins. Prostaglandins cause vasodilatation and reduce platelet aggregation.

Atrial natriuretic peptides (ANPs). These are potent inhibitors of aldosterone secretion and are released by atrial tissue (which is specialized endothelium) in response to changes in chamber distension.

They can also be released by the CNS. It is not yet clear what role they play in the response to injury.

CLINICALLY APPARENT SYSTEMIC EFFECTS OF THE RESPONSE

Hypovolaemia

Most severe injuries cause hypovolaemia, particularly if they are accompanied by blood, gastrointestinal fluid or plasma losses. The acute phase response of vasomotor changes and increased vessel permeability causes fluid loss into the 'third space', the name for a sequestered part of the extracellular fluid (ECF) which includes oedema fluid in the wound, the peritoneal cavity or the lungs. ECF may also shift into cells.

Impaired excretion of water and sodium

Trauma is rapidly followed by a rise in plasma AVP and aldosterone that cannot be suppressed by fluid replacement. During this time there is no free water clearance (so urine osmolality stays higher than plasma osmolality) with impaired excretion of water and sodium. After about 24 hours (depending on the severity of the trauma) these hormones come under normal control mechanisms, so they may stay elevated if there is continuing hypovolaemia. A major but uncomplicated surgical operation with adequate fluid replacement, therefore, is usually followed by 24 hours of impaired free water clearance and about 5 days of impaired sodium excretion. Thus the oliguria which occurs can be increased by increased fluid intake, but only at the expense of an increasing positive balance (i.e. only a proportion of the fluid given will be excreted because part of that fluid passes to the 'third space'). Retention of sodium and bicarbonate may produce a metabolic alkalosis that impairs the delivery of oxygen to the tissues. The diuresis that occurs when this third space fluid mobilizes is a welcome sign of recovery.

Pyrexia

There is usually a 1–2°C increase in body temperature after injury, even in the absence of infection, because the increased metabolic rate is accompanied by an upward shift in the thermoregulatory set point of the hypothalamus. Some of the effects of fever are detrimental, but more are beneficial.

Metabolism after injury

There is an initial 'ebb' phase (Fig. 32.1) of reduced energy expenditure after injury for up to 24 hours. This changes to a catabolic 'flow' phase with increased metabolism, negative nitrogen balance, hyperglycaemia, increased heat production, increased oxygen consumption and weight loss. The increase in metabolic rate ranges from about 10% in elective surgical operations to 50% in multiple trauma and 200% in

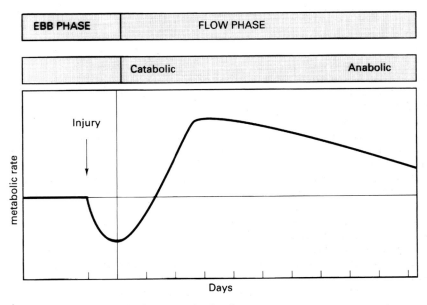

Fig 32.1 Change in metabolic rate relative to preoperative level.

major burns. This may last for days or weeks, depending on the severity of the injury, previous health of the individual and medical intervention; it is less marked at the extremes of age or in previously malnourished individuals. Once started it cannot be stopped rapidly by controlling infection, correcting hypovolaemia, or blocking pain. If recovery occurs it is followed by an anabolic phase in which weight gain is accompanied by restoration of protein and fat stores.

Lipids

Lipids are the principal source of energy following trauma. Lipolysis is produced mainly by catecholamines and increased sympathetic nervous system activity, and also by lower plasma insulin, a rise in ACTH, cortisol, glucagon, growth hormone and, probably, cytokines. Ketones are released into the circulation and are oxidized by all tissue except the blood cells and the CNS. Free fatty acids provide energy for all tissues and for hepatic gluconeogenesis.

Carbohydrates

Hyperglycaemia occurs immediately after injury, because glucose is mobilized from stored glycogen in the liver by catecholamines and glucocorticoids, and because insulin resistance of peripheral tissues impairs their uptake of glucose (the 'diabetes of injury'). It helps to maintain the volume of the ECF, and therefore circulating volume, by shifting water out of cells, and it provides energy for obligate tissue such as the CNS, leucocytes in the wound and red cells (cells not requiring insulin for glucose transport). In major injuries the inflammatory cell infiltrate can account for 70% of glucose uptake.

Body glycogen stores can only maintain blood glucose for about 24 hours. Subsequently it is maintained by gluconeogenesis, stimulated by corticosteroids and glucagon, and this is helped by the initially suppressed insulin levels encouraging the release of amino acids from muscle. Even when insulin levels rise they do not suppress this increased hepatic gluconeogenesis because it is required for clearance of lactate and amino acids which are not used for protein synthesis.

Amino acids

Shortly after injury, skeletal muscle protein breakdown supplies the three- to fourfold increased demand for amino acids (unless there is an exogenous protein source); this reaches a peak after 1 week and may continue for several weeks. The nitrogen loss is proportional to the severity of the trauma, the extent of sepsis and the muscle bulk (so it is greatest in fit young males). A loss of 40% of body protein is usually fatal because it causes the intestinal mucosa to atrophy, resulting in failure of the mucosal barrier to infection. This is probably the main cause of MODS. The mobilized amino acids are used for gluconeogenesis, oxidation in the liver and other tissues, and synthesis of acute-phase reactants. Glutamine is a major energy source for the gastrointestinal tract, for lymphocytes and for fibroblasts during catabolism, and may become an 'essential' amino acid at this time. The catabolic phase is followed by an anabolic phase produced by growth hormone, androgens and 17-ketosteroids.

Albumin

Serum albumin falls after trauma because production by the liver decreases, and loss into damaged tissue increases due to the action of cytokines and prostaglandins on vessel permeability. The accompanying shift of fluid out of the intravascular compartment is a contributing cause of dysfunction in various organs.

Changes in plasma electrolytes

Hyponatraemia is a common occurrence after injury, partly a dilutional effect from retained water (due to AVP), and partly because sodium drifts into cells (impaired sodium pump); it does not indicate sodium deficiency as it occurs at a time when the total body sodium is usually elevated. Serum potassium may rise due to cell death, liberation of potassium by protein catabolism and from impaired potassium excretion.

Acid–base disturbances

The commonest change is a metabolic alkalosis because intense reabsorption of sodium in the distal tubules of the kidney is accompanied by excretion of potassium and hydrogen ions; this impairs oxygen delivery to the tissues because it affects the oxygen–haemoglobin dissociation curve. In more severe injuries a metabolic acidosis is common due to poor tissue perfusion and anaerobic metabolism; this may decrease myocardial contractility and produce arrhythmias as well as decreasing the effect of catecholamines on the myocardium and peripheral vessels.

Other blood changes

A leucocytosis occurs which appears to be due mainly to cytokine-stimulated release of neutrophils from bone marrow. An increase in C-reactive protein and fall in serum albumin are the most easily measured evidence of altered hepatic APR synthesis. Serum iron levels fall.

Wound healing

The systemic responses give 'biological priority' to wound healing, but a wound will still heal more slowly if there are other major injuries.

Immunological responses

Trauma leads to impairment of the immune system, with defects in cell-mediated immunity, antigen presentation, neutrophil and macrophage function, complement activation and bacterial opsonization. This occurs at a time when the initial injury has usually breached mechanical defences, when catabolism impairs the mucosal barrier in the bowel and when many factors contribute to produce pneumonia and other infections.

Cardiac effects

The cardiac index may rise to more than $3.5 \, l \, min^{-1} \, m^{-2}$ after severe trauma, unless there is inadequate preload, previous cardiac disease or acquired cardiac dysfunction.

Pulmonary effects

Areas of lung may be underventilated if secretions obstruct bronchioles and this may lead to shunting of blood and a decreasing P_aO_2 and increasing P_aCO_2. Increased respiratory drive will lead to a respiratory alkalosis and a fall in P_aO_2. Acute lung injury occurs when there is an increasing pulmonary vascular reaction with microemboli, endothelial changes and interstitial oedema.

Coagulation changes

Stimulation of the coagulation cascade and platelets leads to a state of hypercoagulability that may be beneficial at the site of injury but increases the risk of venous thrombi forming. If coagulation is triggered away from the wound, for example by Gram-negative bacteria or hypoxic damage to endothelial cells, then disseminated intravascular coagulation can result.

Systemic inflammatory response syndrome (SIRS)

Severe trauma can lead to this harmful overreaction of the acute-phase response that is defined by set criteria of fever, heart rate, respiration rate, arterial oxygen saturation and white cell count. Bacterial translocation through the bowel is believed to be an important event in this progression. The central problem is impaired extraction of oxygen in the tissues, and this may be due to vasoconstriction and microthrombi impairing the microcirculation, or to a metabolic blockade within individual cells.

Septic shock

Septic shock is a less useful term because the hypotension and perfusion abnormalities with lactic acidosis and oliguria that occur in this condition due to sepsis can also occur in conditions that are not primarily septic.

Multiple-organ dysfunction syndrome (MODS)

SIRS may progress to the multiple-organ dysfunction syndrome (MODS) in which the acutely ill patient has dysfunction of one or more organs, such that intervention is needed to maintain homeostasis. Although the organ dysfunction may be primary and caused directly by the injury it is usually secondary to progressive SIRS. Pulmonary dysfunction is pivotal in SIRS and particularly in MODS and the shunting of blood, reduced compliance and diffuse infiltrates on X-ray are described in milder form as being 'acute lung injury' or in more severe form the 'adult respiratory distress syndrome', which has a 50% mortality. Liver and kidney dysfunction are next commonest and if three organs dysfunction the mortality reaches 90%. The majority of patients who die from burns, trauma or sepsis develop this syndrome.

WAYS OF AFFECTING THE RESPONSE

Although the local response to trauma is beneficial, the systemic response becomes less helpful as the degree of trauma increases, and in a hospital setting it is an advantage to suppress and control the response. In trauma and emergency surgery, pain, bleeding, hypoxia and anxiety have often been present for some hours before surgery starts, whereas in elective surgery it is usually possible to control these stimuli and thereby reduce the systemic response.

 Reduce stimuli causing the response

- **Less trauma**
  - care in handling tissues;
  - minimally invasive surgery
- **Control of infection**
  - antibiotics

– enteral feeding to maintain the mucosal barrier to infection (selective gut decontamination with antibiotic combinations is still being investigated)
- Remove source of toxins
  – debride wounds and drain pus
- Control of pain
  – analgesics, local and regional blockade (given, if feasible, before the noxious stimuli occur)
- Correct hypovolaemia
  – prompt replacement of fluids and electrolytes lost
  – transfusion for haemorrhage
  – colloid for plasma losses
- Correct metabolic alkalosis or metabolic acidosis
- Correct hypoxia
  – attention to airway, breathing or administration of oxygen
- Remove fear and stress
  – give explanations
  – administer analgesics or anxiolytics

Metabolic manipulation

Protein administration to malnourished patients improves their immune function but has no immediate benefit on wound healing. *Enteral feeding* has particular benefits over the parenteral route because it helps to maintain the gut mucosal defence barrier. Increased intake of arginine (which improves weight gain, nitrogen balance, wound healing and immune function) and glutamine (which improves nitrogen balance and prevents the redistribution of body water) can be helpful.

Maintaining ambient *body temperature* at 32°C, especially in burns, may improve nitrogen balance by reducing the need for increased metabolism to replace heat losses.

Drug administration

Ways of manipulating the body's response to trauma are being sought but are still experimental. Many agents are only effective if given before the injury or sepsis occur, and it is difficult to block deleterious responses and still preserve beneficial ones.

Steroids, antiendotoxin antibodies, anti-TNF antibodies, IL-1 receptor antagonists and specific platelet activating factor (PAF) receptor antagonists have increased survival in septic animals but have not yet shown clear advantages in humans, although some are effective if given before the injury. Other agents that have been used are adrenergic blockers (decrease the metabolic rate), aspirin (attenuates cytokine actions), growth hormone (stimulates protein synthesis), mannitol (hydroxyl radical scavenger), propanolol (improves postoperative nitrogen balance), allopurinol (inhibits free radical formation), and atrial natriuretic factor (natiuretic).

Summary

1. Multiple factors in the underlying disease, co-morbidity and the effects of the trauma of a surgical operation cause widespread effects in the body.
2. There may be a wide range of clinically detectable effects.
3. Reducing the stimuli, including trauma, alleviates the effects of surgery.

 Further reading

Beal A L, Cerra F B 1994 Multiple organ failure syndrome in the 1990s. Journal of the American Medical Association 271(3): 226–233

Huljamae H 1993 The pathophysiology of shock. Acta Anaesthesiologica Scandinavica 37(suppl. 98): 3–6

Le Quesne L P, Cochrane J P S, Fieldman N R 1985 Fluid and electrolyte disturbances after trauma: the role of adrenocortical and pituitary hormones. British Medical Bulletin 41(3): 212–217

Mainous M R, Block E F J, Deitch E A 1994 Nutritional support of the gut: how and why. New Horizons 2(2): 193–201

Molloy R G et al 1993 Cytokines, sepsis and immunomodulation. British Journal of Surgery 80(3): 289–297

Woolf P D 1992 Hormonal responses to trauma. Critical Care Medicine 2(2): 216–226

33

Wound healing

S. R. Lakhani, N. Woolf

Objectives

- **Understand the stages of wound healing.**
- **Understand the mechanism of wound contracture, its usefulness and its complications.**
- **Recognize the factors that affect wound healing.**
- **Be familiar with complications that may arise as a result of healing and repair.**

INTRODUCTION

The processes involved in wound healing are some of the most fascinating biological phenomena you are likely to encounter. In this chapter we will examine the processes involved and hopefully appreciate the complex interplay that allows the body to restore the integrity of its tissues. As surgeons, you will be relying on the normal functioning of these processes on a daily basis.

Three fundamental things must happen if wound healing is to occur. Firstly, the circulatory system must be able to control the bleeding (i.e. establish haemostasis). Secondly, the inflammatory response must be effective and provide a defence against microbial infection as well as provide the necessary chemical environment for attracting and stimulating the cells needed for repair. Finally, the process of repair will require many different cells types to proliferate and to synthesize proteins necessary for restoring the integrity and strength to the tissue. Although these three basic processes must occur in the healing of all wounds, you will be aware that not all your patients behave in exactly the same way. The process described above may be modified considerably by the size of the wound, the nutritional status of the patient (and hence their immune competence), the state of the vasculature at the site of injury,

and the metabolic demands of the tissue that has been injured. It is not any one thing but rather a complex interplay between many factors that determines the final outcome.

Wound healing requires

- **Haemostasis**
- **Inflammation**
- **Cell proliferation and repair**

THE PROCESS OF WOUND HEALING

The biological objectives of wound healing are two-fold:

- To restore the integrity of epithelial surfaces if they have been lost and hence protect the underlying tissues against infections and insults from the environment
- To restore the tensile strength of the subepithelial tissue.

Healing by 'primary' and 'secondary intention'

Although the basic mechanisms involved in wound healing are the same, by convention, the healing of cleanly incised wounds, where the edges are in close apposition, is considered separately from those in which there is extensive loss of epithelium, a large subepithelial tissue defect which has to be filled in by scar tissue and where the edges cannot be brought together with sutures. These two circumstances are described as 'healing by primary intention' or 'healing by secondary intention'. These terms first appeared in a surgical treatise published in 1543, although Thomson (1813) in *Lectures on Inflammation*, gives the credit for introducing these terms to Galen.

THE HEALING OF AN INCISED WOUND – 'HEALING BY PRIMARY INTENTION'

Incision involves the division of:

- Epidermis
- Dermal connective tissue fibres and matrix
- Subcutaneous tissue
- Blood vessels.

The very first thing that must be established is haemostasis. Severing of blood vessels obviously leads to haemorrhage with the resulting accumulation of blood within the tissue defect. Injury to blood vessels leads to arteriolar contraction which helps to reduce the bleeding. Platelets and plasma proteins, particularly *fibrinogen* and *fibronectin*, also accumulate. Clotting occurs by both the 'intrinsic' and 'extrinsic' pathways. The former is due to exposure of the collagen and the latter due to release of 'tissue factors' from damaged cells. The platelet plug becomes converted to a clot consisting of polymerized fibrin, which is stabilized by fibronectin binding to it by means of a glutaminase bridge. 'Fibronectin' is the term used for a set of large, extracellular matrix glycoproteins, and the gel formed by fibrin and fibronectin acts in the early stages of healing as a 'glue' which helps to keep the severed edges of the tissue apposed. Thrombin, which is involved in the generation of fibrin, also attracts macrophages and induces fibroblasts to divide. So here we have a molecule that not only has a role in haemostasis but also begins the process of repair. Platelet derived growth factor (PDGF) released from degranulating platelets also has a similar effect on fibroblasts.

At the same time as haemostasis is being established, the process of inflammation is also kicking into action. This involves dilatation of capillaries and the formation of a fluid and cellular exudate. The polymorph leucocytes will attack and remove any bacteria and also scavenge any tissue debris from the cell death. The exudate is responsible for the tissue swelling that occurs. This not only splints and immobilizes the affected area but also the network of fibrin within the exudate forms an infrastructure which helps to localize the microorganisms, hence allowing the polymorphs easy access to them. As mentioned above, one of the biological objectives is to protect the tissues from infectious and environmental hazards and the exudate performs exactly this task by clotting and forming a scab over the wound.

The next important stage is one of cell proliferation and migration. Purely for convenience, the events are divided into those involving the epidermis and those involving the dermis.

Epidermal events

Within a few hours of wounding, a single layer of epidermal cells start to migrate from the wound edges to form a delicate covering over the raw area exposed by the loss of epidermis. The jargon term applied to this spreading process is *epiboly*. Epidermal cell migration across the area of epithelial loss depends on interaction between the keratinocytes at or near the wound edges, fibrin and fibronectin. Fibronectins are present both within plasma and within tissues. Originally they were thought to be cell surface proteins but it is now realized that they constitute part of the extracellular matrix and exert much of their effect by providing sites which act as ligands for receptors on a wide variety of cell types. This ligand–receptor binding mediates cell-matrix adhesion. The binding sites often include the tripeptide arginine-glycine-aspartate (colloquially known as RGD sites). The receptors on cells, which serve as ligands for the RGD sequence, belong to what is known as the *integrin family* of receptors; this includes those surface molecules on phagocytic cells which mediate adhesion to the endothelial cells in the microcirculation. Differences between plasma and tissue fibronectins appear to be mediated by post-translational modifications, differences in splicing being particularly important. In relation to the epidermis in wounds, the type of splicing of fibronectin mRNA resembles that which is found in early embryogenesis. Keratinocytes from normal, unwounded skin do *not* possess receptors which bind to fibronectin, being tightly attached to basement membrane which contains laminin and collagen type IV. Those derived from wounds, however, express a fibronectin receptor which is very similar to a fibronectin receptor expressed on fibroblasts. As already stated, the wound is infiltrated by a gel rich in fibronectin and the activated keratinocytes preferentially adhere to the RGD sequences on the fibronectin and thus migrate across and, indeed, through this matrix. The cells migrate at a rate of approximately two cell diameters per hour.

Epidermal cell movement can provide an initial covering for very small wounds, but in most instances epithelial re-covering cannot be accomplished without proliferation of epidermal cells. The new cells are derived from the stem-cell compartment of the epidermis. From about 12 hours after wounding, there is a marked increase in mitotic activity in the basal cells about three to five cells from the cut edges. This is preceded by an increase in DNA synthesis of about 30% over normal, and similar cycles of increased DNA synthesis and mitosis follow. The new epidermal cells grow under the surface fibrin/fibronectin clot and for a little distance down the gap between the cut edges to form a small 'spur' of epithelium which afterwards regresses. If the wound has been sutured, a similar downgrowth of new epidermis occurs in relation to the suture tracks and, on occasion, these may form the basis of keratin-forming cysts within the dermis – so-called 'implantation dermoid cysts'. This ability of epidermal cells to grow along tracts created by sutures or other foreign material is of course the basis for piercing of tissues for earrings, nose rings, etc.

Dermal events

After the initial arrival of neutrophils to the site of injury, there is recruitment of macrophages into the area (1–2 days after wounding). This is a key event since it is these cells that orchestrate the complex interplay of chemical signs which now takes place. The macrophages are involved in:

• Demolition and removal of any inflammatory exudate and tissue debris.
• Restoring the tensile strength of the subepithelial connective tissue. This is accomplished by: (a) secretion of chemoattractants which recruits cells which synthesize and secrete collagen and other connective tissue proteins (i.e. fibroblasts); (b) expansion of the existing small fibroblast population by stimulating the cells to proliferate, and (c) stimulation of these new fibroblasts to secrete extracellular connective tissue proteins.
• The ingrowth of new small blood vessels (angiogenesis) into the area undergoing repair; this is due to the secretion of TNF-α (tumour necrosis factor) and accumulation of lactate that occurs in anoxic tissues. The angiogenesis involves: (a) budding of new endothelial cells from small intact blood vessels at the edges of the wound, and (b) chemoattraction of these new endothelial cells into the fibrin/fibronectin gel within the wounded area.

In a surgical wound, fibroblasts and myofibroblasts appear in the wound between 2 and 4 days after wounding, and endothelial cells follow about 1 day later. The infiltration of macrophages and fibroblast proliferation are followed, as stated above, by the in growth of new capillary buds which are derived from intact dermal vessels at the margins of the wound. Initially these buds consist of solid ingrowths of endothelial cells, but they soon acquire a lumen. An essential starting step for the ingrowth of new vessels is local degradation of the basement membrane of the existing capillary, this local defect permitting the budding of new endothelial cells. At this stage newly formed capillaries have little basement membrane substance and, compared with a normal capillary, are extremely leaky. This combination of a richly vascularized gel in which both inflammatory cells and collagen-producing fibroblasts are present is known as *granulation tissue*. The term is derived from the observation that the raw surface of a wound shows a granular appearance rather like that seen on the surface of a strawberry. Each of these 'granules' contains a loop of capillaries and hence bleeds easily if traumatized.

The ultimate development of tensile strength in a wound depends on the production of adequate amounts of collagen and on the final orientation of that collagen. Collagen is the only protein which contains large amounts of the amino acids hydroxyproline and hyroxylysine. Within 24 hours of wounding, protein-bound hydroxyproline appears within the damaged area and within 2–3 days some fibrillar material may be seen, though at this time it lacks the dimensions and the typical 64 nm banding of polymerized collagen. Within a few weeks, the amount of collagen in the wounded area is normal, though preoperative tensile strength is not regained for some months. This suggests that replacement and remodelling of the collagen formed early in wound healing is an important part of the whole process. Each type of collagen (there are about ten, of which types I, II and III are the chief fibrillar collagens) consists of three peptide α chains which are wound round each other in a helical pattern. These chains are synthesized in the rough endoplasmic reticulum of the fibroblast. They then undergo post-translational hydroxylation of their proline and lysine moieties and the hydroxylysine is then glycosylated. Linkage of the three chains is accomplished by disulphide bonds. The three chains then become twisted into a helix and the molecule passes to the Golgi zone. Assisted by the microtubules, the soluble procollagen molecules are secreted into the extracellular environment. Solubility is conferred by the presence of an extra peptide. This is removed by a peptidase, and the cleaved molecules then assemble into fibres which gain tensile strength by cross-linking. The typical periodicity of the collagen fibres is due to the assembled molecules having a staggered arrangement. The final result is a scar composed of collagen fibres and very few cells or vessels. The scar therefore changes from pink to white, but this may take many months to occur.

HEALING OF WOUNDS ASSOCIATED WITH A LARGE TISSUE DEFECT – 'HEALING BY SECONDARY INTENTION'

A large volume of tissue loss can occur in cases of severe trauma or extensive burns, or, much less frequently, in relation to certain surgical procedures.

Although qualitatively there are few differences between healing of an incised wound from healing of larger wounds, the most significant problem relates to filling the large defect. Clearly the formation of granulation tissue, and ultimately of scar tissue, occurs, albeit on a far larger scale. One feature, however, that helps to speed up the healing process and which is not seen in relation to healing of incised wounds is wound contraction.

Wound contraction

Two or three days after the formation of large open wounds, the area of raw tissue starts to decrease. This is the expression of a real movement of the wound margins and is quite independent of the rate at which covering by a new epithelial layer can take place. In some fur-bearing animals the raw area may decrease in size by as much as 80% in 2 weeks, and sometimes the degree of contraction may be so great as virtually to close the wound. The wound contraction occurs at a time when relatively little new collagen is being formed in the dermis and subcutaneous tissue, and it therefore seems unlikely that shortening of collagen fibres at the wound margins is responsible for the contraction. Indeed, inhibition of collagen formation does not interfere with the process of wound contraction. There appears to be two mechanisms by which wounds contract. Initially, the scab formed from coagulated exudate containing fibrin contacts. Later, contraction is brought about by the action of cells which appear at the margins of the wound in the first few days and which, on electron microscopy, show features suggesting both fibroblast and smooth muscle differentiation. These cells are called *myofibroblasts*. The cells contain actin, but no smooth-muscle-type myosin within their cytoplasm. For a pulling force to be exerted there must be a connection between the object being pulled and whatever is applying the force. In wound contraction the connection is provided by fibronectin molecules which form bridges between collagen fibres on the one hand and receptors on the myofibroblasts on the other. Thus strips of granulation tissue from healing wounds can be made to shorten in vitro by any pharmacological agents which cause actin fibrils to contract. It has been postulated that a similar mechanism is responsible for the contracture of dermal connective tissue seen in such conditions as Dupuytren's contracture.

Growth factors and cytokines in wound healing

It is clear from what has been said in the previous sections that the cellular events in wound healing must depend on a series of 'instructions' which:

- Facilitate *migration* of fibroblasts and endothelial cells
- Induce these cells as well as the epithelial cells to *proliferate*.

These instructions consist of a set of chemical signals derived from a number of sources. They fall into two principal types: growth factors and cytokines.

Growth factors

Growth factors are peptides which act via one or more of three pathways:

- The *endocrine pathway*, where the growth factors are synthesized at some considerable distance from their targets and are delivered via the bloodstream
- The *paracrine pathway*, where the growth factors are synthesized and released by cells which are in the close proximity of their targets
- The *autocrine pathway*, in which the same cells both synthesize and stimulate their own growth.

The growth factors important in wound healing include platelet derived growth factor (PDGF), epidermal growth factor (EGF) and transforming growth factors α and β (TGF-α and β). We will consider these briefly.

Platelet-derived growth factor (PDGF). Platelet-derived growth factor is a basic protein which has a molecular weight of about 30 000. It consists of two peptides (an A chain and a B chain) which are bound by disulphide bridges. The name 'platelet derived growth factor' is somewhat misleading in two senses. Firstly, while it is certainly stored in the α granules of platelets and released from them when the platelets are activated, the growth factor is also synthesized and secreted from other cells. These include endothelial cells, macrophages, arterial smooth muscle cells and cells from certain tumours. Secondly, PDGF has a number of functions apart from its undoubted powerful mitogenic effect. It is chemotactic for the same cells for which it is a mitogen, it increases intracellular synthesis of cholesterol and also increases binding of low-density lipoprotein (LDL) by increasing the number of LDL receptors expressed on the plasma membrane of the target cell. It increases prostaglandin secretion, initially by making more of the starting material (arachidonic acid) available, and later by stimulating the synthesis of cyclo-oxygenase. It is able to induce changes in cell shape by a reorganization of actin filaments within the cells and it induces increased synthesis of RNA and protein. It is also a potent vasoconstrictor. Thus PDGF can carry out both tasks which were outlined at the beginning of this section. It can attract mesenchymal cells into the wound (with the exception of endothelial cells which do not possess the PDGF receptor) and it acts as a mitogen and stimulator of protein production. PDGF and other growth factors bind to receptors which, after ligand–receptor interaction, act as tyrosine kinases and hence activate the signal transduction pathways for mitogenesis.

Epidermal growth factor and transforming growth factor α. Epidermal growth factor (EGF) is a 53-amino-acid polypeptide which is cleaved from a larger precursor protein. It was discovered by the Nobel laureate Cohen in the course of experiments in which he was engaged in a search for a nerve growth stimulating factor in the salivary glands of baby mice, such a factor having been discovered previously in the salivary glands of snakes. However, extracts of these glands, when injected into baby mice, caused their eyes to open prematurely and their incisor teeth to grow faster, these effects being due to a stimulation of epidermally derived tissues. The factor was purified and is now known as *epidermal growth factor*, though it stimulates mitogenesis in connective tissue as well as in epithelial cells. The salivary glands and the lacrimal glands are storage sites for EGF which can be released in saliva and tears. Thus, licking one's wounds in the literal rather than in the metaphorical sense may be of definite biological advantage, as may be the irrigation of the cornea by tears in corneal abrasion or ulceration. EGF, or a molecule with considerable homology, is also produced in the Brunner's glands in the duodenum and its metabolite, urogastrone, may be measured in the urine. In rodents, EGF may be found in the plasma but in humans, blood-borne EGF is concentrated within the α granules of platelets. Since EGF protein can also be found in the cytoplasm of megakaryocytes in the bone marrow, it seems almost certain that platelet EGF is derived from synthesis within the megakaryocytes rather than by uptake from the plasma. In experimental wounds the application of EGF has been found to significantly accelerate the rate of epidermal regeneration and it has also been shown to have a beneficial effect on the dermal component. In humans, topical application of EGF accelerates the healing of donor sites for skin grafts. There is no evidence that EGF is produced by any of the cells taking part in the healing process, though, as already stated, platelets store EGF. However, there is another factor, known as *transforming growth factor α* (TGF-α), which shows a considerable degree of homology with EGF and which can be produced by both epidermal cells and by macrophages in healing wounds. TGF-α binds to the same receptor on target cells as does EGF and has the same mitogenic effect. In this way TGF-α may be a direct mediator of wound healing.

Transforming growth factor β (TGF-β). Transforming growth factor β (TGF-β) is a polypep-tide, first discovered in culture media conditioned by transformed cells, but produced by almost all cell lines in culture. In the presence of EGF it acts as a mitogen, but in some assays has also been found to inhibit growth. It is possible that these contradictory actions may be a reflection of the different types of assay used and may not tell us much about what is happening in vivo. There is, however, good evidence that macrophages in healing wounds express mRNA for TGF-β as well as for TGF-α. TGF-β has also been shown to be a powerful chemoattractant for monocytes and its release from the first wave of inflammatory cells migrating into the wound may act as a mechanism for recruiting additional monocytes/macrophages.

Cytokines

'Cytokine' is the term used for a group of protein cell regulators which includes such members as lymphokines, monokines, interleukins and interferons. These are low molecular weight proteins (usually less than 80 kDa). They tend to be produced rapidly and locally and can act in either an autocrine or a paracrine fashion. They are produced by a wide range of cells and have many overlapping actions which are mediated by their binding to high-affinity receptors on their target cells. The response of an individual cell to a given cytokine is dependent on the cell type, what other chemical signals are being received at the same time, and the local concentration of the cytokine. Two cytokines which play a significant role in wound healing are interleukin-1 (IL-1) and tumour necrosis factor α (TNF-α) (syn. cachectin).

IL-1. IL-1 (formerly known as endogenous pyrogen) is a small (17 kDa) protein which is produced by a wide variety of cell types, including macrophages and epidermal cells. IL-1 has many biological actions which, in relation to healing, include a proliferative effect on dermal fibroblasts and up-regulation of collagen synthesis by the fibroblasts. It also increases collagenase production and this may be one of the ways in which the collagen in wounds is remodelled so as to achieve maximal tensile strength.

TNF-α. TNF-α is another monocyte/macrophage product which is released following tissue injury or infection. It is the main factor responsible for macrophage-mediated tumour cell killing and is also responsible for the wasting (cachexia) which is seen in certain chronic bacterial and parasitic infections. Its biological activity has a remarkable overlap with that of IL-1, though it does not appear to have the immunoregulatory functions of that molecule. Its receptors, however, are quite distinct from those of IL-1 and presumably the similarities in their actions indicate that they stimulate the same 'second messenger' systems. The expression of TNF-α by monocytes and macrophages requires activation of these cells. This may be brought about by interacting with fibrin (which is always present in wounds), binding of TGF-β, the action of α-interferon and the action of endotoxin.

TNF-α is a potent stimulus for the ingrowth of new blood vessels in healing wounds, being not only chemotactic for endothelial cells but also being the agent responsible for the focal degradation of capillary basement membranes which precedes the migration of endothelial cells into a healing wound.

Important growth factors in healing

- PDGF, EGF, TGF-α and TGF-β

Important cytokines in healing

- IL-1, TNF-α

REPAIR IN SOME SPECIALIZED TISSUES

Bone

The processes involved in the early stages of fracture healing are basically the same as those which have been described in the foregoing sections. Thus the tissue defect created by the fracture is, in the first instance, filled by granulation tissue similar to that in large open wounds. Later, more specific features peculiar to bone are imposed on the basic model of healing. These are necessary because bone, unlike soft tissues, has a mechanical and weight-bearing role. Two types of specialized cell play a central role:

- The *osteoblast*, which lays down seams of uncalcified new bone (osteoid)
- The *osteoclast*, a multinucleated cell probably of macrophage lineage which resorbs bone and which, therefore, remodels the new bone.

Stages of fracture healing

When a bone is fractured, tearing of blood vessels leads to *haemorrhage*, hence the defect between the fractured ends of the bone becomes filled with blood clot and other plasma-derived proteins. As in any other tissue, the injury elicits an *acute inflammatory reaction*, though the degree of neutrophil infiltration is mild. The combined effect of the haemorrhage and the inflammatory oedema causes loosening of the periosteum from the underlying bone ends and this results in a fusiform swelling at the fracture site. Some degree of bone

necrosis is almost inevitable and is due to the blood supply to some areas being cut off as a result of damage to blood vessels. It takes 24–48 hours for the first morphological evidence of bone necrosis to become apparent, the marrow being the site of the first changes. Fat necrosis is seen and if haemopoietic marrow is involved the cells lose their nuclear staining. So far as the bony tissue itself is concerned, the extent of necrosis depends on the anatomy of the local blood supply, and some sites such as the talus, the carpal scaphoid and the head of the femur are particularly likely to show significant ischaemic necrosis after fracture. Empty lacunae, the dead osteocytes having disappeared, are a reliable indication of bone necrosis. *Macrophages* then invade the fracture site and commence the process of demolition. This is followed by the formation of granulation tissue which also extends upwards and downwards within the marrow cavity for a considerable distance from the fracture site. Within the granulation tissue small groups of cartilage cells begin to differentiate from connective tissue stem cells.

Provisional callus is the term used to describe a cuff of woven bone admixed with islands of cartilage which serves to unite the severed portions of bone on their external aspect but not across the gap between the bone ends. The origin of the callus is from two sources, and the relative proportions of these vary depending on a number of factors. The first and more important is the *periosteum*. The cells on its inner aspects proliferate and begin to lay down woven bone (i.e. bone in which the collagenous osteoid tissue is not deposited in a lamellar or 'onion skin' fashion but in series of short bundles of parallel fibres, each bundle having a different orientation). Where the periosteum has been raised from the external surface of the bone the new woven bone fills the gap so that there are two cuffs of new bone around the periosteal aspect of the separated fragments. These cuffs then extend upwards and downwards until they meet, though there is, as yet no direct union across the gap between the separated bone ends. The degree of efficiency with which the external callus formation occurs depends on the adequacy or otherwise of the blood supply around the fracture site. Some of the new blood vessels are derived from the periosteum itself, while others come from the muscle and other soft tissues which abut onto the fractured bone. The amount of cartilage admixed with this periosteal new bone is small in human fractures which are healing well, but tends to be greater in cases where the local blood supply is poor or where the fractured bone ends have not been properly immobilized. The second source of provisional callus is the *medullary cavity* where, following the formation of granulation tissue, fibroblasts and osteoblasts start to proliferate and lay down bone matrix. Some of this is deposited on trabeculae of dead bone while the remainder forms new trabeculae. Well after the provisional callus has been formed, the clot which fills the gap between the fragments is invaded, first by granulation tissue capillaries and then by osteoblasts. Ossification within this gap may occur as a primary event, the osteoblasts being derived from the provisional callus. In some cases the bone ends are united by fibrous tissue and over a period of time this is replaced by woven bone. This takes far longer than direct ossification and is more likely to occur if the fracture has not been properly immobilized or if there is any other factor present which is likely to inhibit healing (i.e. infection or extensive and severe periosteal damage). Occasionally the fibrous tissue filling the gap is not replaced by bone (non-union) and weight bearing by the affected limb is not possible. In cases of delayed or non-union some improvement may be brought about by electrical stimulation, which appears to accelerate ossification at fracture sites. Once union has occurred and the patient is bearing weight, the lumpy new cortical bone gradually becomes resorbed and smoothed out and the excess medullary new bone is similarly removed, with restoration of a normal medullary cavity. Woven bone, which is quite rapidly formed and which is much less efficient at weight bearing, is resorbed completely and is replaced by lamellar bone. This is a lengthy process of *remodelling* and restoration to normal may take up to a year.

Nervous tissue

The central nervous system

Most neurons cannot be replaced once they have been lost, though there is some evidence to suggest that a limited degree of regeneration can take place in the hypothalamic–neorohypophyseal system. In contrast to the peripheral nerves where injury is not associated with any marked tendency towards scarring, necrosis within the central nervous system elicits the proliferation of glial cells which, together with the ingrowth of capillaries, may constitute a physical barrier to the regeneration of new neuronal fibres.

Peripheral nerves

When an axon is severed, the nerve cell shows chromatolysis (i.e. it swells and the Nissl granules which represent zones of the endoplasmic reticulum studded with many ribosomes disappear). The axon swells and becomes irregular, and its lipid-rich myelin sheath splits and later breaks up. The surrounding Schwann cells proliferate and accumulate some of the lipid released from the damaged myelin. Soon new neurofibrils start to sprout from the proximal end of the severed axon and these invaginate the Schwann cells, which act as a guide or template for the new fibrils. The neurofibrils push their way down through the Schwann cells at a rate of about 1 mm per day. Eventually they may reach the appropriate end organ and their myelin sheaths are reformed as a result of the secretory activity of the Schwann cells and, in this way, a degree of functional recovery is attained. In some instances neurofibril sprouting takes place but the fibrils do not grow down existing endoneurial channels, and grow instead in a haphazard fashion. The end result may thus be a tangle of new nerve fibres embedded in a mass of scar tissue. This produces a 'traumatic' or 'stump' neuroma.

FACTORS AFFECTING WOUND HEALING

Failure to heal satisfactorily can be the result of either systemic or local factors.

Systemic factors

Nutrition

The state of nutrition of the patient is a potent factor in determining the success or failure of the healing process. Malnutrition causes depression of the immune system and hence wound infection, and the inflammatory response to this may delay healing. Deficient protein intake may inhibit collagen formation and so inhibit the regaining of tensile strength. In this regard, sulphur-containing amino acids such as methionine seem to be particularly important, and increasing the intake of this amino acid alone can partially offset the effects of a low protein intake on wound healing. Vitamin C has an important role in healing. It has been known since the 17th century that scurvy is associated with poor healing of wounds and fractures. Indeed, there are colourful descriptions of old wounds, acquired honourably or otherwise in combat, breaking down after the onset of scurvy. Vitamin C lack has been found to inhibit the secretion of collagen fibres by fibroblasts and this is due to a failure of hydroxylation of proline in the endoplasmic reticulum of the fibroblast. In addition, Vitamin C concentrations in biological fluids appear to affect the production of galactosamine and hence the deposition of chondroitin sulphate in the extracellular matrix of granulation tissue. Vitamin A has important functions in relation to morphogenesis, epithelial proliferation and epithelial differentiation, and the latter two are believed to be important in wound healing. A role for zinc in wound healing was discovered more or less by accident. In the course of a study on the effects of certain amino acids on wound healing, a phenylalanine analogue which had been expected to impair healing instead accelerated it. Careful study of this analogue revealed that the sample used had been contaminated by zinc. Further studies showed that zinc does indeed accelerate the healing of experimental wounds. Zinc deficiency, such as is found in patients who have been on parenteral nutrition for long periods and in patients with severe burns, is associated with poor healing and this is reversed by the administration of zinc.

Steroid hormones

Many studies show that glucocorticoids have an inhibitory effect on the healing process and on the production of fibrous tissue. Steroids are therefore administered in situations where inappropriate scarring is taking place, such as in interstitial fibrosis in the lung. It is still not clear whether steroids exert their effect indirectly by damping down the inflammatory process or whether they act directly on fibroblasts to alter collagen deposition.

Local factors

The presence of foreign bodies or infection

The presence of infection or of a foreign body will increase the intensity and prolong the duration of the inflammatory response to injury. It is worth remembering that fragments of dead tissue, such as bone, and other elements of the patient's own tissues which have become misplaced, such as hair or keratin, act as foreign bodies.

Excess mobility

The oedema that occurs following tissue injury may lead to immobilization of that part, hence the fifth cardinal sign of inflammation: 'loss of function'. Although this can be troublesome, it also has the benefit of aiding the healing process. It will be clear to everyone that a fractured bone is not going to heal unless it is immobilized. Excess mobility in any tissue will impair healing and prolong the time to full recovery.

Vascular supply

The degree of arterial perfusion and the efficacy of venous drainage play key roles in the healing of injured tissues. Where the arterial perfusion is compromised by

stenosis or occlusion a trivial injury may give rise to a disproportionate degree of tissue damage and healing may be delayed or even completely inhibited. A good example is diabetes mellitus. In patients with long standing disease, trivial injuries develop into chronic, non-healing ulcers. Blood vessel disease affecting both the large muscular arteries of the lower limb (atherosclerosis and its complications) and changes in the walls of arterioles and capillaries probably make the major contribution to failures of healing. These patients are of course also susceptible to infection (particularly if their diabetes is badly controlled) and may also have a sensory neuropathy which makes them more liable to sustain injuries to their extremities.

Adequate venous drainage is also important, and impairment of this may play a part in the genesis of chronic ulcers, which often occur on the anterior surface of the legs in elderly patients. Histological examination of the margins of these lesions suggests that drainage is compromised by the presence of cuffs of polymerized fibrin round the venules. This can, in part, be prevented by administration of the synthetic steroid stanozolol. Suboxygenation of normally perfused tissue, such as may occur in the presence of severe anaemia, will also lead to defective healing.

 Factors modifying healing

- **Nutrition malnutrition, vitamin deficiency**
- **Steroids**
- **Systemic disorders, e.g. diabetes**
- **Vascular supply**
- **Mobility of affected tissues**
- **Infection**

COMPLICATIONS OF HEALING

Although the basic processes involved in healing are designed to be protective, they do occasionally go wrong. This occurs due to a loss of control in the complex interplay between the many varied cellular and chemical processes. Two complications worthy of mention are hypertrophic scar and keloid. Although these haunt all surgeons, they are a particular problem for the plastic surgeon. Hypertrophic scar is simply an overgrowth of scar tissue which causes a raised firm ridge. When the tissue overgrowth is so exuberant that it greatly exceeds the borders of the scar, it is called a keloid. Unfortunately some patients have a tendency to form keloids (more common in black people) and hence excision of the keloid only results in more keloid.

It is worth remembering that due to the contraction

that occurs during wound healing, excessive tissue destruction, especially around joints, may result in contractures and joint deformity.

Summary

1. Wound healing is a complex process relying on the integrated actions of the coagulation system, the inflammatory response and the chemical mediators required to stimulate cell proliferation and protein secretion.
2. The processes are fundamentally the same in cleanly incised wounds and in large open wounds.
3. A similar process also occurs in specialized tissues such as bone, with some changes related to functional demands of that tissue.
4. The healing process can be modified by many factors including nutritional status, steroids, infection and excess mobility of affected parts.
5. Although designed to be protective, complications as a result of contractures and exuberant scar formation produce clinically significant morbidity.

Further reading

Kirsner R S, Eaglestein W H 1993 The wound healing process. Dermatology Clinics 11(4): 629–640

Lakhani S R, Dilly S A, Finlayson C J 1998 Basic pathology: an introduction to the mechanisms of disease, 2nd edn. Edward Arnold, London, pp 78–86

Majno G, Joris I 1996 Wound healing. In: Cells, tissues and disease. Principles of general pathology. Blackwell Science, Oxford, pp 465–485

Waldorf H, Fewkes J 1995 Wound healing. Advances in Dermatology 10: 77–96

34

Postoperative care

J. J. T. Tate

> **Objectives**
>
> - Understand the principles of patient management in the recovery phase immediately after surgery.
> - Understand the general management of the surgical patient on the ward.
> - Consider the initial management of common acute complications during the postoperative period.

INTRODUCTION

Postoperative care of the surgical patient has three phases:

1. Immediate postoperative care (the recovery phase)
2. Care on the ward until discharge from hospital
3. Continuing care after discharge (e.g. stoma care, physiotherapy, surveillance).

The intensity of postoperative monitoring depends upon the type of surgery performed and the severity of the patient's condition.

THE RECOVERY PHASE

Basic management

Immediately after surgery patients require close monitoring, usually by one nurse per patient, in a dedicated recovery ward or area adjacent to the theatre. Monitoring of airway, breathing and circulation is the main priority, but a smooth recovery can only be achieved if pain and anxiety are relieved; monitoring the patient's overall comfort is essential. The nature of the surgery will determine the intensity of monitoring and any special precautions, but children, the elderly, patients with coexisting medical disease and patients who have had major surgery all require special care.

Management of the general comfort of the patient includes:

- Relief of pain and anxiety
- Administering mouthwashes (a dry mouth is common after general anaesthesia)
- The patient's position, including care of pressure points
- Prophylactic measures against
  - atelectasis by encouraging deep breathing, and
  - venous stasis by passive leg exercises.

These steps, including the prophylactic measures, all start in the recovery area and will continue on the main ward.

Airway and breathing

Patients may have an oral airway, a nasopharyngeal airway or, occasionally, may still be intubated on arrival in recovery; all secretions must be cleared by suction and the artificial airway left until the patient can maintain their own. Breathing may be depressed and a patient hypoxic due to three factors:

- Airway obstruction
- Residual anaesthetic gases
- The depressant effects of opioids.

Oxygen is given, ideally by mask, and the oxygen saturation monitored by a pulse oximeter. Special care is needed for patients with a new tracheostomy. If there is concern about vomiting and the risk of aspiration, patients can be sat up or nursed head-up rather than supine.

Circulation

Blood pressure is recorded quarter-hourly or, after major surgery, continuously via a radial artery cannula. The pulse rate is recorded regularly and continuously monitored by a pulse oximeter. The wound and any drains are monitored for signs of reactionary bleeding.

Fluid balance

Before patients are returned to the ward their calculated fluid losses should be replaced with blood, blood products or crystalloids, and, ideally, fluid balance achieved. Monitoring of central venous pressure (CVP) can assist fluid balance management in severely ill patients or after major surgery. Urine output measurement may also provide useful information.

Core temperature

The patient's temperature is monitored as there may be a significant drop during surgery, which should be corrected before they leave the recovery room (e.g. space blanket). As the temperature rises, peripheral vasodilatation may occur; if not anticipated this can lead to hypotension after the patient has returned to the ward.

Special factors

Specific medical conditions and certain types of surgery will require additional monitoring. Some examples are:

- Diabetes mellitus – blood sugar monitoring
- Cardiac disease – electrocardiogram (ECG) monitor
- Orthopaedic surgery – monitoring of distal perfusion in a treated limb, position of limb, maintenance of fracture reduction, examination for peripheral nerve injury
- Neurosurgery – quarter-hourly neurological observations, intracranial pressure monitoring (intraventricular catheter or a transducer in the subarachnoid space)
- Urology – catheter output (after transurethral prostatectomy bladder irrigation is usually implemented and pulmonary oedema can develop if glycine has been absorbed into the circulation; fluid balance is particularly important)
- Vascular surgery – distal limb perfusion.

Pulse oximeter versus arterial blood gas

The pulse oximeter is an essential piece of equipment for the management of the postoperative patient. It monitors three parameters: pulse rate, pulse volume and oxygen saturation. The fingertip sensor contains two light-emitting diodes (LEDs); one red, measuring the amount of oxygenated haemoglobin, the other infrared, measuring the total amount of haemoglobin. The actual amount of oxygen carried in the blood relative to the maximum possible amount is computed – this is the oxygen saturation (S_aO_2). The delivery of oxygen to the tissues depends on:

- Cardiac output
- Haemoglobin concentration
- Oxygen saturation (S_aO_2).

The relationship between oxygen in the blood and S_aO_2 is linear and thus easy to interpret. A fall in oxygen reaching the tissues can be detected far more rapidly with S_aO_2 monitoring than by clinical observation of the lips, nailbeds or mucous membranes for cyanosis (which may only be apparent when the S_aO_2 is 60–70%) or by measuring arterial blood gases. It should be noted that pulse oximetry does not indicate adequate ventilation; the S_aO_2 can be normal due to a high inspired oxygen level.

Blood gases

Arterial blood gases measure pH, arterial oxygen and carbon dioxide tensions (P_aO_2, P_aCO_2), bicarbonate and base excess. These measurements are affected by many variables and can be difficult to interpret. The P_aO_2 has a non-linear relationship to the oxygen content of the blood (the oxygen dissociation curve), and hence oxygen saturation is easier to use in practice.

P_aCO_2 reflects the rate of excretion of carbon dioxide by the lungs and is inversely proportional to the ventilation (assuming constant production of carbon dioxide by the body). The base excess and bicarbonate reflect acid–base disturbances and may be used in conjunction with the P_aCO_2 to distinguish respiratory from metabolic problems.

The recovery phase

- **Management of pain and anxiety is as important as care of airway, breathing and circulation**
- **Restoring body temperature is important for prevention of circulation and clotting problems**
- **S_aO_2 (pulse oximeter) has a linear relationship to the amount of oxygen in the blood giving a sensitive indication of tissue oxygenation**

CARE ON THE WARD

Patients may be discharged from the recovery area when they are able to maintain their vital functions independently (i.e. full consciousness and stable respiratory and cardiovascular observations).

On the ward the aim is to maintain a stable general condition and detect any complications early. Initially, closer and more frequent observation is necessary and the priorities are the same as in the recovery room. Nursing staff perform routine observations; medical staff must undertake additional, clinical monitoring dictated by the nature of the case, including daily review of drug prescriptions (Box 34.1).

General care

General care includes those measures described previously and control of pain. Early ambulation can reduce the risk of thrombotic complications. Patients who cannot mobilize require particular attention to skin care and pressure areas. Appropriate explanation of the results of the operation and the expected postoperative course should be given to the patient and relatives. The nature of the surgery or underlying disease will determine additional specific management (e.g. physiotherapy after orthopaedic surgery, stoma care for a new stoma).

Pain control

It is impossible for a patient to make a smooth recovery from surgery without adequate pain control (see Ch. 35).

Box 34.1   The postoperative ward round – a daily checklist

A fresh assessment of each patient is required at each ward round, often daily but more frequently for seriously ill patients. Only a few factors may change on each occasion but all should be considered.

Look at the **patient**, look at the **charts**, look at the **drug chart** and **communicate**.

Enquire
- General comfort
- Pain control
- Thirst
- Specific symptoms

Examine
- General condition
- Respiration and chest (oxygen saturation if appropriate)
- Surgical wound
- Peripheral circulation/nerves (vascular/limb surgery)
- Drains and tubes (content, kinks or blockage, loss of vacuum)
- Pressure areas
- Drip sites

Box 34.1 (contd.)

Check
- Pulse and blood pressure
- Temperature
- Urine output
- Fluid balance (assess insensible loss, e.g. sweating, diarrhoea)
- Special monitoring (e.g. diabetics – blood sugars)
- Results of blood tests/investigations

Review
- Nutrition/oral fluid and dietary intake
- Analgesia management
- Intravenous fluid prescription (volume, sodium and potassium need)
- Antibiotic prescription
- Other postoperative drugs
- Regular prescription medicines (when to start oral medication)

Inform
- What operation/treatment has been done and result
- Comment on progress over previous 24 hours
- Expected course over next few days
- Results of investigations/histology
- Likely day of discharge (identify any special requirements early)

Communicate
- Receive reports from named nurse, physiotherapist, etc.
- Advise changes of management
- Advise frequency/nature of observations required
- Write in the notes

There has been a general shift from intermittent intramuscular analgesia to intravenous analgesia, either by continuous infusion or patient-controlled bolus, or epidural analgesia after major surgery. An epidural is particularly useful after major abdominal surgery, but insertion of an epidural catheter in patients who have received a preoperative dose of heparin for deep vein thrombosis prophylaxis is controversial and contraindicated if the patient has a coagulopathy.

For day surgery or minor operations oral analgesia is suitable and is most effective when prescribed regularly. Narcotics can still be used if required. Non-steroidal anti-inflammatory drugs (NSAIDs) are popular but must be avoided in some patients, including asthmatics and those with a history of peptic ulcer or indigestion. Rectal administration of NSAIDs to a sedated patient should only be given with preoperative consent.

Fluid balance

Fluid balance is important after major surgery and easier if a urinary catheter is in situ allowing accurate charting of urine output. Visible fluid losses are recorded on a fluid balance chart at regular intervals (e.g. hourly for urine output, 4-hourly for nasogastric aspirations, and 12- or 24-hourly for output into drains) and totalled every 24 hours. Unrecorded fluid losses (e.g. evaporation from skin and lungs, losses into hidden spaces such as the intestine, and diarrhoea) must be estimated and added to the recorded losses to calculate the patient's subsequent fluid requirements (see Ch. 10).

Fluid requirement

For the typical 70 kg patient, intravenous fluid requirement after operation is 2.5 litres per day, of which 0.5 litre is normal saline and the remainder 5% dextrose; potassium is added after the first 24 hours once 1.5 litres of urine have been passed. Typically, the sodium requirement is 1 mmol kg^{-1} (normal saline contains 140 mmol l^{-1} of sodium) and potassium 1 mmol kg^{-1}.

If the dissection area at operation has been large there will be a greater loss of plasma into the operation site and this may need to be replaced with colloid (e.g. Haemaccel) in the early postoperative period. In addition to these basic requirements, gastrointestinal losses are replaced volume-for-volume with normal saline with added potassium. Daily plasma urea and electrolyte measurement are advisable while the patient is dependent on intravenous fluids.

Monitoring

Clinical monitoring should include asking the patient about thirst, assessing central and peripheral perfusion, examination of dependent areas for oedema, and auscultation of the chest. Tachycardia is an important sign that can indicate fluid overload or dehydration, but is also caused by inadequate analgesia.

Patients in whom fluid balance is difficult to manage, or where there is a particular risk of cardiac failure, may require central venous pressure monitoring or even left atrial pressure recording.

Hypovolaemia

Oliguria (defined as a urine output of less than 20 ml h^{-1} in each of two consecutive hours) in postoperative patients is caused by hypovolaemia in the majority of cases, but always consider a blocked catheter or cardiac failure. Hypovolaemia may be due to:

- Unreplaced blood loss
- Loss of fluid into the gastrointestinal tract
- Loss of plasma into the wound or abdomen
- Sequestration of extracellular fluid into the 'third' space.

Blood transfusion

Haemoglobin measurement will be a guide to the need for blood transfusion unless plasma or extracellular fluid loss causes an artificially high measurement; this is most likely in the first 24 hours after surgery and it is generally not necessary to monitor haemoglobin levels more than 72 hours postoperatively. In a stable patient, a top-up transfusion is indicated if the haemoglobin level is less than 8 g% (determined by studies in Jehovah's Witnesses), while above this level patients should be given oral iron. An unstable patient, one who may re-bleed, requires a higher threshold for transfusion of at least 10 g%. If blood transfusion is given, frequent, regular monitoring of pulse, blood pressure and temperature are routine to detect a transfusion reaction.

Complications

A major ABO incompatibility can result in an anaphylactic hypersensitivity reaction (flushing/urticaria, bronchospasm, hypotension). Incompatibility of minor factors is usually less severe and is indicated by tachycardia, pyrexia and possible rash and pruritus. The transfusion should be stopped, some blood sent for culture (both from patient and donor blood) and the remainder of the unit returned to the blood bank for further cross-matching against the patient's serum. However, if the reaction is mild it may be appropriate to give steroids or an antihistamine and to continue the transfusion (see Ch. 9).

Nutrition

Nutrition in postoperative patients is frequently poorly managed and treatment delayed. Dietary intake should be monitored in all patients, but usually only requires specific management in patents undergoing major abdominal surgery or in whom eating or swallowing is impossible. A basic indication for postoperative nutritional support is inability to eat (actual or expected) for more than 5 days. Serum protein is a crude but easily measured index of nutrition, and measurement of weight is useful over a period of time; more specific tests such as skin-fold thickness or estimation of nitrogen balance are used infrequently (see Ch. 11).

If nutritional support is required, enteral feeding is preferable, if possible, because it has a lower complication rate than parenteral nutrition. Fluid balance and electrolyte monitoring are required and treatment should be given to reduce diarrhoea, which may be precipitated by high-calorie regimens. Parenteral feeding requires monitoring of the venous access point for sepsis, plasma and urinary electrolytes, blood sugar, plasma trace elements (e.g. magnesium) and liver function. The patient's fluid balance must be carefully managed.

Surgical drains

Nasogastric tubes

Nasogastric tubes drain fluid and swallowed air from the stomach and should be left on free drainage at all times with intermittent aspiration (4-hourly). There is rarely a need to leave a nasogastric tube spigoted; once drainage has fallen below 100–200 ml per day the tube can be removed.

Chest drains

Pleural drains are attached to an underwater seal because the pleural space is at subatmospheric pressure. If the lung does not expand fully, then low-pressure, high-volume suction may be added. When a drain is bubbling it should not be clamped because there is a danger of tension pneumothorax if the clamp is forgotten or left too long; however, it is essential that the bottle is never raised above the level of the patent's chest since there is a risk that fluid will syphon back into the pleural cavity.

The drain is removed when:

- Bubbling has stopped for 24 hours
- There is no bubbling when the patient coughs
- The daily chest X-ray shows that the lung is fully expanded.

Check X-rays should be taken at 24 and 48 hours after removal of the drain.

Drains at the operative site

Drains at the operative site are used for the removal of anticipated fluid collections, not as an alternative to adequate haemostasis, and are usually simple tube drains or suction drains (check daily that the vacuum is maintained). Such drains should be removed early; if left in place they will not reduce the risk of a subsequent abscess and may introduce infection, if there is a chronic collection of fluid (such as an abscess or empyema) the drain may be left for several days to create a track. This type of drain is often removed a few centimetres at a time over several days (shortening) in an attempt to prevent the track closing too quickly; a sinogram may be used to confirm that the abscess cavity is shrinking.

Complications

All drains have similar potential complications:

- Trauma during insertion
- Failure to drain adequately due to
  - incorrect placement
  - too small size
  - blocked lumen
- Complications due to disconnection
- Introduction of infection from outside via the drain track
- Erosion by the drain of adjacent tissue
- Fracture of drain during removal (retained foreign body).

DAY-CASE SURGERY

After day-case operations the postoperative period is inevitably short, but management should follow the same basic principles outlined above. Special considerations are:

- Is the patient being discharged to a suitable environment?
- Can adequate, non-parenteral pain control be achieved?
- Possible side-effects of sedation and anaesthesia.

Patients who have had a general anaesthetic or sedation must be accompanied home and should not drive for at least 24 hours. Written advice and instructions should be given both to the patient and to their accompanying relative or friend.

Local anaesthetic

The main problems with local anaesthesia are systemic toxicity of the anaesthetic agent and reactionary haemorrhage if adrenalin has been employed.

Toxicity

All the commonly used local anaesthetics (lignocaine, bupivicaine and prilocaine) are cardiotoxic. Initial symptoms are paraesthesiae around the lips, tinnitus and/or visual disturbance. These are followed by dizziness, which may progress to convulsions and cardiac arrhythmia and collapse. Such complications are prevented by strict adherence to maximum dosage schedules (Table 34.1).

Treatment of systemic toxicity is directed firstly towards maintaining ventilation (hypotension is uncommon in the absence of hypoxia):

- Give 100% oxygen and maintain the airway (by intubation if necessary)
- Control convulsions with intravenous diazepam
- Establish an ECG monitor; various arrhthymias can occur
- If cardiac arrest occurs, start with high energy (360–400 J) DC shock and continue resuscitation attempts for at least 1 hour.

Sedation

For sedoanalgesia or sedation alone (e.g. endoscopy patients) particular attention is paid to monitoring respiration. During upper gastrointestinal endoscopy, delivery of oxygen by nasal spectacles is mandatory. All sedated patients should have a pulse oximeter attached during the procedure and until they are fully awake. The use of the antagonist flumazenil to reverse the sedative effects of benzodiazepines can be associated with delayed respiratory depression as the reversal agent may have a shorter half-life than the sedative itself. Midazolam, with a shorter half-life, is preferred to diazepam. All patients given sedation should be observed for at least 2 hours before being sent home.

CARE AFTER HOSPITAL DISCHARGE

The key is good communication. The patient should understand what treatment they have had, its effect, the

likely time period required to complete their recovery and special restrictions on normal activity. Whenever appropriate, the relatives should also have this information. As many complications (e.g. wound infection) occur in the first week or two after hospital discharge, it is essential that the patient's GP is aware of the diagnosis and treatment given and also what information the patient has received. Ensure arrangements are made to communicate histology results to the patient and plans for additional investigation or treatment have been made and explained to the patient.

Postoperative care

- **Adequate management of postoperative pain is essential**
- **Poor management of fluid balance is probably the greatest cause of avoidable morbidity after major surgery**
- **It is essential to know the maximum dosage for local anaesthetic agents and how to manage toxicity**
- **Clear and concise communication with the patient and other health professionals involved in care will prevent problems and confusion**

PROBLEMS IN THE POSTOPERATIVE PATIENT

The incidence and nature of postoperative complications depends upon the nature and extent of the operative intervention (see Ch. 36). Many are self-evident, but some specific problems are discussed below.

Cyanosis/respiratory inadequacy

The time between onset of respiratory problems and surgery may suggest the cause. In the recovery phase, it may be due to inadequate reversal of anaesthesia or excess opiates and the anaesthetist should be called.

Opiate overdosage usually presents in a drowsy patient with shallow, infrequent breaths, while airway obstruction is associated with obvious efforts to breathe, undrawn intercostal muscles and agitation.

Airway obstruction

If a patient is in respiratory distress give verbal reassurance and 100% oxygen by mask. If cyanosed, check the pulse as the most common cause is cardiac arrest.

Table 34.1	Maximum doses of anaesthetic agents	
	Plain solution	With adrenalin
Lignocaine	200 mg (20 ml of 1%)	500 mg (50 ml of 1%)
Bupivacaine	150 mg (30 ml of 0.5%)	200 mg (40 ml of 0.5%)
Prilocaine	400 mg (80 ml of 0.5%)	600 mg (120 ml of 0.5%)

If breathing appears obstructed, call for anaesthetic help and:

- Inspect the mouth for foreign bodies (e.g. vomit, slipped denture and surgical swab after surgery in the mouth)
- Extend the neck and pull the jaw forward to clear the tongue from the back of the mouth and get an assistant to maintain the position
- Insert an oral airway
- If the patient has had a thyroidectomy, open the wound (skin and deep fascia) at the bedside
- If the patient has had surgery in the mouth, throat or neck, or if there is no improvement with an airway in place perform a cricothyroidotomy without delay
- Check that the patient can exhale
- Monitor the oxygen saturation and obtain blood gases and chest X-ray as soon as possible.

Do not attempt to intubate a patient after surgery in the mouth or neck unless experienced – do a cricothyroidotomy and call an anaesthetist. In an emergency, a large-gauge intravenous cannula can be used for cricothyroidotomy but requires jet ventilation, whether the patient is breathing or not, because of the small lumen (attach rigid oxygen line to cannula via the barrel of a 5 ml syringe). During insertion, check that the needle is in the trachea, which may be displaced, by aspiration of air and be careful not to pass it straight through the back. The cannula can kink or displace and should be replaced as soon as possible with a purpose-made device.

Normal breathing

Cyanosis in a patient who appears to be breathing normally may be due to a problem in the lungs or circulation. Listen to the chest for bronchospasm (wheeze is absent in severe bronchospasm) and for uniform air entry. Is the patient asthmatic? Is this a hypersensitivity reaction? Loss of air entry in the upper chest suggests pneumothorax and in the dependent part of the chest, haemothorax or pleural effusion. Has the patient had attempts at intravenous line insertion in the neck?

Acute circulatory problems which can cause cyanosis are loss of venous return (massive sudden blood loss), pump failure (myocardial infarct) and obstruction (massive pulmonary embolism). Check the blood pressure and get an ECG. Other possible causes include severe adverse drug reaction and severe sepsis (air hunger).

Hypotension

The commonest cause of hypotension in a postoperative patient is hypovolaemia, either due to inadequate fluid replacement or to bleeding. Myocardial infarction needs to be considered and excluded. Poor management of pain control, either too much or too little analgesia, may be a factor and hypotension is a side-effect of an epidural (local anaesthetic drugs may cause dilatation of the main capacitance vessels). It is difficult to confirm that an epidural is responsible without turning it off; however, treatment by volume replacement is the same whether hypotension is caused by hypovolaemia or the epidural.

An assessment of the overall clinical situation may suggest an obvious cause of hypotension in a given patient. If not:

- Increase the rate of intravenous fluids
- Elevate the legs
- Give oxygen up to 50% by mask
- Obtain an ECG (dysrhythmia, acute ischaemia, signs of pulmonary embolus).

If the ECG is normal, place a central venous pressure line whilst giving additional intravenous fluid. Listen to the chest to exclude tension pneumothorax (chest trauma, chest surgery, surgery around the oesophageal hiatus, or failed neck line) and consider pulmonary embolus and septicaemia. If no cause is apparent, and the blood pressure responds to volume infusion, hidden blood loss is likely.

Hypertension

This may be dangerous in patients with ischaemic heart disease, cerebrovascular disease or following vascular surgery. Obtain anaesthetic assistance with the management of such patients if a cause cannot be found; the commonest causes of hypertension are inadequate control of pain and/or anxiety, urinary retention and shivering.

Postoperative infection

The patient's temperature is a basic, but crude, observation for infection. Clinical monitoring includes examination of the chest and inspection of the wound. The upper limit of normal temperature is 37°C, but there is considerable variation and occasionally a patient may be pyrexial despite a temperature below this 'magic' figure. The timing of postoperative pyrexia may suggest a cause (e.g. after a large bowel resection: pyrexia within the first 48 hours – chest infection; fifth or sixth day – an anastomotic leakage or wound infection; tenth day – venous thrombosis).

If a patient develops a pyrexia, a routine 'infection screen' is carried out:

1. Examine the chest – chest X-ray; sputum for culture; ECG (if? pulmonary embolism)

2. Examine the wound – wound swab for culture
3. Enquire about urinary symptoms – urine culture
4. Examine for signs of deep vein thrombosis
5. Examine intravenous sites (phlebitis) and other catheter sites (epidural)
6. Examine pressure areas
7. If a child – look in the ears and mouth
8. If cause uncertain – send blood cultures; measure white cell count
9. Consider the underlying disease (e.g. pyrexia of malignancy)
10. Consider hidden infection (e.g. subphrenic or pelvic abscess).

Delayed gastric emptying/aspiration

Abdominal surgery is frequently associated with delayed gastric emptying and impaired colonic motility, even though small bowel activity, and hence bowel sounds, may return relatively early. If there is intra-abdominal sepsis, metabolic disturbances, or retroperitoneal haematoma or inflammation there may be prolonged inactivity of the small bowel also (paralytic ileus). Colonic pseudo-obstruction occurs most often in elderly patients confined to bed (e.g. after fracture or orthopaedic surgery) and postpartum. Reintroduction of diet too soon can lead to gastric dilatation with vomiting and the risk of aspiration. Monitoring nasogastric aspirates, abdominal distension and the passage of flatus determines the timing of reintroduction of normal diet. However, a restricted intake of oral fluids (30 ml h⁻¹) is permissible almost without exception, and increases patient comfort.

Gastric aspiration can be life-threatening:

• Place the patient head-down in the recovery position
• Suction out the mouth
• Give 100% oxygen by mask
• Pass a nasogastric tube to empty the stomach
• Examine for bronchospasm – if present give nebulized salbutamol ± intravenous aminophylline and consider intubation and ventilation

• Obtain chest X-ray
• Arrange early chest physiotherapy.

Steroids are not thought to be helpful.

Summary

1. Postoperative care is divided into three phases.
2. The recovery phase is the immediate care of patients after surgery until they can maintain all vital functions independently.
3. The second phase is care on the ward during which the three most important general considerations are pain control, fluid balance management and nutrition.
4. The third phase of care follows discharge from hospital and includes consideration of appropriate follow up and/or surveillance.
5. The intensity of monitoring in the postoperative phase depends on the severity of disease and/or the nature of surgery.
6. Many specialized features of postoperative care are determined by the type of operation.
7. Good communication is essential throughout postoperative care to ensure the best outcome.

 Further reading

In addition to the chapters in this book referred to in the text, several pocket-sized texts aimed at trainee anaesthetists are available and provide useful guidelines on the management of acute postoperative problems, for example:
Eaton J M, Fielden J M, Wilson M E Anaesthesia action plans. Abbott Laboratories Ltd., Abbott House, Norden Road, Maidenhead, Berks SL6 4XE

35

The management of postoperative pain

R. Fernando, K. D. Hunt

Objectives

- **Define the pathophysiology of pain.**
- **Define the effects of pain on the postoperative patient.**
- **Discuss pharmacological and non-pharmacological methods of analgesia.**
- **Discuss the assessment of postoperative pain.**
- **Discuss the causes and treatment of postoperative nausea and vomiting.**

Pain relief after surgery is still inadequately managed despite the development of new drugs and more effective techniques to control postoperative pain. The traditional approach to postoperative pain is the use of a fixed dose of intramuscular opioid on an intermittent pro re nata (PRN) schedule (e.g. morphine 10 mg, prn, 3-hourly). This approach is simple, cheap, requires no special equipment and sometimes it may actually work. A standard dose of intramuscular opioid such as morphine (10 mg) can result in a five-fold difference in peak plasma concentrations of morphine among different patients, with the time taken to reach these levels varying by as much as seven-fold. In addition, the plasma concentrations of opioid needed to provide analgesia, the minimum effective analgesic concentration (MEAC), may vary by up to four-fold between patients. Therefore the 'standard' dose prescribed is only optimal for a few patients and the PRN ('as needed') part of the order is often interpreted by nursing staff to mean 'as little as possible'.

Additional problems with postoperative pain are:

- The management of postoperative pain is often delegated to the most junior doctor

- The fear of drug addiction and side-effects such as respiratory depression lead to nursing staff withholding medication
- The time delay between the request for analgesia and the final administration of a drug may increase the amount of a patient's pain.

HOW DOES POSTOPERATIVE PAIN ARISE?

Pain is defined as an unpleasant sensory or emotional experience associated with actual or potential tissue damage. Pain involves four physiological processes: transduction, transmission, modulation and perception. Pain begins when local tissue damage, a noxious stimulus, occurs during surgery; this causes the release of inflammatory substances (prostaglandins, histamine, serotonin, bradykinin and substance P). This leads to the generation of electrical impulses (transduction) at peripheral sensory nerve endings, or nociceptors. These electrical impulses are conducted by nerve fibres (A-delta and C fibres) to the spinal cord (transmission). Further relay to the higher brain centres can be modified within the spinal cord (modulation) before an individual perceives a painful stimulus (perception). Therefore pain can, in theory, be *blocked* at various levels in this complex chain. Non-steroidal anti-inflammatory drugs (NSAIDs) can reduce the peripheral inflammatory response by reducing prostaglandin production. Local anaesthetic drugs injected into the epidural or subarachnoid spaces can block impulses to the spinal cord by acting on spinal nerve roots. Opioids can produce analgesia through modulation by binding to opioid receptors in the spinal cord and other higher brain centres such as the periaqueductal grey, the nucleus raphe magnus and the thalamus, whereas binding to opioid receptors in the cerebral cortex can affect the perception of pain (Fig. 35.1).

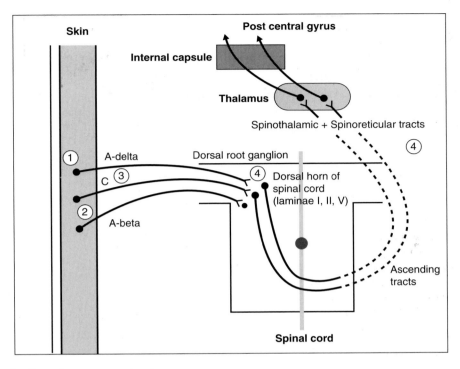

Fig 35.1 Sites of action of common analgesics

Site of action	Analgesic/effect
1. *Nociceptors in skin and subcutaneous tissues* These receptors are stimulated by inflammatory substances, e.g. prostaglandins.	NSAIDS, e.g. diclofenac, ibuprofen, ketorolac, block pathways involved in the formation of inflammatory agents.
2. *A-beta fibres* Stimulation of these fibres inhibits transmission of pain to higher centres.	Transcutaneous electrical nerve stimulation (TENS); stimulates A-beta fibres.
3. *Primary afferent neurones (A-delta, C fibres)* Transmit impulses from nociceptors to the spinal cord.	Local anaesthetics, e.g. lignocaine, bupivacaine, prilocaine, ropivacaine. Block the transmission of impulses along neurones.
4. *Dorsal horn of spinal cord and higher centres* Further relay/transmission of painful stimuli to the cerebral cortex.	Opioids, e.g. morphine, pethidine diamorphine, fentanyl, act as agonists at opioid receptors. [Also ketamine]

WHY SHOULD WE TREAT POSTOPERATIVE PAIN?

Apart from the humanitarian aspect, there are several physiological reasons for treating postoperative pain.

Respiratory effects

Surgery involving the upper abdomen or chest reduces vital capacity, functional residual capacity and the ability to cough and deep breathe. This in turn can lead to retention of secretions, atelectasis and pneumonia.

Inadequately treated pain aggravates these changes, while analgesia improves respiratory function.

Cardiovascular effects

Pain causes an increase in sympathetic output (tachycardia, hypertension and increasing blood catecholamines) which leads to increasing myocardial oxygen demand, which may in turn increase the risk of postoperative myocardial ischaemia, especially in those patients with pre-existing cardiac disease.

Neuroendocrine effects

The stress response to surgery and pain includes the secretion of catecholamines and catabolic hormones. This increases metabolism and oxygen consumption and promotes sodium and water retention.

Effects on mobilization

Mobilization of a patient in the postoperative period may be delayed if the patient is experiencing pain. This may in turn increase their risk of developing a deep vein thrombosis and also prolong hospital stay.

METHODS AVAILABLE TO TREAT POSTOPERATIVE PAIN

Non-pharmacological

Preoperative counselling

The management of postoperative pain does not begin after the completion of surgery. Patients who are well informed as to the nature of the operation, the nature of the postoperative pain and the methods of analgesia available to them may be able to cope better with postoperative pain. Ideally each patient would be assessed jointly by the surgeon performing the operation, the anaesthetist and a member of the nursing staff. The site and nature of the surgery (Box 35.1), the extent of the incision and the physiological and psychological make-up of the patient will all be relevant in planning intraoperative and postoperative analgesia. Once these things have been ascertained, the various methods available for postoperative analgesia (including opioids, non-steroidal anti-inflammatory agents, isolated nerve blocks and epidural and spinal anaesthesia and analgesia) can be discussed between the patient and medical staff in order to reach a mutually agreeable postoperative treatment plan.

> **Box 35.1 Pain associated with different surgical procedures (decreasing order of severity)**
>
> - Thoracic surgery
> - Upper abdominal surgery
> - Lower abdominal surgery
> - Inguinal and femoral hernia repair
> - Head/neck/limb surgery

TENS

A TENS machine (transcutaneous electrical nerve stimulation) is made up of a pulse generator, an amplifier and a system of electrodes. It acts by stimulating afferent myelinated (A-beta) nerve fibres at a rate of 70 Hz. This activates inhibitory circuits within the spinal cord that reduce the transmission of painful nerve impulses to the higher cortical centres, thereby reducing the level of postoperative pain. TENS has been shown to have maximal benefit in neurogenic pain which is experienced in nerve damage and phantom limb pain.

Opioids

Opioids act at opioid receptors in the spinal cord and higher brain centres to produce analgesia. They act by mimicking endogenous opioid peptides, causing activation of opioid receptors within the central nervous system. The activation of these receptors modulates the activity of the dorsal horn relay neurons that transmit painful stimuli, thereby reducing the transmission of these stimuli to higher centres and producing analgesia. Activation of the receptors also causes the unwanted side-effects of opioids, namely, sedation, respiratory depression, nausea and vomiting, and euphoria or dysphoria (Table 35.1). The opioids such as morphine and pethidine are agonists, i.e. they bind to and activate the opioid receptors producing the maximal desired response. Drugs such as naloxone are antagonists at the opioid receptor, i.e. they bind to the receptor but fail to activate it. Drugs such as pentazocine are partial agonists. Pentazocine acts as an agonist at the kappa receptor but as an antagonist at the mu receptor producing weak analgesia but also producing hallucinations, thought disorders and bad dreams.

Oral opioids. These include codeine, dihydrocodeine and dextropropoxyphene. For example:

- Codeine phosphate, 30–60 mg, 6-hourly
- Codydramol (= dihydrocodeine 10 mg + paracetamol 500 mg), 1–2 tablets, 6-hourly

Table 35.1 Opioid receptor classification

Receptor	Agonist effect	Agonist	Antagonist
Mu-1	Spinal and supraspinal analgesia, meiosis, ileus	Morphine Meptazinol	Naloxone Pentazocine
Mu-2	Hypoventilation, bradycardia, dependence, euphoria	Pethidine	Nalbuphine
Delta	Modulate mu receptor activity	Leu-enkephalin (endogenous CNS transmitter)	naloxone
Kappa	Analgesia, sedation, diuresis, meiosis, dysphoria	Pentazocine Buprenorphine	Naloxone
Sigma	Dysphoria, tachycardia, tachypnoea, mydriasis	?	Naloxone

- Coproxamol (= dextropropoxyphene 32.5 mg + paracetamol 325 mg) 1–2 tablets, 6-hourly.

The oral route for opioids is not recommended initially after major surgery for the following reasons:

- The use of opioids during general anaesthesia can lead to postoperative nausea and vomiting and delayed gastric emptying
- Intra-abdominal surgery can result in postoperative ileus
- Orally absorbed opioids from the gut reach the liver via the splanchnic blood flow where they are highly metabolized (first-pass metabolism) causing insufficient plasma concentrations of drug e.g. 70% of orally administered morphine is eliminated through first pass metabolism.

Despite this, oral opioid combinations with paracetamol (codydramol or coproxamol) are adequate for treating mild pain after day-case surgery or 3–4 days after major surgery when parenteral opioids are no longer needed. Pethidine, morphine and methadone are also available as oral preparations:

- Pethidine hydrochloride tablets are available as 50 mg tablets, and the dose for adults is 50–150 mg, 4-hourly
- Morphine is available as Oromorph solution or morphine sulphate tablets, and the dose is 5–20 mg, 4-hourly for adults
- Methadone is available in 5 mg tablets, and the dose is 5–10 mg, 6–8-hourly.

Intramuscular opioids. These include morphine, diamorphine, pethidine and papaveretum. For example:

- Morphine, 10 mg, 3-hourly
- Pethidine, 75 mg, 3-hourly.

This is the most common route used today, for the reasons given above. It is convenient and is associated with few side-effects, although the degree of analgesia varies between patients. Up to 40% of patients on a PRN intramuscular opioid regimen may have inadequate pain relief. Care needs to be taken when multiple doses of intramuscular opioids are administered to shocked patients with poor peripheral perfusion. In such cases a large depot of opioid can accumulate intramuscularly to be later released into the bloodstream when the peripheral circulation is restored with unpredictable and often dangerous results.

Intravenous opioid continuous infusions. These include morphine and pethidine. For example:

- Morphine, 50 mg in 50 ml saline (1 mg ml^{-1}), infusion rate 1–10 ml h^{-1}
- Pethidine, 250 mg in 50 ml saline (5 mg ml^{-1}), infusion rate 1–8 ml h^{-1}.

A continuous infusion of opioid through an intravenous cannula can abolish wide swings in plasma drug concentration found with the intramuscular route and allow adjustment of the rate to the individual needs of a patient. An initial intravenous loading dose of opioid is usually needed before an infusion is started, otherwise it may take several hours for the drug to reach the patient's MEAC to achieve pain relief. Unfortunately, plasma drug concentrations may continue to increase with such regimens, leading to sedation and respiratory depression. Regular monitoring is therefore essential, with the infusion rate being changed as necessary. Naloxone should be available to reverse opioid side-effects such as excessive sedation and respiratory depression.

Intravenous opioid patient-controlled analgesia. These include morphine, diamorphine and pethidine.

For example:

- Morphine, 50 mg in 50 ml saline (1 mg ml^{-1} morphine)
  Bolus = 1 ml (1 mg morphine)
  Lock-out time = 5 min
  4-hour limit = 30 mg morphine

- Pethidine, 250 mg in 50 ml saline (5 mg ml^{-1} pethidine)
  Bolus = 2 ml (10 mg pethidine)
  Lock-out time = 5 min
  4-hour limit = 300 mg pethidine

Intravenous opioid patient-controlled analgesia (PCA) is superior to both intramuscular and continuous infusion routes because it allows the patient to self-administer small doses of opioid when pain occurs. PCA is administered using a special microprocessor-controlled pump which is triggered by depressing a button held in the patient's hand. When triggered, a pre-set amount (the bolus dose) is delivered to the patient, usually via a separate intravenous line. A timer prevents the administration of another bolus for a specified period (the lock-out interval). Before a PCA is started, a loading dose of opioid must be given to achieve adequate analgesia. Background infusions of opioid are no longer used with PCA because of increasing side-effects. The theoretical basis of PCA is that, since individual patients require different plasma opioid concentrations to achieve an MEAC, each patient will control the frequency of opioid boluses to achieve good pain relief with minimal side-effects. From a safety aspect, if the patient becomes oversedated on PCA, they cannot give themselves another bolus. This will lead to a fall in plasma opioid concentration to safer levels. Regardless of this, regular monitoring of patients with PCA is essential. Naloxone should once again be available to treat respiratory depression and excessive sedation.

Miscellaneous routes of opioid administration.

Transdermal. Fentanyl, a potent short-acting opioid, has been used in a drug-containing patch which adheres to the skin. The drug diffuses through the skin and into the bloodstream. Unfortunately, the dose cannot be titrated to the patient's needs and it takes several hours to achieve an MEAC.

Sublingual. Since the drug is delivered directly into the bloodstream via the sublingual route, first-pass metabolism is avoided. Sublingual buprenorphine, a partial agonist, is available, but has a 20% incidence of nausea and vomiting and a 50% incidence of sedation or drowsiness.

Rectal. The rectal route is useful for providing a high systemic bioavailability of drugs that have a low oral bioavailability. Absorption, however, is slow, with peak concentrations being reached 3–4 hours after administration. Pethidine and pentazocine are commonly administered by this route in Europe.

Subcutaneous. Morphine is commonly administered by the subcutaneous route in cancer patients and is occasionally used for postoperative pain. This route is tolerated better than the i.m. route of administration but the entry site must be changed every 24–48 hours to avoid infection, and rapid titration of the dose of drug against patient response is difficult to achieve.

Nebulizer. Morphine, diamorphine and fentanyl have all been administered as nebulized solutions with the advantage that the lungs can provide a large surface area onto which the opioids can be rapidly absorbed; however, systemic absorption is variable, probably because an indeterminate amount of the agent is swallowed by the patient.

Intra-articular. In orthopaedic surgery, morphine may be of benefit by binding to opioid receptors that are present in inflamed tissue formed after injury within the joint spaces.

Epidural. This route is discussed below.

Local anaesthetics

Local anaesthetic (LA) drugs (e.g. bupivacaine, lignocaine and prilocaine) block the conduction of nerve impulses when applied to peripheral nerves or nerve roots. Sensory and sympathetic nerve fibres are blocked by smaller amounts of LA compared to motor nerves. In the treatment of postoperative pain, LA drugs injected close to a peripheral nerve (digital nerves in a ring block) or a plexus of nerves (brachial plexus in an axillary block) will block painful stimuli arising from an area supplied by those nerves. Bupivacaine is the most commonly used LA drug due to its long duration of action (2–3 hours).

All LA drugs can cause toxic effects if given in large doses or if accidental intravascular injection occurs. Central nervous system and cardiovascular toxicity can result in restlessness, convulsions, hypotension and cardiorespiratory arrest. Suggested safe maximum doses of LA are 2 mg kg^{-1} for plain bupivacaine and 3 mg kg^{-1} for plain lignocaine. LA solutions are also available with small amounts of adrenaline (e.g. 1 in 200 000) which, acting as a vasoconstrictor due to its action on alpha-1 receptors, reduces the absorption of the LA, thereby allowing larger amounts of LA to be given. Adrenaline has also been found to act on alpha-2 receptors in the spinal cord which helps to potentiate the analgesic effect of local anaesthetics at spinal cord level. Injection of adrenaline-containing solutions is absolutely contraindicated in areas supplied by end arteries, such as the fingers, toes and the penis, since prolonged ischaemia may lead to tissue necrosis.

Local infiltration to wound

For example:

- Bupivacaine, 0.25%, 10–20 ml, after inguinal hernia repair.

Catheters can also be used to constantly infuse LA into the wound to provide analgesia.

Nerve blocks

For example:

- Bupivacaine, 0.5%, 1–4 ml, penile block for circumcision
- Bupivacaine 0.25%, 10 ml, ilioinguinal/iliohypogastric nerve block for hernia repair.

These blocks can be performed by the anaesthetist while the patient is anaesthetized.

Epidural block

For example:

- Single-shot caudal epidural for paediatric circumcision using bupivacaine, 0.25%, 0.5 ml kg^{-1}
- Continuous epidural infusions for abdominal or thoracic operations:
  - (a) Bupivacaine 0.25%, 30 ml + diamorphine 5 mg + saline 30 ml
    Concentration: bupivacaine 0.125% + diamorphine 0.008%
    Infusion rate = 2–8 ml h^{-1}
  - (b) Bupivacaine 0.5%, 10 ml + fentanyl (50 mcg ml^{-1}) 2 ml + saline 38 ml
    Concentration: bupivacaine 0.1% + fentanyl 0.0002%
    Infusion rate = 2–12 ml h^{-1}

Plain LA solutions such as bupivacaine 0.25% can be administered into the epidural space intermittently through an epidural catheter or, more usually, continuously via an infusion pump to block nerves within the spinal canal. Excellent analgesia can be obtained with this technique, especially for thoracic and major abdominal operations. Side-effects of LA used in epidural blocks include hypotension (sympathetic block), muscle weakness of the legs (motor block) and urinary retention.

Most hospitals in the UK nowadays use epidural infusions consisting of combinations of low-dose LA (e.g. bupivacaine 0.1%) and opioid (e.g. fentanyl 0.0002%). Such low-dose combinations are synergistic. Side-effects related to epidural opioids alone include nausea and vomiting, pruritus, sedation and delayed respiratory depression. Low-dose mixtures, by reducing the amount of both LA and opioid, actually reduce the side-effects of both drugs. However, monitoring of the patient is still important. Naloxone should once again be available to reverse opioid side-effects such as excessive sedation and respiratory depression. Typically, patients receiving low-dose LA + opioid epidural infusions have superior analgesia, improved cardiovascular stability, and the ability to move about due to a reduction in motor block.

Ropivacaine

Ropivacaine is a new local anaesthetic agent similar in structure to bupivacaine. It is prepared in the S-isomer form as opposed to commercially available bupivacaine which is prepared as a racemic (R + S) mixture. Because of this, ropivacaine is less cardiotoxic than its parent drug and exhibits a more selective blockade on A delta and C fibres, producing less motor blockade. These effects are due to its lower lipid solubility and may be advantageous in treating obstetric patients and patients suffering from both acute and chronic pain.

NSAIDs

For example:

- Mefenamic acid, 500 mg, orally, 8-hourly
- Diclofenac sodium, 100 mg, rectally, 12–15 hourly (oral preparation also available)
- Ketorolac trometamol, 10 mg, intravenously/intramuscularly, 4–6 hourly.

NSAIDs block the synthesis of prostaglandins by inhibiting the enzyme cyclo-oxygenase (prostaglandin synthetase). Prostaglandins mediate several components of the inflammatory response, including fever, pain and vasodilation.

NSAIDs are usually only suitable for the treatment of mild to moderate postoperative pain. However, if used in conjunction with opioids, they may also reduce the amount of opioids used to treat postoperative pain. In this way opioid side-effects such as nausea and vomiting can also be reduced. This is the concept of 'balanced analgesia'. Diclofenac sodium (Voltarol) is widely used in the UK, usually in suppository form to provide analgesia after many minor day-case operations, including gynaecological laparoscopy. Due to its long duration of action (12 hours) diclofenac can be given preoperatively to provide analgesia into the postoperative period. Diclofenac is also generally safe to administer to patients with stable asthma who have *no* history of allergy or worsening asthma with aspirin or other NSAIDs. Other problems with diclofenac apply to NSAIDs in general:

- Gastric ulceration – avoid NSAIDs in patients with a history of gastric ulceration
- Nephrotoxicity – renal function can be altered by NSAIDs secondary to prostaglandin inhibition, but only usually in patients with pre-existing renal problems
- Impaired haemostasis – due to the inhibition of the prostaglandin thromboxane A_2 within platelets, NSAIDs may also increase the risk of bleeding.

Pre-emptive analgesia

A hypothesis exists that surgery, which produces a barrage of pain signals to the spinal cord, is a 'priming' mechanism which sensitizes the central nervous system. This is said to lead to enhanced postoperative pain. The rationale behind several studies is that by providing presurgery, or pre-emptive, analgesia using parenteral opioids, regional blocks or NSAIDs, either individually or in combination, these sensitizing neuroplastic changes can be prevented within the spinal cord, leading to diminished postoperative pain requirements. Therefore the concept of pre-emptive analgesia may have implications in reducing not only acute postoperative pain, but also chronic pain states such as post-thoracotomy chest-wall pain and postamputation lower limb stump pain. Taken to an extreme, a single dose of analgesic drug administered before surgery could theoretically abolish postoperative pain. Unfortunately, no current study proves the existence of pre-emptive analgesia in humans.

Methods of treating postoperative pain

- **Preoperative patient counselling and education**
- **Administration of opioids by various routes**
- **Wound infiltration and regional blockade with local anaesthetics**
- **Non-steroidal anti-inflammatory agents**

MONITORING OF POSTOPERATIVE ANALGESIA

The effectiveness of any postoperative analgesic regimen, as well as any side-effects, needs to be assessed regularly. Pain scores, sedation scores and respiratory monitoring should be used to optimize any form of analgesia.

Monitoring of pain

The simplest method of monitoring pain is through observation of the behaviour of the patient, for example the time taken for the patient to sit or stand or the ability of the patient to cough. One can also monitor the analgesic requirements of the patient (e.g. the total dose of analgesia administered over a 24-hour period or the number of demands of a PCA pump). Other methods of monitoring available include:

- *Visual analogue score (VAS)* – patients are asked to mark their pain score on a 10-cm scale ranging from 0 = no pain to 10 = worst pain imaginable
- *Verbal rating score (VRS)* – patients rate their pain as 1 = no pain, 2 = mild pain, 3 = moderate pain, 4 = severe pain.

Pain scores can be difficult to interpret since individual patients vary in their perception of pain. VAS and VRS are the most commonly used methods when adjusting analgesic regimens such as opioid PCA or epidural infusions. Most pain scores only measure pain when the patient is resting. Obviously such a score will change when, for example, a patient after upper abdominal surgery attempts to cough to clear secretions or receives chest physiotherapy. Therefore pain scores on coughing or moving will be just as important as those at rest.

Monitoring of sedation and respiration

For example, a *sedation score* may be:
0 = No sedation (patient alert)
1 = Mild sedation (occasionally drowsy; easy to arouse)
2 = Moderate sedation (often drowsy; easy to arouse)
3 = Severe sedation (difficult to arouse).

The major fear with opioids, administered by any route (intravenously, intramuscularly or epidurally) is that of respiratory depression. Epidural opioids have the added risk of delayed respiratory depression. This risk is extremely small. Highly lipid-soluble opioids such as fentanyl have a lower risk of this complication, administered epidurally, than does morphine which is less lipid soluble. Of course the general medical condition of the patient must also be considered, since elderly patients with cardiorespiratory disease are at a higher risk of this potentially dangerous complication. Traditionally it has been assumed that intermittent observation of a patient's respiratory rate by a ward nurse is adequate to detect respiratory problems. The development of pulse oximetry, which allows a patient's blood oxygen saturation (S_pO_2) to be measured non-invasively using a simple finger probe, has shown that episodes of hypoxaemia may occur despite a normal respiratory rate with any form of opioid analgesia. In fact an increasing level of sedation may precede respiratory depression. Therefore it is important to regularly monitor not only pain scores but also sedation scores and respiratory rate. A sedation score of 3 or a respiratory rate less than 8 breaths per minute should be treated immediately with intravenous naloxone.

If pulse oximetry is used, a S_pO_2 of less than 94% in a patient breathing air should be treated with supplemental oxygen through nasal cannulae or a face mask.

Measurement of S_pO_2 using pulse oximetry is already a minimum monitoring standard during anaesthesia and the immediate recovery period. Several studies which have extended the use of pulse oximetry to the postoperative period on the ward have detected periods of hypoxaemia 3–4 days after major surgery. The relationship of these events to the risk of myocardial ischaemia is a subject of ongoing research. In the future, the gold standard of patient monitoring could well be the pulse oximeter which will be allocated to patients scheduled for surgery when they first arrive in hospital. Continuous monitoring of S_pO_2 will then occur

preoperatively (to obtain baseline values) and postoperatively. On this basis the use of postoperative oxygen therapy on the ward could be extended to more patients at risk of hypoxaemia. Note, however, that pulse oximetry alone gives no information about the adequacy of respiration or the level of sedation. As such it can only be useful if used in combination with regular nursing observations.

Monitoring patient analgesia

- **Observe the patient**
- **Measure pain scores**
- **Monitor the degree of sedation and the respiratory rate**

POSTOPERATIVE NAUSEA AND VOMITING (PONV)

The vomiting centre is found in the reticular formation of the medulla. It receives afferent impulses from vari-

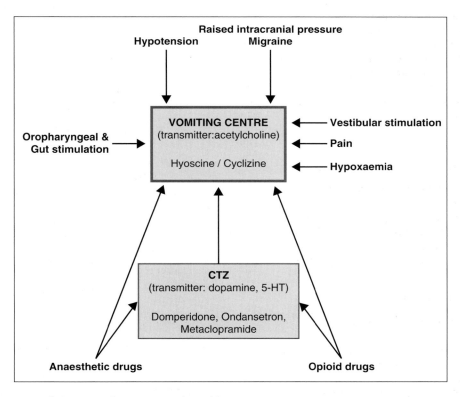

Fig 35.2 Management of postoperative nausea and vomiting.

ous pathways, including the chemoreceptor trigger zone (CTZ). This area is located within the floor of the fourth ventricle and itself is activated by various stimuli. Risk factors associated with postoperative nausea and vomiting include obesity, past history of postoperative nausea and vomiting, the female sex, a history of motion sickness or migraine, prolonged starvation or recent oral intake. PONV is commonly associated with gastrointestinal, ENT, ophthalmic, gynaecological, orthopaedic and emergency surgery. Drugs, including anaesthetic gases, thiopentone and opioids, may also stimulate PONV. The following may be useful in treating PONV:

- anticholinergic agents, e.g. hyoscine (300 μg QDS)
- antidoperminergic agents, e.g. domperidone (10–20 mg, 4–8-hourly, orally; or 30–60 mg, 4–8-hourly, rectally); and metaclopramide (10 mg TDS p.o, i.m, i.v.)
- 5-HT3 antagonists, e.g. ondansetron (4–8 mg, 12-hourly orally or intravenously; or 16 mg, 12-hourly, rectally).

ACUTE PAIN SERVICE (APS)

Each hospital should have an APS team as recommended in 1990 by the Royal College of Surgeons of England and the Royal College of Anaesthetists. The establishment of an APS requires a multidisciplinary approach using medical, nursing and pharmaceutical expertise. Anaesthetists have a major role to play, since they not only initiate postoperative analgesic regimens such as PCA and epidural infusions, but also are familiar with the drugs and equipment used in such cases. Many hospitals have an acute pain team consisting of a dedicated pain nurse, consultant anaesthetist, and sometimes junior anaesthetic staff. The role of the acute pain team involves devising, implementing and auditing pain protocols, reviewing patients in whom postoperative analgesia is proving difficult and those with epidural and intravenous infusions, and treating patients with chronic pain. Protocols or standing orders for PCA and epidural regimens for the ward staff are recommended (Boxes 35.2 and 35.3).

CONCLUSION

Currently, in the treatment of postoperative pain there is no single analgesic therapy which can treat all aspects

---

Box 35.2 Intravenous opioid PCA standing orders

1. PCA drug concentration: morphine 1 mg ml^{-1}
2. Bolus dose: morphine 1 mg (= 1 ml)
3. Lock-out interval: 5 minutes
4. 4-hour limit: 30 mg morphine
5. If pain not controlled after 1 hour, **increase** bolus dose to: ... ... mg = ... ml of morphine
6. If pain still not controlled after 1 hour, **reduce** lock-out interval to: ... ... min
7. If pain still not controlled, call acute pain service (APS) (bleep ... ...) for further advice
8. No systemic opioids or other CNS depressants to be given
9. Monitor: heart rate/blood pressure/pain score/respiratory rate/sedation score Monitor hourly for the first 8 hours, then 2–3-hourly
10. SIDE-EFFECTS:
    (a) Sedation score = 3. **Action:** Call APS (bleep ... ...)
    (b) Respiratory rate < 8 min^{-1}. **Action:** Call APS (bleep ... ...)
    (c) Sedation score = 3 + respiratory rate < 8 min^{-1}. **Action: Give intravenous naloxone 0.4 mg STAT and fast bleep APS**
    (d) Nausea and vomiting: **Action:** Metoclopramide, 10 mg, i.v./i.m. *or* Ondansetron, 4 mg, i.v./i.m.
    (e) Pruritus:
    Mild **Action:** Give chlorpheniramine (Piriton), 10 mg, i.m., 8-hourly (or 4 mg orally)
    Severe **Action:** Give naloxone, 40 μg, i.v. bolus (repeat if needed)
    (f) Urinary retention: **Action:** In/out bladder catheter.

---

of pain without causing side-effects. The emphasis should be on a 'balanced analgesic' technique, especially after major surgical procedures, using NSAIDs in combination with other drugs such as opioids or local anaesthetics. Using such principles, we may be able not only to improve analgesic efficacy, but also to reduce analgesic-induced side-effects.

Box 35.3   Epidural opioid/local anaesthetic infusion standing orders

1. Drugs: **fentanyl** (50 µg ml⁻¹, 2 ml) + **bupivacaine** (0.5%, 10 ml) + **saline** (38 ml) Concentration = fentanyl 0.0002% + bupivacaine 0.1%
2. Infusion rate: 2–12 ml h⁻¹
3. If in pain, increase rate by 2 ml h⁻¹ each hour, until maximum rate
4. If pain still not controlled, call APS (bleep … …) for further advice
5. If epidural bolus given by APS, check blood pressure every 5 minutes for 30 minutes
6. No systemic opioids or other CNS depressants to be given
7. Monitor: heart rate/blood pressure/pain score/respiratory rate/sedation score Monitor hourly for the first 8 hours, then 2–3 hourly
8. SIDE-EFFECTS:

    (a) Sedation score = 3. **Action:** Call APS (Bleep … …)

    (b) Respiratory rate <8 min⁻¹. **Action:** Call APS (Bleep … …)

    (c) Sedation score = 3 + respiratory rate <8 min⁻¹. **Action: Give intravenous naloxone 0.4 mg STAT and fast bleep APS**

    (d) Nausea and vomiting: **Action:** Metoclopramide, 10 mg, i.v./i.m. *or* Ondansetron, 4 mg, i.v./i.m.

    (e) Pruritus:

    Mild   **Action:** Give chlorpheniramine (Piriton), 10 mg, i.m., 8-hourly (or 4 mg orally) Severe   **Action:** Give naloxone, 40 µg, i.v. bolus (repeat if needed)

    (f) Urinary retention. **Action:** In/out bladder catheter.

Summary

1. Pain can be treated by various methods which affect the transmission of a painful stimulus at different levels along its pathway to the central nervous system.
2. Treatment of pain may reduce the incidence of some postoperative complications and hence reduce hospital stay.
3. Opioids, given i.v. or i.m., remain common analgesics for the treatment of postoperative pain. Regional blockade using a low dose combination of local anaesthetic and opioid is also now popular. The concurrent use of NSAIDs may be useful in reducing opioid requirements.
4. The degree of analgesia and sedation must be carefully monitored on the ward.
5. In most hospitals an acute pain service is available to advise on the methods available for the treatment of postoperative pain and potential complications associated with such methods.

Ferrante F M, Vade Boncouer T R 1993 Postoperative pain management. Churchill Livingstone, Edinburgh

Liu S, Carpenter R L, Neal J M 1995 Epidural anesthesia and analgesia, their role in postoperative outcome. Anesthesiology 82: 1474–1506

McQuay H J 1992 Pre-emptive analgesia. British Journal of Anaesthesia 69: 1–3

Ogilvy A J, Smith G 1994 Postoperative pain. In: Nimo W S, Rowbotham D J, Smith G (eds) Anaesthesia. Blackwell, pp 1570–1602

Ready L B 1990 Acute postoperative pain. In: Aitkenhead A R, Smith G (eds) Anesthesia, 3rd edn. Churchill Livingstone, Edinburgh, pp 2135–2145

Rowbotham D J 1994 Gastric emptying, postoperative nausea and vomiting and antiemetics. In: Nimo W S, Rowbotham D J, Smith G (eds) Anaesthesia. Blackwell, pp 350–371

Sabanathan S 1995 Has postoperative pain been eradicated? Annals of the Royal College of Surgeons 77(3): 202–209

Souter A J, Fredman B, White P F 1994 Controversies in the perioperative use of nonsteroidal antiinflammatory drugs. Anesthesia and Analgesia 79: 1178–1190

Tighe S Q M, Bie J A, Nelson R A, Skues M A 1998 The acute pain service: effective or expensive care? Anaesthesia 53: 397–403

Further reading

Commission on the Provision of Surgical Services 1990 Report of the working party on pain after surgery. Royal College of Surgeons of England and the College of Anaesthetists, London

Deakin C D 1996 Clinical notes for the FRCA. Churchill Livingstone,

Complications

36

Complications – prevention and management

J. A. R. Smith

Objectives

- **Accept that complications are best anticipated and avoided.**
- **Recognize the incidence of comorbidity.**
- **Understand the importance of matching the procedure to the associated risks.**
- **Appreciate the importance of recognizing complications early and treating them vigorously.**

RISK FACTORS

- General – applicable to all procedures, *or*
- Specific to the operation and/or the complication concerned.

Old age

In older age, some conditions are encountered more commonly:

1. Neoplastic conditions.
2. Peripheral and cardiovascular disease. The incidence of cardiovascular disease rises with age (Table 36.1) and this is associated with an increased risk of postoperative myocardial infarction. Over age 50 years the risk is 6% with a 70% mortality rate. There is also an increased incidence of atrial fibrillation and hypertension and therefore of serious dysrhythmia and death.
3. Respiratory disease. Several changes occur in the elderly. These include reduced arterial oxygen tension, especially over 80 years of age. There are also: increased physiological dead space; decreased lung capacity, vital capacity, maximal breathing capacity, forced expiratory volume and peak expiratory flow rate.
4. Renal function deteriorates with age because of peripheral vascular disease, loss of nephrons, and impaired cell function. Therefore fluid overload and

Table 36.1	Risk of cardiovascular disease with age
Age (years)	Incidence of cardiovascular disease (%)
40–50	6
60–70	41
70–80	100

disturbance of both acid–base and electrolyte balance are more common in the elderly.

5. Medication. Elderly patients are more likely to be on regular medication for a number of disorders. The risk of drug interaction is therefore increased.

Neonatal period

At the other end of the age spectrum, neonatal surgery is also hazardous:

1. Tolerance of intravenous fluids is poor.
2. GI losses by vomiting and diarrhoea are common and can be life threatening. There is increased susceptibility to disturbance of acid base balance, and accurate replacement of fluid and electrolytes and correction of disturbance of pH is much more difficult.

Thermal regulation is poor, resulting in an increased risk of hypothermia. Enzyme systems are immature so that jaundice is more common, and both general and drug metabolism may be impaired. Congenital abnormalities are often multiple and major, and surgery is more demanding because of the physical size of the patient and the delicacy of the tissues.

Obesity

Patients may be overweight (up to 10% above their ideal body weight), obese (10–40% above), or morbidly obese (greater than 40% above their ideal).

Anaesthetic difficulties include difficulty in intubation, and in the placement of intravenous lines. Chest wall compliance is reduced, with consequent difficulties with ventilation. Positioning the patient on the operating table while avoiding pressure injuries requires considerable skill. In morbidly obese patients, cardiomyopathy and respiratory dysfunction may be severe enough to be life threatening. In some series, mortalities of 10–25% because of anaesthetic risks alone have been reported.

Surgery is complicated by technical difficulties; these can include limited exposure, adipose tissue obscuring the view and making trauma to associated structures more likely, and problems in minimally invasive surgery because of difficulty in gaining access to the peritoneal cavity.

In addition, blood vessels are less well supported and tend to retract if divided. Control of haemorrhage is therefore more difficult and haematoma formation more common. As a consequence, wound infection and impaired wound healing are encountered more often. The risk of venous thromboembolism is increased because fat patients tend to be less mobile, their weight exerts greater pressure on the calf veins during surgery, and there is an increased likelihood of endothelial trauma. In some obese patients there is an association with atherosclerosis and therefore with peripheral vascular disease.

In orthopaedic practice, obesity increases the incidence of arthritis, makes joint replacement more difficult from a technical view point and places an extra strain on lower limb prostheses. Indeed such patients may require bariatric surgery such as vertical banded gastroplasty to allow weight loss before joint replacement. A reduction of between 50 and 75% of the excess body weight over 12 months can be anticipated.

Key point

In general terms, there is no scientific evidence that weight reduction is rewarded by a reduction in the incidence of postoperative complications.

Cardiovascular disease

Myocardial infarction. A recent infarct is the most serious predisposing factor (Table 36.2). The more recent the infarct, the greater the risk of a further infarct. The risk remains higher than normal even after an interval of 3 years. The mortality from recurrent infarcts is also time related, being 75% in the first 6 months and falling to 25% after 1 year. Therefore, defer operations with a low risk of morbidity and mortality for at least 6 months post infarct.

Table 36.2 Risk of myocardial infarction with time

Time since infarct	Incidence of further infarction after surgery (%)
0–6 months	55
1–2 years	22
2–3 years	6
>3 years	1
No infarct	0.66

Angina. The severity of angina dictates the risk of cardiovascular complications in general and myocardial infarction in particular.

Dysrhythmias. Dysrhythmias such as atrial fibrillation and heart block carry the worst prognosis. Correction of the dysrhythmia reduces but does not abolish the risk of cardiovascular complications.

Cardiac valve disease. The presence of an artificial valve causes a major risk of bacterial colonization following surgery. Administer prophylactic antibiotics for all procedures. Mitral valve disease increases the risk of atrial fibrillation and of atrial thrombosis. Significant valve disease impairs cardiac responses to surgery and to infused fluids.

Cardiac pacemakers. These are 'foreign bodies', therefore prophylactic antibiotics are indicated. If a pacemaker is at a fixed rate, an inability to increase heart rate renders the patient vulnerable to hypovolaemia. Take care when using diathermy, especially if it is unipolar.

Atherosclerosis The incidence of atherosclerosis tends to increase with age, e.g. at age 50 the incidence is 23% with a 0.7% risk of myocardial infarction, while at age 70 the incidence of arteriosclerosis is 100%. The risk of cardiovascular complications shows a similar pattern to the incidence of atheroma.

Hypertension. This does not increase the risk of myocardial infarction in abdominal surgery, but there is an increased risk as a result of cardiac surgery. Remember that surgery for phaeochromocytoma and sometimes for carcinoid disease can be associated with wide fluctuations in blood pressure. This increases the risk of cerebral vascular accident.

Key points

- **The combination of respiratory and cardiovascular disease is more serious than one of them alone. A combination results in arterial hypoxaemia and is more common in older patients.**

- If renal function is also impaired, the risk of fluid overload is greatly increased.
- Down to a haemoglobin level of 10 g dl a *normal* myocardium can compensate well. Below this level, or if there is myocardial disease, peripheral hypoxaemia is more likely. Even at this level subendocardial ischaemia and fibrosis may occur.

Respiratory disease

There is an increased risk of respiratory complications in: smokers, in patients with bronchiectasis and emphysema, and if surgery is undertaken in the presence of tonsillitis, bronchitis or even coryza. In this group postpone elective surgery until the infection has cleared.

As indicated above, with advancing years there is a reduction in arterial oxygen tension and various changes in lung physiology. This results in a greater difference in alveolar–arterial oxygen and thus any respiratory complication produces more severe hypoxemia.

Key point

A combination of cor pulmonale and ischaemic heart disease produces a mortality of about 50%.

Diabetes mellitus

Insulin dependent diabetics are high risk patients for a number of different reasons:

Metabolic factors

The metabolic response to surgery results in hyperglycaemia. Maintenance of blood sugar can be difficult in the perioperative period and even non-insulin dependent diabetics may require insulin for a short time. If complications such as infection arise, both hyperinsulinaemia and hyperglycaemia may coexist – so called insulin resistance. The major danger is the development of severe ketoacidosis. This is seen most commonly in poorly controlled diabetic patients or indeed in those who are previously undiagnosed.

Infection

In diabetes mellitus, polymorphonuclear phagocyte function is impaired. There is an increased incidence of peripheral vascular disease affecting both medium and small vessels. Diabetic neuropathy reduces sensation to touch and to pain. Skin ulceration commonly acts as a nidus for infection. Where diabetes is poorly controlled there may be a higher sugar level in blood and tissues; this also encourages bacterial growth.

Wound healing

The disease in medium and small vessels reduces blood supply to healing tissue. The impaired polymorph phagocyte function interferes with the acute inflammatory reaction. As described, there is an increased risk of infection. All of these factors contribute to impaired wound healing.

Peripheral vascular disease

The increased risk of atheroma affecting both medium and small arteries increases the risk of gangrene. Neuropathic ulcers are more common. If infection does occur in the presence of gangrene, wet gangrene is more likely to be encountered.

Renal disease

If diabetes mellitus has been present for 20 years there is a 15% incidence of glomerulosclerosis. This impairment of renal function makes fluid and electrolyte balance more complex. Diabetic patients are more sensitive to protein depletion, and are at increased risk of severe ketoacidosis during a surgical illness.

DRUG THERAPY

Antibiotics

Misuse of antibiotics is said to be a major cause of litigation in the United States of America. Anaphylactic reactions are rare but can be life threatening. Hypersensitivity reactions, however, are slightly more common and only marginally less serious. It is vital to ask about drug allergy during the systematic enquiry of every patient.

Misuse of antibiotics may result in the development of resistance. The most serious from the point of view of the patient and the surgical department is the methicillin resistant *Staphylococcus aureus* (MRSA). It is important to have a hospital antibiotics policy, with clear indications for the use of antibiotics. Use them for a specific period only and take advice from the microbiologist for complex infections or immunocompromised patients.

Pseudomembranous colitis

This may present as a surgical emergency. Exposure to antibiotics combined with a period of hypovolaemia or hypotension are joint factors in pathogenesis. Diagnosis is made on the basis of a frozen section biopsy taken at sigmoidoscopy and confirmed by the demonstration of the *Clostridium difficile* toxin in the faecal fluid. Intravenous vancomycin or metronidazole are usually effective in treatment. Occasionally total colectomy is required for resistant cases.

Aminoglycocides

Gentamicin causes ototoxicity in 3% of patients. The elderly and those with impaired renal function are at increased risk. It causes nephrotoxicity in 2% of patients. For that reason peak and trough blood levels must be monitored in all patients receiving this therapy.

Corticosteroids

The greatest risk of complications occurs in patients on high dosage or on long courses of therapy.

The actions of the corticoids are to interfere with the mobility and phagocytic activity of polymorphonuclear leucocytes. This means that acute inflammation and the handling of bacteria are impaired, including the inflammatory reaction which is an essential part in the repair of wounds. Therefore deficient wound healing and wound infection are more common.

The production of ground substance is reduced. Therefore capillary and fragility is increased and wound haematoma is more common. This will contribute to impaired wound healing and will also provide a nidus for infection. It should be noted, however, that in experimental circumstances the short term use of methylprednisolone has not been associated with impaired healing of colonic anastomoses.

Stress response

Steroid therapy within the 6 months before surgery depresses the endogenous production of glucocorticoids. The output of endogenous glucocorticoid is an essential part of the response to surgery and anaesthesia. In order to avoid this complication the patient should receive 100 mg of hydrocortisone intravenously at the induction of anaesthesia and at 6 hourly intervals for 48 hours. Over the next 5–7 days reduce the intake of glucocorticoid either to zero or to the preoperative level.

Delay in diagnosis

Because of the depression of the acute inflammatory reaction, steroid therapy may delay the diagnosis of postoperative complications. It may also render some complications more likely to occur. For example, if a peptic ulcer perforates in someone on steroid therapy the diagnosis may be delayed with resulting increase in morbidity and mortality.

There is some evidence that glucocorticoids in dosage used for immunosuppression may encourage the development of certain virally induced tumours. In transplant patients there is evidence that the incidence of head and neck tumours and the virally induced tumours may be increased. This has not been reported in more common tumours of lung, breast or gastrointestinal tract.

Orthopaedic practice

Patients who are on steroid therapy in general, and those on steroids for rheumatoid arthritis in particular, have an increased risk of osteoporosis, which makes them more prone to suffer pathological fractures. Joint replacement is more difficult in such patients because of bone thinning and because of the general complications mentioned above.

Cytotoxic agents

Patients on cytotoxic chemotherapy have well recognized problems of gastrointestinal upset and hair loss. Depression of the white cell count and white cell function interfere with acute inflammation. This produces an increased incidence of wound infection and of impaired wound healing. Bone marrow depression is common. This also increases the risk of infection, especially with opportunistic organisms. It also risks purpuric eruption and frank bleeding. The expected reduction in cell mediated immunity increases the risk of developing a second neoplasm. For example, in patients successfully treated for primary lymphoma there is a 3% risk of a second tumour developing.

Cyclosporin

Cyclosporin A carries all the risks of depressing immune responses. More specifically it can result in depression of renal function. This is the usual reason for having to discontinue therapy with this agent.

Blood transfusion

Incompatibility

Major incompatibility reactions are now rare even with emergency cross-matching. Minor group incompatibility is more common, especially in patients who have had repeated transfusions. This involves, in order of importance, Kell Duffy or Kidd systems. It is common to attribute febrile reactions to incompatibility. Remember that transfusion of pyrogens or antibodies to white cells are alternative explanations for a febrile reaction.

Consequences of storage

The life span of red cells is finite and therefore lysis is an inevitable consequence of storage. This may produce transient jaundice but this is not of dire consequence. More importantly there is a potential for hyperkalaemia after massive blood transfusion because of the release of that intracellular ion. Careful monitoring of such patients by regular assessment of urea and electrolytes and of ECG changes which begin to occur above a level of 6 mmol/l are essential.

Acid citrate dextrose

This is the most commonly used anticoagulant. Transfused citrate may bind free calcium resulting in hypocalcaemia. Careful monitoring of the ECG is essential. Both platelets and clotting factors are consumed within some hours of storage. As a consequence, transfused stored blood cannot be relied upon to correct haemorrhagic tendencies and transfusion of fresh platelets or fresh frozen plasma may be required. The level of 2,3-diphosphoglycerate falls in stored red cells. This produces a shift of the oxyhaemoglobin dissociation curve to the left, resulting in an increased affinity of haemoglobin for oxygen. Delivery of oxygen at tissue level is therefore reduced. Stored red cells become more rigid. This impairs capillary circulation and encourages sludging.

Transmission of disease

In the past, both syphilis and hepatitis B were transmitted by transfusion (see Ch. 21). These diseases have been virtually abolished by stringent screening methods. Hepatitis C, however, remains a significant risk, although it is likely that screening for this will be widely available in the near future. More recently, the human immunodeficiency virus (HIV) has been transfused, mainly to haemophilic patients, with disastrous consequences.

Alteration in immunity

In transplantation surgery it is clear that the risk of renal rejection is reduced after blood transfusion. In patients undergoing resection for colonic cancer, perioperative transfusion results in a poorer prognosis, even when groups are matched for stage of disease, degree of operative trauma, age, sex and other factors. This is attributed to a reduction in cell mediated immunity. Other neoplastic processes and the relevance of blood transfusion to prognosis remain under investigation. In colorectal surgery, the use of blood transfusion is also associated with an increased risk of infective complications in the postoperative period. This risk has not been identified in patients undergoing joint replacement in orthopaedic practice.

Types of pathology

Obstructive jaundice

1. Effect on coagulation. Patients with obstructive jaundice have an increased risk of haemorrhage in the perioperative period. The absorption of the fat soluble vitamin K is impaired in the absence of bile salts. This interferes with the production of the vitamin K dependent factors II, VII, IX and X. The liver manufactures most clotting factors and therefore back pressure from obstruction may interfere with the synthesis of these factors and also factors V, XI, XII and XIII. The liver also clears activated coagulation factors such as fibrin degradation products (FDPS). When there is severe impairment of liver function there may also be disseminated intravascular coagulation.

All patients with obstructive jaundice should have a full clotting screen. Depending on the results of that screen, patients should be given systemic vitamin K_1 and/or fresh frozen plasma. The intravenous route for vitamin K_1 is recommended as it reduces the risk of intramuscular haematoma.

2. Effect on wound healing. Back pressure interferes with hepatocellular function and therefore disturbs protein metabolism. There is clear evidence that where obstructive jaundice is due to a malignancy there is impairment of healing of wounds and anastomoses. It is also taught that the same problem occurs in all patients with obstructive jaundice. The evidence for this is less clear. However, sufficient doubt remains for all patients with obstructive jaundice to be considered at high risk of wound failure.

As already indicated an increased incidence of wound haematoma and infection will also interfere with wound healing.

3. Effect on infective complications. Stasis within the biliary system increases the risk of infection, particularly with Gram-negative organisms. It is well established that opening the common bile duct produces a three-fold increase in the incidence of wound infection

relative to cholecystectomy alone. Where obstructive jaundice is secondary to stones or to postoperative stricture, the incidence of infected bile is at least 75%. With malignant obstruction, incidences of infection of 25% have been reported. The more often the bile duct is operated upon the more likely there is to be infected bile with consequent increase in postoperative infective complications.

The whole picture is complicated by the fact that there is reduced efficacy of the reticuloendothelial (Kupffer) cells in the liver. This means that the incidence of septicaemia and endotoxinaemia is increased. Increased mortality and morbidity result, particularly from ascending cholangitis.

4. Effect on renal function. Following surgery for obstructive jaundice, patients are at risk from acute renal failure – the 'hepatorenal syndrome'. There are a number of theories as to aetiology.

Acute renal failure is also a complication of Gram-negative septic shock, believed to be caused by the effects of endotoxins. The effects include activation of complement by the alternative pathway, the release of a number of cell mediators, including tumour necrosis factor and interleukins, and inappropriate disseminated intravascular coagulation (DIC). DIC results in microthrombi being found in the renal parenchyma, thus interfering with renal function.

It is also said that at least some part of renal failure occurs because the tubules are blocked by excess bilirubin. Histological evidence of this is variable and at most it is likely to be no more than a contributing factor.

The hormones responsible for maintaining fluid and electrolyte balance (ADH aldosterone and natriuretic factors) are metabolized in the liver. Disturbance of hepatic function may interfere with the activities of these hormones. Because of the increasing problems of haemorrhage, patients with obstructive jaundice are at greater risk of hypovolaemia. Protection against the effects of obstructive jaundice on renal function are to ensure adequate perioperative fluid infusion and a good diuresis, e.g. by the use of the osmotic diuretic mannitol. Give prophylactic antibiotics.

5. Effects on drugs and metabolism. It is assumed that general drug metabolism is altered in the presence of obstructive jaundice. The evidence in support of this is not strong. However, a particular problem does arise for drugs which are oxidized in the liver. In surgical practice great caution is required with analgesic and sedative therapy with, for example, morphine-like agents.

6. The specific problem relating to warfarin and interference with the INR with certain antibiotics must be remembered.

Neoplastic disease

Venous thromboembolism

The association between superficial thrombophlebitis migraines and pancreatic carcinoma is well established. However, it seems likely that malignant tumours secrete factors such as thromboplastins which affect the thrombotic cascade. In general terms, oncological procedures tend to be prolonged, they are associated with greater operative trauma, and they often require blood transfusion; all of this increases the incidence of deep vein thrombosis. Both in urology and in gynaecology major procedures in the pelvis are at particular risk of this complication. In addition to the factors mentioned above, pressure on the iliac veins is a significant problem.

Wound healing

It is generally accepted that patients with carcinoma are at increased risk both of primary wound failure and later incisional herniation. This relationship has been most clearly confirmed in malignant obstructive jaundice. In this condition malnutrition is combined with impaired protein metabolism in the liver.

The whole concept of cancer cachexia is complex and in patients who have lost greater than 10% of their premorbid body weight, or who present with a serum albumin of less than 30 g /l^{-1}, there is impaired healing both of wounds and anastomoses.

Patients with ovarian cancer have a high incidence of ascites with omental and peritoneal deposits. In contrast to gastrointestinal malignancy, radical surgery in these patients can be rewarding. However, this involves the rapid loss of protein-rich fluid. If the ascites reaccumulates rapidly in the postoperative period there will be associated abdominal distention and leaking through the wound. Both of these factors also impair wound healing.

TYPE OF SURGERY

Minimally invasive surgery

No field of surgical practice has escaped the introduction of minimally invasive procedures. The picture is most clearly established in laparoscopic cholecystectomy where there is evidence of more rapid recovery from surgery, earlier discharge from hospital, and earlier return to normal activities. The operation of mini cholecystectomy has been compared to the laparoscopic route with no clear benefit of the latter being proven.

The learning curve for this new form of operation can be long. This is because hand/eye coordination is different from conventional surgery and because the handling of tissues at a distance means that tactile sensitivity is reduced. Visual fields are limited, which is of particular importance when diathermy, laser or intracorporial suturing are being applied. Great care must be taken to visualize probes and needles and to keep them within the visual field at all times.

A particular problem exists when diathermy is used when capacitance coupling may occur, resulting in burn injuries at the trocar sites. Initially there was a vogue for the use of laser-assisted dissection; this has largely been overtaken by diathermy. However, if a laser is used all the normal precautions for the use of lasers have to be taken. It is also important to have a clear understanding of the characteristics of the different forms of laser in current use.

With specific reference to cholecystectomy, it is clear that there is at least a five-fold increase in the incidence of bile duct injury. Great care must be taken clearly to identify the anatomy and to have a low threshold for conversion to open cholecystectomy should there be any doubt or should the visual field be obscured.

Orthopaedic

Thromboembolism

Operations on the hips and pelvis have an increased risk of DVT, such that warfarin is often used for prophylaxis. Recent reports have demonstrated the value of low molecular weight heparin. The risk is higher if surgery is performed after major trauma. Blood transfusion also increases the risk of DVT.

Wound infection

Most orthopaedic procedures are classified as clean. Therefore the incidence of wound infection is low. However, the consequence of infection (e.g. after joint replacement) is catastrophic. If a foreign body such as a joint prosthesis becomes infected the chance of eradicating the infection by antibiotics is minimal. Removal of the prosthesis is required.

Use of tourniquets

In orthopaedic surgery tourniquets are widely used and it is recognized that tourniquet time must be kept to a minimum. However, it is vitally important that the vascular supply, especially to the lower limbs, is assessed. If this is not done the potential hazard of, for example, knee replacement is greatly increased. It also must be remembered that skin ischaemia may complicate badly planned incisions.

Steroid therapy

The problem with steroid therapy has already been mentioned. Especially in patients on steroids for rheumatoid arthritis, surgery is more difficult and anaesthetic problems may be faced, for example if the cervical spine is involved.

Gynaecology

In operations in the pelvis, particularly those lasting over 45 minutes, there is increased risk of trauma to the pelvic veins. This increases the risk of ileofemoral thrombosis. Extensive oncological eradication carries all the risks relevant to cancer surgery (see above).

Thoracic and upper abdominal procedures

Incisions used for this type of surgery are usually more painful. This makes respiratory movement more likely to be restricted, increasing the risk of atelectasis and infective complications. This is of particular importance in the elderly.

Prolonged operations

Traditional teaching is that prolonged operations increase the risk of respiratory difficulties, fluid and electrolyte imbalance and deep vein thrombosis. Experience with prolonged keyhole operations by the laparoscopic route have proved them relatively free of complications. This seems likely to be related to reducing the influence of such factors as:

- Intraoperative trauma
- Need for blood transfusion
- Loss of fluid and heat from exposed cavities
- Minimal damage to tissues.

It must be remembered that although the incidence of complications may be lower in minimally invasive surgery they are not abolished. Deep vein thrombosis, wound infection and wound hernia at port sites do occur. Therefore prophylactic measures must be taken and careful observation of patients be ensured in the postoperative period.

COMPLICATIONS AND THEIR MANAGEMENT

Venous thromboembolism

Risk factors

These include obesity, old age, and malignant disease. Long operations, pelvic and hip surgery, a past history of DVT or pulmonary embolism and varicose veins increase the risk. Other provoking factors are pregnancy and the oral contraceptive pill.

Incidence

The incidence varies with the type of operation and the risk factors mentioned. Overall it is estimated that for every 1000 operations there will be 100 DVTs, ten pulmonary emboli and one death. Pelvic and hip surgery, prolonged procedures and operations for neoplasia carry the highest risk of venous thrombosis.

Diagnosis

Early diagnosis is difficult and clinical diagnosis inaccurate. Experimentally, I^{125} fibrinogen scanning is sensitive in detecting developing thrombi but is of no value for established thrombosis. The new D-dimer assay is a very sensitive screening test which can be done at the bedside. Validation is still required but it seems likely that if the test is negative then deep vein thrombosis is not present. In inpatients some caution must be exercised in interpreting the result as it may be positive, for example, in the presence of an inflammatory process. Doppler ultrasound scans are valuable for peripheral sites. However, isolated calf vein thromboses are probably of no significance.

For suspected iliofemoral thrombosis a colour duplex scan is the investigation of choice. Where this is negative, repeating the scan in 1 week is probably preferable to venography. Venography has been the gold standard for diagnosis in the past but colour duplex appears to be more accurate and is clearly less invasive.

Prophylaxis

Because of the difficulties of diagnosis, prophylaxis is the cornerstone of management. Such risk factors as obesity, contraceptive pill, etc. should be corrected if clinically possible. The time of maximum risk of a thrombosis developing in surgical practice is during the operation when the three factors of stasis, endothelial trauma and increased coagulability are most prevalent.

Electrical methods of stimulating muscle function and thereby maintaining blood flow have been superseded. Mechanical methods, such as intermittent pumping of the calves by air insufflation of below knee stockings, are again more popular.

Subcutaneous calcium heparin (5000 units), injected 2 hours before surgery and continued postoperatively 12-hourly until the patient is fully mobile is well established in reducing the incidence of DVT. Calcium heparin causes less bleeding than sodium heparin. More recently, the low molecular fragment heparin has been shown to be at least as effective in general, gynaecological and orthopaedic surgery. It may reduce the risk of perioperative bleeding, although this is still debated. A once per day dosage regimen saves nursing time, decreases patient discomfort and is cost effective. Some orthopaedic surgeons favour full anticoagulation with warfarin as prophylaxis for major joint replacement, especially for revision surgery. Shorter operating times and earlier mobilization have contributed to the decreased risk.

Treatment

If the thrombus can be shown to be confined to the calf and is less than 5 cm long, no anticoagulation is indicated. Analgesics and support stockings may well be helpful. Take care when actively treating patients with a dyspeptic history or with a history of cerebrovascular accident.

Most patients require intravenous heparin, a loading dose of 10 000 units being followed by continuous intravenous infusion to prolong the activated partial thromboplastin time (APTT) by twice the control level. Thereafter, continue anticoagulation with warfarin for at least 3 months. Especially in hip replacement, the risk of DVT persists for several weeks. Low molecular weight heparin by subcutaneous injection is being used increasingly for established DVTs.

Complications

Pulmonary embolism may be fatal or multiple, producing pulmonary hypertension. Diagnosis is on the basis of a radioisotope ventilation/perfusion lung scan. If surgery is contemplated, as for a major embolism in a specialist centre, pulmonary angiography should be performed if time allows. Alternatively, thrombolysis with streptokinase or urokinase may be used. The alternative is full anticoagulation, as described for DVT.

Postphlebitic limb is more likely to follow an occlusive iliofemoral thrombosis. Treatment is symptomatic with support stockings and analgesics or aimed at treating the venous ulcers which can complicate this condition, probably secondary to liposclerosis.

Respiratory complications

Respiratory complications are the most common following surgery but because of the various risk factors involved a true incidence is difficult to establish.

Risk factors

Arterial oxygen tension falls gradually with age, more rapidly over age 80. The reduction with age in vital capacity, lung capacity, peak expiratory flow rate and post expiratory volume has been mentioned. Cardiovascular disease is more common with advanced years and a combination of cardiovascular and respiratory problems is particularly serious.

The risk of respiratory complications is increased with obesity, excessive sedation, immobility, pre-existing lung disease and myocardial disease, and following cardiothoracic, upper abdominal and vertical wounds, all of which reduce expiratory movements.

Pathology

The commonest problem after surgery is atelectasis. Small plugs of mucus block minor air passages and cause localized collapse. The plugs can usually be coughed clear by physiotherapy, but if they are not, superinfection may result. Pulmonary embolus (see below) may also predispose to infection. Pulmonary effusion often complicates pulmonary pathology such as infection, infarct or metastatic disease. An effusion may also result from a subdiaphragmatic abscess or pancreatitis. An effusion may also complicate congestive cardiac failure and hypoalbuminaemia. Pneumothrorax can result during ventilation. This complication can also be caused by cannulation of central veins, either for monitoring central venous pressure or for parenteral nutrition.

Adult respiratory distress syndrome (ARDS) is the most serious pulmonary complication in surgical practice. It may complicate severe sepsis, fluid overload, chest trauma, fat emboli, burn injury and inhalation pneumonitis. The cause is unclear but contributing factors are:

- Changes in type I and II alveolar cells, resulting in loss of surfactant and alveolar collapse
- Impaired capillary to alveolar diffusion
- Arteriovenous shunts
- The effects of endotoxin resulting in complement activation by the alternate pathway and disseminated intravascular coagulation (DIC)
- Consequent upon the effects of endotoxin numerous mediatory cytokines are released which contribute to pulmonary damage (e.g. tumour necrosis factor or interleukins)
- The effects of hyperoxide radicals.

Management

Where possible correct clinical risk factors such as obesity and smoking habit prior to surgery. In all patients it is essential to ensure adequate analgesia without excessive sedation. Encourage regular physiotherapy administered both by the therapist and by the nursing and medical staff. It is important to time physiotherapy when the patient is free of pain and not overly sedated.

It is important carefully to monitor the pulse, respiratory rate and temperature. Appropriate antibiotics are administered to patients who are pyrexial despite conservative measures, clinically ill, at high risk, especially if there is combined myocardial and pulmonary disease, and all patients who have features of ARDS.

Key point

Supplementary oxygen by mask is required. If, despite that, the P_aO_2 falls below 75 mmHg, consider ventilatory support.

Infective complications

Risk factors

Alimentary surgery not only has a higher incidence of infection but this is often associated with endogenous organisms. In 'clean' surgery, infection is usually secondary to exogenous agents. Wounds may be classified as:

- Clean, such as thyroid or hernia surgery
- Potentially contaminated, as in elective gastrointestinal surgery
- Contaminated, as following bowel perforation
- Dirty, where there is faecal contamination.

The incidence of infection, morbidity and mortality increases from clean to dirty. The risk of infection is greater in all categories if surgery is performed as an emergency.

In clean surgery, infection is usually secondary to exogenous agents such as *Staphylococcus aureus*. Where there is a series of infections in one unit following clean procedures seek a source of carriage of such organisms. In alimentary surgery the infecting organisms are usually endogenous. These are usually Gram-negative aerobes. Where surgery is performed in the lower ileum and in the large bowel, remember the importance of anaerobic infection. It cannot be emphasized too strongly that, although the incidence of wound infection after clean procedures is low, the consequences of such infection may be catastrophic (e.g. following joint replacement or after valvular heart surgery).

The risk of wound infection is increased in the presence of obesity, in haematomas and in patients with diabetes mellitus. Other factors are glucocorticoid therapy, immunosuppression, malnutrition and obstructive jaundice.

Prophylaxis

Identify the patients at risk. This includes those in whom the incidence of infection is higher and those for whom infection is particularly hazardous. Reduce or control risk factors if possible. Ensure that your surgical technique is as perfect and as meticulous as possible, with particular reference to haemostasis, avoiding excessive use of diathermy, leaving dead space or traumatizing tissues by rough handling.

Select the appropriate antibiotic to give the greatest protection and tissue penetration at the time of surgery. Remember to take account of possible patient allergies and the cost involved. It is sufficient to give one dose intravenously at the time of induction. Alternatively, one dose intramuscularly can be given with the premedication. Give more than one dose only if the operation lasts longer than 4 hours or if there has been contamination during gastrointestinal surgery. In this case treatment rather than prophylaxis is being practised.

Remember the value of mechanical bowel preparation which reduces loading at the time of large bowel anastomosis but which does not remove pathogens from the gastrointestinal tract.

There is continuing controversy about the need for and timing of shaving the operative area. There is some evidence that shaving increases the number of potential pathogens on the skin. There is also controversy about the agent used for skin preparation. Chlorhexidine in spirit or aqueous Betadine are both acceptable. Debate continues about the value of intracavity antibiotics or antiseptics and these have probably been superseded by prophylactic antibiotics.

In potentially contaminated surgery there is no value in the use of plastic drapes; these tend to increase the number of pathogens on the skin. The use of danger towels, separate knives for incising skin and deeper tissues and changing gloves after performing anastomoses are now of historical interest only.

Key point

Antibiotics are no substitute for gentle handling of tissues, careful haemostasis, judicious use of diathermy and avoiding strangling tissues with ligatures and sutures.

Treatment

Wound infection.   Open the wound to allow adequate drainage. Obtain pus for culture, to establish the infecting organism(s) and antibiotic sensitivity. Irrigate the wound for adequate drainage and debridement.

Formally reopen and surgically debride dirty wounds. If clean wounds become infected, consider cross-infections and investigate the likely sources.

Use antibiotics only if specifically indicated (for cellulitis or septicaemia) or if the consequences of infection would be disastrous (see above).

If the wound infection is chronic, consider the possibility of specific organisms such as *Actinomyces*, a foreign body, such as a suture in the wound, an associated fistula as may occur in Crohn's disease, or associated factors such as irradiation and perineal wounds. Remember the danger of synergistic infections and dermal gangrene.

Postoperative abscess. These are usually intraperitoneal but can be found deep in the wound. Localize the abscess and attempt drainage, if necessary under ultrasound or computed tomography (CT) control. Monitor resolution of the cavity radiologically if necessary. Exclude anastomotic leakage as a cause (see below).

If the patient remains toxic or the cavity fails to resolve, proceed to operative drainage and definitive treatment of any underlying cause.

Septicaemia and septic shock.   The septic complications mentioned above may progress to septicaemia and septic shock in patients who are debilitated by disease or drug therapy, such as steroids or cytotoxic chemotherapy. However, some organisms may be particularly virulent from the outset.

After surgery it is vital to remain alert for all septic problems. In terms of recognizing the more serious conditions remember the danger signs, which are:

- Persistent, often swinging pyrexia with tachycardia
- Signs of toxicity – flushed warm skin, glazed eyes, tachypnoea
- Falling urinary output – less than 40 ml h^{-1}
- Hypoxaemia.

Key point

Treat suspected septic shock effectively to avoid low-output septic shock with its associated high mortality (>50%).

The nature of death in such patients is multiple organ failure, and while a patient may survive failure of a single organ system such as the kidneys, the more organs which fail the higher the mortality (Table 36.3).

This problem is most likely to be encountered when diagnosis and localization of a septic focus is delayed, and when inadequate initial treatment is instituted.

Table 36.3	Multiple organ failure—rates of survival
1	90%
2	40–50%
3	5–10%

Principles of treatment are:

1. Ensure adequate circulating blood volume using a mixture of crystalloid and colloid fluids, aiming for a central venous pressure of 10–15 cmH_2O in a ventilated patient.
2. Oxygen supplementation.
3. Broad spectrum intravenous antibiotic(s).
4. Ventilatory support if the P_aO_2 is less than 75 mmHg.
5. Cardiac support with such drugs as dopamine, dobutamine, digitalis and catecholamines, as indicated.
6. Attention to renal function with dialysis for established renal failure.
7. Early recognition and treatment of any evidence of multiple organ failure.

More controversial are the methods used in some centres to ensure gastrointestinal decontamination. This involves a combination of enteral antibiotic and antiseptic agents, combined with a parenteral antibiotic, and this is gaining popularity. The value of enteral glutamine and/or α-ketoglutarate is considered vital in several intensive care units. This is yet to be proven in a controlled trial. However, enteral nutritional support is preferable to the parenteral route.

Anastomotic leakage

Anastomotic leakage may complicate any anastomosis, but is seen most commonly following oesophageal and colorectal surgery. In the latter group, leakage results in a three-fold increase in operative mortality.

Colonic anastomoses below the pelvic peritoneal reflection are associated with an increased risk of leakage, both clinical and radiological (Table 36.4). The clinical rate always underestimates the true incidence of leakage, as detected by gastrograffin or barium enema.

Predisposing factors

The general factors are similar to those which apply to wound healing in general, such as nutritional deficiencies (particularly protein, vitamin C and zinc), old age and impaired local blood flow from general conditions such as arteriosclerosis and cardiac disease.

Table 36.4 Rates of clinically evident and radiologically detected leaks following colonic anastomoses performed above and below the pelvic peritoneal reflection		
Location of anastomoses	Detected leaks (%)	
	Clinical	Radiological
Above pelvic peritoneum	1.2	18.3
Below pelvic peritoneum	16	33

Local factors include tension at the anastomosis and poor surgical technique with regard to preparing the bowel ends, handling of tissues, excessive use of diathermy and the insertion and ligation of sutures. Contamination of the anastomosis with liquid faeces prejudices healing, as does an inadequate vascular supply to one or both sides of the anastomosis. Less important factors are the suture material, the number of layers employed, and whether a stapling or suturing technique is used. However, there is preliminary evidence that tumour recurrence is lower in experimental studies when stainless wire is used for the anastomosis and, in clinical work, if the anastomosis is stapled.

Presentation

Gastrointestinal contents may be identified in the wound or at a drain site. An intra-abdominal abscess or more serious septic complication may develop. There may be prolonged ileus, unexplained pyrexia or tachycardia, sudden collapse postoperatively or development of an internal fistula.

Where there is any doubt, confirmation can often be obtained from a gently performed X-ray using a contrast medium. In this regards gastrograffin which is water soluble, is preferable to barium since leakage of barium has much more serious consequences if present free in the peritoneal cavity.

Management

If the patient is adversely affected by peritonitis, shock or infection, interventional treatment is indicated:

1. Adequate resuscitation
2. Antibiotic cover
3. Surgery.

The surgical procedure depends on the operative findings, but the principles are:

1. Thorough peritoneal lavage with tetracycline and warmed saline (1 gl 1^{-1})

2. Identification of the leak and any associated pathology such as Crohn's disease
3. Resection of the affected area (never try to insert a few extra sutures)
4. Be prepared to establish a proximal stoma and a distal mucous fistula or carry out a Hartmann's type procedure of closing the distal rectal stump
5. Very occasionally, if contamination is slight, and conditions are satisfactory, an expert surgeon may elect to excise the margins and re-form the anastomosis
6. As a rule, after restoring the patient's health and nutritional status over a minimum of 6–12 weeks the bowels ends may be reanastomosed.

In the presence of a fistula, management depends on the state of the patient and the volume draining. When the volume is small (i.e. less than 500 ml per 24 hours) and the patient is well, the initial treatment should be conservative:

1. Restricted oral intake
2. Intravenous fluids
3. Correct fluid, protein, electrolyte, acid–base and vitamin deficiencies
4. Treat associated sepsis
5. Institute nutritional support
6. Consider the somatostatin analogue octreotide to reduce gastrointestinal secretion and motility. If such treatment fails or the output is high (>500 ml day^{-1}) or there is associated sepsis, intervention along the lines described above will be required.

Problems with the wound

Failure of wound healing may result (in descending order of importance) in: wound dehiscence, incisional hernia or superficial wound disruption. Wound dehiscence should now be less than 0.1%. Incisional hernia is more common but should occur in less than 10% of abdominal wounds.

Risk factors

General risk factors include respiratory disease, smoking, obesity, obstructive jaundice (especially secondary to malignant disease), nutritional deficiencies of protein, zinc and vitamin C, malignant disease, steroid therapy, and following emergency procedures.

Local risk factors include wound infections, impaired blood supply, foreign body in the wound and following irradiation to the area. Clean incised wounds heal better than ragged traumatic wounds. The site of wound is important (the anterior tibial area is notorious for wound breakdown and inappropriate length-to-

width flap wounds heal less well). Another important factor is poor surgical technique.

Prevention

As in all complications, the cornerstone of success is to recognize risk factors, correct those which can be corrected and use an appropriate surgical technique for all wounds. For closing the abdominal wall, the best results are obtained by suture with a non-absorbable material such as nylon or an absorbable suture with prolonged tensile strength such as polydioxanone.

Management of superficial disruption

- Evacuate haematoma and/or pus
- Excise and remove slough
- Remove any foreign body
- Irrigate with, for example, hydrogen peroxide and povidone–iodine
- Pack gently to avoid too rapid healing over of the skin, but avoid trauma to granulation tissue
- Carefully monitor healing by secondary intention
- Use newer materials such as Kaltostat or Sorbsan which help clean sloughy wounds and are well tolerated by patients.

Management of wound dehiscence

The mortality reported following abdominal wound rupture varies from 24% to 46%.

- Recognize the problem early
- Do not overlook premonitory serous discharge from the wound, a prolonged ileus or low-grade pyrexia
- Resuscitate the patient
- Re-explore the abdomen and perform adequate peritoneal lavage
- Proceed to resuture the abdomen under general anaesthetic, using an adequate length of non-absorbable suture without tension
- Use 1 cm bites about 1 cm apart
- Avoid pulling the suture tightly in the tissues
- It may be helpful to decompress the small bowel in retrograde fashion to reduce intra-abdominal tension.

Recurrence is uncommon, but incisional herniation complicates approximately 25% of cases.

Management of incisional hernia

The indications for surgical intervention are obstruction, pain or increasing size making control difficult. First spend time reducing such risk factors as obesity, smoking, constipation and prostatism. Assess the overall prognosis. Not all patients require or want surgical repair. Where there is unresected neoplastic disease, repair is usually contraindicated. In elderly and high risk patients an abdominal support will control symptoms in the majority of cases.

Historically a number of options are available as regards surgical technique including Mayo or Keel repairs. However, except where the hernia is very small a mesh repair is now the treatment of choice. Following the repair the mortality should be less than 1% and the recurrence rate 5–10%. If a patient is morbidly obese at the time of repair a satisfactory result is less likely. The main problem with mesh repair is if infection supervenes. Under those circumstances it is most unusual that the repair will heal because of the presence of a foreign body. It is usual to have to remove the mesh and to start all over again.

Hypertrophic and keloid scarring

Hypertrophic scars are limited to the wound area and do not advance after 6 months. Keloid scars are more extensive and continue to expand beyond 6 months, but fortunately are much less common. Predisposing factors are pigmented skin, burn trauma, wounds on posterior aspects, younger age groups, and a past history of keloid scarring.

There is excessive production and contraction of fibrous tissue. The synthesis of collagen is increased but the scar contains embryonic or fetal collagen. Only in hypertrophic scars is there an increased lysis of collagen. The main complication is joint deformity, but the cosmetic problems can be considerable in exposed sites and with younger patients.

Successful treatment is difficult, and should not be contemplated until 6 months from injury. There is no treatment for hypertrophic scars, and keloid scars should not be approached until they are mature. Re-excision with and without pressure or plastic procedures are as disappointing as radiotherapy. Greater success has been claimed for injection of steroid into the wound. The mode of action appears to be increased collagen lysis, with depression of the proliferation of fibroblasts. Injection of triamcinolone can be repeated at intervals of 1 or 2 weeks, depending on the result achieved.

Haemorrhage

Incidence

The incidence and severity of haemorrhagic complications are not easy to quantify. Re-exploration of a wound to evacuate haematoma and to secure haemostasis is uncommon. Wound haematoma and local bruising are sufficiently common to make it difficult to differentiate a complication from a normal sequel of surgery.

Where bleeding complicates intra-abdominal surgery, warning signs are haemodynamic instability with rising pulse and falling blood pressure, reduction in hourly urine volume to less than 40 ml per hour, and excessive volume draining from the abdominal drain.

Predisposing factors are obesity, long-term steroid therapy, and jaundice. Recent transfusions of stored blood, coagulation diseases, platelet deficiencies, and anticoagulant therapy may result in haemorrhage and in old age there is increased capillary fragility. Severe sepsis may result in disseminated intravascular coagulation.

Pathology

It is conventional to consider primary haemorrhage within 24 hours of surgery. This is usually a technical problem of haemostasis. The operative area appears dry but with restoration of normal blood pressure or continuous infusion of intravenous fluids a vessel may dilate and bleed. In secondary haemorrhage bleeding usually occurs 5–10 days after operation. It is due to local infection, sloughing of a clot or erosion of a ligature.

Prevention

It is vital to recognize patients at risk and to reverse risk factors whenever possible. In patients on long term warfarin it is relatively straightforward to convert the anticoagulation to intravenous heparin, which can be reversed more rapidly than warfarin by the injection of protamine.

Cooperation with a haematologist is essential in managing patients with coagulation disorders (see Ch. 9). Specific factors can be infused as required. Timing is vital – for example, if fresh platelets are required for patients undergoing splenectomy it is essential they are given after the spleen has been removed. Give vitamin K by intravenous route to reverse the problems associated with the obstructive element of jaundice. Control of infection is essential. Surgical technique must be meticulous.

Management

The need for intervention is dictated by the patient's symptoms and vital signs. Where haemorrhage is overt it is usually easier to decide whether exploration of the wound and cavity is indicated or not. When bleeding is internal reliance cannot be placed on any intracavity drain.

- Check a clotting screen to assess any established and to identify any new problem.
- Correct any deficit appropriately with vitamin K by injection for problems with the clotting mechanism, expressed as the international normalized ratio (INR). Use specific factors for deficiencies, fresh frozen plasma, and fresh platelets as indicated by the results of the coagulation study.
- Do not undertake surgical exploration until any deficit has been corrected at least in part.
- It is unusual to identify a specific bleeding point at exploration.

The principles of surgery are to evacuate the blood and clot, identify any bleeding point or points, and control them appropriately. If a troublesome ooze persists, try the effect of a haemostatic agent such as Spongistan, or a collagen derivative. If control remains difficult, pack the raw surface for 24–48 hours. Consider leaving the superficial wound open, and give thought to the benefits of laparostomy (leaving the main wound open, packed with sterile packs) when a deeper source is suspected and recurrent bleeding is feared, as after pancreatic surgery – this facilitates re-exploration.

Summary

1. The combination of cor pulmonale and ischaemic heart disease, or low output septic shock, carry up to 50% mortality.
2. Correct co-morbidity factors before operation whenever possible.
3. There are many complications common to all types of operation.
4. In addition, each form of surgery carries its special risks.

 Further reading

Cuschieri A, Giles G R, Moossa A R 1988 Essential surgical Practice. Wright, Bristol

Pollock A V 1991 Postoperative complications in surgery. Blackwell Scientific, Oxford

Smith J A R (ed) 1984 Complications of surgery in general. Bailliere Tindall, London

Tayfor I, Karran S J (eds) 1996 Surgical principles. Edward Arnold, London

37

Intensive care

J. Jones

Objectives

- **Appreciate the value and limitations of intensive care.**
- **Understand the specific indications for admission to intensive care units.**

An intensive care unit (ICU) (also sometimes called an intensive therapy unit (ITU)) provides a safe environment for treating the critically ill. It is reasonable to believe (though it has never been proved), that a hospital's sickest patients, whatever the nature of their disease, will benefit from being managed in a separate area, specially equipped for their needs. It must also be cost-effective to concentrate the resources necessary for the care of the very sick into a single space. The Department of Health recommends that 1–2% of the acute beds in a hospital should be allocated to intensive care, a figure increasingly regarded by people who work in ICUs as too low.

Of all the resources an ICU must be able to command, the most important is staff. The best bedside monitor is a competent nurse, and every ICU worthy of the name should have a nurse at each bedside for all the time that the bed is occupied. There should, in addition, be a senior nurse in charge of the unit. Shortages of suitably qualified nurses, and of the money with which to pay them, limit the availability of intensive care.

There must be a doctor always on duty within the ICU and free from commitments elsewhere. He or she does not have to be an anaesthetist, but must be able to intubate patients. A consultant should be immediately available. Although 75% of ICUs in the UK are run by anaesthetists, successful intensive care requires the cooperation of specialists of many disciplines (Intensive Care Society 1990). It is vital to the successful management of very sick patients that specialist colleagues be called in whenever necessary. Microbiologists can give immensely helpful advice on antibiotic therapy and infection control. A renal physician should be involved early in the care of a patient with suspected renal failure. 'Does the patient have renal failure?' is a better question than, 'How soon can you dialyse the patient?'.

The Intercollegiate Committee on Intensive Care proposes that senior house officers (SHOs) in medicine, surgery and anaesthetics should all spend 3 months of their training in intensive care. Some years are likely to pass before suitable training programmes can be set up and recognized. Until they are, surgical SHOs should involve themselves as heavily as possible in the management of their firm's patients when they pass through the ICU.

INDICATIONS FOR ADMISSION

It should be clear from the above that intensive care is expensive, and should be offered only to patients who really need it, and who may be expected to benefit from it. Such patients fall, in descending order of priority, into three categories: those who need

1. *Mechanical support of a vital function.* In practice, the mechanical support most frequently employed is a ventilator. It may also be an intra-aortic balloon pump to augment cardiac output, a machine for haemofiltration or haemodialysis, or even an extracorporeal oxygenator. None of these can safely be used anywhere but in an ICU.

2. *Close monitoring.* Patients who need intensive monitoring always require the continuous attention of a specially trained nurse, and often need frequent medical interventions such as blood transfusions or infusions of drugs that improve myocardial contractility (inotropic drugs).

3. *'Heavy' nursing.* Under this heading fall patients (nearly always surgical) who need scrupulous care of skin, wounds and drains, and whose fluid balance and

nutrition call for careful attention. Such patients need a great deal of nursing time, but a less sophisticated level of nursing skill than patients in the first two categories.

It is now fashionable to point out that patients in the second two categories may, perhaps, be effectively, and more cheaply, managed in a high dependency unit (HDU) leaving the scarce and expensive facilities of the ICU more readily available to patients with organ failure, i.e. those in the first category.

It is not reasonable to refuse admission to the ICU to a patient simply on the grounds that he or she is old. Old people can be very resilient, and have been shown to respond to intensive care just as well as younger ones with similar disorders. Equally, it is not good practice to make the ICU a final common pathway to the mortuary. For example, patients with respiratory failure due to diffuse metastatic infiltration of the lungs should not, as a rule, be supported with artificial respiration in the hope that chemotherapy will grant them a few more months of life.

Scoring systems in intensive care

A number of scoring systems have been used in intensive care (see Box 37.1) with various aims:

- Assessment of the severity of the patient's illness
- Prediction of the outcome of the patient's illness
- Comparison of the performance of different ICUs in treating patients (with similar disorders of similar severity; it is meaningless to compare mortality rates in units with vastly different patient populations)
- Estimation of the cost of treating patients.

In the UK, the APACHE II scoring system is the most popular for quantifying the severity of a patient's illness. APACHE is an acronym signifying Acute Physiology, Age and Chronic Health Evaluation, and the roman numeral II indicates that it is a modification of the original APACHE system published in 1981 and found to be too complicated for routine use. The acute physiological derangement is calculated by computer from the worst values of a dozen parameters (such as blood pressure and haemoglobin concentration) obtained in the first 24 hours of intensive care, plus the Glasgow Coma Score, and weighted by the patient's age, general health, and diagnosis. The more severe the patient's illness, the higher the APACHE II score will be, and higher APACHE II scores are associated with higher mortality rates. However, neither the APACHE II scoring system nor any other scoring system yet devised has been established as an accurate predictor of outcome in the individual case. (The APACHE III system, which is more refined, but which involves the collection of more complicated data than APACHE II, has not achieved great popularity in the UK).

If consistently performed, APACHE II scores, together with data on hospital mortality, could be a useful tool for audit purposes. The ratio of hospital mortality rate actually observed to that predicted by the APACHE II score is known as the standard mortality ration (SMR). An SMR greater than unity suggests that patients are succumbing more frequently than the APACHE II score would lead the observer to expect, and an SMR of less than unity would suggest the reverse. Unfortunately, great variation has been demonstrated in the way ICUs collect their APACHE II data, and the system itself has limitations; for example, it should not be used for patients under 18 years old, nor for those who have burns or who have undergone cardiac surgery.

The Intensive Care National Audit and Research Centre (ICNARC) has begun to collect data from many (eventually, it is hoped, from all) ICUs in this country in a standardized way. ICUs collaborating with ICNARC are able to compare their SMRs with those of other units treating patients in the same diagnostic categories.

Numerous other scoring systems have been introduced (see Box 37.1) some for general ICUs and some for specialist units. The adoption of the APACHE II system by ICNARC would seem to guarantee the future of that system in this country. The Intensive Care Society has recommended that the Nursing Dependency score and Therapeutic Intervention Scoring System points should be recorded as well.

The Therapeutic Interventions Scoring System (TISS) allocates points from 1 to 4 for 76 different therapeutic interventions, which are, for the most part, nursing procedures. Although the authors thought it a useful way to quantify severity of illness, TISS is really a reflection of nursing workload, and might thus be the basis of a system to determine the 'pay' element of an

---

Box 37.1   Some scoring systems used in intensive care

- Acute Physiology, Age and Chronic Health Evaluation (APACHE)
- Simplified Acute Physiology Score
- Organ Failure Score
- Sickness Score
- Therapeutic Intervention Scoring System (TISS)
- Mortality Probability Models (MPM)
- Nursing Dependency Score

individual patient's ICU cost. However, it takes no account of the 'non-pay' element of the cost of intensive care, i.e. the cost of equipment and disposables, and fixed costs, such as heating and lighting.

OXYGEN DELIVERY AND
OXYGEN CONSUMPTION

The amount of oxygen available to the tissues is given by the equation:

| Oxygen delivery Do_2 | = | Cardiac output CO | × | Arterial oxygen content C_aO_2 |

Normal values (Nunn & Freeman 1964):

$$1000 \text{ ml min}^{-1} = 5000 \text{ ml min}^{-1} \times 20 \text{ ml dl}^{-1}$$

Also:

| Arterial oxygen content | = | Hb concn | × | O_2 carried (ml/g Hb) |

Normal values at full saturation:

$$20 \text{ ml dl}^{-1} = 15 \text{ g dl}^{-1} \times 1.34 \text{ ml/g Hb}$$

An adequate supply of oxygen to the tissues thus depends on:

- Cardiac output (CO)
- Hb concentration
- Percentage saturation of Hb (S_aO_2).

The volume of oxygen consumed by the tissues at rest is given by:

| Oxygen consumption Vo_2 | = CO × (Arterial oxygen content − Mixed venous oxygen content) |
| | = CO × $(C_aO_2 - C_vO_2)$ |

Normal values:

$$250 \text{ ml min}^{-1} = 5000 \text{ ml min}^{-1} (20 \text{ ml dl}^{-1} - 15 \text{ ml dl}^{-1})$$

In normal circumstances, therefore, oxygen delivery exceeds consumption by a comfortable margin. In very sick patients, however, oxygen delivery may fall because of:

- A low cardiac output
- Anaemia
- Respiratory disorders causing the S_aO_2 to fall.

Unfortunately, especially if they have sepsis, such patients may also have a higher than normal oxygen consumption. If oxygen delivery is inadequate to supply the tissues' needs, the consequences will be:

- Lactic acidosis

- A low C_vO_2
- Organ failure.

Direct estimations of the adequacy of tissue oxygen supply are not easy to make. It is possible to measure both serum lactate and mixed venous oxygen saturation levels, but both are difficult to interpret. It has been suggested that the intracellular pH of the mucosa lining the gastrointestinal tract is a good indicator of the adequacy of the oxygen supply to the bowel. The pH of saline sampled from an intragastric balloon may mirror the pH within gastric mucosal cells, but doubt has been expressed as to the usefulness of such measurements.

It is, therefore, crucial in intensive care:

- To monitor and support the cardiovascular and respiratory systems in order to maintain a satisfactory tissue oxygen supply. The belief that manipulation of oxygen delivery to supranormal levels improves survival in patients in intensive care units no longer seems sustainable (Consensus Report 1996).
- To monitor and support the function of the vital organs which demand adequate perfusion with oxygenated blood.

SHOCK

Shock can be defined as inadequate tissue perfusion due to acute circulatory failure. It may be classified as hypovolaemic, cardiogenic, anaphylactic or septic (see Table 37.1). Oxygen delivery to the tissues is always reduced, sometimes critically.

1. *Hypovolaemic shock.* Hypovolaemic shock is due to a reduction in the circulating volume, after haemorrhage, plasma loss (as in burns) or loss of water and electrolytes (e.g. intestinal obstruction, diabetic ketoacidosis and Addisonian crisis). The venous return to the heart is reduced, and the cardiac output and blood pressure fall. Tachycardia and peripheral vasoconstriction, reflexly mediated by the baroceptors, partially compensate for the hypotension. Splanchnic vasoconstriction and underperfusion of the gut may be associated with an increased permeability of the intestinal mucosa to bacteria or endotoxin. Hypovolaemia may thus be a precursor of sepsis.

2. *Cardiogenic shock.* In cardiogenic shock, the primary defect is a fall in cardiac output. Causes include myocardial infarction and cardiac compression (tamponade). In the elderly, impaired myocardial perfusion secondary to hypovolaemia may cause acute cardiac failure. Hypotension, tachycardia and vasoconstriction are again seen, but the cardiac filling pressure (central

Table 37.1

	HR	BP	CO	Extremities	CVP
Hypovolaemic	↑	↓	↓	Cold	↓
Cardiogenic	↑	↓	↓	Cold	↑
Anaphylactic	↑	↓	↓	Rash sometimes; warm at first	↓
Septic	↑	↓	↑ at first Then ↓	Warm at first Cold later	↓

venous pressure (CVP)) will be raised because the heart is unable to eject all the blood that is returned to it.

3. *Anaphylactic shock.* The clinical features of anaphylactic shock are those of acute histamine release. This is often secondary to the administration of drugs to which the patient is sensitive, of plasma substitutes or of contrast medium. Profound vasodilatation causes hypotension with a fall in venous return and cardiac output. Urticarial rashes, bronchospasm and spasm of the gut also occur. There is an increase in capillary permeability, which may add an element of hypovolaemia.

4. *Septic shock.* Septic shock is due to overwhelming infection. The clinical features, which may be caused by the release of a variety of vasoactive substances such as bacterial endotoxin, are at first vasodilatation, opening of arteriovenous shunts and increased capillary permeability. The extremities are initially warm, and the cardiac output high. Later, loss of fluid from the circulation brings about the signs of hypovolaemia. Impaired organ function due to inadequate perfusion and oxygen delivery may occur in all forms of shock, but multiple organ failure, with the development of coagulopathy and the adult respiratory distress syndrome (ARDS), is a particular feature of continued sepsis.

The treatment of all forms of shock is, in part, supportive, and careful monitoring of the patient (see below) is essential if support is to be appropriate. Support must be promptly given if organ failure is not to supervene. However, support is not all-important. Prompt treatment of the cause of shock may be crucial to the patient's survival. There is no point in relying simply on massive blood transfusion, attentively monitored, in a patient whose hypovolaemia is due to a ruptured ectopic pregnancy or to a leaking aortic aneurysm. Similarly, supportive treatment will not cure a patient with septic shock due to a ruptured bowel or to an empyema. Early surgery, after initial resuscitation, is the best treatment for patients of this sort.

CARDIAC SUPPORT

Monitoring the cardiovascular system

The measurement of cardiac output (CO) is an invasive procedure and, fortunately, is not essential in every patient in the ICU. Estimates of the adequacy of cardiac output can be made by monitoring other variables which are easier to measure. These include:

- Electrocardiogram (ECG)
- Blood pressure (BP)
- Core–peripheral temperature gradient
- Central venous pressure (CVP).

In addition, estimates of the adequacy of tissue perfusion can be made from simple clinical observations. A patient who is alert and passing urine must be supplying his brain and kidneys with enough oxygenated blood for them to function.

ECG

Since:

$$CO = \text{Heart rate} \times \text{Stroke volume}$$

continuous monitoring of the ECG provides reliable information of one determinant of the CO. The ECG will also demonstrate any arrhythmias; depression or elevation of the ST segments may be a warning of inadequate myocardial oxygenation.

Blood pressure

The blood pressure may be measured intermittently using a cuff or displayed continuously on a monitor after arterial (usually radial) cannulation. Since:

$$CO = \frac{BP}{\text{Systemic vascular resistance (SVR)}}$$

the blood pressure is often a reliable guide to the adequacy of the cardiac output. However, in the presence of vasoconstriction, which may be secondary to inadequate filling of the circulation or to primary cardiac failure, a normal blood pressure can be associated with a low cardiac output. Further information on the state of the circulation can be obtained from the peripheral temperature.

Peripheral temperature

The core (rectal or oesophageal)–peripheral temperature gradient has been shown to be a reliable guide to the cardiac output (Joly & Weil 1969). Clearly, a patient with warm, pink feet cannot be vasoconstricted.

Central venous pressure

Clinical estimation of the jugular venous pressure is made by observing the level of the external jugular veins above the angle of Louis in a patient propped up to 45°. Cannulation of a central vein (usually the subclavian or internal jugular) enables the CVP to be measured, either intermittently using a water manometer or continuously using a transducer. Zero is taken from the level at which the right atrium is presumed to be (the midaxillary line if the patient is lying flat). Because the zero level is somewhat arbitrary, and, in any event, alters when the patient moves to a different position, single measurements of the CVP are not very helpful. However, a low CVP (normal range 5–10 mmHg) which rises only transiently on the rapid administration of 200 ml intravenous fluid is strongly suggestive of an empty circulation. A persistently elevated CVP with a normal venous waveform (i.e. the high value is not due to a blocked cannula) in the presence of peripheral vasoconstriction suggests myocardial failure (Sykes 1963) (Fig. 37.1).

Measurement of CVP is an invasive procedure. The complications are:

- Pneumothorax
- Accidental arterial puncture causing haematoma or haemothorax
- Misplacement (check the position of the catheter with a chest X-ray)
- Air embolism if the catheter is opened to the atmosphere with the patient sitting up
- Infection – especially if the catheter is handled frequently or left in for too long.

If we monitor all the variables above, then in many patients we will be able to infer:

- Whether or not the cardiac output is adequate
- Whether a low cardiac output is due to
  (a) insufficient filling of the circulation, or
  (b) impaired myocardial function.

Furthermore, we will be guided as to whether matters may be improved by infusing intravenous fluids, or using drugs to improve cardiac performance. Finally, we will be able to follow the results of whatever therapy we institute. In only a few patients will it be necessary to monitor any further variables.

Pulmonary artery catheterization

The CVP is a reliable indicator of cardiac filling (or preload) if both right and left ventricles are functioning similarly. Although the right and left ventricles function similarly in most patients, there are circumstances in which the performance of one may be impaired while the other continues to work normally.

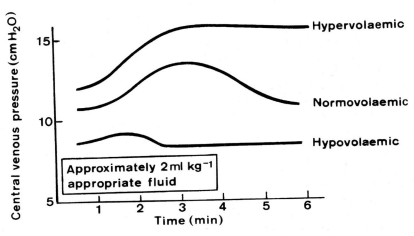

Fig 37.1 Effect of rapid infusion of intravenous fluid on central venous pressure (Sykes 1963).

The left ventricle is usually the one afflicted by ischaemic heart disease, with or without myocardial infarction. Left ventricular ischaemia, especially in the elderly, may follow hypovolaemic or septic shock. Some cardiac valvular lesions and cardiomyopathies affect solely or predominantly the left ventricle. Right ventricular performance may be impaired in the presence of normal left ventricular function in pulmonary hypertension of any cause. In all these circumstances, it is desirable to measure the left atrial pressure as well as the right. It is also useful, in some patients with hypoxaemia and diffuse pulmonary shadowing, to monitor the left atrial pressure to ascertain whether the underlying cause is left ventricular failure or primary pulmonary disease, such as ARDS.

The least invasive way to measure left atrial pressure is to float a balloon-tipped catheter (often known as a Swan–Ganz catheter) into the pulmonary artery through an introducer placed in a central vein. The catheter is advanced until, with the balloon inflated, it 'wedges' in a branch of the pulmonary artery. The pressure at this point, the pulmonary capillary wedge pressure (PCWP), corresponds in most circumstances to the left atrial pressure. Deflation of the balloon reveals a pulmonary artery pressure tracing.

Pulmonary artery catheterization carries the risks of central venous catheterization, as listed above, and, in addition, those of:

- Dysrhythmia during passage
- Knotting and misplacement
- Trauma to cardiac valves
- Pulmonary infarction if the balloon is kept inflated all the time
- Pulmonary artery rupture
- Problems with the balloon:
  (a) rupture
  (b) leakage
  (c) embolism
- Thrombosis and embolism of the catheter.

The septic complications of pulmonary artery catheterization include bacterial endocarditis, and it is recommended that, to minimize this risk, the catheter should be withdrawn after 72 hours.

A recent observational study (Connors et al 1996) has suggested that the use of pulmonary artery catheters is associated with increased mortality. Although the study provided no explanation for the raised mortality rate, it has provoked considerable debate, and may be regarded as a warning against the indiscriminate use of pulmonary artery catheterization.

Measurement of the cardiac output

Once a pulmonary artery catheter is correctly placed, it is possible to measure the cardiac output. If the catheter incorporates a thermistor, the method of thermal dilution may be employed. This is the method most commonly employed in ICUs. (Other methods employ the Fick principle or indicator dilution.)

Cardiac output computers are often programmed to calculate additional physiological variables. For example, if the cardiac output and blood pressure are measured, the systemic vascular resistance (SVR) can be calculated. Such more sophisticated information is extremely useful in patients with complicated disorders. For instance, the circulatory derangements in patients with trauma and sepsis may combine hypovolaemia with cardiac dysfunction; these patients may also have respiratory problems which further reduce oxygen delivery. The more information we have about cardiac performance, the better we shall be able to choose drugs which may improve it.

Improving cardiac performance

General measures

1. Ensure that an optimal degree of cardiac filling has been achieved.
2. Correct any coexisting abnormalities such as hypoxaemia (see respiratory support), acidosis (lactic acidosis occurs if oxygen delivery is impaired), hyper- or hypokalaemia and hypocalcaemia.
3. Correct any dysrhythmias. (Apart from specific antidysrhythmic drugs, atropine raises the cardiac output in sinus brachycardia.)

Drugs which increase cardiac output

Sympathomimetic drugs. These agents act on α- or β-adrenergic receptors or both (see Table 37.2). Dopamine in low doses improves renal perfusion through a direct effect on dopaminergic receptors (see section on Renal support). All these agents can increase cardiac output at the cost of increased myocardial oxygen consumption. The α-agonists cause vasoconstriction, which may be of benefit in septic shock when SVR may be very low, but which increases cardiac work.

Vasodilators. (Examples, nitroglycerine, sodium nitroprusside.) These drugs bring about a fall in SVR, and reduce the work and oxygen consumption of the heart. Some of them act predominantly on the capacitance vessels and reduce CVP (or preload), which may improve the performance of the failing heart. Because the use of vasodilators is associated with a fall in BP, patients receiving these drugs must be closely monitored.

Table 37.2 Properties of some sympathetic amines

	α-Receptors (agonists→ vasoconstriction rise in BP)	β-Receptors (agonists→ tachycardia, improved contractility, vasodilatation)	Other receptors
Adrenaline	α-agonist at high doses	β-effects at low doses	
Noradrenaline	α-agonist	Some β_1 effects	
Isoprenaline		β-Agonist	
Salbutamol		β_2-Agonist	
Dopamine	Resembles noradrenaline at high doses		Agonist at dopaminergic receptors → enhanced renal perfusion at low doses
Dobutamine	Closely resembles dopamine; believed by some to cause less tachycardia and to be a more effective inotrope		

Phosphodiesterase inhibitors. (Examples: enoximone, milrinone.) Drugs in this recently introduced category increase cardiac output and reduce SVR. Unlike β-adrenergic agonists, they do not cause tachycardia or a rise in myocardial oxygen consumption. They would appear to be most useful in cardiac dysfunction associated with peripheral vaso-constriction.

RESPIRATORY SUPPORT

Arterial oxygen saturation (S_aO_2)

To recapitulate the equations given earlier (p. 355), oxygen delivery to the tissues depends on:

- Cardiac output (discussed in cardiac support)
- Haemoglobin concentration
- S_aO_2.

S_aO_2 is related to arterial oxygen tension (P_aO_2), as shown by the oxygen dissociation curve (Fig. 37.2).
Note that:

- The normal P_aO_2 in a healthy young person at sea level is 100 mmHg (13.3 kPa), and corresponds to an S_aO_2 of almost 100%.
- The PO_2 of mixed venous blood (p_vO_2) is 40 mmHg (5.3 kPa), which is associated with an S_aO_2 of 70%.
- The normal P_aO_2 falls with advancing age. The normal P_aO_2 for an 80-year-old is 60 mmHg.
- At a P_aO_2 of 60 mmHg, Hb is 90% saturated.

Measurement of arterial oxygen saturation

S_aO_2 may be continually and non-invasively monitored using a pulse oximeter. A sensing probe is attached to a finger or earlobe and the pulse rate and S_aO_2 are digitally displayed. The device is generally reliable, although it may fail in the presence of intensive peripheral vasoconstriction, and can give inaccurate figures for S_aO_2 if the patient has methaemoglobinaemia or jaundice. The pulse oximeter is an excellent simple guide to the adequacy of tissue oxygenation. If a patient has a peripheral pulse which can be sensed and an S_aO_2 of 90% or more, he must be perfusing at least his finger or earlobe with oxygenated blood.

Arterial blood gas analysis

Most machines measure the pH, pO_2 and pCO_2 of a sample of blood directly, and will derive values for variables such as bicarbonate and base excess. It is essential to obtain a sample of arterial blood if P_aO_2 is to be estimated, but an 'arterialized' capillary specimen from the back of the hand will give a reasonable idea of the arterial pH and P_aCO_2. Normal values are shown in Table 37.3.

Blood gas analysis thus yields information on:

- Whether or not the patient is hypoxaemic
- Whether the patient is underventilating (P_aCO_2 elevated) or overventilating (P_aCO_2 low) their alveoli
- Whether the patient is acidotic or alkalotic, and whether the acid–base disturbance is respiratory or metabolic.

End-tidal carbon dioxide analysis

At the beginning of expiration, gas from the respiratory dead space leaves the airways first, with alveolar gas

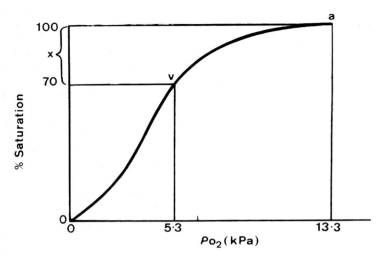

Fig 37.2 The oxygen dissociation curve: a = arterial point; v = venous point; x = arteriovenous oxygen content difference.

Table 37.3	Blood gas analysis: normal values
pH	7.35–7.45
P_aO_2	75–100 mmHg, 10–13.3 kPa (see text)
P_aCO_2	36–44 mmHg, 4.8–6.0 kPa
S_aO_2	95–100%
Base deficit	± 2.5
HCO_3-	22–26 mM l^{-1}

emerging at the end. Continuous monitoring of the expired carbon dioxide concentration (using infra-red absorption) will therefore display a peak concentration of carbon dioxide at the end of each expiration. Since alveolar and arterial carbon dioxide tensions are closely matched, measurement of end-tidal carbon dioxide tension provides a guide to P_aCO_2. Like pulse oximetry, end-tidal carbon dioxide analysis is a continuous and (in a patient connected to a breathing system) non-invasive method of assessment of respiratory function. An end-tidal carbon dioxide analyser is also a good warning of disconnection from a ventilator.

Hypoxaemia (low P_aO_2)

General causes

- Low inspired oxygen tension:
  (a) high altitude
  (b) negligent anaesthesia
- Hypoventilation – (see Ventilatory failure, Table 37.4)
- 'Shunting' of venous blood into the arterial system:

(a) pulmonary disease causing venous admixture (see Hypoxaemic failure, Table 37.4)
(b) low cardiac output
(c) congenital cyanotic heart disease with right-to-left shunts.

In most patients, hypoxaemia has a respiratory cause.

Hypoxaemia in the postoperative period

Immediately after surgery, a patient is liable to under-ventilate because of pain, or because of the residual effects of drugs used in anaesthesia (especially opiates and muscle relaxants). For reasons not fully under-stood, general anaesthesia causes a degree of venous admixture (ventilation/perfusion mismatch). If the patient's temperature has been allowed to fall during the operation, he will start shivering as he wakes up and will consume an excess of oxygen.

If satisfactory pain relief is not achieved the patient will not breathe or cough properly, nor will he cooper-ate with physiotherapy. Retained respiratory secretions, pulmonary collapse and infection may follow. Obviously, the patient's prospects are worse if surgery has been major or if he has pre-existing chest disease, usually due to smoking. It has been explained elsewhere (Ch. 35) that poisoning the patient with large doses of opiates in the hope of providing pain relief will, in its turn, produce respiratory depression. More sophisti-cated analgesic techniques have complications of their own.

It may be helpful to admit a patient who is at high risk of chest complications to the ICU for a night or two

Table 37.4   Causes of respiratory failure

Ventilatory failure ($P_a\text{CO}_2 \uparrow$; $P_a\text{O}_2\downarrow$)
   Deranged mechanics
      Obstructive airways disease
      Chest wall lesions
         Kyphocoliosis
         Chest trauma – flail chest
   Deranged control
      Depression of the respiratory centre
         Drugs
         Trauma
         Increased intracranial pressure
      Spinal cord lesions
         Trauma above C3.4
         Motor neuron disease; poliomyelitis
      Peripheral neuropathy
      Neuromuscular lesions
         Myasthenia gravis
         Botulism
         Relaxants
Hypoxaemic failure ($P_a\text{O}_2 \downarrow$; $P_a\text{CO}_2 \downarrow$ or normal)
   Collapse
   Consolidation
   Contusion
   Oedema
      LVF
      ARDS
   Pulmonary emboli

after his operation. The ICU staff can provide the close supervision that a patient with, say, an epidural infusion requires. They can also monitor his $S_a\text{O}_2$ and $P_a\text{O}_2$, and maintain his oxygenation with controlled oxygen therapy. Chest physiotherapy always seems to be better performed in the ICU, possibly because the nursing staff here have a good understanding of it. It must be more economical to keep a patient for a short, elective period in the ICU than to admit him as an emergency with respiratory failure due to pneumonia a few days later and to ventilate him artificially for (perhaps) weeks.

Artificial ventilation (intermittent positive pressure respiration (IPPR))

Indications

- Respiratory failure, which may be ventilatory or hypoxaemic
- Cerebral oedema
- Prophylaxis.

Respiratory failure.   A detailed list of the causes of both types of respiratory failure is given in Table 37.4.

Ventilatory failure is the consequence of inadequate movement of gas in and out of the lungs. Failure to excrete carbon dioxide causes the $P_a\text{CO}_2$ to rise (hypercarbia), and the $P_a\text{O}_2$ falls proportionately. The physical signs of hypercarbia are tachycardia, hypertension and vasodilatation in the cutaneous and cerebral circulations. The resultant rise in intracranial pressure may cause headache, confusion and papilloedema. Ventilatory failure is usually due to deranged respiratory mechanics or to disordered respiratory control (see Table 37.4). Excessive carbon dioxide production due to intravenous feeding has also been incriminated (Ashkenazi et al 1982).

Hypoxaemic failure occurs when large quantities of venous blood pass through the pulmonary circulation without participating in gas exchange, i.e. when nonventilated or underventilated alveoli remain perfused. Ventilation/perfusion mismatch of a minor degree is normal; severe derangements occur if large numbers of alveoli are collapsed, or are filled with blood, pus or fluid instead of gas (see Table 37.4). The $P_a\text{CO}_2$ does not rise in hypoxaemic failure; overventilation of the remaining functional alveoli keeps it at a normal level. If the $P_a\text{O}_2$ falls below 60 mmHg, hypoxaemia reflexly stimulates the respiratory centre, and the $P_a\text{CO}_2$ will fall below 40 mmHg. The physical signs of hypoxaemia are cyanosis and confusion.

Cerebral oedema.   If the intracranial pressure is raised, hyperventilation can bring about a temporary fall in cerebral blood flow and in intracranial pressure. Artificial ventilation is also indicated in patients with cerebral oedema to prevent hypoxaemia or hypercarbia, both of which may cause the intracranial pressure to rise even further.

Prophylaxis.   In a number of patients, respiratory failure may fairly confidently be predicted, and elective ventilation will prevent the development of dangerous hypoxaemia and/or hypercarbia. It has already been mentioned that some postoperative patients may benefit from a period of respiratory monitoring in the ICU. In others, usually those in whom the cardiac output, haemoglobin concentration and $S_a\text{O}_2$ may all be erratic, artificial ventilation may be continued after surgery until the patient's condition has stabilized. Cardiac and major vascular surgery almost invariably demand a period of elective postoperative artificial ventilation.

Benefits of artificial ventilation

In all the circumstances mentioned above, artificial ventilation will ensure:

- The elimination of carbon dioxide
- Improved oxygenation by:

(a) reducing respiratory work and oxygen consumption by the respiratory muscles

(b) enabling very high inspired concentrations of oxygen to be administered

(c) recruiting collapsed or oedematous alveoli (especially if positive end-expiratory pressure is employed) in hypoxaemic respiratory failure.

Management of artificial ventilation

1. Establish an artificial airway with
   (a) Endotracheal tube (oral or nasal)
   (b) Tracheostomy.

This must subsequently be properly cared for. The inspired gases must be humidified to prevent drying of respiratory secretions, and great care must be taken not to introduce infection.

2. Suppress the patient's drive to spontaneous respiration:

(a) Unless the patient is comatose or weak, it will probably be necessary to use drugs for the purpose, initially at least:

Opiates – provide analgesia as well as depression of the respiratory centre, and are the first choice for most surgical patients

Benzodiazepines – reduce anxiety and cause amnesia

Muscle relaxants – are inhumane in the conscious patient, and particularly hazardous if the patient is accidentally detached from the ventilator. Their place is extremely limited.

(b) Once artificial ventilation is established, a moderate degree of hypocarbia or the choice of a mode of artificial ventilation which permits some spontaneous respiratory effects (e.g. synchronized intermittent mandatory ventilation (SIMV) may keep the patient 'settled' on the ventilator with minimal sedation).

3. Monitor the patient and the machine.

Hazards of artificial ventilation

- Complications of the artificial airway:
  (a) trauma from the endotracheal or tracheostomy tube
  (b) obstruction due to inspissated secretions
  (c) misplacement
- Accidental disconnection of the patient from the ventilator
- Barotrauma from positive pressure to the respiratory tract:
  (a) pneumothorax
  (b) surgical emphysema

- Circulatory embarrassment – positive intrathoracic pressure may impede venous return to the heart
- Acute gastric dilatation
- Sodium and water retention
- Introduction of microorganisms into the respiratory tract.

Weaning from artificial ventilation

It may not be possible to wean a patient from his ventilator until he has recovered from the condition which brought him to it. This is a very simple point, but is constantly forgotten or ignored. For example, a patient with hypoxaemic respiratory failure due to a chest infection should be apyrexial, with clear sputum, resolution of the physical signs in the chest, a falling white cell count and some radiological improvement. It is not enough to demonstrate that the blood gases conform more closely to the ideal since IPPR was instituted. The longer the patient has been artificially ventilated, the more protracted the weaning process will be. Malnutrition, especially if associated with hypophosphataemia (Aubier et al 1985) can make weaning difficult.

A patient may be weaned by separating him from his ventilator for short periods of spontaneous respiration, which are gradually extended. Alternatively, the gradual and progressive reduction of support using a technique such as SIMV may be tried.

Extubation can be considered when the patient has demonstrated:

- A capacity to breathe spontaneously for an indefinite period
- An ability to cough effectively

The longer the time of weaning has been, the longer the tube will have to be left in place after weaning is over.

RENAL SUPPORT

Renal failure is a frequent occurrence in ICUs. An episode of hypotension, of any cause, may result in renal hypoperfusion and failure. Patients with sepsis may develop multiple organ failure, coagulopathy and ARDS, and in this group renal failure is often a terminal event. Generally, however, acute renal failure (acute tubular necrosis) is reversible, and the patient will recover if he is supported through his illness.

A patient who develops acute tubular necrosis will come to no immediate harm if his renal failure is diagnosed and promptly treated. Acute renal failure usually presents as oliguria, and it is crucial not to confuse it with oliguria due to some other cause. In a surgical patient in the ICU, the other causes of oliguria are:

- Obstruction to the flow of urine, most commonly due to a partially blocked catheter (N.B.: there are only two causes of anuria: renal cortical necrosis, which is irreversible, and a completely blocked catheter, which can be changed at once)
- Sodium and water retention occurring:
  (a) as part of the 'stress response' to surgery
  (b) in response to an episode of renal hypoperfusion, past or present
  (c) in response to an inadequate fluid intake.

Once obstruction and hypovolaemia have been excluded, the urine osmolality should be measured. An osmolality close to that of plasma (280–320 mOsm l^{-1}) is suggestive of renal failure, and the patient should, until the skilled advice of a specialist in renal medicine has been obtained, be treated as if the diagnosis were certain. There is little to do except:

- Restrict the basic fluid intake to 20 ml h^{-1} plus the previous hour's output
- Watch the serum potassium, checking the level 4-hourly. If it is above 6 mmol l^{-1} it may be controlled, for some hours at least, with 50% glucose (50 ml boluses or 20 ml h^{-1}) with soluble insulin (1 unit for each 2–4 g glucose)
- Check blood gas measurements 4–6 hourly, to see if metabolic acidosis develops
- Measure and keep all the urine which is passed for 24 hours. Send 24-hourly aliquots for electrolyte and creatinine estimations. The serum creatinine level must be measured daily.
- Consider the infusion of dopamine at 3 $\mu g\ kg^{-1}\ min^{-1}$ to improve renal perfusion. Although dopamine will usually increase the urine output, it has not been demonstrated to prevent renal failure (Cuthbertson & Noble 1997).

The other causes of oliguria are associated with a concentrated urine of high osmolality. As long as adequate renal perfusion is ensured, the patient will not develop renal failure. Attempts may be made to increase the urine volume by giving more fluid. They will not necessarily be successful in the presence of the stress response, but a good flow of urine is comforting to the doctor.

It is absolutely essential *not* to treat the patient who is passing isosmotic urine – i.e. a patient who may have renal failure – with repeated 'fluid challenges' amounting to several litres over a few hours. Remember the words of a wise nephrologist: 'No patient with renal failure ever died of dehydration, but, every day, one dies of pulmonary oedema'.

Of course, it is also essential to obtain expert advice as soon as possible. It is usual to persist with conservative treatment unless:

- It is difficult to control the serum potassium
- The serum creatinine is rising steeply
- Fluid restriction is undesirable because of the need to feed the patient intravenously.

Active treatment, haemofiltration, or haemodialysis, is indicated in the above circumstances. Peritoneal dialysis is an alternative if the patient has not had recent abdominal surgery.

ALIMENTARY SUPPORT (see also Ch. 11)

The importance of feeding

It has been pointed out elsewhere in this book that patients who are starved break down their own tissues to meet their energy requirements. The catabolic response to surgery, trauma and sepsis promotes the breakdown of protein as well as of fat, so that many patients in the ICU are liable to sustain substantial nitrogen losses. Loss of muscle bulk in patients on ventilators may make weaning more difficult (Larca & Greenbaum 1982).

Enteral feeding is preferable to intravenous because it is:

- Cheaper
- Less fraught with complications
- Protective against stress ulceration of the stomach (Pingleton & Hadzima 1983)
- Protective of gut wall integrity and thus protective against the translocation of Gram-negative bacteria from the lumen.

Unfortunately, many surgical patients in the ICU are unable to absorb enteral feeds, and intravenous feeding must be resorted to. In some ICU patients, nutritional requirements are so large that only intravenous feeding can meet them. It has already been mentioned that intravenous feeding, especially if glucose is the main source of calories, increases carbon dioxide production, which can be a respiratory embarrassment.

Prevention of stress ulceration

Very sick patients are liable to acute peptic ulceration, with consequent gastrointestinal haemorrhage. Routine prophylaxis is recommended, but it is uncertain which method is the best. The choices are as follows:

1. Enteral feeding, when it is feasible, is simple, safe and reliable.

2. Elevation of the gastric pH using one of the following:

(a) Antacids, which may be instilled through a nasogastric tube, are effective, although large doses are required to raise the gastric pH above 4. Antacids containing magnesium may cause hypermagnesaemia in patients with renal failure.

(b) H_2-receptor blockers (cimetidine or ranitidine) can be administered parenterally. These drugs are, however, expensive and have side-effects which include (i) interference with the metabolism of other drugs, notably benzodiazepines, (ii) thrombocytopenia and (iii) arrhythmias.

The neutralization of gastric acidity, unfortunately, permits the colonization of the stomach by Gram-negative microorganisms, which may go on to infect the lungs.

3. Sucralfate, which has to be enterally administered, appears to have a protective effect on the gastric mucosa with very little effect on the pH of gastric juice. It has yet to be shown conclusively that its use in the prophylaxis of stress ulcers is associated with a lower incidence of hospital-acquired (nosocomial) pneumonia than is the use of H_2-receptor blockers. It is certainly cheaper.

Selective decontamination of the digestive tract

Because the Gram-negative organisms which normally colonize the digestive tract have such deadly effects if they migrate, attempts have been made to decontaminate the bowel itself by the prophylactic administration of non-absorbable antibiotics. Routine selective decontamination has been claimed to reduce the incidence of infection in patients with trauma (Stroutenbeck et al 1984). The universal pursuit of the practice would certainly add to the cost of intensive care and might promote the emergence of resistant bacterial strains.

References

Ashkenazi J, Weissman C, Rosenbaum S H et al 1982 Nutrition and the respiratory system. Critical Care Medicine 10: 163–172

Summary

1. The most important resource of an ICU is expert staff.
2. Scoring systems are valuable for audit but cannot be used as reliable predictors in individual cases.
3. ICUs offer outstanding facilities in monitoring and supporting cardiorespiratory, renal and alimentary systems.

Aubier M, Murciano D, Legogguic Y et al 1985 Effect of hypophosphataemia on diaphragmatic contractility in patients with acute respiratory failure. New England Journal of Medicine 313: 420–424

Connors A F, Speroff T, Dawson N V et al 1996 The effectiveness of right heart catheterisation in the initial care of critically ill patients. Journal of the American Medical Association 276: 889–897

Consensus Report 1996 Tissue hypoxia. Intensive Care Medicine 22: 1250–1257

Cuthbertson B H, Noble D W 1997 Dopamine in oliguria. British Medical Journal 314: 690–691

Intensive Care Audit 1990 Intensive Care Society, London

Intensive Care Society 1984 Standards for intensive care unit. Biomedica, London

Intensive Care Society 1990 Intensive care service in the UK. ICS, London

Joly H R, Weil M H 1969 Temperature of the great toe as an indication of the severity of shock. Circulation 39: 131–138

Larca L, Greenbaum D M 1982 Effectiveness of intensive nutritional regimes in patients who fail to wean from mechanical ventilations. Critical Care Medicine 10: 297–300

Nunn J F, Freeman J 1964 Problems of oxygenation and oxygen transport during haemorrhage. Anaesthesia 19: 206–216

Palazzo M, Patel M 1993a The use and interpretation of scoring systems in the ICU: Part I. British Journal of Intensive Care 3: 111–113

Palazzo M, Patel M 1993b The use and interpretation of scoring systems in the ICU: Part 2. British Journal of Intensive Care 3: 115–118

Pingleton S K, Hadzima S K 1983 Enteral alimentation and gastrointestinal bleeding in mechanically ventilated patients. Critical Care Medicine 11: 13–16

Stroutenbeck C P, van Saene H K F, Miranda D R et al 1984 The effect of selective decontamination of the digestive tract on colonisation and infection rate in multiple trauma patients. Critical Care Medicine 10: 185–192

Sykes M K 1963 Venous pressure as a clinical indication of adequacy of transfusion. Annals of the Royal College of Surgeons 33: 185–197

Further reading

Hinds C J 1995 Intensive care: a concise textbook. Baillière
    Tindall, London

Dialysis

J. E. Scoble

Objectives

- **Understand the principles of the renal replacement therapies available.**

INTRODUCTION

Renal function maintains the 'internal environment' of the body as described by the early physiologists. Changes or failure of renal function can often occur in context of illnesses requiring immediate surgical treatment. This chapter seeks to analyse the mechanisms that can be applied if these fail.

INDICATIONS

Dialysis therapy replaces the excretory functions of failed kidneys in patients with acute or chronic renal failure.

> As with all illnesses prevention is vital, encompassing optimal fluid, drug and infection management in acute renal failure and treatment of exacerbating factors, especially hypertension, in chronic renal failure.

It is important to realize that with most renal replacement therapies, excretory function equivalent to only 10% of normal renal function, and of course no endocrine functions are provided by the artificial kidney. Dialysis therapy uses two principles to imitate the kidney and provide effective renal therapy.

PRINCIPLES

Diffusion

The first principle is diffusion of a solute from a region of high concentration to a region of low concentration (Fig. 38.1). In renal failure, waste products such as urea or creatinine are present in high concentrations in the blood. Dialysis fluid (either peritoneal or haemo)

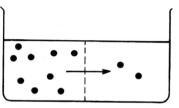

DIFFUSION OF SOLUTE (MEMBRANE PERMEABLE TO SOLUTE)

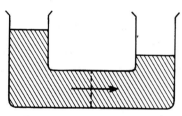

ULTRAFILTRATION DUE TO HYDROSTATIC GRADIENT

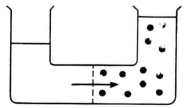

ULTRAFILTRATION DUE TO OSMOTIC GRADIENT (MEMBRANE IMPERMEABLE TO SOLUTE)

Fig 38.1 Diffusion of a solute from a region of high concentration to one of low concentration.

contains neither and, provided the membrane between the two is permeable to these solutes, net movement will occur from the blood to the dialysis fluid. In peritoneal dialysis the membrane is the peritoneum and in haemodialysis it is an artificial membrane. It is important to note that some substances such as calcium and bicarbonate are present in low concentrations in the blood but in high concentrations in the dialysis fluid. Provided the membrane is permeable to these, net movement will occur from the dialysis fluid to the blood.

Ultrafiltration

The second principle is ultrafiltration in which solvent moves through a membrane driven either by a hydrostatic or osmotic pressure difference (Fig. 38.2). The glomerulus in the kidney uses the hydrostatic pressure difference between the glomerular arteriole and the renal tubule to ultrafiltrate 180 litres per day under normal circumstances! Similarly, in haemodialysis a pressure difference, which can be varied at will, can be exerted between the blood and the dialysis fluid by a blood pump. This results in net fluid movement. In fact under certain circumstances the dialysis fluid can be disconnected and pure ultrafiltration occurs from the blood to the perimembrane space in the artificial kidney. In peritoneal dialysis where the 'blood pump' is the heart, ultrafiltration would be extremely slow if it were not for the fact that increased osmotic pressure is exerted on the dialysis-fluid side of the peritoneal membrane by increasing the concentration of glucose in the dialysis fluid. Thus both haemodialysis and peritoneal dialysis as conventionally used rely on both diffusion and ultrafiltration.

DEVELOPMENT OF METHODS

Although the principles of dialysis appear relatively simple, the practical problems are very large. Kolff in Holland was the first to devise a practical haemodialysis machine and use it to dialyse a woman with acute renal failure. It is interesting to note that the patient was 69 years old, underlining the fact that since the beginning of dialysis the majority of patients have been in the older age group. The major problems with the early dialyses were the large extracorporeal volume of blood and poor access to the vasculature. Scribner transformed haemodialysis by inventing a semipermanent arteriovenous external shunt which could be regularly disconnected and attached to a machine. This enabled regular dialysis for patients with chronic renal failure rather than, as previously, once or twice on patients

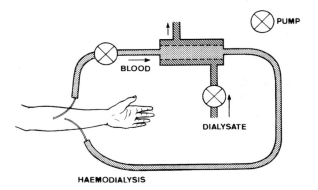

Fig 38.2 Ultrafiltration.

with acute renal failure. An arteriovenous shunt can be placed in the leg or arm, providing immediate vascular access for dialysis, but since it involves the placement of foreign material in the body, infections are not uncommon. There is also a danger of accidental disconnection and patients with shunts are limited in their ability to swim or bathe. The arteriovenous shunt still remains a useful form of access for acute renal failure although present practice is to insert a central venous double lumen catheter which can be tunnelled if required. These tunnelled lines can give good medium term access as discussed below.

The next step forward was the introduction of the Cimino–Brescia arteriovenous fistula formed either in the fore or mid-arm by side-to-side anastomosis of an artery and vein. The vein is then exposed to arterial blood pressure, enlarges, and arterializes over a period of 4–6 weeks. The advantages are that repeated punctures by large-bore needles are relatively simple and the veins do not clot. Very high dialysis blood flows can usually be achieved, increasing the efficiency of dialysis and shortening time on the machine. Once the needles are removed after dialysis there is no foreign material present and the patient can easily bathe or swim. The disadvantages are that steal syndromes can occur in the hand, aneurysms can form on the fistula and, if the arteriovenous flow through a more proximal fistula is very large, heart failure may be precipitated. The arteriovenous fistula is now the preferred form of vascular access in haemodialysis patients. There are, however, patients in whom it is impossible to form fistulae, perhaps because previous venous access has caused clotting of forearm veins, or the veins are thin walled and of very small diameter.

Urgent access may be achieved by a tunnelled subclavian catheter or, more temporarily, by direct subclavian access. When required, catheters may be placed in the internal jugular, subclavian or femoral veins. When suitable arteries and veins are not available or have already been used, some centres use a Goretex graft to link an artery and vein. The graft itself can be needled, but if infection occurs it may prove impossible to eradicate.

Peritoneal dialysis has been used for the management of acute renal failure using a hard catheter inserted percutaneously midway between the umbilicus and pubic symphysis, care being taken to avoid the aorta by directing the point of the obturator towards the pelvis. This has the advantage of easy and rapid placement in a unit not having access to haemodialysis. The disadvantages are that after 48 hours infection may occur and in many patients previous abdominal surgery makes placement of the catheter impossible. Although initially used on a weekly basis for chronic renal failure it came to be used only for acute renal failure until the late 1970s. Tenkhoff developed a soft catheter which needs to be placed surgically; it has one to three cuffs on it which stimulates a local fibrous reaction. This seals the catheter track and stops both leakage and passage of infection around the catheter. The advantage of this system is that it can be used long term as chronic ambulatory peritoneal dialysis (CAPD). In this system the peritoneal fluid is changed four times a day. The advantages are that the patient is independent of any machine and is permanently undergoing dialysis, making fluid balance easier. The disadvantage is that it is relatively inefficient and peritonitis may occur, necessitating stopping treatment.

AVAILABLE DIALYSIS TREATMENTS

The dialysis treatments on offer seem confusing, with a large number of different names. The principles though are those already outlined. A glossary of what is available follows.

Haemodialysis

In haemodialysis, blood is pumped through the centre of the fibres of an artificial kidney and dialysate is pumped around the fibres in a countercurrent direction (Fig. 38.2). The dialysate may contain either bicarbonate or acetate as a pH buffer. High-flux dialysers use a very permeable membrane, but this requires specialized monitoring equipment because of potential large fluid fluxes. This method may enable shorter dialysis periods and may prevent dialysis amyloid by depletion of circulating β_2-microglobulin. It is now rare to use intermittent haemodialysis in the management of acute renal failure, but management of fluid balance is more difficult using this method than the haemodiafiltration

described below. In the intensive care unit (ICU) setting, acute haemodialysis has been replaced by haemofiltration.

Peritoneal dialysis

This may be acute with a hard catheter or chronic with a Tenkhoff catheter (Fig. 38.3). Chronic ambulatory dialysis requires peritoneal dialysis solution to be changed four times a day with the fluid dwelling in the abdomen between changes. Intermittent peritoneal dialysis is usually controlled by a machine; the patient is attached for a period of 6–8 hours and the cycle of fluid-in/dwell/fluid-out takes approximately 30 minutes.

Haemofiltration

This is used mainly in the intensive care unit (ICU) and depends on an ultrafiltrate being produced from blood driven through a filter, usually by the patient's arteriovenous pressure difference; it does not require the complicated air detectors required in a pumped system (Fig. 38.4). The filters used have very low resistance to the passage of fluid from the blood through the membrane. If, in addition to this, a dialysate solution is passed around the filter, both dialysis and ultrafiltration can occur. With this method a clearance of approximately 20–30 ml min^{-1} can be achieved. It is in essence a slow haemodialysis, but does not require a haemodialysis machine and can continue for many hours or even days at a time, facilitating intravenous drug and nutrition administration in the ICU setting.

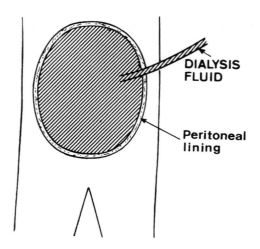

Fig 38.3 Peritoneal dialysis.

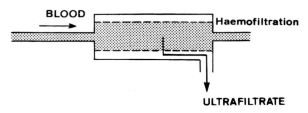

Fig 38.4   Haemofiltration.

PROBLEMS WITH DIALYSIS

Compared with a well-functioning transplant dialysis, therapy with an artificial kidney of any kind is always second best. There are many patients, however, either awaiting transplantation or who have rejected a number of transplants, who need long-term dialysis therapy. The aim of dialysis is to maximize the well-being of the patient on the therapy. The quality of life on dialysis has been dramatically improved by erythropoietin. This treats the severe anaemia seen in many patients on dialysis and improves their exercise tolerance. Erythropoietin deficient anaemia due to renal atrophy, however, is only one of a number of long-term complications of dialysis, of which the first recognized was renal osteodystrophy, a combination of osteoporosis, hyperparathyroidism and osteomalacia. Early use of phosphate binders, vitamin D administration of 1,25-dihydroxycholecalciferol (or an analogue) and, later, total parathyroidectomy has meant that severe bone disease is seen much less often. The second major complication is a specific form of amyloid caused by the non-excretion of β-microglobulin. This eventually may cause severe arthropathy and may affect other organs. It is thought that some of the modern high-flux artificial kidneys for haemodialysis may decrease this problem. The third major problem is cystic changes which occur in the kidneys of patients on long-term dialysis. This may lead to haemorrhage or, occasionally, malignancy. This condition has been termed 'acquired multicystic kidney disease', to differentiate it from the inherited polycystic kidney disease which predates dialysis.

Summary

1. Dialysis therapy replaces sufficient renal function to avoid death but it does not in any way provide normal renal function.
2. The aims of dialysis treatment are to maximize the well-being of the patient until recovery occurs in acute renal failure, or transplantation in chronic renal failure.

Further reading

Bellomo R, Boyce N 1993 Acute continuous haemofiltration: a prospective study of 110 patients, with a review of the literature. American Journal of Kidney Disease 21: 508–518

Davenport A, Will E J, Davidson A M 1993 Improved cardiovascular stability during continuous modes of renal replacement therapy in critically ill patients with acute hepatic and renal failure. Critical Care Medicine 21: 328–338

Golper T A 1992 Indications, technical considerations and strategies for renal replacement therapy in the intensive care unit. Journal of Intensive Care Medicine 7: 310

Comprehensive Reference

Davison A M, Cameron J S, Grunfeld J P, Kerr D N S, Ritz E, Winearls C G (eds) 1998 Oxford textbook of clinical nephrology, 2nd edn. Oxford University Press, Oxford

39

Chronic illness, rehabilitation and terminal care

A. C. Kurowska, A. Tookman

> **Objectives**
> - **Recognize the importance of effective communication.**
> - **Understand the principles of pain and symptom control.**
> - **Prescribe analgesics appropriately (especially opioids).**
> - **Be able to manage the process of dying.**

In patients with chronic illness and advanced disease effective symptom control forms the basis of management. For such patients the primary aim of treatment is not necessarily to prolong life but to make life as comfortable and meaningful as possible (Box 39.1). Effective palliative care will enable this to happen. A significant number of patients experience functional limitations because of their disease or its treatment. Many of these can be treated by rehabilitation techniques which enable them to develop to their maximum potential.

Patients with malignancy will form a large proportion of the case-load of patients with chronic and terminal illness who are seen by general surgeons. Since patients with incurable illness present with complex problems, an approach which focuses on the whole patient, rather than simply on the disease, is needed. It should:

- Address the psychological, social, sexual, spiritual and financial needs of the patient as well as their physical symptoms
- Provide effective symptom control
- Offer control, independence and choice. This will enable the patient to participate in decisions about the management of his problems. For the terminally ill patient this would include negotiating the most appropriate place for the patient to die (home, hospice or hospital)

Box 39.1   Important definitions

- A *terminally ill* patient is one in whom an accurate diagnosis has been made and cure is impossible. Usually prognosis is of the order of months or less. Treatment is aimed at relief of symptoms. The majority of such patients have far advanced cancer, but patients with non-malignant disease also fall under this definition, e.g. the end-stage of diseases such as renal failure, chronic obstructive airways disease, multiple sclerosis, acquired immunodeficiency syndrome (AIDS) and motor neurone disease.
- A *chronically ill* patient has a longer and less predictable prognosis. Many of these are likely to have non-malignant disease, e.g. inflammatory bowel disease, peripheral vascular disease and post-trauma. However, some malignant conditions have a protracted course, e.g. breast and prostatic cancer.
- The *palliative care approach* aims to promote both physical and psychosocial well-being. It is a vital and integral part of all clinical practice, whatever the illness or its stage, informed by a knowledge and practice of palliative care principles.*
- *Specialist palliative care* is those services with palliative care as their core speciality. Specialist palliative care services are needed by a significant minority of people whose deaths are anticipated and may be provided directly through specialist services ... or indirectly through advice to a patient's present professional advisers/carers.*

*National Council of Hospices and Palliative Care Services 1995 Specialist palliative care: a statement of definitions. Occasional Paper 8.

- Support 'the family' (i.e. all those who are important to the patient) as well as the patient
- Provide bereavement counselling for the terminally ill patient's 'family'.

To achieve these aims an interdisciplinary team approach is essential. The team includes the patient and their 'family'.

The proportion of all deaths occurring in hospital has increased over the last 15 years. The development of specialist palliative care support teams, based in the hospital and/or the community, has led to changes in this trend in certain areas. Effective use of these teams will enable patients to choose the most appropriate place to spend their terminal illness. Such teams exist to provide support and expert advice to the professionals and other carers involved in the patient's management. It is therefore important that the surgeon be familiar with the local teams both within the hospital and in the community.

COMMUNICATION

Communication with patients who have advanced incurable illness is always difficult. Chronic and terminal illness can be seen as a failure and may generate feelings of inadequacy, fear and despair in the doctors. These fears lead to the use of certain tactics (see below) in order to keep patients at a safe emotional distance (see also Ch. 46).

Distancing tactics used by doctors

Premature reassurance.   The doctor reassures the patient that he has the ability to control physical symptoms when the real issue is the patient's underlying emotional fears. For example, when a patient complains of pain a quick reassurance is given that it can be got rid of rather than exploring the significance of the pain to the patient.

Selective attention.   A patient may complain of losing weight and constipation and say 'I am worried'; the doctor ignores the worry expressed and proceeds to discuss the constipation. This tactic avoids a doctor addressing the emotional issue by selecting out the physical problem for attention.

Changing the topic when emotional issues are raised.
Closed questions.
Physical avoidance by walking past the end of the patient's bed.

As well as avoiding the use of distancing tactics, clear explanations of the physical and functional outcome of surgery should be given. Understanding of the rationale

for treatment helps patients handle side-effects better and enhances trust in the physician. Patients who are given accurate facts about their diagnosis and treatment adapt better to radical surgery. The opportunity to prepare psychologically for the major physical changes associated with procedures such as radical mastectomy, colostomy and head and neck surgery facilitates postoperative adaptation.

When patients have radical surgery, especially when associated with cosmetic deformity, issues surrounding 'loss' need to be explored. Such issues include altered body image, sexuality, social role and anxieties related to death and dying. The professionals involved must be sensitive to the psychological needs of patients and educate these patients in order to ease their acceptance of their new image and readjust their goals. Often these issues are not discussed at all. The rehabilitation process should start as soon as the diagnosis is made. Clinical nurse specialists (e.g. breast, stoma, incontinence advisors) can play a key role.

There are some fundamental principles of good communication:

- The patient's concerns should be dealt with before professional concerns
- Each topic should be fully covered before proceeding to the next
- All the problems should be elicited before giving advice or attempting any solution
- Non-verbal cues are very important
- It is helpful to clarify and summarize what the patient reports and the proposed plan of action.

Remember it is not always a question of 'What should the patient know?' but rather 'What does the patient want to know?'

COMMON EMOTIONAL REACTIONS TO LIFE-THREATENING ILLNESS

Anxiety

This is a normal reaction to a serious illness. One of the commonest emotional reactions to a life-threatening illness is fear (Box 39.2). It is important to find out precisely what the patient fears since many anxieties are based on fears that can be resolved (see below). Normal levels of anxiety should be acknowledged and accepted; however, the patient must be assessed for signs of clinical anxiety. Anxiolytics may be helpful in this group of patients.

Signs of clinical anxiety include:

- Persistently anxious mood which is subjectively different from normal worrying
- Difficulty in distracting the patient from his worries
- Feelings of tension and restlessness
- Insomnia
- Autonomic hyperactivity (e.g. palpitations, sensation of choking)
- Panic attacks.

Despair/depression

Despair is a normal reaction to a life-threatening illness which should be recognized and acknowledged. However, it is important to look for signs of clinical depression.

The classical somatic symptoms of depression, e.g. weight loss, anorexia and lethargy, carry less importance in the assessment of patients with terminal illness as they are often a manifestation of cancer. Important clues are:

- A persistently depressed mood which is subjectively different from normal sadness
- Difficulty in distracting the patient
- A lowering of interest in and enjoyment of social activities
- Crying, irritability, etc
- Insomnia
- Feelings of guilt
- Suicidal ideas may be present.

These patients should be treated with antidepressants.

Denial

It is important to assess whether the denial is causing harm (e.g. refusal of necessary medication, psychological turmoil). In many patients it represents a successful coping strategy, in which case breaking down the denial may cause unnecessary distress.

Anger

This can be displaced onto staff and/or onto the relatives. It is important not to react with anger but to try to accept and understand. It needs to be explained to the relatives that the patient is not really angry with them, but is displacing the anger he/she feels towards the disease onto them.

UNDERLYING PRINCIPLES OF SYMPTOM CONTROL

A positive but realistic attitude should be encouraged and assurance given that a considerable amount can be achieved. A problem-oriented individualized approach is the key to effective symptom control. For each symptom:

1. Diagnose the cause and treat appropriately. An accurate diagnosis is important for good symptom control. A careful history and examination can be more revealing than extensive investigations, which are often impractical and distressing. Investigations may be important but should only be carried out if they alter subsequent management.

The treatment of a symptom varies considerably depending on the underlying pathology. For example, in a patient with cancer, vomiting may be due to:

- Raised intracranial pressure
- Drugs
- Hepatomegaly
- Intestinal obstruction, etc.

Each of the above requires specific management.

Since many symptoms are multifactorial in origin it is important to recognize the contributory factors and address each as far as possible. Other intercurrent illnesses are common in debilitated patients, hence it is vital to consider non-malignant as well as malignant causes. It is easy to make assumptions that the symptom is caused by the primary diagnosis and this can lead to inappropriate management.

If the diagnosis is tentative but it is not appropriate to investigate further, symptomatic relief must be given. Very often a therapeutic trial will indicate the cause; for example, a trial of steroids in a confused patient with suspected cerebral metastases who is too unwell to undergo a computed tomography (CT) scan.

2. Explain symptom to the patient. Fear is an important contributory factor in the patient's interpretation of any symptom. The fact that the doctor acknowledges the problem, understands the symptom, can explain its cause and can offer treatment is reassuring.

3. *Discuss the treatment options.* Patients should be given accurate and balanced information that is appropriate to the stage of their illness. This will allow the patient to make informed choices about their treatment and possible options. This enhances the patient's sense of control. Treatment with a palliative intent need not be limited to drugs. Other measures, such as radiotherapy, nerve blocks, physiotherapy, psychological therapies (counselling, hypnotherapy), etc., may be appropriate.

4. *Set objectives that are realistic.* It is frustrating for both patient and staff alike if expectations are set that will never be achieved.

5. *Anticipate.* In patients with advanced illness symptoms (Box 39.3) may change rapidly. If such changes are anticipated much distress may be avoided. For example, deterioration in a patient's condition with a progressive, advanced cancer may make it impossible for them to continue with oral medication. Such deterioration should be anticipated and injectable preparations should be available. This particularly applies in the home care setting and can avert an unnecessary crisis.

6. *Ensure relatives remain informed and supported.* It is important to treat the 'whole family'.

Box 39.3 Approximate incidence of common symptoms in patients with advanced cancer

Physical

Weakness	80%
Pain	70%
Anorexia	70%
Dyspnoea	50%
Cough	50%
Constipation	50%
Nausea and vomiting	40%

Psychological

Depression	30%
Anxiety	30%

PAIN

Pain is a common symptom in chronic and terminal illness and one that is particularly feared by cancer patients. Pain can be alleviated or modified in all patients. Proper pain assessment leads to effective management. The principles outlined here have been developed in the context of management of patients with advanced cancer, but are applicable to patients who have non-malignant pain secondary to chronic disease.

Diagnose the cause of the pain

The majority of patients with far advanced disease have pain at more than one site. Each pain should be evaluated individually.

In order to establish the cause of any pain it is essential to take a careful history, particularly noting:

- The site of pain and any radiation
- The type and severity of pain
- When the pain started and any subsequent changes
- Exacerbating and alleviating factors
- Analgesic agents already used.

Physical examination often confirms the diagnosis. On occasion it may be appropriate to investigate the patient with X-rays, isotope bone scans, CT scans, etc.

Pain may be due to a malignant or non-malignant cause. In one-third of patients with advanced cancer who complain of pain the underlying pathology is non-malignant.

It is always important to assess how significant the pain is for the individual patient – how does it affect him and alter his lifestyle?

Common causes of pain in cancer patients

Pain in patients with advanced disease is often complex since it can be due to multiple pathologies. An accurate assessment of the cause of the pain will lead to more effective management.

Bone pain

Due to metastatic disease or local infiltration by adjacent tumour. It is characteristically a deep gnawing pain made worse by movement. The bone is often tender on percussion.

Visceral pain

Due to tumour mass in the lung or internal organs of the abdomen and pelvis. The tumour causes pain by a variety of mechanisms:

1. *Soft tissue infiltration.* Deep-seated pain which is due to complex pathology. The tumour invades and/or

stretches pain-sensitive structures (e.g. parietal and visceral pleura, peritoneum, nerve plexuses, and local bony structures).

2. *Stretching of a capsule.* The capsule of an organ is sensitive when stretched. The most common example of this is right hypochondrial pain due to stretching of the liver capsule. The pain can be very severe, and a sudden exacerbation of liver pain may be due to a bleed into a local deposit.

3. *Stretching of a hollow organ.* Distension of hollow viscera (small and large intestines, bladder, ureters, etc.) can cause severe spasmodic colicky pain.

Nerve pain

Nerves can be irritated, infiltrated and/or compressed. Nerve compression pain is often a deep ache. Nerve destruction pain may be burning, lancinating, and associated with abnormal sensations (e.g. hyperaesthesia). When there is destruction of nerve plexuses, nerve roots or peripheral nerves de-afferentation pain may result. This type of pain is not uncommon and often coexists with visceral and somatic pain. Deafferentation pain is characterized by unpleasant pain that is difficult to describe. It is often associated with sensory changes in the painful area and patients complain of allodynia (pain that is produced by a non-painful stimulus – e.g. stroking skin lightly can be exquisitely painful). Pain of central origin (brain or spinal cord) is often unilateral and manifests itself as spontaneous pain and hypersensitivity, including dysaesthesiae of a disagreeable kind.

Myofascial pain

Musculoskeletal pains are common in chronically ill patients. They radiate in a non-dermatomal pattern. Typically there are localized hypersensitive areas of muscle known as trigger points, which are tender to pressure.

Superficial pain

In weak, debilitated patients bedsores may be unavoidable and give rise to distressing pain.

Realistic objectives

In nearly all patients pain can be significantly modified and in many patients total freedom from pain can be achieved. In a few patients pain can prove to be an intractable symptom, unresponsive to most treatments. It is these patients who provide the greatest challenge and in whom all avenues of achieving pain relief must be explored.

Realistic goals

- Freedom from pain at night – should always be achievable
- Freedom from pain at rest – usually achievable
- Freedom from pain on mobility – may not be achievable.

Treat appropriately

This clearly depends on the cause – not all pain requires analgesia (e.g. the pain of constipation is best treated with laxatives, not analgesics!). However, when indicated, analgesics must be prescribed correctly.

Analgesic treatment of pain

The variety of analgesics available for use in the treatment of pain can be daunting. It is better to use a few drugs really well than many badly. The following 'three-step' regimen is effective in the majority of situations:

STEP 1 – Non opioid +/– adjuvant
e.g. paracetamol
If pain not relieved with 2 paracetamol 6-hourly move on to:
STEP 2 – Weak opioid +/– adjuvant
e.g. paracetamol/dextropropoxyphene, paracetamol/codeine, tramadol
If pain not relieved with 2 coproxamol (or equivalent) 6-hourly move on to:
STEP 3 – Strong opioid +/– adjuvant
e.g. morphine sulphate immediate release, morphine sulphate slow release, diamorphine (subcut.).

Principles of prescribing opioids

- Morphine should be given orally unless the patient cannot tolerate oral medication.
- It must be prescribed regularly to pre-empt pain. (Use on an as-required basis will result in poor pain control, increased incidence of side-effects and the use of higher doses overall).
- It must be given an adequate trial at an adequate dose.
- Extra doses for breakthrough and incident pain must be co-prescribed to be used as necessary (p.r.n.). (See key points box opposite.)
- Side-effects should be anticipated so that they can be prevented.

Prescibe p.r.n. doses of analgesic for:

- **Pain that breaks through the background analgesia. Daily use of breakthrough analgesics implies the regular dose of analgesic is not adequately controlling the pain and should be increased accordingly.**
- **Pain that is precipitated by painful incidents, e.g. dressing changes. Using p.r.n. analgesics in this way does not imply that the background pain is inadequately controlled by regular medication. There is therefore no need to increase the regular analgesic dose. Indeed any such increase would result in increased side-effects**

Strong opioids of choice

Morphine sulphate (tablets or solution). Quick-acting preparations. Prescribe 4-hourly (day and night). The short duration of action means there is rapid response to alterations of dose. They are therefore used when the patient first starts on opioids in order to estimate the overall opioid requirement of that individual.

Morphine sulphate slow release. Long-acting preparation. Prescribe 12-hourly. When the patient's pain is stable on 4-hourly morphine they should be converted to the equivalent dose of morphine sulphate slow release in order to simplify their regimen.

In certain circumstances it is possible to start patients on morphine sulphate slow release straight away (e.g. outpatients with moderate pain where urgent control of pain is not necessary).

The above two morphine preparations will be suitable for virtually all needs. There are other strong opioids that may have a role in pain management (see Box 39.4). However, their precise role is yet to be determined. Currently their use is based on clinical experience rather than scientific evaluation. These drugs are generally used when opioid sensitive pain has become resistant to morphine, when morphine has been unexpectedly ineffective or when morphine is causing too many side effects. They are generally second line agents, though on occasion they may be indicated first line.

Choosing the dose

The dose depends on previous analgesic requirements.

- If not on any previous analgesic, start with 2.5 mg morphine 4-hourly or 10 mg morphine sulphate slow release 12-hourly.

Box 39.4 Alternative opioids

- **Fentanyl.** This is available in a transdermal preparation, the patch being changed every third day. It takes several days to reach steady state (biological half-life of 17 hours). It is therefore not indicated in patients who need quick titration nor in the opioid naïve. It is particularly useful in patients who cannot swallow, who have absorption problems or who are poorly compliant with oral medication. It is metabolized in the liver to inactive metabolites and is therefore useful in patients with renal dysfunction. It is said to cause less constipation than morphine. Switching between transdermal fentanyl and other opioids can be difficult, conversion tables are only a guide
- **Hydromorphone.** Similar to morphine but 7.5 times more potent. Anecdotal reports suggest metabolites may be less active.
- **Methadone.** Long acting opioid which may have a useful role in neuropathic pain. (Although opioids are said to be ineffective in neuropathic pain, clinical experience challenges this.) Its long half-life makes it a difficult drug to use since accumulation can occur.
- **Phenazocine.** Clinical experience suggests this is a useful drug in patients with drowsiness on morphine sulphate.

- If on weak opioid (e.g. coproxamol) start with 5–10 mg morphine 4 hourly or 30 mg morphine sulphate slow release 12-hourly.
- If on other strong opioid, use Table 39.1 to convert to equivalent dose of morphine 4-hourly. Titrate the dose as indicated by the level of pain control achieved.

Summary

If a patient has significant pain then adequate, effective analgesics should be started early.

Valuable time can be wasted using an array of ineffective moderate analgesics. In particular this can mean that the terminally ill patient may spend a substantial portion of his remaining life with uncontrolled pain. Opioids are the most effective strong analgesics.

Routes of administration

If the patient is able to swallow use the oral route. However, at times it may be necessary to give opioids

Table 39.1 Relative potency of opioids

Opioid	Relative oral potency (for repeated dosing)	Typical starting dose	Equipotent morphine dose (approx. – great individual variation)
Morphine	**1**	**10 mg**	**10 mg**
Codeine	0.1	30 mg	3 mg
Dihydrocodeine	0.1	30 mg	3 mg
Pethidine	0.125	50 mg	6.25 mg
Tramadol	0.2	50 mg	10 mg
Methadone	4–5	5 mg	20–25 mg

transdermally or parenterally (opioids can be given rectally, but this route is rarely necessary).

Indications for transdermal/parenteral opioids

- In the last few hours/days of life when the patient is unable to swallow
- Dysphagia
- Nausea and vomiting
- Gut obstruction
- Unable to tolerate taste/number of tablets.

Parenteral opioids. Diamorphine hydrochloride is highly soluble (1 g in 1.6 ml). It is the drug of choice for parenteral use because of the small volume needed. *Subcutaneous* injections are effective and this is the route of choice. Diamorphine undergoes first-pass metabolism in the liver, hence the subcutaneous dose should be half to one-third the oral dose.

If the patient is going to require more than two or three injections a subcutaneous infusion pump should be considered. This is a small battery-driven device that will inject the contents of a syringe over a 24-hour period. It can be used in the home as well as in the hospital. (See Box 39.5.)

Transdermal opioids. Fentanyl patches may occasionally be used in preference to subcutaneous infusion (see above under alternative opioids).

Fears of prescribing opioids

Fears about prescribing opioids are common and may lead to patients having effective analgesia withheld. Both professionals and patients have unfounded anxieties about opioids. An understanding of these myths will lead to improved communication, more appropriate analgesic prescribing and better compliance.

Box 39.5 Equivalent dose of opioids

Equivalent doses of opioids
(Dose of oral morphine: Dose of injected diamorphine = 2:1 or 3:1)
10 mg morphine sulphate orally 4-hourly
(60 mg oral morphine in 24 hours)
is equivalent to
30 mg slow release morphine twice a day
(60 mg oral morphine in 24 hours)
is equivalent to
5 mg of diamorphine s.c. 4-hourly
(30 mg s.c. diamorphine in 24 hours)
is equivalent to
30 mg diamorphine in a 24-hour s.c. infusion
(syringe driver)

Fear of addiction

It has been shown in many studies that psychological addiction does not occur. Patients reduce and/or stop their opioid if their pain is controlled by another method (e.g. nerve block, surgical fixation). Since chemical dependence occurs (as is the case with many drugs) morphine should be gradually reduced. It must never be stopped abruptly.

Fear of tolerance

Tolerance occurs only to a minor degree and for practical purposes is not relevant. If the dose of opioid needs to be increased it is as a result of an increase in pain secondary to disease progression.

Fear of respiratory depression

With careful attention to dosage this does not occur. In fact opioids are used in palliative care to alleviate dyspnoea by reducing ventilatory demand and hence the sensation of breathlessness.

Fear of hastening death

Opioids do not hasten death when correctly prescribed. The exhaustion caused by unrelieved pain may do so.

Fear that a morphine prescription signals that death is imminent

This is a common anxiety for the patient. The patient may believe that a morphine prescription is only given when the doctor feels that death is imminent and has kept this information from them.

Predictable side-effects of morphine/diamorphine

- *Constipation occurs in >95% of patients.* Regular prophylactic laxative should always be prescribed.
- *Nausea and vomiting occur in approximately 30% of patients.* An antiemetic should be prescribed if nausea or vomiting occurs but it is not necessary to prescribe antiemetics prophylactically unless the patient is primed to vomit (e.g. gastrointestinal tumour, already nauseated). The antiemetic of choice for opioid-induced nausea is haloperidol. Nausea due to opioids is usually self-limiting so the antiemetic can be withdrawn after 10–14 days.
- *Drowsiness occurs in about 20% of patients.* This side-effect wears off after approximately 5 days on a stable dose.
- *Other side-effects.* These include: dry mouth, which is very common and should be treated with simple local measures; confusion and hallucinations are extremely rare (<1% of patients) and other causes should be excluded; twitching can occur on high doses. Morphine and its metabolites are dependent on the kidney for excretion. Dose adjustments **must** be made if a patient has renal dysfunction or toxicity can result.

Opioid-resistant pain

Some pains are either partially sensitive or insensitive to opioids. These pains will need to be managed with an additional or alternative drug or some other technique.

Bone pain. Although partially sensitive to opioids, bone pain frequently requires the addition of a non-steroidal anti-inflammatory drug. Localized bone pain can often be treated with radiotherapy. Surgical fixation may be indicated if there is a pathological fracture. Prophylactic fixation should be considered (if >75% of the cortex is eroded spontaneous fracture is highly likely). Generalized bone pain in malignancy may need systemic therapy with chemotherapy or hormone therapy. Hemibody radiation, strontium 89 (a therapeutic systemic radiopharmaceutical) and bisphosphonate therapy all have a role in the management of bone pain.

Nerve pain. This is very often opioid insensitive; however, a trial of opioid is usually indicated. Methadone seems to be particularly effective. Steroids are useful in nerve compression. Nerve infiltration/irritation/destruction pain may respond to drugs which alter neurotransmission (e.g. low-dose tricyclic antidepressants, anticonvulsants, membrane stabilizers). Radiotherapy and nerve blocks may also be indicated.

Liver capsule. This pain is partially opioid sensitive. Steroids are very useful in this context as they may reduce the liver swelling and relieve capsular stretching.

Colic. If due to constipation treat with laxatives. Drugs causing hyperperistalsis should be stopped. If due to tumour obstruction then this will need appropriate treatment and antispasmodics may be required.

Meningeal pain/raised intracranial pressure. Steroids are the drug of choice. Radiotherapy should be considered.

Lymphoedema. Non-steroidal anti-inflammatory drugs and steroids can be helpful. Physical treatment plays an important role (massage, compression hosiery and intermittent pneumatic compression).

Muscle spasm. Benzodiazepines or baclofen can be used.

Infection. It may be appropriate to treat infections in order to relieve pain.

Joint/myofascial pain. Non-steroidal anti-inflammatories should be used in conjunction with opioids. Local injections of steroid into joints and trigger points may be of value. Physiotherapy can also be helpful.

Superficial pain. Patients with bedsores need to be kept off the pressure areas with regular turning. An effective mattress to support the patient is essential.

Psychological pain. If management is solely directed at physical factors, one may fail to control pain adequately in some patients. It is important to treat coexistent depression or anxiety, and if appropriate offer counselling, diversionary activities, etc.

Complementary therapies

Although scientifically unproven, these seem to benefit some groups of patients. If the patient perceives these therapies as adding to their overall well-being then one should support the patient, provided the treatment does not harm the patient or interfere with their conventional management.

Injection techniques in cancer pain

Nerve blocks have a place in palliative care. They are highly effective when used in a selected group of patients (approximately 4% of patients with pain will benefit). Various 'injection techniques' can be used. Although some of these techniques need expertise and specialized equipment to perform, simple techniques can be performed at the bedside.

Nerve blocks

Nerve blocks can be considered when there is:

- Unilateral pain
- Localized pain
- Pain due to involvement of one or two nerve roots
- Abdominal pain arising from 'upper' gut
- Rib pain.

The patient needs careful assessment as to the cause of the pain before a block is carried out. This assessment will determine the exact site at which the pain pathways should be interrupted.

Many procedures can be performed using local anaesthetics and steroids. These blocks can give good pain relief outlasting the effect of the anaesthetic and are safe procedures. The pain relief from a nerve block may be transient and repeated blocks may be necessary. Careful patient selection is vital. A nerve block should not be offered as a 'last resort' but only if there is a reasonable chance of success. In addition to neural blockade, spinal analgesics have an important role in selected cases. Epidural and intrathecal administration of opioids (and local anaesthetics) by a catheter system are particularly useful in patients with opioid sensitive pain who are experiencing side-effects with systemic therapy.

Major neurolytic procedures may carry the risk of serious side-effects. For example:

- Intraspinal neurolysis for nerve root pain can produce urinary and faecal incontinence
- Coeliac plexus block for upper abdominal pain can cause postural hypotension.

Once again careful patient assessment is vital.

WEAKNESS AND IMMOBILITY

Weakness is a common and distressing symptom in patients with advanced illness. When due to general debility it is very difficult to treat. Reversible causes such as cord compression and cerebral metastases must be excluded.

It is important to acknowledge the problem and explain to the patient that it is a result of the illness. This allows realistic goals to be set, which in itself can reduce the patient's distress. Even very sick patients need to feel a sense of control. Simple measures such as a wheelchair can help them achieve this.

Steroids improve weakness in a proportion of patients. The response, however, is often short lived and side-effects, such as proximal myopathy and poor wound healing, must be taken into consideration. Therefore patients must be carefully selected and the time at which steroids are introduced has to be carefully assessed.

A patient who is immobile and confined to bed will lose muscle strength. A normal person loses 10–15% of his muscle strength when completely rested for 1 week and it takes 60 days to restore that strength. It is therefore not surprising that muscle weakness quickly develops in the immobile cancer patient, especially in the common situation where protein catabolism is increased. If immobility continues contractures can develop, leading to impaired ability to self-care. Contractures are more likely when soft tissue damage is present and with improper positioning in bed. Good nursing care and regular physiotherapy are essential for these patients.

When patients are debilitated and immobile, pressure sores can rapidly develop. This is aggravated by increased protein catabolism and negative nitrogen balance as well as other factors (e.g. diabetes, steroids). Damage can be minimized if pressure on the skin is intermittent. Early prophylaxis with scrupulous nursing attention and the use of effective patient support systems (e.g. special mattresses, low-loss airbeds) will limit damage and help prevent distressing pain.

Autonomic dysfunction and impaired peripheral circulation are the cardiovascular consequences of immobility. There is an increased likelihood of deep venous thrombosis and pulmonary embolism.

Atelectasis as a result of reduced aeration of the posterior lungs predisposes patients to chest infection.

Urinary retention and urinary infection are more common in immobile patients.

Immobility, anorexia and weakness lead to reduced peristalsis and constipation.

Loss of proprioceptors in skin of feet will lead to an inability to balance which can take many weeks to recover.

ANOREXIA

This symptom is common. It occurs in approximately 70% of patients with advanced cancer. It is important to decide whose problem it is – the patient's or the carers'. The family need to understand that as death approaches it is normal to lose interest in food. At this stage the goal of eating is enjoyment, not optimal nutrition.

Causes

- Tumour bulk and associated biochemical abnormalities (hypercalcaemia, uraemia, etc.)
- Oral problems (e.g. thrush, oral tumour)
- Constipation
- Drugs, radiotherapy
- Depression or anxiety.

It must be remembered that fear of vomiting may lead to avoidance of food (as opposed to true anorexia). Psychological factors such as anxiety and depression can manifest as lack of appetite. Presentation of food is important – it should be in small portions and well presented.

If the above factors have been attended to and it is still felt to be a problem for the patient, steroids can be tried as an appetite stimulant.

DYSPHAGIA

Site of dysphagia

The site of dysphagia can be predicted from the symptom complex. Drooling, leaking of food and retention of food in the mouth indicate a buccal cause; nasal regurgitation, gagging, choking and coughing suggest pharyngeal pathology; a sensation of food sticking behind the sternum and pain between the shoulder blades imply oesophageal obstruction.

Management

It is important to explain the cause (Table 39.2) to the patient so that any dietary adjustments are understood. Restriction to liquids or soft foods may be necessary.

Any associated pain should be treated. Mucaine is useful for the local pain of *Candida* or radiotherapy, but many patients require opioids for satisfactory pain relief. *Candida* should be actively treated with topical or systemic antifungals. If patients are unable to swallow even liquids, drugs should be given by another route. A subcutaneous infusion of drugs (analgesics, etc.) is both effective and well tolerated.

If it is appropriate to attempt to relieve the obstruction, then possibilities include radiotherapy, endo-oesophageal tubes, stents, dilatation and laser therapy. Steroids, by reducing oedema, may palliate dysphagia for a significant period. They can be particularly useful

Table 39.2 Common causes of dysphagia in patients with advanced disease

Problem	Implication	Example of cause
Solids then liquids	Obstruction	Tumour mass. External compression
Solids and liquids simultaneously	Neuromuscular cause	Terminal neuromuscular dysfunction in very weak patients. Perineural tumour infiltration with head and neck tumours which damage cranial nerves (V, IX, X). Bulbar palsy
Painful	Mucosal causes	*Candida* (N.B.: only 50% of patients with oesophageal *Candida* have clinically apparent oral *Candida*). Post-radiotherapy

in the management of dysphagia syndrome associated with head and neck tumour.

Endo-oesophageal tubes and stents should be considered in patients who are relatively independent and active, but are not appropriate for the moribund. Gastrostomy may be an option in patients with incurable malignant obstruction, however, it does not solve the problem of saliva aspiration. In patients with carcinoma of the stomach or oesophagus, by the time severe obstruction occurs the prognosis is very short. Gastrostomy does have a significant morbidity and mortality and can even contribute to terminal discomfort.

However, with the advent of percutaneous techniques, gastrostomy now has an established role in selected patients. Nasogastric tubes and gastrostomies may be appropriate for patients with a longer prognosis (e.g. those with neurological problems, certain malignancies of the head and neck and cerebral tumours).

In irreversible total obstruction or terminal neuromuscular dysfunction secretions must be reduced to a minimum using hyoscine.

Dehydration should be looked on as a natural process in the last few days of life. It can help relieve a number of symptoms. Intravenous fluids may exacerbate discomfort by increasing bronchial secretions, gastrointestinal fluid (thereby increased likelihood of vomiting), urine flow (leading to need for catheter), etc. However, hydration is appropriate in selected patients, e.g. if a patient is complaining of thirst/dryness. Usually these patients can be managed with subcutaneous fluids preventing the repeated trauma of cannulation.

NAUSEA AND VOMITING

Nausea and/or vomiting occur in approximately 40% of patients with far-advanced cancer. The cause must be found in order that rational treatment can be offered (Table 39.3)

If an antiemetic is needed, most nausea and vomiting in patients with advanced illness can be controlled using the antiemetic drugs in Table 39.4. Most antiemetics act at one of the sites shown in the table. Sometimes more than one antiemetic will be necessary. If this is the case it is common sense to combine drugs which act at different sites, i.e. a neuroleptic with an antihistamine.

The antiemetic must be delivered by a suitable route. There is little point giving a drug orally if the patient is vomiting! Rectal or parenteral routes should be chosen in these situations. A 24-hour subcutaneous infusion by means of a syringe driver is a simple and effective method of drug delivery. (Syringe drivers are discussed in more detail later.)

BOWEL OBSTRUCTION

Gastrointestinal obstruction occurs in approximately 4% of patients with advanced cancer. It occurs more commonly in those with colonic primary (10%) and ovarian primary (25%).

Surgical management in patients with known malignancy is indicated if the patient's general condition is good, they have low-bulk disease and an easily reversible cause seems likely. Previous laparotomy findings must be taken into consideration. Surgery remains the primary treatment because in selected patients 10% of obstructions prove to be non-malignant, 10% represent a new primary and approximately 60% will not reobstruct.

With conservative treatment (drip and suck) 30% of obstructions resolve spontaneously. Therefore this management should be considered prior to proceeding to surgery.

Neither of these strategies should form part of the primary management of irreversible obstruction in patients with far-advanced cancer. The majority of such patients have obstruction at multiple sites. The aim is symptom control with drugs. Intravenous fluids and nasogastric tubes are rarely needed.

Medical management of bowel obstruction
(Box 39.6)

Obstruction may be proximal, in which case the predominant symptom is vomiting, or distal, when the pre-

Table 39.3	Common causes of nausea and vomiting in advanced cancer
Cause	Symptomatic treatment
Drugs	If possible withdraw the drug
Metabolic (hypercalcaemia, uraemia etc.)	Treat with centrally acting antiemetic
Bowel obstruction	Centrally acting antiemetic (see below)
Squashed stomach syndrome*	Prokinetic antiemetic, H_2 antagonist/proton pump inhibitor
Gastric irritation (e.g. NSAIDs, gastric ulceration)	Prokinetic antiemetic, H_2 antagonist/proton pump inhibitor/misoprostol
Constipation	Laxatives
Liver metastases	Centrally acting antiemetic/steroids
High bulk disease	Steroids Centrally acting antiemetic/ondansetron
Raised intracranial pressure	Steroids

NSAIDs – non-steroidal anti-inflammatory drugs
*Squashed/small stomach syndrome is a constellation of alimentary symptoms seen in patients with large epigastric mass/gross hepatomegaly. It is manifested as early satiation, epigastric fullness, flatulence, hiccoughs, nausea, vomiting and heartburn.

Table 39.4 Sites of action of antiemetic drugs

Main site of action	Class of drug	Example
Central		
Chemoreceptor trigger zone	Neuroleptic	Haloperidol
Vomiting centre	Antihistamine	Cyclizine
5HT3 receptors	5HT3 receptor antagonists	Ondansetron
All central sites	Phenothiazine	Methotrimeprazine
Peripheral	Prokinetic	Domperidone

Box 39.6 Medical management of bowel obstruction

Diet	No restrictions but small meals appropriate
Nausea and vomiting	Cyclizine 150 mg/24 hours via syringe pump. If partial/no success combine with haloperidol 5–10 mg/24 hours in syringe pump. Octreotide via subcutaneous route has a role in high volume vomiting.
Reverse obstruction	If constipated attempt to clear with softeners. Docusate 100 mg–200 mg t.d.s. Consider dexamethasone 16 mg/24 hours by subcutaneous infusion to reduce oedema. In certain cases, e.g. cancer of ovary, chemotherapy may be effective.
Pain	Diamorphine in appropriate dose in syringe pump according to previous analgesic requirement and level of pain. Halve the oral dose to calculate the equivalent subcutaneous dose.
Colic	If colic persists despite the above, add hyoscine butylbromide 60–120 mg/24 hours to pump. Octreotide is helpful by decompressing the bowel and reducing the distension.

Gastrokinetic antiemetics such as metoclopramide or domperidone are contraindicated – they will exacerbate vomiting.

Baines et al (1985) reported on this form of management in 38 patients with advanced malignant disease. They found that nausea and vomiting was well controlled in 90% of patients, colic in 100% and pain relief was total in 90% with only mild residual pain in 10%. The median survival was 3 months and 24% survived >6 months.

CONSTIPATION

The need to treat constipation is usually a consequence of failing to use prophylactic laxatives (virtually all patients on opioids should have a regular laxative). A rectal examination is essential on any patient complaining of constipation or diarrhoea to assess for impaction. Use a laxative that combines a softener and stimulant (e.g. co-danthramer).

SYRINGE DRIVERS IN SYMPTOM CONTROL

Syringe drivers delivering subcutaneous infusions of analgesics, antiemetics, anticholinergics and tranquillizers are commonly used in patients who would require regular parenteral medication (Table 39.5). The subcutaneous route is simple, safe, effective and acceptable to most patients. Indications for the use of such syringe drivers have already been discussed above in the context of pain control.

THE MANAGEMENT OF THE TERMINAL PHASE OF THE ILLNESS

When a patient who has advanced illness enters into the terminal phase (normally a day or so prior to death) *all* medication should be reviewed. All drugs should be stopped apart from those aimed at symptom control. Communication is vital and explanation should be

dominant symptom is colicky pain. Nausea is often more distressing than vomiting. The aim is to eliminate nausea, reduce vomiting to a maximum of once or twice a day and treat associated pain.

Table 39.5 Drugs commonly used in a continuous 24-hour subcutaneous infusion pump

Reason for drug	Drug	Dose in 24 hours
Analgesia	Diamorphine	According to need
Colic	Hyoscine butylbromide	30–60 mg
Antiemetic	Haloperidol	5–10 mg
	Cyclizine	150 mg
	Methotrimeprazine	12.5–25 mg
Bronchial secretions	Hyoscine hydrobromide	1.2–1.8 mg
Anxiolysis	Midazolam	5–10 mg
Terminal agitation	Midazolam	15–60 mg
	Methotrimeprazine	100–200 mg
Other drugs	Dexamethasone	0.5–16 mg
	Octreotide	300–1200 µg

given to the patient and their carers about anticipated changes in the patient's condition. Reassurance should be given that symptoms will remain controlled and the patient kept comfortable. Often it is appropriate to use a syringe driver to administer medications.

Analgesia. This should be continued even if a patient becomes unconscious. The patient may still perceive pain and in addition abrupt withdrawal of opioids can result in an unpleasant physical withdrawal reaction. If a patient is on regular opioids they will need to be continued at an equivalent dose subcutaneously. If the patient will require more than a few injections a syringe driver should be started.

Agitation. Causes must be looked for and treated appropriately, e.g. retention of urine requires catheterization. However, it is not uncommon for patients to become agitated and confused shortly before death. If a tranquillizer is indicated, use subcutaneous midazolam (5–10 mg, 4–6-hourly). Midazolam (20–60 mg per 24 hours) can be combined with diamorphine in a syringe driver.

Bronchial secretion. This can be controlled using subcutaneous hyoscine hydrobromide (600 µg 4-hourly) as required. It can also be added into the syringe driver together with diamorphine and midazolam. If this symptom does not respond to repeated doses of hyoscine, try bumetanide 2 mg intramuscularly.

Crises. In some circumstances it may be appropriate to prescribe drugs for a crisis. For example, if it is likely that the patient may have a major bleed (haemoptysis, haematemesis, etc.) prescribe diamorphine and midazolam as a 'crisis pack' to be given in the event of such an emergency. Such crises can be of great distress to the patient and the family and need to be handled with speed and sensitivity.

The rules of symptom control should always be followed, even at this stage of the illness. Symptoms should be evaluated and appropriate treatment instituted. It is important to anticipate problems and to communicate well with all concerned. It has been shown that a 'peaceful' death leads to far fewer bereavement problems in the family.

BEREAVEMENT

Support offered to the family both during the patient's illness and at the time of the patient's death not only helps them to cope better but reduces the likelihood of future complications. Evidence suggests there is higher physical and psychiatric morbidity and possibly increased mortality in those recently bereaved.

People avoid grieving individuals because they feel helpless, awkward, embarrassed, they do not wish to feel sad themselves and they fear releasing strong emotions.

Normal stages in the process of grief

Denial

Death represents an enormous threat to the individual. Even if the death is anticipated the reaction of the bereaved person is often one of shock and disbelief. They feel numb and immobilized. The response of the individual depends very much on the circumstances of the death. Religious beliefs and cultural background will influence their reactions.

Developing awareness

Gradually an awareness of the reality of the loss develops and various emotional reactions can emerge such as depression/sadness, anger, guilt, loneliness. In addition, outbursts of grief, with episodes of anxiety and anguish associated with crying, restlessness and preoccupation with the dead person are common. A strong sense of the physical presence of the deceased, at times amounting to a visual awareness, should not be misinterpreted as abnormal. It is during this phase that the bereaved often present to their GP with physical and psychological symptoms. Stress, irrational behaviour, lethargy and physical illness which mimics the symptoms of the deceased are common complaints.

Resolution

Ultimately the individual gains a new sense of self-identity and adjusts to their new role in society. Gradually there develops a resolve that they will cope, and a feeling that it is now appropriate to develop new social contacts.

Bereavement counselling

It is important to interpret normal reactions to loss. Many people who are undergoing a normal grief reaction interpret their symptoms as evidence of psychiatric illness. For example, they may feel the dead person is present or actually see the dead person. Reassurance can be given that such reactions are expected and will resolve with time.

The survivor will need to accept the reality of the loss in order to deal with its emotional impact. It is vital that they have time to talk about the dead person so that they can identify and express their feelings. Anger and guilt are common emotions. Anger may be directed at the deceased, other family members, professionals involved in the patient's care, God, etc. Such anger needs ventilating. Depression may result from self-directed anger (guilt), thus it is important to check for clinical depression and suicidal ideas. Feelings of anxiety and helplessness may make the survivor feel unable to cope. Exploring the resources the bereaved person utilized before the loss will enable them to see that they can indeed cope. When sadness occurs the bereaved person needs to be given permission to cry.

The recently bereaved person needs to adjust to their new role. Major life-changing decisions in the immediate bereavement period should be actively discouraged. As time passes a degree of emotional withdrawal from the deceased and the formation of new social contacts should be encouraged.

It is important to identify those who are likely to have a difficult bereavement since they are at risk of developing psychiatric illness in the bereavement period (e.g. psychosis, clinical depression, extreme anxiety states). Some individuals may resort to alcohol, drugs, denial, idealization, etc., as a way of coping with loss. They should be referred early to the appropriate agency (psychiatrist, bereavement counsellor, etc.).

Important risk factors for abnormal bereavement reaction

Those at increased risk of difficult bereavement include those:

- With a close, dependent or ambivalent relationship
- Undergoing concurrent stress at the time of bereavement
- With memories of a 'bad' death (e.g. uncontrolled symptoms)
- Who have a perceived low level of support (the carer's perception is more important than the actual support in determining outcome)
- Experiencing strong feelings of guilt/reproach
- Unable to say goodbye, who feel there are things left unsaid (e.g. sudden or traumatic deaths or absence at the time of death).

 References

Baines M, Oliver D J, Carter R L 1985 Medical management of intestinal obstruction in patients with advanced malignant disease: a clinical and pathological study. Lancet ii: 990–993

Summary

1. Clear effective communication is essential.
2. Treat the whole patient not just the disease.
3. Fully assess each symptom before prescribing treatment. Constantly review symptom management in the light of progressive disease.
4. You should be able to control or modify pain in the majority of patients. If strong analgesia is indicated, morphine sulphate is the first line choice.
5. When the patient enters the terminal phase ensure you continue to provide good symptom control with adequate analgesia, sedation and antisecretory drugs for excessive respiratory secretions.
6. Remember to use the expertise of your local palliative care team/hospice.

Further reading

Buckman R 1992 How to break bad news: a guide for health care professionals. Papermac

Directory of hospice and palliative care services in the United Kingdom and Republic of Ireland 1995 Hospice Information Service, St Christopher's Hospice, London

Doyle D, Hanks W C, Macdonald N 1998 Oxford textbook of palliative medicine. Oxford University Press, Oxford

Kaye P 1996 Breaking bad news. (Pocket Book) EPL Publications, Northampton

Faulkner A, Maguire P 1994 Talking to cancer patients. Oxford Medical Publications, Oxford

Parkes C M 1972 Bereavement: studies of grief in adult life. Tavistock and Pelican, London; International Universities Press, New York

Regnard C, Davies A 1986 A guide to symptom relief in advanced cancer. Haigh & Hochland, Manchester

Stedeford A 1985 Facing death. Heinemann, London

Twycross R G, Lack S A 1986 Control of alimentary symptoms in far advanced cancer. Churchill Livingstone, Edinburgh

Twycross R G 1997 Symptom management in advanced cancer. Radcliffe Medical Press, Abingdon Oxon

General considerations

40

Genetic aspects of surgery

K. D. MacDermot, M. C. Winslet

Objectives

- **Recognize genetic disorders which may produce life-threatening complications during surgery and anaesthesia:**
  - **defects of haemoglobin and haemostasis**
  - **defects of muscle**
  - **defects of connective tissue**
  - **skeletal dysplasias.**
- **Become familiar with the disorders leading to a genetic susceptibility to cancer.**

RELEVANCE OF CLINICAL GENETICS TO SURGERY

In certain genetic disorders life-threatening complications may occur during surgery and anaesthesia. The recognition of clinical signs or family history suggestive of these genetic disorders is important for diagnosis so that appropriate perioperative management of the patient is undertaken. Furthermore, the study of the molecular basis of genetic disorders, human development, carcinogenesis and many other biological events is now possible due to exciting advances in laboratory techniques for the analysis of human genome.

Genes involved in the control of cell proliferation and transcription of genetic information have been shown to cause increased susceptibility to cancer if their function is defective. Thus, genetic analysis and the development of new methods for clinical diagnosis, monitoring of cancer progression and treatment are being reported in medical literature and incorporated in clinical medicine. These advances clearly illustrate the link between basic sciences and clinical practice and an understanding of basic genetic concepts is now required to keep abreast of new developments.

BASIC GENETICS CONCEPTS AND TERMINOLOGY

Genes are units of genetic information which are passed on from generation to generation. Biochemically, genes are stretches of *DNA* (deoxyribonucleic acid) which direct the synthesis of a specific protein. DNA is tightly coiled and packaged in *chromosomes*, which are visible under the light microscope in the nucleus of dividing cells. *Somatic cells* (non-germline tissue) have 23 pairs of chromosomes (*diploid* number 46), one chromosome from each pair is inherited from each parent. Chromosome pairs 1–22 are called *autosomes*, whilst the 23rd pair are the *sex chromosomes*, XX in females and XY in males. In the ovum or sperm (*germ cells* or gonadal tissue cells) one set of autosomes and a sex chromosome are present (*haploid* set), so on fertilization, a diploid set of chromosomes is restored. It can be seen that males determine the sex of the offspring. When viewed under the microscope, each chromosome has a visible constriction (*centromere*). The part of the chromosome above the centromere is usually shorter and is referred to by standard nomenclature as the short arm or *p* (from petite), the long arm is termed *q*. Each arm of the chromosome is further divided into bands for easy reference. Thus, 5q21 is the position of the adenomatous polyposis coli gene on the long arm of chromosome 5. *Mutation* is a change in the gene function which either results in activation (more protein is produced) or, more often, inactivation of the gene with reduction or loss of function.

Mendelian inheritance refers to the mode of transmission of genetic information from generation to generation as proposed by Mendel. *Dominant inheritance* (autosomal or X linked) is clinically expressed when only one copy of the mutated gene is present. In *recessive inheritance* the clinical signs of the disease is only clinically evident when both copies of the gene have the mutation. *Oncogenes* are genes present in normal cells, which promote cell growth and proliferation. *Tumour suppressor genes* (or antioncogenes) have the opposite function.

An essential aid for establishing the diagnosis of genetic disorder is, of course, a *family history* of the same disease or clinical signs in relatives. The drawing of a family tree (pedigree) is straightforward and shows in graphic form the mode of genetic transmission (Fig. 40.1). When a complex of symptoms and signs occur together in a particular disorder, this is referred to as a *syndrome*, usually named after the author(s) of the first report (e.g. Li–Fraumeni syndrome) or by an anagram which describes the clinical signs (e.g. HNPCC, hereditary non-polyposis colon cancer).

GENETIC DIAGNOSIS FOR PREOPERATIVE ASSESSMENT AND PERIOPERATIVE MANAGEMENT OF SURGICAL PATIENTS

The genetic disorders discussed in this section will concentrate on those which the trainee surgeon should be familiar with since they may result in serious complications during surgery and anaesthesia.

These genetic disorders can be divided into four groups: defects of haemoglobin and haemostasis; defects of muscle; connective tissue defects; and skeletal dysplasias.

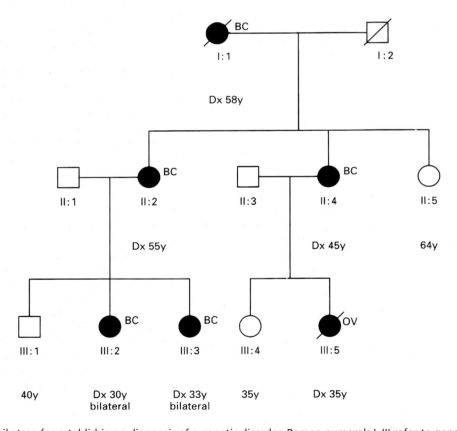

Fig 40.1 A family tree for establishing a diagnosis of a genetic disorder. Roman numerals I–III refer to generations; arabic numerals refer to the individual (e.g. III:5, fifth individual from the third generation shown on the pedigree). (○) female; (□) male; shaded symbols = affected; crossed symbols = dead; BC = breast cancer; OV = ovarian cancer; Dx = diagnosed; y = years (present age or age at diagnosis).

Defects of haemoglobin and haemostasis

Enquire about history of anaemia, bleeding tendency or recurrent venous thrombosis in the patient or their relatives. The development of sickle cell crisis due to hypoxia during surgery and the need for factor VIII infusion in haemophilia A are well known. Most rare defects of other clotting factors will be diagnosed on a routine screen, when a suggestive history is obtained. For example, in Noonan syndrome with a birth frequency of 1 : 2000, factor XI and XII deficiency and thrombocytopenia occur in 60% of patients. The clinical signs include short stature, neck webbing and congenital heart defects.

Patients with thromboembolic disease due to inherited protein C or S deficiency may give a history of superficial and deep vein thrombosis, thrombosis of the mesenteric, cerebral, renal and axillary veins, portal veins and pulmonary embolism.

Muscle defects

Enquire about the development of hyperthermia, acute renal failure and tonic spasms during previous surgery or anaesthetic death in relatives. Malignant hyperthermia is the most serious genetic disorder of muscle presenting in the operating theatre. It consists of acute onset of skeletal muscle rigidity, metabolic acidosis and malignant hyperpyrexia. If not immediately reversed, these episodes can lead to tissue damage and death. The mainstay of treatment is dantrolene, given either prophylactically or immediately a hyperthermic episode is suspected. Malignant hyperthermia is estimated to affect approximately 1 : 15 000 paediatric patients and 1 : 40 000 adult patients. It is triggered by halogenated anaesthetic agents with or without depolarizing muscle relaxants. The inheritance is autosomal dominant or recessive and approximately 50% of families have a mutation in the calcium ion channel gene on chromosome 19.

Hand-grip weakness and difficulty in walking are symptoms of myotonic dystrophy and a positive family history is usually present. Myotonic dystrophy affects approximately 1 : 10 000 individuals and the clinical expression is very variable. Myotonic dystrophy and the other less common myotonias are due to defects in the chloride and sodium channels of the muscle membrane. Patients show undue sensitivity to various anaesthetics and sedative agents including opioids, barbiturates and benzodiazepines. Tonic spasms during operation, prolonged recovery from anaesthetic and depression of the respiratory centre necessitating prolonged ventilation have been reported. Cold and shivering also induces myotonia. Myotonic dystrophy usually presents between the ages 15–35 years. The most noticeable clinical signs are facial and neck weakness with ptosis. Patients usually notice weakness of hand grip, inability to open clenched fist and difficulty in walking due to weakness of foot dorsiflexion. This is a multisystem disorder; heart block frequently develops in adults and patients should be fully evaluated before surgery. Anaesthetic management may be difficult and regional anaesthesia should be used whenever possible.

Connective tissue defects

Enquire about poor wound healing, paper thin scar tissue, joint dislocations and the diagnosis of aortic aneurysm in relatives.

Connective tissue abnormalities may cause difficulty during suturing resulting in a high incidence of anastomotic and wound dehiscence. In Marfan's syndrome, the clinical signs are usually obvious; the patient has tall thin stature, long slim fingers, chest deformity, scolisis and dislocated optic lens. Preoperative cardiac assessment is mandatory, as there is high incidence of dissecting aortic aneurysm with aortic valve insufficiency at a young age.

Ehlers–Danlos syndrome, particularly the arterial type IV, is characterized by friable arteries and veins and spontaneous arterial rupture has been reported. Paper thin scars, joint dislocation and spontaneous colonic perforation may also occur. Arteriography and vascular surgery is particular hazardous; varicose vein surgery, if absolutely necessary, should be performed with the utmost care!

Skeletal dysplasias

Patients with such disorders may have odontoid dysplasia or C1–C2 subluxation due to ligamentous laxity. The patient is of short stature, with some body disproportion. The most commonly encountered conditions are achondroplasia and Down syndrome, which are easily recognized. Skeletal dysplasia due to mucopolysaccharidosis, an inborn metabolic storage disorder (such as Hurler's syndrome), are characterized by 'coarse' looking face and mental retardation. During surgery, head and neck manipulation should be limited, as cervical medullary compression has been reported. In certain cases, elective cervical vertebral fusion may be required.

Congenital malformations and genetic disorders may indicate the presence of unsuspected anatomical abnormalities of obvious importance to the surgeon. Patients with Sturge–Weber syndrome have a port wine stain on the skin which, if present over the face or cranium, is associated with epilepsy or mental retardation. Multiple arteriovenous malformations may be encountered during surgical manipulation of tissues beneath the port wine stain. Similarly, hypoplasia of the lesser wing of the sphenoid bone is a developmental abnormality associated with peripheral neurofibromatosis type 1. The operative reduction of raised intracranial pressure in such patients may be associated with enophthalmos.

GENETIC MECHANISM OF CANCER DEVELOPMENT

Cancer development is the result of accumulation of mutations in a number of genes (4–5 in colorectal cancer) over time in somatic tissues. Each mutation results in step-wise clonal proliferation of cells with the next mutation giving rise to further expansion. The mutations are present in two types of genes which regulate cell growth. There is a mutational activation of oncogenes and mutational inactivation of tumour suppressor genes. A genetic model for colorectal tumourigenesis has been particularly well studied (Fearon & Vogelstein 1990). Early mutations in the bowel epithelium in the oncogene ras and the tumour suppressor genes on 5q and 18q give rise to a colon adenoma. Additional mutation of the tumour suppressor gene p53 (localized at 17p) result in progression to carcinoma. Further tumour growth results from the accumulated loss of suppressor genes on additional chromosomes. This correlates with the ability of the carcinomas to metastasize and cause death.

GENETIC SUSCEPTIBILITY TO CANCER

The great majority of malignant tumours are sporadic (in one individual in the family) and develop in older age. Cancer is a common cause of death in the population, but cancer occurring in successive generations in a family is rare. Features which suggest the probability of the presence of a genetic predisposition to cancer are shown in Table 40.1.

As molecular genetic analysis methods have become available, attention has focused over the last 10 years on unusual families where a particular type of cancer (breast/ovary, colorectal) has developed in many relatives, over several generations and at a young age. Significantly, the tumours were often bilateral or multifocal. This clinical presentation could be explained by an inherited mutation of a tumour suppressor gene (which is present in all tissues). Subsequent mutations of further genes results frequently in multiple tumours at a young age of onset. This mechanism of genetic sus-

Table 40.1 Features which increase the probability of the presence of genetic predisposition to cancer

- The development of specific (e.g. breast/ovary) or uncommon tumours (e.g. adrenal/ rhabdomyosarcoma)
- Unusually early onset of cancer (<45 years)
- Multiple primary cancers in one individual
- Relatives with cancer (maternal or paternal side)
- Associated phenotypic or developmental abnormalities (rare)

ceptibility to cancer was initially proposed by Knudson in 1986 (Knudson hypothesis) and has recently been confirmed. Among the first genes to be localized were those causing clinically well characterized disorders such as familial retinoblastoma, Wilms' tumour and adenomatous polyposis coli (APC). Table 40.2 shows the gene localization and clinical presentation of some of the more common cancer susceptibility genetic disorders. One disorder will be described in more detail to illustrate the clinical presentation, surgical management and impact of diagnosis on the family. Adenomatous polyposis coli is a serious autosomal dominant disorder presenting in late childhood/early teens with abdominal pain or bleeding per rectum due to multiple large bowel polyps. At colonoscopy numerous polyps, almost replacing the bowel mucosa, will be identified. Polyps in the rest of the gastrointestinal tract may be also present. The frequency of progression of such polyps to the adenoma–carcinoma sequence is high. The procedures of choice are proctocolectomy with ileoanal pouch or, in the young, initial total colectomy with ileorectal anastomosis and surveillance of the rectal stump to minimize psychosexual sequelae. Another serious complication occurring in approximately 10% of patients with APC are desmoid tumours arising mainly from the peritoneum or abdominal wall; these are highly vascular and difficult to resect in their entirety. When the clinical diagnosis of APC is made, the patient's close relatives have to be informed and counselled about their increased cancer risk. They will have to make a decision whether to have regular colonoscopy, as in some gene carriers the polyps appear later, or to opt for a predictive genetic test. Such potentially predictive tests may carry social stigma or be potentially misused by insurance and employment agencies. At the same time, for the patients and their families, the knowledge of cancer risk and subsequent need for major surgery is stressful. Mutation analysis in the APC gene has to be performed on a sample from the affected family member, as many

Table 40.2 Gene localization and clinical presentation of disorders with a genetic susceptibility to cancer

Disorder	Mode of inheritance	Gene localization	Tumour susceptibility
Retinoblastoma	Autosomal dominant	13q14	Retinoblastoma, osteogenic sarcoma
Wilms' tumour	Autosomal dominant	11p13	Nephroblastoma
Adenomatous polyposis coli	Autosomal dominant	5q21	Colorectal, gastrointestinal tract
Li–Fraumeni syndrome	Autosomal dominant	17p12	Rhabdomyosarcoma, leukaemia, glioma, breast cancer
Breast and ovarian cancer	Autosomal dominant	BRCA1–17q21 BRCA2–13q12	Breast and ovarian Breast? Pancreas
Hereditary non-polyposis colon cancer	Autosomal dominant	hMSH2–2p12 hMLH1–3p21 hPMS1–2q31 hPMS–7p22	Colorectal and gastrointestinal, ureteric, endometrial, ovarian cancer
Neurofibromatosis 1	Autosomal dominant	17q11	Benign schwannoma, brain tumours (rare)
Neurofibromatosis 2	Autosomal dominant	22q13	Optic neuroma, acoustic neuroma, meningioma, glioma
von Hippel–Lindau syndrome	Autosomal dominant	3p25	Meningioma, renal
Peutz–Jeghers syndrome	Autosomal dominant	19p	Hamartoma, gastrointestinal tract

different mutations from different families may be found spanning the whole length of the gene. When the mutation is identified in a family, prenatal diagnosis is of course also possible, with all its associated problems regarding the decision to terminate pregnancy for late onset disorder.

Recently, the cloning of breast/ovarian cancer susceptibility genes (BRCA1 and BRCA2) has been accomplished (Miki et al 1994, Wooster et al 1995). This constitutes a major advance in the study of these common cancers. Mutations have been identified in all areas of these large genes. For practical clinical application, less expensive and less laborious methods of gene analysis will have to be developed. Genetic susceptibility to breast and ovarian cancer is impossible to diagnose clinically in the absence of convincing pedigree suggestive of autosomal dominant inheritance. Several mutations occur more frequently in the Ashkenazi Jewish population; the knowledge of the patient's background may facilitate mutation detection. The population risk for breast cancer in a woman aged 30–39 is 4 in 1000. Whilst the numbers of cases analysed to date are relatively small, and with only preliminary data available, the percentage of breast cancer due to BRCA1 within that age range has been estimated at 5%.

A number of cancer syndromes have been described showing a characteristic combination of cancers (Table 40.2). As relatively small numbers of families have been analysed to date, it is likely that a more accurate clinical spectrum will be available in the future.

The study of families with a high frequency of site specific colorectal cancer and colorectal cancer associated with malignant tumours of the genitourinary tract, uterus, breast cancer and other malignancies has facilitated the recent discovery of several new genes. These syndromes were initially described by Lynch (Lynch et al 1988), but have subsequently been termed 'hereditary nonpolyposis colon cancer' and 'cancer family syndrome'. The colorectal cancer is of early onset with a proclivity to the proximal colon and an excess of synchronous/metachronous lesions. It is often, but not always, preceded by the development of colonic polyps. Colonoscopy is advocated every 3–5 years, with an increasing frequency in the presence of polyps. The surveillance for the associated cancers is problematic as again clinical diagnosis is difficult. Genetic diagnosis is now possible, but methodological problems will have to be overcome for potential clinical application, as is the case with BRCA1/2 genes.

It has been noted that tumours from these affected individuals contain a large number of DNA replication errors. The normal function of these newly discovered genes is to survey the fidelity of DNA replication and repair. Mistakes are frequently introduced during normal DNA replication and DNA repair has to take place, especially when the cell is exposed to carcinogens, ionizing radiation or alkylating agents. The clinical expression of mutations in these genes is compatible with their function as tumour suppressor genes. The frequency of these gene mutations in the population is unknown, but in patients with colorectal cancer, genetic susceptibility has been estimated to account for 5–10% of cases.

Advances in molecular genetics continue at an intense pace. With the current study of oncogene amplification to tumour stage and ultimately to prognosis, the further development of tumour drug targeting and gene therapy, major practical advances in cancer prediction, detection and therapy should be forthcoming in the foreseeable future.

References

Fearon E R, Vogelstein B 1990 A genetic model for colorectal tumourgenesis. Cell 61: 759–767

Lynch H T, Lanspa S J, Bonan B M, Smyth T, Walson P, Lynch J F (1988) Hereditary non-polyposis colorectal cancer, Lynch syndromes I and II. Gastroenterology Clinics of North America 174: 679–715

Miki Y, Swensen J, Shattuck-Eidens D et al 1994 A strong candidate for the breast and ovarian susceptibility gene BRCA1. Science 266: 66–71

Wooster R, Bignell G, Lancaster J et al 1995 Identification of the breast cancer susceptibility gene BRCA2. Nature 378(6559): 789–792

Summary

1. Genetic disorders may predispose to life-threatening complications during surgery or anaesthesia and also may be the cause of increased susceptibility to cancer. Salient features in the history and examination suggestive of defects in haemoglobin, haemostasis, muscle, connective tissue and the skeleton should be noted.

2. Cancer develops following the accumulation of mutations in oncogenes and in tumour suppressor genes. Whilst the great majority of cancers are sporadic, early age at the development of colon or breast/ovarian cancer (<45 years) and similarly affected relatives may indicate the presence of an inherited predisposition. Genetic mutations in specific tumour suppressor genes were identified in approximately 20% of individuals with early onset and family history of cancer.

3. Exciting recent developments include predictive genetic testing for relatives at high risk for developing cancer by mutation analysis. Clinical trials directed towards early cancer detection and chemoprevention in this group will provide statistically significant outcome data in shorter time than other general population trials.

41

Screening for surgical disease

T. Bates

Objectives

- Identify essentials for justifying a screening programme.
- Appreciate the practical requirements.
- Recognize the cost-benefits including mortality and quality of life.

INTRODUCTION

At first sight, screening the population for the common forms of surgical disease seems a good idea since it should then be possible to cure the condition before it becomes symptomatic. Cancer of the lung, which is still the commonest malignancy (22 700 male, 11 000 female deaths in England and Wales per year) (Office of Population Censuses and Surveys 1994) has such a poor prognosis that screening the population by mass miniature chest X-ray failed, whereas prevention by a public health programme to stop smoking has reduced death rates. Screening programmes have been set up for carcinoma of the colon, stomach, breast and cervix and more recently the prostate and ovary. It is possible that screening for non-malignant conditions such as abdominal aortic aneurysm may reduce the number of deaths in elderly men from leaking aneurysm. To be effective, early detection and treatment must lead to fewer deaths from the disease or have a major impact on the quality of life in the screened population but in some of these conditions there are still doubts that this can be achieved. An increased survival time from diagnosis to death could well be due to earlier, and therefore more prolonged observation, of the natural history of the disease which might be unaffected by the treatment. This situation is known as *lead-time bias*.

The acid test for a screening programme is to compare a screened population with an identical non-screened population and this should ideally be set up as a randomized controlled trial (RCT) to avoid unrecognized biases (Shapiro 1981, Hardcastle et al 1996). If the disease carries a relatively good prognosis when adequately treated at an early stage, it may take many years of observation to show a difference in the number of deaths between the screened and non-screened groups; this will require considerable resources.

There are many questions which should be answered before considerable amounts of time, money and effort are committed to a screening programme. These questions must be addressed by several disciplines – clinical scientists in the relevant speciality, epidemiologists with expertise in screening, social scientists and economists.

Is the burden of the disease in the population sufficient to warrant an intervention? Is the screening test accurate in detecting cases in the population to be screened, and is the subsequent treatment effective in curing the disease? In trying to answer these three critical questions the following specific issues must be considered.

THE REQUIREMENTS FOR A SCREENING TEST

1. Is the screening test sensitive (i.e. does it detect most of the cases with few false negatives)?
2. Is the test specific (i.e. does it only detect cancer cases with few false positives)?
3. The test must be safe, relatively inexpensive and capable of achieving adequate compliance in the population to be screened.

There are many examples of screening where these criteria have not been met: *O*-tolidine-based dyes for detecting occult blood increased the risk of bladder cancer in laboratory staff and the dose of irradiation used for the first breast screening mammograms is no longer regarded as safe. Investigation and treatment of false-positive cases may lead to psychological or physical morbidity.

THE POPULATION TO BE SCREENED

The at-risk population must be defined. To screen young people for cancer does not make sense but cancer of the cervix has become more common in younger women; this has led to a reduction in the age at which screening is offered. It is essential to have an accurate register of the population to be screened and in city areas this must be frequently updated if the client is to receive the invitation for screening. Screening the very elderly is likely to show poor compliance and the cost–benefit ratio will therefore be less favourable. Screening high risk groups, e.g. those with a strong family history, poses special problems and different criteria must be used.

COLORECTAL CANCER (8750 MALE, 8650 FEMALE DEATHS PER YEAR)

Colonoscopy is the gold-standard test for detecting colonic cancer or polyps with both specificity and sensitivity nearing 100%, but high price and low compliance rule this out as a screening test unless a very high-risk population such as a family with familial adenomatous polyposis is being examined. Colorectal cancer should be an ideal candidate for screening since it seems that many cancers are preceded by benign adenomatous polyps and, furthermore, early cancer (Dukes A) has a 5-year survival of 90% with conventional operative treatment. However, the best available test is poor. The guaiac-based Haemoccult test is probably the best available test for faecal occult blood but it has a relatively low sensitivity, especially for right-sided and rectal tumours. Immunologically-based tests are more sensitive but less specific and give rise to false-positive cases which require expensive and unnecessary investigation.

Randomized controlled trials of faecal occult blood screening have shown a reduced number of deaths from colorectal cancer in the screened group (Hardcastle et al 1996) but doubts about the overall number of deaths in each group, the low compliance and the cost of implementation remain (Ahlquist 1997).

CANCER OF THE BREAST (13 700 DEATHS PER YEAR)

There have been four randomly allocated trials of population screening for breast cancer by mammography; of these, only the Swedish Two-Counties study has shown a significant reduction in mortality (Tabar et al

1989). However, a recent overview of these trials and other non-randomized studies shows that all report fewer deaths in the screened versus the non-screened population (Wald et al 1991). There has been a recent reduction in the number of deaths from breast cancer in many countries but this trend preceded screening and may be related to the increased use of adjuvant therapy. There has been an unexpectedly high number of cancers presenting between 3-yearly screens (interval cancers) in the UK National Breast Screening Programme which has led to the adoption of 2-view instead of single-view mammography for the first screen (Blanks et al 1997) and to studies of 2- versus 3-yearly frequency of screening (Woodman et al 1995). There are also pilot studies to increase the upper age limit from 64 to 69 years since compliance in this age group seems better than was expected. Screening women under the age of 50 is not of proven benefit and remains highly controversial.

CARCINOMA OF THE CERVIX (1650 DEATHS PER YEAR)

Unfortunately no randomized trial of cytological screening for carcinoma of the cervix has been carried out and although death rates for this disease have fallen in many countries, this fall has often preceded the introduction of screening (Williams 1992).

Up to 60% of women who have developed cervical cancer in the UK had never been screened and the false-negative rate for examination of the smears is about 10%. Not all smears are adequate and cytoscreening is very labour intensive which has led to problems with quality control. This situation has been unsatisfactory since the outcome of adequate treatment in cervical intraepithelial neoplasia (CIN) is highly successful. However, there is now an efficient mechanism for the re-call and treatment of patients with positive smears based on general practice and compliance has reached 83% (Austoker 1994a).

CARCINOMA OF THE STOMACH (5000 MALE, 3300 FEMALE DEATHS PER YEAR)

The incidence of cancer of the stomach seems to be falling as colon cancer rises but these changes may be confounded by the vagaries of death certification.

Cancer of the stomach is much more common in Japan where screening for early gastric cancer seems to be effective with the use of barium studies, gastroscopy and, more recently, serum pepsinogen. In the UK the search has been less successful and screening by gastroscopy should be confined to symptomatic patients over the age of 55 (Hallissey et al 1990).

CARCINOMA OF THE PROSTATE (8700 DEATHS PER YEAR)

Screening for carcinoma of the prostate is controversial since the disease mainly affects an elderly population and 30% of men over the age of 50 have histological evidence of prostatic cancer at necropsy but in only 1% of these is there clinically active disease (Austoker 1994b). The available screening tests, apart from rectal examination, are prostatic specific antigen and transrectal ultrasound. Neither the sensitivity nor the specificity of these tests is high, either alone or in combination, and the treatment of localized prostatic cancer is also controversial. Radical prostatectomy, radiotherapy, hormonal manipulation and a watch-policy are all used in this situation but there is no randomized trial to indicate survival benefit and it must be important not to cause unnecessary morbidity in elderly men with asymptomatic disease.

CANCER OF THE OVARY (3900 DEATHS PER YEAR)

Evidence for survival benefit from screening is lacking but a large randomized controlled trial has been set up. The main screening tests are antigen marker CA 125 and transvaginal ultrasound, but other tumour markers and colour Doppler are being evaluated. The sensitivity of CA 125 for early ovarian cancer may be as low as 50%. There must, however, be a strong case for screening a high risk group with family ovarian cancer syndrome (Austoker 1994c).

SCREENING FOR NON-MALIGNANT SURGICAL DISEASE

Neonatal screening

Congenital disease is increasingly diagnosed as a result of routine antenatal ultrasound screening but postnatal clinical examination should be carried out for evidence of congenital cardiac and renal abnormalities as well as orthopaedic, sexual and anorectal malformations. Most congenital abnormalities will normally present as a

clinical problem in the first few days of life but it is important to recognize silent conditions such as congenital dislocation of the hip where delay in diagnosis may worsen the outcome.

Abdominal aortic aneurysm (2900 male, 1040 female deaths per year)

There are several population screening studies from the UK and the USA and in men over the age of 65 ultrasound screening of the aorta shows a prevalence of aneurysm of about 5% depending on size criteria. This rate may be twice as high in men with hypertension or vascular disease and the lifetime prevalence in first-degree male relatives may be as high as 50% (Collin 1994). It seems likely that deaths from leaking abdominal aortic aneurysm could be reduced by screening men at age 65 years with a policy of elective surgery for fit patients with an aortic diameter of about 5 cm or more. Randomized trials of screening are in progress but it remains a controversial issue (Cheatle 1997).

WHAT COMPLIANCE IS TO BE EXPECTED?

Compliance varies with the social acceptability and public awareness of the disease, the screening test and the perceived effectiveness of the treatment. Screening for breast cancer by mammography achieves 80% in areas with a stable population but this may be less than 50% in inner city areas. Compliance is also sensitive to media exposure in the short term.

In screening for colorectal cancer, the acceptability of the faecal occult blood test is very low which leads to poor compliance unless considerable efforts are made to increase public awareness at the time that screening is offered. There are many reasons why people decline screening invitations but failure to receive the letter is a common cause. The true refusers are an unusual group of people who have a poor outlook from both a health and a social standpoint. They neglect or abuse their health in many respects and it is therefore important not to use them as a control group for comparison with the accepters of screening since whatever comparison is made the refusers will be disadvantaged. Compliance for cervical screening is worst in the low socioeconomic group most at risk from the disease (Segnan 1997)

THE INTERVENTION TO BE USED

It has already been noted that an operation for early bowel cancer has a high cure rate but we cannot be sure this is the case for breast cancer. Screen detected breast cancer has many features known to indicate a good prognosis (Klemi et al 1992) but ductal carcinoma in situ is diagnosed in up to 20% of screened cases and the best treatment for this condition is still in doubt. It is possible that fear of overtreatment by mastectomy may lead to a sacrifice of survival advantage by inadequate surgery. Severe dysplasia of the cervix (CIN III) has an extremely good outlook with local treatment and close surveillance. Node positive carcinoma of the stomach has a 5-year survival rate of less than 10% but in situ tumours carry a good prognosis if treated with adequate surgery. The Japanese have pioneered more radical surgery for gastric cancer than has been the norm in the West and clinical trials are currently in hand to try and repeat their excellent results in the UK. The place of radical prostatectomy in the treatment of screen detected prostatic cancer remains uncertain.

WHAT IS THE COST?

The economist will want to know the cost per case detected, the cost per case treated and per life saved. The sociologist will want to know the psychosocial cost to those false-positive cases investigated unnecessarily and the quality of life in those patients who have cancer detected sooner than it otherwise would have been.

Summary

1. A screening test for cancer must be able to detect the disease at a stage when earlier treatment will lead to fewer deaths.
2. To achieve this the test must be sensitive, specific and acceptable: the treatment must be effective.
3. The overall cost of a life saved may be difficult to quantify but this should be taken into account.

References

Ahlquist D A 1997 Fecal occult blood testing for colorectal cancer. Can we afford this? Gastroenterology Clinics of North America 26: 41–55

Austoker J 1994a Screening and self-examination for breast cancer. British Medical Journal 309: 168–174

Austoker J 1994b Screening for cervical cancer. British Medical Journal 309: 241–248

Austoker J 1994c Screening for ovarian, prostatic and testicular cancers. British Medical Journal 309: 315–320

Blanks R G, Moss S M, Wallis M G 1997 Use of two view mammography compared with one view in the detection of small invasive cancers: further results from the NHS breast screening programme. Journal of Medical Screening 4: 98–101

Cheatle T R 1997 The case against a national screening programme for aortic aneurysms. Annals of the Royal College of Surgeons of England 79: 90–95 (subsequent comments 79: 310, 385–386)

Collin R 1994 Abdominal aorta: epidemiology. In: Morris P J, Malt R A (eds) Oxford textbook for surgery. Oxford University Press, New York pp 377–378

Hallissey M T, Allum W H, Jewkes A J, Ellis D J, Fielding J W L 1990 Early detection of gastric cancer. British Medical Journal 301: 513–515

Hardcastle J D, Chamberlain O, Robinson M H et al 1996 Randomised controlled trial of faecal occult blood screening for colorectal cancer. Lancet 348: 1472–1477

Hisamichi S, Sugawara N 1984 Mass screening for gastric cancer by X-ray examination. Japanese Journal of Clinical Oncology 14: 211–223

Klemi P J, Joensuu H, Toikkanen S, Tuominen J, Rasanen O, Tyrkko J, Parvinen I 1992 Aggressiveness of breast cancers found with and without screening. British Medical Journal 304: 467–469

Office of Population Censuses and Surveys 1994. Series DH2, No. 19. Mortality statistics for 1992. Cause. HMSO, London

Segnan N 1997 Socioeconomic status and cancer screening. IARC Scientific Publications 138: 369–376

Shapiro S 1981 Evidence on screening for breast cancer from a randomised trial. Cancer 39: 618–627

Tabar L, Fagerberg F, Duffy S W, Day N E 1989 The Swedish two counties trial of mammographic screening for breast cancer: recent results and calculation of benefit. Journal of Epidemiology and Community Health 43: 107–114

Wald N, Frost C, Cuckle H 1991 Breast cancer screening: the current position. British Medical Journal 302: 845–846

Williams C 1992 Ovarian and cervical cancer. British Medical Journal 304: 1501–1504

Woodman C B J, Threlfall A G, Boggis C R M, Prior P 1995 Is the three year breast screening interval too long? Occurrence of interval cancers in NHS breast screening programme's north western region. British Medical Journal 310: 224–226

42

Audit

B. W. Ellis, J. Simpson

Objectives

- **Appreciate what audit is and its link with clinical effectiveness.**
- **Understand the basic methods of audit and the need for confidentiality.**
- **Recognize that changing clinical practice is not straightforward.**

DEFINITIONS

Clinical audit is defined by the Department of Health (DoH) as: 'The systematic, critical analysis of the quality of medical care, including the procedures used for diagnosis and treatment, the use of resources, and the resulting outcome and quality of life for the patient', and states that 'an effective programme of medical audit will also help to provide reassurance to doctors, their patients, and managers that the best quality of service is being achieved, having regard to the resources available' (DoH 1989). The efficient and effective use of resources is important (Ellis et al 1990), but it is not the first priority of clinical audit.

Clinical audit is the responsibility of clinicians and must be led by them (Standing Committee on Postgraduate Medical Education 1989). The terms 'clinical audit' and 'medical audit' are sometimes used interchangeably, but a consensus has developed whereby *medical audit* refers to the assessment by peer review of the medical care provided by the medical profession to the patient, and *clinical audit* refers to an assessment of the total care of the patient by nurses, professions allied to medicine (such as physiotherapists) as well as doctors. The multiprofessional team has an essential role in patient care and the quality of health care cannot be determined by doctors alone. Most hospitals have now focused their audit activity around clinical rather than medical audit.

A revised position statement on clinical audit (NHSE 1996a) describes the development of audit so far and identifies future goals. Audit should aim to achieve:

- A clear patient focus
- Greater multiprofessional working
- Patient care managed across primary, secondary and continuing care
- Closer links with education
- Better integration of effectiveness information.

This document also stresses the important role of clinical audit in improving the clinical effectiveness of services.

HISTORY AND BACKGROUND

While modern-day concepts of audit may be new to many, a critical appraisal of the care dispensed by clinicians is by no means new. There have been many examples of audit activity in a number of guises over the last few centuries. Our forefathers in surgery very often had no option but to learn by trial and error. The openness of their writing, especially in their descriptions of surgical disasters, makes fascinating reading when we can look back with the benefit of hindsight and with our current state of knowledge:

> The patient had complete retention. I was induced at length to try forcible catheterisation with a straight instrument – an operation which has been recommended by excellent surgeons, especially Dupytren. My attempt was unsuccessful; the instrument bent and did not penetrate the prostate gland. Retroperitoneal infiltration of urine followed and the patient died. I do not advise anyone to follow my example. In such a case puncture of the bladder by the rectum would have been the proper proceeding [sic]. (Bilroth 1881)

Nor were these expositions confined to the anecdotal. In the same book, T. H. Bilroth, who was then professor of surgery in Vienna, noted:

Of 118 operations on the breast alone, eight were fatal; the cause of death in all cases being erysipelas. Of 187 operations on the breast and axillary glands ... forty patients died from various causes; three deaths occurred from severe secondary haemorrhage, but many of the other cases, who were attacked with septicaemia, pyaemia or erysipelas had also haemorrhage from the axilla.

There then follows a critical appraisal of the various techniques of ligature of veins and the use of antiseptics and caustics.

The improvement in standards of care in surgery as a whole and in the practices of individual surgeons has, until recently, relied on the apprenticeship of the training years, and the dissemination of new learning and good practice through the medium of the book, the journal and the lecture by the 'expert'. Those who were prepared to listen and read were able to change practice where appropriate. Even now many surgeons rely on the annual meetings of the various 'craft' associations for education in current surgical practice.

The roots of modern audit lie in the regular morbidity and mortality meetings held in many hospitals in the UK and the USA in the 1950s and 1960s. The value of these meetings as a means of learning was recognized and formed the basis of broader audit activities.

In the early 1980s, microcomputers made their first appearance on the audit scene and this made it possible to collect and analyse large amounts of information very swiftly. This then gave the clinician a powerful tool to assist in the interpretation of types of work done, throughput and complications. Audit systems are now very powerful, and can rapidly highlight areas of high risk of complication, death, cost, etc. However, there is the danger that some surgeons believe ownership of an 'audit' system to be synonymous with the successful practice of audit. They must appreciate that such systems are merely tools with which we can get a grasp and some understanding of the activity for which we are responsible.

Every hospital in the UK is responsible for ensuring the development of clinical audit in which all doctors participate (DoH 1989). Whereas before audit was practised on a voluntary basis, and thus predominantly by enthusiasts, the requirement for audit is now written into the job descriptions of all new medical staff. By 1995, a survey by the National Audit Office confirmed that more than 80% of doctors were involved in audit and that clinical audit was generally accepted to have become embedded in the NHS as part of routine clinical practice (NAO 1995). However, the effectiveness of this activity in securing worthwhile and lasting improvements in the quality of care for patients is still very variable (Walshe & Spurgeon 1997). These authors have developed a clinical audit assessment and improvement framework to enable both audit programmes and individual audit projects to improve their effectiveness (Walshe & Spurgeon 1997).

Until 1990 there was no funding or allocation of time for audit activity. Funds were available centrally for several years. Since the transfer of funding responsibility in 1995, health authorities must agree plans for audit addressing local service and clinical priorities with trust managers and audit groups. As part of the audit contract with hospitals, health authorities can request audit of specific clinical areas.

ATTITUDES TO AUDIT

Many clinicians will argue that audit is practised already; that ward rounds, clinical presentations, research and morbidity and mortality meetings fulfil this function. However, there are differences between these and clinical audit. Audit must be seen as a systematic approach to the review of clinical care to highlight opportunities for improvement and to provide a mechanism for bringing them about. As such, it endeavours to get away from the 'single interesting case' and look for patterns of care that should ideally be evaluated against research based evidence or accepted best practice. Audit should initiate investigation into those areas of clinical care that are considered as high risk, high cost, or very common. Audit investigation is also suitable for resolving issues of contention or local interest. The rare and clinically interesting case should be left for the clinical conference.

Many feel that the time spent on audit could be much better spent on other activities, such as treating more patients. This is not a wholly spurious argument; audit was introduced without any prior evaluation and although there have been several subsequent evaluations, the results have, to date, failed to demonstrate clear value for money or effort expended (Walshe 1995). There is, none the less, general agreement that a regular review of his or her own practice by a clinician against agreed standards of best practice can lead to improved delivery of care for the patient. It is important that we do not lose sight of the fact that the principal beneficiary of the process should be the patient. Furthermore, clinical audit can improve care of our patients not only through direct changes in clinical practice but also through indirect effects such as professional education and team development.

With the implementation of the internal market in health care from 1991, and the split between purchasers (hospitals and general practice fund holders) and providers (trusts), there was a need to specify the quality of the service provided and to link quality of care with quantity and cost. An effective clinical audit programme can give the necessary reassurance to patients, clinicians and managers that an agreed quality of service is being given within available resources (NHS Confederation 1997). Information is now requested on the arrangements for clinical audit, the level of participation by doctors and other professional staff, the topics examined and improvements generated. Clinicians and managers share audit information within agreed rules of confidentiality. Many deficiencies revealed by audit relate to the organization of care and although audit must remain clinically-led, support from NHS board directors and management is vital if it is to achieve the necessary changes in practice.

The Labour government which came into office in 1997 abolished the internal market whilst retaining the separation between the planning of hospital care and its provision. Clinical audit is expected to take a central role in the requirement for hospitals to deliver high quality patient services.

CLINICAL EFFECTIVENESS

There is a growing need to base clinical practice on the knowledge obtained from rigorous research into the effectiveness of health care interventions. Clinically effective interventions maintain and improve health and secure the greatest possible health gain from the available resources (NHSE 1996b). Clinical audit has a crucial role to play in this; in assessing current practice, identifying and bringing about the necessary changes in practice and monitoring that the expected outcomes have been achieved. Clinical staff are encouraged to review care against agreed clinical standards, evidence-based clinical guidelines, and systematic reviews of research (NHSE 1996b). Clinicians are increasingly being asked to develop evidence-based guidelines for the delivery of care and to audit care against locally developed or nationally commended guidelines (NHSE 1996c) (see also Criterion audit, p. 401). However, it is acknowledged that the freedom of clinicians to determine the treatment of individual patients must be preserved (NHSE 1993). An important part of the national research and development strategy is to make information on research findings easily available to clinical and managerial staff, both in printed form (e.g. Effective Health Care bulletins) and electronic media (e.g. the Cochrane Library). All hospital libraries should have easy access to this information with trained staff to help in its use.

THE IMPLEMENTATION OF CHANGE

If audit is to be effective, it must lead to change. Audit may be considered as a cycle, the first component of which is the observation of existing practice to establish what is actually happening. Then, standards of practice are set to define what ought to happen and a comparison made between observed practice with the standard. Finally, change is implemented. Clinical practice is observed again to see whether what has been planned has been achieved. A decision can then be made as to whether practice needs to change further, or whether the standards were unrealistic or unobtainable. This process has become known as the 'cycle of audit' (Royal College of Physicians 1989) and the achievement of change has been termed 'closing the audit loop'.

The provision of information on clinical activity, without any evaluation or suggestions for improvement, has been judged to have almost no effect on clinical practice (Mitchell et al 1990), unless it is targeted at decision-makers who had already agreed to review their practice (Mugford et al 1991). A systematic review of 160 interventions directed at changing clinical behaviour or health outcomes showed that effects were small to moderate (Davis et al 1995). Effective strategies were outreach visits, opinion leaders, patient-mediated interventions and physician reminders. Variable results were found for audit with feedback. The most commonly used approach involves the publication of guidelines, which has been shown to change practice and affect outcomes. Guidelines are more likely to be effective if they have local involvement and take into account local circumstances, are supported by active educational interventions and use patient-specific reminders, for example, in the medical notes (Effective Health Care 1994). Guidelines need to be reviewed regularly to establish 'ownership' and to incorporate the latest research findings.

THE EDUCATIONAL COMPONENT

The educational benefits of clinical audit have been considered in depth by Batstone (1990). It is now seen as vital that doctors in training are taught the basic principles of audit. Equally, conclusions drawn from the audit process should be seen as an important feeder into education.

There can be little doubt that the critical review of current practice and comparisons against predefined standards encourages the acquisition and updating of knowledge. The audit process also enables the identification of important features of clinical practice which should help to make teaching more explicit. Doctors involved in audit are taking part in an active process of review. 'Passive' recipients, who are unclear whether their current practice is inappropriate, are unlikely to respond to information through traditional channels such as journals or continuing medical education (Lomas 1993).

Through audit, it is possible to identify particular areas where knowledge could be improved or is deficient, suggesting the need for research. It must be remembered that audit itself will not lead to new clinical knowledge. Research aims to identify 'the right thing to do' while audit assesses whether 'the right thing has been done' and whether further improvement is required. Self-evaluation and peer review, common activities in audit, are important components of postgraduate education. In order fully to realize the educational potential of audit it is essential that the lessons arising from previous audit meetings are reviewed and the conclusions acted upon.

STAFF FOR AUDIT

Most hospitals in England now have an audit officer and/or audit coordinator. It is their task to enable the implementation of audit and to assist where possible in the execution of the audit process.

While much still rests on the clinical staff to prepare for audit exercises, the audit staff should be able to provide support in:

- Helping to prepare audit programmes
- Helping to plan audit studies
- Literature searching
- Screening case records against clinically determined criteria
- Computer assistance with databases/graphics and forms
- Preparing audit reports.

COMMITTEES FOR AUDIT

The hospitals have a clinical audit committee reporting to their unit management. An audit committee should draw members from a range of clinical backgrounds so that a wide perspective can be used in the planning of audit at a local level. The chairman needs to be well motivated and prepared to devote time on a regular basis. There should be representation from the nursing profession, primary health care (general practice), education (usually the clinical tutor) and the doctors in the training grades, plus other clinical staff such as

pharmacists and physiotherapists. The audit staff should also sit on the committee.

Hospital audit committees have the following functions. They should:

- Coordinate and foster clinical audit for everyone involved in patient care
- Attempt to minimize the perception that audit is a threat
- Highlight the benefits of the audit process for patients and the clinical staff
- Determine existing practice of audit
- Assist clinicians in the implementation of audit methods
- Monitor the results and conclusions of the audit process and check the validity of data and reporting
- Ensure that changes, where indicated by the outcome of audit, are implemented
- Ensure that the outcome of audit is perceived as educational and that all clinical staff are educated in the practice and process of audit
- Train and direct audit officers
- Ensure effective liaison with GPs and management
- Maintain confidentiality
- Estimate funding required for audit
- Prepare annual report and forward programme.

Some audit committees have extended their role to integrate actively audit with clinical effectiveness, clinical risk management or complaints monitoring.

GUIDANCE ON AUDIT

The Royal College of Surgeons of England has published guidance on audit, *Clinical Audit in Surgical Practice* (1995) as well as a number of clinical guidelines.

A National Centre for Clinical Audit (NCCA) was established in 1995. Publications include the *NCCA Clinical Audit Action Pack* (NCCA 1996), a regular newsletter and a series of fact sheets. The centre runs an information service and has its own web site on the Internet.

TECHNIQUES IN AUDIT

Donabedian (1966) identified three main elements in the delivery of health care: structure, process and outcome.

Structure. This includes the quantity and type of resources available and is generally easy to measure. It is not a good indicator of the quality of care but should be taken into account in the assessment of process and outcome.

Process. This is what is done to the patient. It includes consideration of the way an operation was performed, what medications were prescribed, the adequacy of notes, and compliance with consensus policies. There is an underlying assumption that the activities under review have been previously shown to produce an optimal medical outcome. This is the area of patient care that is most open to change by the clinician.

Outcome. This is the result of clinical intervention and may represent the success or failure of process. For example, outcome could be measured by studies of surgical fatality rates, incidence of complications, or patient satisfaction. It can be considered to be the most relevant indicator of patient care, but it is the most difficult to define and quantify. Mortality and length of stay in hospital are very easily measured outcome indicators, but variations in these outcomes are rarely related directly to the quality of the service being delivered. It may be more important to consider whether patients perceive that their problems have been solved, their quality of life improved and, where appropriate, the duration of their survival.

A number of audit techniques have evolved and found a place in the regular assessment of clinical practice. These are as follows.

Basic clinical audit. This entails an analysis of throughput, a broad analysis of case type, complications and morbidity and mortality. It is suggested that review of such data is undertaken by each clinical firm at intervals of approximately 3 months. The essential ingredient is to distil out of the data any notable deviations from an accepted 'norm' and then to investigate the reason for this observation.

Incident review. This involves the discussion of strategies to be adopted under certain clinical scenarios. An incident may be taken to be anything from a patient suffering from a leaking aortic aneurysm to the use of a department for an investigation (e.g. emergency intravenous urography). It is expected that such discussions would lead to clear policies for future use and may result in the production of local guidelines. This audit method is particularly suitable for multidisciplinary or interdisciplinary audit.

Clinical record review. A member of another firm of the same or similar speciality is invited to review a random selection of case notes. Where possible, criteria should be established for this review purpose. Clinical record audit has the advantage of simplicity and requires relatively little additional time or other resources. However, there is a potential disadvantage in that discussion might concentrate too much on the quality of record keeping and not enough on patient care – these two are distinct facets of the clinical process, although related.

Criterion audit. A more advanced and structured form of incident audit. Retrospective analysis of clinical records is made and judged against a number of carefully chosen criteria. These criteria should encapsulate the key elements in management of a particular topic which should be capable of unambiguous interpretation from the medical record by a non-medical audit assistant. All cases falling within the scope of the topic in question are screened and those that fail to meet any of the criteria are brought forward for further clinical review. The criteria may relate to administrative elements (e.g. waiting time), investigations ordered, treatments given, outcome, follow-up strategies, etc. Criteria for adequate management of a particular condition can be easily derived from clinical guidelines. Clinical time is necessary in the preliminary discussion, but the majority of the work can be done by audit assistants. It is applicable to a variety of circumstances and allows the comparison of data between different hospitals (Shaw 1989). The criteria can be used for the setting of standards, with targets identifying the proportion of patients in whom the criterion should be met. After review, new targets can be set to stimulate improvement. An example would be to reduce infection rates in colorectal surgery to the levels obtained in other published studies (Hancock 1990).

Adverse occurrence screening. A clinical firm decides on a shortlist of events that are worthy of avoidance (e.g. wound infections, unplanned readmissions, delay or error in diagnosis). Details of occurrences are recorded and complex or serious occurrences are reviewed by clinicians. A database is built up which can then be interrogated to identify trends, perform comparative analyses, etc. Cases can be selected by considering all admissions or a sample of them. This technique can also be used for risk management (Bennett & Walshe 1990).

Comparative audit. In any one hospital, the number of departments undertaking similar work is often very small. Even between two firms of general surgeons the case mix may be sufficiently different to make comparisons difficult. In other specialities, there may not be anyone else in the hospital with whom to compare results. Comparative audit implies the collection of data and its comparison across units, health authorities and even through a whole region (Gruer et al 1986, Black 1991). In 1991, the Royal College of Surgeons set up a comparative audit service in which all surgeons are requested to supply information under a confidential number for comparison with their peers at regular meetings (Royal College of Surgeons 1991). Techniques in data presentation allow such sensitive information to be widely disseminated and discussed, while maintaining an individual clinician's confidentiality (Emberton et al 1991). In Scotland, a regional computerized audit system maintained by general surgeons over 15 years, recording clinical data which is regularly reviewed in a peer-group setting, has given clear evidence that regional audit can significantly influence and improve surgical practice (Aitken et al 1997).

National studies. These were first used over a decade ago to address the question of perinatal mortality in obstetric units. The report of the first confidential enquiry into perioperative deaths (CEPOD) (Buck et al 1987) considered the factors involved in the deaths of patients who died within 30 days of surgery in three regional health authorities. Much was learnt from that exercise, especially the need for doctors in the training grades to be given adequate support and supervision. It was clear that disaster frequently arose when surgeons attempted procedures for which they possessed insufficient skill or training. The enquiry has since developed into a national review (NCEPOD) to which data is submitted on a voluntary confidential basis by surgeons and anaesthetists. Reports are published annually (Gallimore et al 1997). The findings can identify remedial actions and indicate appropriate topics for local audit, such as out-of-hours surgery (Campling et al 1997).

Outcome audit. Outcome will depend on the whole of the process of health-care delivery during a patient's episode in hospital. It is thus a measure of the spectrum of the skills of the medical and nursing staff, the hospital administration and indeed, every person or department with whom the patient comes into contact. There will inevitably be a contrast between the perspectives on outcome between the patient, the GP and the clinician, and much work remains to be done to evolve satisfactory measures. Studies on outcome, especially in the surgical specialities, are likely to be seen as an important measure of the quality of care.

ETHICS AND CONFIDENTIALITY

Information used in audit about patients must protect the confidentiality of individual patients and also that of the professionals involved.

With regard to patient confidentiality, the same principles are involved as in the clinical conferences which form part of any academic programme. It is important to secure an undertaking from all those involved not to talk about what was discussed in an audit meeting outside that meeting. Unless an explicit and convincing case can be made for inclusion of identifying details of a patient in verbal or written presentations, such details should be excluded.

The confidentiality of the professionals involved also requires protection. This is likely to prove difficult in some types of audit, for example where one consultant reviews the clinical records of another consultant's patient. Nevertheless, this type of audit can be successful if the necessary atmosphere of trust and collaboration is fostered. It is always necessary to obtain permission from all consultants involved before starting an audit exercise.

It is important to consider what should happen if audit reveals problems of deficiencies in a given individual's clinical practice. Such a situation is likely to occur infrequently, if at all, but this makes it the more important to anticipate such an eventuality and to make explicit provision for it (Ellis & Sensky 1991). The Joint Consultants Committee has recently recommended that clinicians develop a local protocol for action, and has published a suggested course of action (DoH 1996a).

Ethical committee permission before interviewing patients is occasionally required, but this is usually a local requirement which needs to be checked. In general, audit projects need not involve ethical committees.

COMPUTERS

The surgical trainee should have a good working knowledge of the basics of computing. Many postgraduate medical centres now offer the use of a microcomputer for the production of graphics and for word processing. Some centres have also installed CD-ROM drives to enable enquiry on databases published in CD format. The best known, and most useful, medical publication in this format is MEDLINE. Compared to searching through numerous volumes of the *Index Medicus*, computer-based searching is a great deal faster and permits searching in many different ways. For those trainees with access to a CD-ROM, a 'download' facility allows the export of selected papers with or without abstracts into a database on a personal computer. The Internet is also finding a place as a reference source including access to systematic reviews of the effectiveness of health-care interventions (Booth 1996).

Computing skills are best acquired by practice on the computer itself. A number of programs are available as clinical information systems, which usually have outputs configured to help in the process of audit. Despite some pioneering ventures into the realms of clinical decision-making systems and artificial intelligence, there is still a great deal to be learned about the clinical as opposed to the administrative capabilities of computing in medicine.

Hospital information systems

The DoH has never been keen to prescribe rigid solutions, with the result that every hospital has the potential to find a different configuration of computer to manage and monitor its activity.

A few hospitals have a completely integrated 'hospital information system' covering every function from the recording of clinical data, the scheduling of clinics, to the provision of financial and manpower reports, etc. At the other end of this computing spectrum are those hospitals which have a patient administration system (PAS), including the 'master index' (patients' demographic details) and records of admissions and diagnostic codes. This represents the minimum upon which a hospital manager can rely for information. PAS systems regularly pass aggregated patient-level data according to a national minimum data set to the local health authority. This, together with contract activity information, enables local planning of services.

In hospitals with this minimum configuration there are bound to be clinical departments which have implemented their own information systems, and these may provide sufficient information on which to draw patient samples for audit projects and some limited clinical data.

Current trends seem to favour the integration of all these disparate systems so that key patient specific information, once entered, is available throughout the organization. The surgical trainee will almost certainly be involved in the gathering of information for the production of a discharge summary to the GP and for clinical audit.

THE NEW NHS

The government white paper *The New NHS: Modern, Dependable* (Cmnd 3807 1977) outlines a new 'ten year' structuring and modernization programme. The internal market is replaced by a system of integrated care based on a partnership between health and social care. The split between planning and providing care is maintained, with cooperation replacing competition. The quality of care is a priority for everyone.

Chief executives of trusts will be held accountable for the quality of services they provide. This responsibility for 'clinical governance' covers quality improvement including clinical audit, evidence-based practice, clinical risk reduction, adverse incidents, etc., and includes encouraging good practice and correcting poor clinical performance. At national level, there will be a new National Institute of Clinical Effectiveness. A Commission for Health Improvement will oversee the quality of care and can intervene when necessary, working with the organization to put things right.

The importance of clinical audit, led by clinicians, in improving the quality of care for patients was recognized in the last NHS reorganization in 1989. The new framework signals a more directed, but integrated role for audit within the organization. This can be seen as an opportunity for audit to deliver the necessary changes in practice which have been identified, and fulfil its potential in improving patient care.

Summary

1. Analysis of our medical care, to maintain and improve standards, in the responsibility of each one of us.
2. It is fruitless to record our performance unless we use the knowledge to bring about change.

References

Aitken R J, Nixon S J, Ruckley C V 1997 Lothian surgical audit: a 15-year experience of improvement in surgical practice through regional computerised audit. Lancet 350: 800–804

Batstone G F 1990 Educational aspects of medical audit. British Medical Journal 301: 326–328

Bennett J, Walshe K 1990 Occurrence screening as a method of audit. British Medical Journal 300: 1248–1251

Booth A 1996 The SCHARR guide to evidence-based practice. Sheffield Centre for Health and Related Research, Sheffield

Bilroth T H 1881 Clinical surgery: reports of surgical practice, 1860–1876. New Sydenham Society, London

Black N 1991 A regional computerised surgical audit project. Quality Assurance in Health Care 2: 263–270

Buck N, Devlin H B, Lunn J N 1987 Report of a confidential enquiry into perioperative deaths. London

Campling E A, Devlin H B, Hoile R W, Ingram G S, Lunn J N 1997 Who operates when? A Report of The National Confidential Enquiry into Perioperative Deaths. London

Davis D A, Thomson M A, Oxman A D, Haynes R B 1995 Changing physician performance: a systematic review of the effect of continuing medical education strategies. Journal of the American Medical Association 274(9): 700–705

Department of Health 1989 Working for patients (Paper No. 6). HMSO, London

Department of Health 1997 The new NHS; modern, dependable (Cmnd 3807). Stationery Office London

Donabedian A 1966 Evaluating the quality of medical care. Millbank Memorial Federation of Quality 3(2): 166–203

Effective Health Care 1994 Implementing clinical practice guidelines. University of Leeds, Leeds, vol. 1: 8

Ellis B W, Sensky T 1991 A clinician's guide to setting up audit. British Medical Journal 302: 704–707

Ellis B W, Rivett R C, Dudley H A F 1990 Extending the use of clinical audit data. British Medical Journal 301: 159–162

Emberton M, Rivett R C, Ellis B W 1991 Comparative audit: a new method of delivering audit. Bulletin of the Annals of the Royal College of Surgeons 73: 117–120

Gallimore S C, Hoile R W, Ingram G S, Sherry K M 1997 The report of the national confidential enquiry into perioperative deaths, 1994–5. London

Gruer R, Gordon D S, Gunn A A, Ruckley C V 1986 Audit of surgical audit. Lancet i: 23–26

Hancock B D 1990 Audit of major colorectal and biliary surgery to reduce rates of wound infection. British Medical Journal 301: 911–912

Lomas J 1993 Diffusion dissemination, and implementation: who should do what? Annals of New York Academy of Sciences 703: 226–235

Mitchell M W, Fowkes F G R 1990 Audit reviewed: does feedback on performance change clinical behaviour? Journal of Royal College of Physicians 19: 251–254

Mugford M, Banfield P, O'Hanlon M 1991 Effects of feedback of information on clinical practice: a review. British Medical Journal 303: 398–402

National Audit Office 1995 Clinical audit in England. National Audit Office, London

National Centre for Clinical Audit 1996 NCCA clinical audit action pack: a practical approach. National Centre for Clinical Audit, London

NHS Confederation 1997 Clinical audit: the role of the board. NHS Confederation, Birmingham

NHS Executive 1993 EL (93) Improving clinical effectiveness. Department of Health, Leeds

NHS Executive 1996a Clinical audit in the NHS: a position statement. Department of Health, Leeds

NHS Executive 1996b Promoting clinical effectiveness: a framework for action in and through the NHS. Department of Health, Leeds

NHS Executive 1996c Clinical guidelines: using clinical guidelines to improve patient care within the NHS. Department of Health, Leeds

Royal College of Physicians 1989 Medical audit. A first report – what, why and how? Royal College of Physicians, London

Royal College of Surgeons 1991 Royal College of Surgeons Confidential Comparative Audit Service. Bulletin of the Annals of the Royal College of Surgeons 73: 96

Shaw C D 1989 Medical audit: a hospital handbook. King's Fund, London

Standing Committee on Postgraduate Medical Education 1989 Medical audit: the educational implications. SCOPME, London

Walshe K 1995 Evaluating clinical audit: past lessons, future directions. Royal Society of Medicine Press, London

Walshe K, Spurgeon P 1997 Clinical audit assessment framework. Handbook Series 24. HMSU, University of Birmingham, Birmingham

Further reading

National Centre for Clinical Audit 1996 NCCA criteria for clinical audit. NCCA, London

Royal College of Surgeons of England 1994 Guidelines for clinicians on medical records and notes. Royal College of Surgeons, London

Royal Society of Medicine 1990 Computers in medical audit: a guide for hospital consultants to personal computer based medical audit systems. Royal Society of Medicine Services, London

Trent Regional Health Authority 1993 Guidelines on confidentiality and medical audit. Sheffield

43

Economic aspects of surgery

R. W. Hoile

Objectives

- **Understand some basic principles behind economic considerations in surgical practice.**
- **Recognize the potential conflict between clinical freedom, medical ethics and the logic of health economics.**
- **Examine areas where surgeons, by good clinical practice, can influence the costs of surgery.**

INTRODUCTION

This is probably a subject which, up to now in your surgical career, you have not needed to think about or understand. Before you progress much further you will undoubtedly be exposed to economic considerations and the consequences of your actions, so it is worthwhile discussing some of the principles used when addressing this topic.

The National Health Service was developed on the principle of fairness and that health care was free to the patient at the point of delivery, but with the rising costs of health care, limited resources and the heightened expectations of our patients it is inevitable that a debate about costs will occur. Will the economic arguments take over and conflict with good patient care, or can good economic strategies mean better patient care? At all times the outcome for the patient must be central to this debate.

Key points

Clinical freedom allows you to choose the best treatment for a patient (based on clinical knowledge and understanding) but this choice should be tempered by an appreciation of the resources available. For example, triage in the accident and emergency department is based on the need to use resources efficiently.

WHERE DO SURGEONS GO WRONG?

Looked at from the standpoint of health-care economics (and accepting the conflict between caring for an individual and considering the wise use of resources for the good of all), we make mistakes. These include:

- Using resources inefficiently or inappropriately
- Using investigative or operative techniques which are outdated
- Not acting in the patient's interests but perhaps in the interest of academia or research
- High complication rates
- The poorly considered introduction of new techniques which demand expensive technological back-up or instrumentation for an unproved gain.

How can we address these issues?

THE MEASUREMENT OF COST-EFFECTIVENESS

The measurement of cost-effectiveness can be considered, in simple terms, as synonymous with economic evaluation. The cost of surgery is not just monetary but also personal and social. For the patient there is pain, suffering, time spent in hospital and the economic consequences of the disease, hospitalization and time off work. Whilst we should be striving to deliver a cost-effective health-care system, we should not lose sight of these personal costs. Measuring cost-effectiveness is an unfamiliar process to clinicians, but it is important in evaluating and practising modern surgery. Before the cost-effectiveness of any surgical management is understood, it is necessary to understand some of the principles, definitions and accounting practices which are applied to problems of health care and the way in which they may affect clinical decision-making. Health economists refer to *direct costs* (in that they are borne by the health care system, community and family in directly addressing the problem), *indirect costs* (mainly loss in productivity and time spent in dealing with the illness which is borne by the individual, family, society or employer) and *intangible costs* (such as pain, grief, anxiety, suffering and loss of leisure time). In the event of a death after surgery the cost of that life is often considered, in health economics language, as an intangible loss.

'Costs' of surgery

- **Direct (due to dealing with the disease)**
- **Indirect (loss of productivity due to the illness and operation)**
- **Intangible (pain, suffering, anxiety and grief)**

WHAT DOES
COST-EFFECTIVENESS MEAN?

There are four ways of interpreting cost-effectiveness in clinical practice:

- Cost savings
- Effectiveness in improving health care
- Cost savings with an equal (or better) health outcome
- Having an additional benefit worth the additional cost.

The first of these, cost savings, can also be considered as avoided costs. This involves estimating the costs caused by the disease process which are avoided by surgical intervention. These avoided costs are sometimes known as benefits. An example might be the benefits (or avoided costs) of appropriate treatment for venous insufficiency in the leg, thus avoiding burdensome and costly (in all senses of the word) venous ulceration in the patient's later life. However, it is the last two of these four interpretations of cost-effectiveness which are used most in evaluating surgical practice. It should be noted that the third option requires no compromise by accountants, financial directors or clinicians, i.e. it is a 'win–win' situation. Both of the last two categories in the list require judgment to decide whether additional cost is worth the anticipated benefit and to select the

course of action with the least cost at the most probable benefit.

MEASURING COSTS AND BENEFITS

Cost–benefit and cost-effective analyses measure and compare the significant gains and losses associated with different methods of patient management. One could try to equate the value, in financial terms, of a year of healthy life. One such method is the calculation of quality-adjusted-life-years (QALYs, pronounced 'Qualys'). The benefits used in any calculation might include:

- Cure
- Increase in life expectancy
- Increased quality of life.

Some of the costs to be considered might include:

- Medical and surgical risks
- Operative or hospital mortality
- Disability
- Anxiety, pain and suffering
- Financial cost.

Imagination and a critical attitude often result in an improvement in cost-effectiveness. The intensive care unit (ICU) is a good example of a high cost–benefit area where carefully thought through policy changes can result in proven cost savings without changes in the quality of care.

CLINICAL 'PROFIT'

This is what primarily interests the patient because it could be described as the gain to be expected from a clinical decision once the patient has paid the price of pain, disability and financial loss whilst under treatment. Similarly, a consultation or clinic visit should be of benefit to the patient and/or clinicians. Consultations are often expensive, worthless and overused (e.g. follow-up appointments after routine surgical procedures).

CLINICAL RELEVANCE

Clinical decisions and the tests that support those decisions will be relevant in terms of cost-effectiveness depending upon their potential for clinical benefit. For instance, a test which, with great accuracy, confirms a diagnosis of extensive pancreatic cancer is less relevant than a test which would confirm gallstones with the same accuracy. One test has a small potential for prolonged benefit. The other will probably result in cure.

Benefit to patients should be proven for high-cost supportive treatments and services (e.g. nutritional support is of proven benefit). Minimal evidence of benefit requires a re-evaluation of the therapy in question.

HOW CAN SURGEONS INFLUENCE HOSPITAL COSTS?

The introduction of day surgery as a low-cost/high-throughput service reduces the cost of procedures without increased morbidity. Similarly, short stay, 5-day wards and low-dependency units (or hotels) also reduce costs without detriment (or even with advantage) to the patient. Preadmission clinics, which may avoid last-minute cancellations, are also proven to be cost-effective.

Laboratory tests

'Routine' investigations for all admissions are an example of uncritical and inefficient use of laboratory tests. Costs of laboratory tests constitute a significant part of the cost of health care. The effectiveness of a test is a measure of how the test findings influence the subsequent diagnostic or surgical strategy. Many tests are expensive and overlap others and, while being prestigious and impressive, may constitute poor medical practice. The best surgeon orders the fewest tests – in an appropriate order – that will provide the speediest diagnosis. Try to become familiar with the sensitivity, specificity and broad costs of the tests which are commonly used in your practice.

New technologies

Advances always emerge with benefits and limitations. Following evaluation, appropriate use of these new techniques will allow replacement of some costly procedures; for example, fine needle aspiration biopsies of the breast and aspiration of abscesses may, under some circumstances, replace open procedures. Some new techniques, although being considered as high-cost/high-yield procedures, are adopted because they revolutionize the management of certain conditions; for example, if successful, ileoanal anastomosis after colectomy for ulcerative colitis and angioplasty for peripheral or coronary arterial disease can have immense gains in terms of quality of life for the patient. The danger is in accepting new glamorous ideas without adequate evaluation. For instance, laparoscopic cholecystectomy is associated with a significantly reduced length of hospital stay, shorter recovery and a significantly shorter

back-to-work time than the open counterpart. The hospital costs are also lower but on the other side of the balance sheet there may be the costs produced by a higher incidence of bile duct injury and the sequelae. Similarly, when laparoscopic hernia repair is investigated from the economic point of view the costs are, at best, comparable to the open approach and, in some hospitals, higher. Audit, however, suggests that endoscopic hernia repair is preferred by patients and this knowledge highlights the clash between economic logic and clinical knowledge. You could probably make considerable cost reductions and feel more at ease with resource implications if you and your clinical colleagues could agree 'best practices' for selected procedures, develop local protocols and adhere to them. For example you might agree to perform laparoscopic procedures but define circumstances when it would be acceptable to use the more expensive disposable pieces of equipment.

Complications

Postoperative complications are expensive and can spoil any attempt to improve the cost effectiveness of surgery. The impact can be minimized by the use of clinical audit, specialization, abandoning outdated unproved procedures, using appropriate prophylactic regimens (e.g. antibiotics and thromboembolic prophylaxis), cautiously adopting new proven techniques and recognizing individual performance limitations. A single postoperative complication can completely wipe out the advantages and savings of careful, well thought out preoperative diagnosis and operative surgery. The main burden of a complication falls, of course, on the patient, but inevitably the knock-on effect will have consequences for your departmental budget. A wound infection, reoperation for infection, bleeding or anastomotic breakdown, pulmonary embolus and cardiac or renal failure are but a few of the complications which we could all list and which happen within our practice and have implications for labour and resources. If you think of the prolonged hospitalization and expensive investigations involved and translate these into monetary terms, it will demonstrate to you how the overall costs of surgery within your department will rise in the presence of complications; this could eventually double or triple the costs of uncomplicated surgery. Obviously, a certain level of complications should be built in when costs are calculated, but this will usually assume fairly minimal rates of incidence of complications. We all have complications sooner or later and they are all detrimental to the patient, the hospital and the budget! Your objective should be to minimize the incidence of such complications and, when they occur, to limit their duration, extent and cost (in all senses of the word).

Even as a trainee surgeon you should appreciate the economic consequences of your own behaviour; careful clinical decision-making and operative technique will help you to reduce your own personal complication rates. This will be for the good of the patient (which is, after all, your first concern), your reputation and also for the good of the department within which you work, as it will reduce the expense of surgery. This expense is something which not only you should be concerned about; it will also be of concern to your managers and those who must eventually foot the bill for health care (i.e. the public at large).

The detection of metastases

The detection of metastases in malignant disease must be analysed carefully and the value of commonly performed clinical procedures questioned. Is there a proven benefit? Similarly, playing 'hunt the primary' may be of no value to the patient in terms of palliation or survival, while having a considerable cost implication for the health care organization (i.e. your hospital).

Diagnosis

Staging for ovarian malignancy involves inherently high costs but has great clinical value when properly performed. It is inappropriate if done routinely or when the attempt at staging is poorly designed. In situations with a high cost and low yield, especially if there may be disabling side-effects, then ethical considerations may also come into play. Consider projectile vomiting in infancy. A clinical finding of hypertrophic pyloric stenosis would be a low-cost/high-yield diagnosis, whereas duodenal atresia might be a high-cost/low-yield condition.

Screening

There is much discussion about screening. Does the expense of setting up population screening (e.g. for breast cancer, colonic cancer and aortic aneurysms) produce better survival figures and quality of life for the patients? Can the health services cope with the increased elective workload? Is the subsequent treatment cheaper? Certainly for abdominal aortic aneurysm the outcome is better for elective surgery and the treatment is cheaper. Many of these issues are for society to decide; discrimination with regard to sex and age and the influence of pressure groups all play their part in decisions about the provision of health care.

Operations

Some procedures are of low benefit with a slight chance of cure (e.g. surgery for oesophageal carcinoma). However, the palliative benefits may be high; this is an area where careful clinical judgement is required. The open surgery of adult inguinal hernia is an example of a relatively well accepted low-cost/high-yield treatment with an accumulative economic importance in view of the disease frequency. Laparoscopic surgery may not have the same benefits. Similarly, total hip replacement is a high-cost/high-yield procedure. In emergency surgery (e.g. appendicitis) costs can be minimized by attempting to avoid negative laparotomies and complications.

 Using resources wisely

- **Recognize that the benefit and outcome for the patient are the most important factors**
- **Choose relevant investigations**
- **Take precautions to minimize complications**
- **Only adopt new techniques after proper evaluation**

CONCLUSIONS

Thinking about the economics of health care raises questions which are sometimes uncomfortable. Questions about waste, the inappropriateness of investigations and operations, rationing, cost-containment, ethics, etc. The response to these questions needs to be well thought out and workable. It is possible to set professional standards and deliver appropriate care whilst eliminating the unwarranted use of medical resources. It is easy to 'do something', particularly when faced with an individual patient, but perhaps we should stand back, take a broader view and consider whether an action for the individual patient is appropriate and/or cost-effective. A multitude of tests and procedures does not necessarily produce an accurate or speedy diagnosis, a lower morbidity or mortality, or 'better' health care. Professional guidelines and clinical audit may sometimes help us when it is necessary to say 'no'.

We have not found all the answers yet but you must begin to address these difficult questions.

Summary

1. You should recognize that the costs of surgery (and health care in general) are rising but resources are limited.
2. Health economics provides a logical framework on which to base decisions about the allocation of resources.
3. You can reduce costs without compromising clinical freedom and patient care by investigating wisely, keeping complications low and evaluating new techniques carefully.
4. You may perceive a conflict between your medical ethics and the economic logic applied by your hospital accountants and trust financial director. However, having read this chapter, you will appreciate that the aim of both disciplines is to promote health and alleviate suffering. The surgical economic argument is just one more tool for you to use when making decisions about the care of your patients.

Further reading

Eiseman B, Stahlgren L 1987 Cost-effective surgical management. Saunders, Philadelphia

Gray A J, Hoile R W, Ingram G S, Sherry K M 1998 The report of the national confidential enquiry into perioperative deaths 1996/97. NCEPOD, London

Hicks N R 1994 Some observations on attempts to measure appropriateness of care. British Medical Journal 309: 730–733

Hodgson K, Hoile R W 1996 Managing health service contracts. W B Saunders, London

Jefferson T, Demicheli V, Mugford M 1996 Elementary economic evaluation in health care. BMJ Publishing Group, London

O'Brien B 1986 'What are my chances doctor?' A review of clinical risks. Health Economics Research Group, Brunel University

44

Science, logic and the surgeon

M. Hobsley

Objectives

- **Appreciate the value of scientific logic and statistics in surgery.**
- **Become familiar with the terms used in scientific assessment of surgical phenomena.**
- **Recognize that in biological matters there is no certainty, only probability.**
- **Become equipped to assess submitted evidence logically.**

DEFINITIONS

Science can be defined for our purposes as intelligent forecasting – the clinician has to decide what to do in order to heal the patient. *Scientific logic* allows the clinician to forecast the likely outcome of treatment in the given situation.

CAUSE AND EFFECT

Physically, some phenomena are always *associated*, that is they are observed to be present at the same time. However, it is not always possible to determine whether one is causing the other – and which one is the cause and which is the effect, whether a third, as yet unrecognized factor is responsible, whether the relationship is indirect via a third factor (Fig. 44.1), or whether they are merely coincidental. If B can be seen definitely to follow A (i.e. B is only seen after A has been seen), then the natural presumption is that A is the cause, B the effect. How long is the time-interval between A and B that can be permitted without destroying the idea of a causal relationship? Birth is inevitably followed by death, but only after a lifetime: can we accept that birth is the *cause* of death? There is no satisfactory answer to this question.

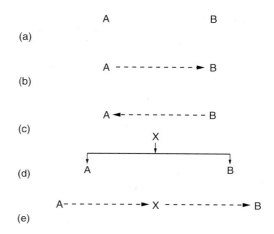

Fig 44.1 **(a)** Whenever we observe A, we also observe B. This defines a *relationship* or *correlation*. **(b)** Whenever we observe A, we know that we are about to observe B. This defines a *causal* relationship but leaves undefined the acceptable duration of 'some' time. **(c)** If we observe a *correlation*, as in (a), we are not entitled to assume that A causes B, just because that fits in with our ideas. It may be that B causes A. **(d)** Apparent, or 'spurious' correlation between A and B might result from their sharing a common cause, X. **(e)** Apparent correlation can also be due to indirect relationship, as in the case illustrated here. A causes X and does not itself cause B. However, X does cause B.

Impurities

A difficulty with cause and effect relationships is that it is usually impossible to isolate two phenomena from the many other possible factors that could exert an influence. The ideal is a controlled experiment in which all confusing factors are excluded if possible, but if they cannot all be excluded then they are as far as possible identical in both trial and control groups (Fig. 44.2).

Occasionally it is possible to dispense with the control group because the results produced by chance

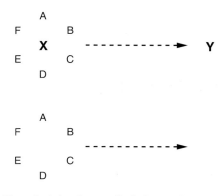

Fig 44.2   The principle of controlled observations. **X** may be the cause of **Y**, but so may A, B, C, D, E or F. If **X** is removed and **Y** disappears, then this evidence strongly suggests that **X** is causing **Y**. Remember, however, that this is not *proof* of the causative relationship: there is no such thing as proof.

alone are so obvious (see section The nature of chance below).

QUANTIFICATION

Relationships between phenomena take various forms including *occurrence, proportional occurrence, differences in magnitude, mathematical correspondences in magnitude, factors demonstrably affecting the chance of observing the event*, and *ranking*.

Occurrences

If a relationship is recognized between the occurrences of two phenomena, how many times must the experiment be repeated in order to establish that they are related? The great scientific philosopher Karl Popper pointed out that this can never be *proved*; at best it can be considered highly probable. He used the example of the fact that our swans are usually white. Even if every inspected swan is white, it can never be stated, 'All swans are white'. It takes but a single black swan to refute the assumption.

The mathematical method of demonstrating the probability, as opposed to the certainty, of a relationship is by means of *statistics* (Greek: *status* = state – tabulated facts, originally relating to a state, condition or set of circumstances). Properly used, statistics allow the likelihood of a relationship between phenomena to result from chance, as opposed to a causal relationship, to be defined in numerical terms. The figure usually quoted is the *probability* that the observed relationship

occurred by chance, expressed as a fraction or percentage. P or p = 0.1 or 10% means that we might on average expect the observed result in one of every ten runs of the experiment.

Discussion of the other possible types of relationship is deferred until later.

THE NATURE OF CHANCE

If a coin is tossed, it has a 50 out of 100, or 50% chance of landing 'heads' or 'tails' up. However many times it has landed heads up, the chance of the next toss landing heads up remains 50 : 50, since the previous throw has no effect on the next one. The result is, therefore, completely random, i.e. uncontrolled, the result only of chance (Latan: *cadere* = to fall, as, for example, how a coin or a die falls). It is unlikely that all the factors that determine the fall of the coin could be so controlled that the result could be predicted for every toss.

PROBABILITY AND CONFIDENCE

If a coin is tossed and falls down heads, the chance of falling heads again is 1 in 2 (1/2) and the chance of coming down heads a third time is again 1/2 and so on. To find the likelihood of heads resulting on each of five consecutive throws is $1/2 \times 1/2 \times 1/2 \times 1/2 \times 1/2 = 1/32$ – once in 32 trials, approximately 3 times in 100, or 3%. If 5 consecutively tossed coins all land heads, we know that there is only a 3% chance (p = 0.03) of this having happened by coincidence.

In everyday life, we need to know about a possible future event not precisely the chance that it will occur, but whether it would be reasonable to arrange our lives on the assumption that it will or will not occur. If I reasonably rely on catching a train by leaving 1 hour to get to the station, I believe that there is no *significant* chance of missing the train. Also, when we consider a measurement (such as the length of time that the journey to the station would take), we need a yardstick of the variability of the measurement so that we can express a range about the average that we are reasonably likely to meet on any one occasion. This yardstick is often termed a *confidence interval*.

By convention, in medicine a phenomenon is considered unlikely to have arisen by chance if its probability of occurring is less than 5%, although a stricter threshold of 1% is adopted in some circumstances. In statistical jargon, five tossed coins coming down heads is *significant* at the 5% level (sometimes stated as the 95% level of confidence). This is, to reiterate an argument previously given, because $1/2 \times 1/2 \times 1/2 \times 1/2 \times$

1/2 is 1/32 or only slightly greater than 3%, i.e., smaller than the benchmark of 5%.

DISTRIBUTION

One can work out the chance, not only that all four coins come down heads, but also the chances of all the other possible results. Figure 44.3 shows the calculations for eight throws. This array of the frequency of all possible results is termed a *distribution*. When the number of coins tossed, n, is very large, a smooth distribution curve results. It is possible to calculate that only 5% of the results will lie more than twice √n away from the mean value. Thus if 200 coins are tossed, the number coming down heads is unlikely to be below the aver-

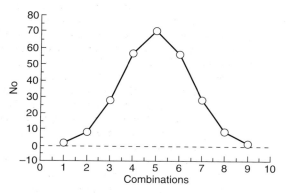

Fig 44.3   A distribution. Along the (horizontal) x-axis, the numbers 1–9 (ignore 0 and 10 which have been put in only to make the graph easier to read) express 1 + the numbers of coins that have fallen in the heads position when eight coins have been tossed. Thus the point 1 specifies that no coin had landed heads, all eight having landed tails; the point 7 that six had landed heads and two tails. The (vertical) y-axis is proportional to the chance of any particular combination of heads and tails being met in any simultaneous tossing of the eight coins. For example, 5 heads and 5 tails would be met on 70 occasions, no head on only one occasion. It is important to understand that these are the *average relative proportions* in which the different combinations would be met, provided that a sufficiently large number of tossings had been performed. The actual numbers represented on the x-axis for the nine combinations are 1, 8, 28, 56, 70, 56, 28, 8, 1. These total 256. Of every 256 occasions that eight coins are tossed, one would expect to find 5 heads and 5 tails on about 70 occasions, but the exact number would probably differ a little from that theoretical value of 70/256 or 27%. The greater the number of times the experiment is performed, the more likely is any observed number of times a distribution is encountered to tally exactly with its theoretical value.

age of 100 (the mean value) – 2 × 10 = 80; or above the value 100 (average) + 2 × 10 = 120.

The figure √100 is known as the *standard deviation* as it is a measure of the *spread of observations around the commonest observation*. The commonest observation is called the *mode*. In a symmetrical distribution like this *binomial distribution*, the mode is also the *mean* (or *average*), and the *median*, the observation with the same numbers of observations higher and lower than itself.

OTHER TYPES OF CORRELATION

Proportional occurrences

Suppose we wish to know whether inguinal hernias are more common in England than in Scotland. The corresponding numbers might prove to be, say, 10 million in England, 2 million in Scotland. Should we conclude that inguinal hernias are commoner in England than in Scotland? Surely not: there are about 40 million people in England and only about 5 million in Scotland. The *proportion* of English hernias is 1 in 4 or 25%, but in Scotland it is 2 in 5 or 40%. If these figures were accurate rather than fictional, we should conclude that inguinal hernias are commoner in Scotland.

There are several tests for determining the significance of differences in proportions: the most commonly used is called the χ (pronounced Kai)-*squared test*.

Until now we have dealt with whether some phenomenon occurred or did not occur – an all-or-none matter. Often we need to consider measurements, usually referred to as *continuous variables*. Examples are height and weight They are *continuous* in the sense that between 72 inches and 73 inches one can always measure a subject to be 72.5 inches, 72.1 inches, 72.01 inches, and so on.

Differences in magnitude

To determine whether the difference in magnitude between two groups of variables is significant, one needs to know not only the averages of the groups but also the extent of dispersion of the measurements in each group. The so-called *normal distribution* is important because it represents the variability of *measurements*, such as the height of the population, when there are at least 60 observations. Figure 44.4 is a diagram of the normal distribution. The percentage of observations lying between any two points on the x-axis have been calculated. The lines representing two standard deviations on either side of the mean enclose between them 95% of the observations and are called the *tolerance limits* of the population. Any measurement lying

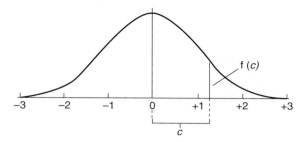

Fig 44.4 The normal (also called Gaussian) distribution. (after Diemk K, Lentner C (eds) 1973 *Geigy Scientific Tables*, 7th edn., p. 162 © Novartis AG, Basel, Switzerland, with permission. Macclesfield).
The x-(horizontal) axis displays the magnitude of a variable, expressed in terms of its standard deviation c as unit. Thus the point 0 represents the mean value of the variable, and the point + 1c represents a value which is one standard deviation greater than the mean. The y-(vertical) axis represents the proportion of occasions on which, if the measurement is made on many occasions, a particular value of the measurement will be seen. The vertical line labelled f(c) is thus the proportion of times one expects to find the measurement has the value of one standard deviation greater than the mean. The commonest observation, in a symmetrical distribution like this, is the mean itself, and the curve representing f(c) (these symbols imply 'function of c', meaning that the curve is related to the value of the point along the x-axis) diminishes from that maximum to tail away to being immeasurably small at about 3 standard deviations away (both + and –) from the mean. The zone between – and + twice the standard deviation contains about 95% of the observations, i.e. any individual observation of the mean is likely to lie, with 95% confidence, between the values of true mean ± two standard deviations. Tables exist that allow the proportion of expected observations to be calculated that lie between *any* two points along the x-axis.

outside those limits is unlikely to come from a normal member of the population. The mean estimated from a number, n, of observations, itself has a *standard error*, the standard deviation divided by √n. A deviation from the mean of twice the standard error of the mean defines the upper and lower *confidence limits* of the estimate of the mean.

If the number of observations is smaller than 60, the distribution known as *Student's 't'* can be used. The distribution has a thinner peak and longer lateral tails. It is more difficult to conclude that an observation is outside tolerance limits, or a mean outside confidence limits.

Differences between means (e.g. is the average height of one group significantly different from the average height of another) are tested to see whether they are *significantly* different by formulae specific for the distribution being used.

Mathematical comparisons between magnitudes

Instead of comparing the means of two groups, *regression* measures whether there is a quantitative relationship between one set of measurements and another. For example, is height related to weight?

In Figure 44.5 the data are set out as points on a graph. The x-axis measures height in inches, the y-axis indicates weight in kilograms. Weight tends to be greater in taller individuals.

This relationship is usually expressed as *weight increases with height*, and is called a *positive correlation*. Had weight increased while height decreased, the relationship would have been called a *negative correlation*. A number represented usually as *r* and called the *correlation coefficient* expresses the extent of the correlation. If the relationship were 100% so that all points lay on a single line such as AA', then *r* = 1. Had the correlation been negative, the perfect relationship would give *r* = –1. If there were no relationship, so that the data points were scattered randomly over the diagram, *r* = 0. The greater the value of *r*, whether positive or negative, the less likely is the relationship to have arisen by chance. Assessing the significance of any given value of *r* requires that the number of pairs of observations needs to be taken into account: the fewer the observations, the greater the value of *r* needed to attain significance.

A line, AA', the *regression line*, can be drawn to represent the average behaviour of the relationship (Fig. 44.6). The dotted lines BB' and CC' have been drawn by calculation to include (with 95% confidence) 95% of the total population of sample measurements of weight with height. The significance of these *95% tolerance limits* is that if a particular individual lies above BB' it is 95% likely that he is abnormally heavy, and a similar deduction about lightness can be made if the individual lies below CC'.

The regression line can be represented by an algebraic equation of the form $y = mx + c$ where *y* represents weight, *x* height, and *c* is a constant, the value of *y* if the straight regression line is prolonged back to the y-axis, i.e., to the imaginary point where *x* = 0, and the individual has no height. The value *m* is the slope of the line, in other words the amount by which weight increases for each inch of height.

This description refers to correlations analysed as straight line relationships between two variables. There are techniques available to analyse one variable as dependent on several others (y against x_1, x_2, x_3 ..., *multiple linear regression*) or dependent on some relationship

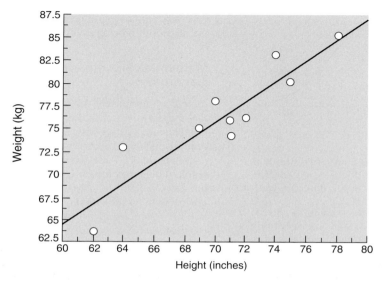

$$Y = -1.721 + 1.107 \times X; R^\wedge 2 = .833$$

Fig 44.5 This graph shows a correlation between two variables: height along the x-axis and weight along the y-axis. One thinks of height as not being under the control of the individual. Thus, since on average a tall person is likely to be heavier than a short one, it seems reasonable to call height an independent variable, weight a dependent one, even though weight, at least to some extent, is also under the individual's control, depending on how much or little that individual eats. It is conventional to plot the independent variable on the x-axis, the dependent on the y. The plotted points, which represent ten hypothetical people, show a tendency for weight to increase with increasing height, a positive correlation. The straight line has been drawn to provide a 'best-fit' approximation to the average relationship between height and weight. The spread of points around this so-called regression line indicates how well (or poorly) the observed individuals conform to the average behaviour of the group. The statistic that describes the degree of dispersion is the correlation coefficient, r or R. Its meaning can be thought of in terms of its square, R^2 – in this case 0.833 as indicated after the equation below the graph. This means that one can approximately assign 83% of the variations in weight of these individuals to the effect of height: the 17% remaining is due to other factors such as food intake and exercise. However, these are statistical hypotheses that require further direct confirmation, e.g. by changing the food intake of a number of people and showing that there is no change in height despite a change in weight.

other than a straight line (*non-linear regression*), but the principles involved are no different.

FACTORS AFFECTING
THE CHANCE OF AN EVENT

Regression of the type considered above relates the magnitude of a variable to the magnitude or magnitudes of one or more other variables. The method can, however, be adapted to all-or-none variables. One can think of this type of analysis, called *logistic regression*, as similar to an ordinary linear regression except that the dependent variable y either happens or does not happen and that the y-axis represents the chance that it happens instead of its size. The independent variables can be quantitative or all-or-none, or any mixture of the two types.

To illustrate this concept, aetiological factors in duodenal ulcer disease are thought to include cigarette smoking, gastric acid production, blood groups, gastric metaplasia in the duodenum and *Helicobacter pylori* infection. Cigarette smoking and gastric acid production can be quantified, but not the other factors. This statistical technique enables a logistic regression equation to be developed relating the chance of a man having a duodenal ulcer to whether he has one or other blood group, whether his duodenum shows evidence of gastric metaplasia, whether the stomach is infected with *H. pylori*, and also how many cigarettes he smokes and how much acid his stomach secretes.

Non-parametric statistics

This term is confusing because it suggests that it does not depend on measurements. A better term is *distribution-free statistics*.

Many distribution-independent methods are available. They all depend on knowing the chance of an

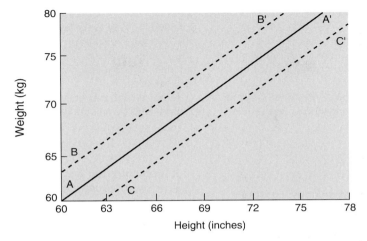

Fig 44.6 This is another diagram based on the relationship of the dependent variable, weight, to the independent variable, height. No individual observation is shown, but AA' represents the regression line, i.e. the line which describes the average relationship between the two variables. BB' and CC' are lines that represent the 95% tolerance interval of the regression line. In other words, the two outer lines represent the limits of the readings obtained from individuals whom we can accept as members of the 'normal' population from which the lines were derived.

event occurring or not occurring (50% in the standard sign test, but if the odds are not 1:1 but some other ratio the appropriate calculations can still be made). The various ranking tests are good examples. If two groups, A and B, are measured and the observations are ranked by size in a single set, the total of the rank numbers (1 for the smallest, 10 for the highest of ten observations) in group A should total much the same as the total of the rank numbers in group B if the two groups do not differ significantly, but should differ significantly if the two groups are different.

For example, suppose that the heights of ten individuals are measured in inches and the results ranked in ascending order.

Group A:	60, 62, 63,		66, 70				
Group B:		65,		71, 72, 74, 76			
Rank:	*1 2 3*	*4*	*5 6*	*7 8 9 10*			

Group A includes ranks 1, 2, 3, 5 and 6, totalling 17. Group B includes ranks 4, 7, 8, 9, 10, totalling 38. Tables are available to calculate the significance of the difference between 17 and 38, given that this difference between the ranks was obtained in ten cases. You may feel that this result seems most unlikely to have arisen by chance and the tables indeed confirm this (p 0.05), but only just!

CLINICAL APPLICATIONS

Every time a clinician interacts with a patient, the aim is always to save life, limit and repair damage, and relieve symptoms, in that order of priority. The doctor intervenes in some way (including sometimes a decision *not* to intervene) which it is hoped will produce the desired effect reliably and speedily. This is an experiment, because even when the clinical picture is very familiar and the treatment to be applied is simple, no one can forecast exactly what will happen in an individual case.

On what rules or guidelines does the doctor base his treatment? The *empirical* approach depends on experience that a particular remedy works although the reason is unknown.

A second approach is nowadays dignified by the term *heuristic*, although some would call it playing a hunch. The doctor does not know precisely the cause of the clinical situation yet he somehow (and rapidly and reliably) makes the right choice of effective treatment. My opinion is that the doctor who acts heuristically has analysed a familiar, or at least well-remembered clinical situation so rapidly that the steps of reasoning were performed subconsciously.

The third approach is irrational – that is, there is no logical reason for that particular treatment in those particular clinical circumstances but there is a theory based on the phases of the moon or the conjunctions of the planets or the magical properties of a herb. One hopes there is not much of such irrationality left in medicine today.

The fourth approach is the *scientific*: the doctor attempts rationally to forecast what will happen in a given situation, i.e. the clinical picture modified by the treatment he is about to give.

Most doctors believe they use the scientific approach, with a bit of the empirical, but evidence gained in truly scientific investigations at present covers less than 10% of everyday problems. To keep abreast of the literature is an enormous task. Being familiar with the results of those studies in ones own field is not enough: it is necessary to recognize the good studies and reject the bad.

What advice can one give for the 90% of our work not covered by reliable information?

Summary

1. Beware the argument of analogy. Especially beware the advice that starts: 'It stands to reason ...'. Arguments from similar, but not identical situations often break down because reasoning is only reliable when *all* the relevant facts are known.
2. Be prepared to respond to a changing situation, and give yourself time to do so. In correcting body fluid disturbances, aim at achieving half the correction rapidly, and then reassess – you may not need to give any more, or it may become obvious that you have underestimated the problem.
3. Keep your pathways of logic working smoothly. Having previously avoided defining cause and effect, the following definition is now offered.

   A cause and effect relationship between two phenomena exists when the effect is always associated with the cause and never occurs in the absence of the cause

   It is obvious that this rigorous definition is of little use because *always* and *never* are impossible to prove. The clinician needs to know whether a difference is *significant*, what size of difference is *meaningful*. For example, an antipyretic that significantly lowered a patient's temperature by 0.1°C would not be useful in the everyday commonsense world.
4. Commonsense is uncommon. The best ways to develop clinical commonsense are to be meticulous and accurate in history-taking and physical examination, to record in the patient's notes at all decision-making points exactly what decisions were made, to include in that record when the next decision-making point is to be reached, and – above all – to review all errors as soon as possible after the event. No one can exclude errors from clinical practice, but everyone should be determined to learn from mistakes.

Further reading

Campbell M J, Machin D 1995 Medical statistics. A commonsense approach, 2nd edn. John Wiley, Chichester

Diem K, Letner C (eds) 1973 Scientific tables, 7th edn. Geigy Pharmaceuticals, Macclesfield

Dunn G 1995 Clinical biostatistics; an introduction to evidence-based medicine. Graham Dunn and Brian Everitt

Gardner M J, Altman D G (eds) 1993 Statistics with confidence – confidence intervals and statistical guidelines. British Medical Journal, London

Hill A B, Hill I D 1991 Principles of medical statistics 12th edn. The Lancet Ltd, London

Siegel S, Castellan J Jnr 1988 Nonparametric statistics for the behavioral sciences, 2nd edn. McGraw-Hill, New York

Swinscoe T D V 1990 Statistics at square one, 8th edn. British Medical Journal, London

45

Critical reading of the literature

R. M. Kirk

Objectives

- **Have self-confidence. Do not accept received opinions – make up your own mind.**
- **Recognize that surgery is not standing still – you must keep up to date.**

Even as late as the turn of the 20th century many surgeons could learn from their masters and thereafter add to their knowledge only as a result of experience.

The rate of change of surgical practice has gradually increased so that now it would be considered negligent for a surgeon to fail to keep up to date with the literature.

Textbooks are in part out of date before they are published, since the time from writing to being put on sale is often 2 years. Some annuals contain reviews of the literature contributed by experts in the field. They offer a digest of many papers, interpreted by a single, albeit authoritative, author.

In each subject there are a few 'core' journals which publish important papers that have been refereed by at least two experts. Competition to publish in these prestigious journals is severe so the editors are able to select only the best articles. As a rule the research or investigation that has led to the publication has been well authenticated. Many of us accept without question the findings and conclusions of the articles we read in these journals. This is sometimes a dangerous assumption.

Key points

Literature (Latin: from *litera* = a letter) is not confined to books and journals but also to other media (intervening means, agencies or channels for communication). If opportunity allows, exploit the many computer-generated sources of generalized information such as Medline and the World Wide Web and the facility of e-mail to contact primary sources of information directly.

LOGIC OF SCIENCE

Advances in science are made in many ways and by many different people. There are no identifiable characteristics of successful originators of discoveries. Very often advances result from attempts to solve a problem. Sometimes, in a blinding flash, an idea strikes out of the blue. Ideas bounced between people working in the same or different fields may be productive. Louis Pasteur stated, 'Dans les champs, le hasard ne favorise que les esprits préparés' (In the field of observation, chance favours only the prepared minds). This emphasized the fact that many of us have the opportunity to make discoveries but may fail to recognize them unless we are receptive. Those of us engaged in any form of medical practice meet unusual circumstances but only a few pick up those that give fresh insights.

Chance observations, juxtaposition of circumstances that suggest an association, and attempts to solve problems may throw up questions. These may stimulate provisional solutions or possible methods of achieving them. Such suppositions are termed 'hypotheses'. These require to be tested.

The great scientific philosopher, Karl Popper, pointed out that it is not possible to prove a statement but it is possible to disprove it. He used as an example a possible statement about the colour of swans. Most of the swans we see are white, and one might deduce that all swans are white. It is impossible to *prove* that all swans are white because it is impossible to be sure one has seen every swan. However, it is possible to disprove the hypothesis by merely seeing a single swan that is not white. And, of course, there are famous black swans on the Freemantle River in Western Australia.

Popper stated that an investigator who constructs a hypothesis should try to falsify it, not to prove it. If the hypothesis cannot be disproved, then it is reasonable to adopt it for use until a better hypothesis emerges or the present one proves to be fallacious.

Unfortunately, although we pay lip service to Popper's views, in practice they are rarely applied. Pick up any scientific journal and you will find the authors marshal their evidence to prove their hypothesis. It becomes the duty of readers to identify the defects in the evidence presented.

CONSTRUCTION OF SCIENTIFIC PAPERS

Scientific reports can be expressed in many ways. The famous, Nobel prize winning discovery by Crick and Watson that DNA exists as a double helix was reported in a short letter to *Nature*.

However, when an investigation has been carried out, it is conventional to construct the report in a standardized way for easy reference. The article is traditionally now published in a journal that will be read by others interested in the subject. We scan the contents list looking for articles of particular interest, read the summary of perhaps one or two, read excerpts of perhaps one, and from time to time avidly read every word of an article of particular interest.

Title: states as succinctly as possible what the paper is about. It is chosen so that key words can be included in the great American contribution to science, the *Index Medicus*. In this way, the work can be easily traced.

Summary: should, as briefly as possible, state what was done, what was found and the conclusion that was reached. In this way a reader scanning the journal, seeing the title, can quickly decide whether the work is sufficiently relevant to be worth reading further.

Introduction: states why the work was done. It gives the background facts that define the question that the authors wish to answer.

Methods: tells what was done, giving all the relevant information.

Results: states what was found.

Discussion: what does it mean. It places the results in the context of previous work.

Conclusion: is not essential if the summary is well expressed but in some cases there is need of an expansion or rearrangement of the end statement of the discussion, perhaps pointing the way to future work.

References: to published work give corroboration to statements made in the text that are not specifically investigated in the reported work.

CRITICAL READING

There is insufficient time to read every paper on any subject of interest and check the authenticity of the references. It is of great educational value to critically read an article on a topic of personal interest to you.

Introduction: may start with the wrong premise, or one with which you do not agree. Read at least some of the papers referred to by the authors in constructing their hypothesis.

Method: the design of experiments and investigations may be poorly described. It is important that the authors give full information so that you can judge whether it is logical and well conducted.

Results: do they provide full, reliable information on which you can base a judgement?

Discussion: do the authors read more into their results than is justified by the findings?

WHAT DO YOU LEARN?

1. Most importantly, you practice making up your own mind about the 'facts' that are presented to you on the basis of the evidence placed before you. You are not just a passive accepter of the opinions of others. This gives you the confidence to reject evidence you consider unreliable, and confidence in your own good sense rather than relying unthinkingly on 'experts'.

2. You may not know the fine points of statistics (see Ch. 44) but you can decide whether they have been properly applied. Too often, when reading statistical comparisons of like groups that we are told differ in one respect only, this is not so. Biological variation is so great that too much cannot be read into small differences. Sometimes you can identify these. Ignoring differences between compared populations is often said to be 'comparing apples with pears'. You may also detect imperfections in the way in which two populations have been compared. The clear demonstration of claimed 'prospective, double blind,' clinical trials is sometimes fudged. 'Follow-up' is used without making clear who carried it out and how it was performed. Sometimes the raw data are not given but are displayed in an indirect manner in derived data or graphs, so you cannot see individual results.

3. When comparing diagnostic methods or treatments, authors may make erroneous claims that one is better than another. For example, earlier diagnosis and treatment of a malignant tumour may appear to improve life expectancy when compared with diagnosis and treatment at a later stage. In fact the progress of the disease may be unchanged and the apparent life expectancy improvement following early treatment may

represent the 'lead time' that it would take for an early tumour to develop to the stage it has reached when detected later.

4. Because it is usual for authors to provide only the evidence in support of their hypothesis – and contradictory evidence they can demolish – we rely upon independent investigations to support or challenge the findings and conclusions. Therefore do not accept uncritically a single paper, especially if it runs counter to the accepted views.

5. If you read the literature you will discover that the results of investigations do not always agree. By selectively quoting the literature, support for the authors' views can be corroborated. Always look for other articles on the subject not quoted by the authors.

6. During your career you will see patients with unusual, perhaps unique, conditions. If you have kept up with your reading you may recognize those that should be investigated or reported to your colleagues. Your familiarity with the surgical literature will have prepared you for creating a logically argued and acceptable publication.

WHY NOT JUST READ REVIEWS?

There are two well-recognized methods of finding out the 'truth' that are used in the judicial systems of different countries. In the UK we have an adversarial system (Latin: *ad* = to + *vertere* = to turn [from]), in which two advocates offer opposing arguments and views and attempt to destroy the arguments of each other. In France, for example, the system is inquisitorial (Latin: *in* = in + *quaerere* = to seek) in which the prosecutor is also the judge; the magistrate 'enquires' into the facts and reaches a judgment. At its best, the second method is less theatrical than the adversarial system but does it uncover all the facts and counter-arguments?

When you read a review by an expert it is inevitable that he or she already has a view. In spite of the intention to be scrupulously fair we all select from proffered facts, consciously or unconsciously, which are valid, which can be demolished and which should be ignored.

If you wish to acquire a view on a subject, you should read as many original papers as possible, as critically as possible, so the opinion you reach will at least be yours and you can repeat the arguments that led you to your position.

Summary

1. We are fortunate to live in an era in which information is available to guide us in surgical practice. Use it.
2. Whatever the prestige of the journal or the distinction of the writer, your common sense is your best guide.
3. We are all supposed to submit our hypotheses to attempted falsification. How many authors do so? You will find the most testing arguments in the writings of those with opposing views. Read them.

 Further reading

Popper K R 1959 The logic of scientific discovery. Hutchinson, London (3rd edn 1972). *This is a translation of a book written in German in 1934. It is a very difficult book to read but there are many simplified accounts of his contributions*, e.g.
Magee B 1974 Popper. Fontana Modern Masters. Collins, London

46

Communication skills

R. M. Kirk, M. Lloyd

Objectives

- Good communication is essential in all areas of activity, not just in relation to patients.
- Recognize non-verbal as well as verbal communication.
- Empathasize with the listener, especially when giving bad news.

'Communication skills' sounds like yet another facility to be learned, like operating. However, most of us already have inbred and acquired competence since it pervades our contact with all other people.

VERBAL COMMUNICATION

The words we use, the tone of voice, the speed with which we speak, the pauses that we interject, all have an effect on the listener. If we are giving similar information to two different people, we usually do not attempt to employ the same words to each of them. Some people adopt the word patterns of those to whom they are speaking; others, wishing to impress, may use abstruse or jargon words or acronyms (words formed from the initial letters of other words).

The tone of voice and rhythm add a layer of meaning. Terse, staccato speech is sometimes commanding or threatening or signifies tension in the speaker. Quietly spoken words may be soothing or, if given in a sibilant (hissing) manner, may suggest potential threats.

Face to face communication is much richer than writing. Words have defined meanings and the writer is limited to choosing the ones nearest to the intended meaning plus a few symbols such as exclamation and question marks or underlining. The writer has to guess at the response to the message and cannot modify it if the receiver reacts unexpectedly. The words do not have to be cast on tablets of stone to be irrevocable in their effect. In contrast the tone of voice, the emphasis placed on certain words and the reaction to the listener's responses help to guide the speaker to know how to proceed and estimate the effect of the words.

Telephone conversations are mid-way, containing vocal overtones but lacking the non-verbal expression and gestures that add a layer of meaning to the words.

It is self-evident that if you wish to communicate with someone over an important or delicate matter, you should always choose to do so face to face.

NON-VERBAL COMMUNICATION

This is a very deeply ingrained way of informing others of our mood and intentions. Our dress may indicate that we are relaxed and informal, or we may wish it to register professionalism and formality. Posture indicates depression and humility or confidence and command. Most revealing are our facial expressions. The giving out of signals and the reading of them is often unconscious.

Most of us acquire a social awareness of non-verbal communication. When one person is speaking and the listener wishes to interject a remark, he or she signals the wish or intention, perhaps by a movement to attract the speaker's attention, a raising of the hand, a seeking of eye contact with the speaker. The speaker responds, sometimes by returning the eye contact, by smiling and bringing the statement to a close, or resists by raising a hand with palm towards the person wishing to speak or raising the voice, to indicate resistance to stopping. The giving and receiving of signals can be confused and confusing. A smile and a sneer are not dissimilar – indeed one may change into the other. A gentle touch is a subtle method of conveying sympathy, a firm grip can convey authority and trust, but a push or a blow are threatening.

Actors, salesmen and confidence tricksters have always recognized, sometimes instinctively, the fundamentals of what is often called 'body language'. In recent years, non-verbal communication has been studied and brought to notice by those claiming to advise salespeople, job applicants, interviewers and interviewees.

COMMUNICATING WITH PATIENTS

Remember that you are familiar with clinical surroundings but patients associate them with anxiety and sometimes dreaded import. They are apprehensive and often confused. Because most patients are in later adult life, and often, therefore, more conventional, they expect to see doctors dressed and behaving reasonably formally.

Note that colleagues may adopt a serious and grave manner, others try to appear cheerful and light-hearted. There is no standard pattern; sometimes we are serious with one patient and jovial with another. Avoid attitudes and speech that denote overbearing and curt superiority, or the overcasual 'jokeyness' that suggests we take the patient's problems light-heartedly. The tendency to informality in dress and speech, and the use of first names, is not welcomed by many older patients raised in an era of more formality. Similarly, casual exposure of their bodies and clinical features are resented. We owe it to them to respect their wishes if we are to obtain their cooperation and trust.

When you wish to discuss important information with a patient, ensure that the surroundings are quiet, that you will not be disturbed or distracted. Hand your 'bleep' to someone who can answer it for you. In appropriate circumstances suggest that a relative or friend of the patient is present.

Angry or threatening patient

- **Anticipate aggression – but do not behave like a 'victim'.**
- **Do not contradict or respond to aggressive behaviour.**
- **Stay calm, do not interrupt, be willing to listen.**
- **If all else fails, summon help from 'Security.'**

Questioning

When taking a medical history (see Ch. 3), allow the patients time to speak. Do not make them feel that what they have to say is of little account. If they are stuck for words allow them time to choose a suitable one; do not immediately feed one that fits your prejudice. However, we must control the interview, so that

our timing when we interject a question for clarification, or to ask a new question, must be sensitively judged.

Choose words suited to the patient before you. A simple person needs simple language spoken slowly, and repeated or rephrased without signs of impatience. For example, ask one person where is the pain in the belly if that was the term he or she employed to you. A professional person may resent the avoidance of the more formal 'abdomen'.

The ability to communicate is severely tested if the patient is a young child, deaf, has a speech defect, a behavioural anomaly, or has difficulty with the language. It can be impossible to communicate rationally with those under the influence of alcohol or other drugs, with people who are hysterical or violent, or with those suffering from diminished consciousness, whether it is the result of injury or disease.

Key points

If you have difficulty in communicating, consider whether you need help from a senior colleague, an interpreter, or should you defer action if the patient's cooperation is likely to return later?

Telling and discussing

First find out what is already known, what that information signifies and how should the additional information be presented. As a rule it is best to start by asking questions such as, 'Would you like to talk about the [problem]? I am not sure how much you know.' Later, you may ask questions in order to evaluate the patient's appreciation of the information they already have, including what you have told them.

In many circumstances do not try to say too much all at once. Give the patient time to absorb what has already been said; wait for him or her to indicate readiness to continue. From time to time ask questions to check that the patient really understands what has passed between you by asking, for example, 'Can you tell me then, how you see the situation?'

Especially when discussing important problems, be extremely sensitive to the listener's reactions and signals. In some cases it may be better to defer the interview to a later date to allow the patient to absorb and react to what has already been said.

Patients anticipating bad news frequently demonstrate by their body language, or by suddenly ceasing to ask questions, that they do not wish to be told anything more at present.

Advising

Discuss with patients what options are available, what are the advantages and disadvantages of each. This is not always easy to do, since not many treatment choices can be scientifically justified. In biology there are few areas that are either black or white; most are shades of grey. This explains the differing advice that patients receive when they ask for a second opinion.

Surgeons have a reputation for being decisive and in practice most of us are in no doubt about the advice we wish to give. Our advice is based on our professional experience – what we have encountered, read about and talked about. The patient needs to be encouraged to ask questions, and when there is no urgency, to go away, think about the advice, come back and discuss it again. However, I believe it is a rejection of professional responsibility to merely lay before our patients the pros and cons of each course of management and leave it to them to decide which one to follow. Patients are often not in a suitable state of mind to make the best decision, especially when the doctor has just told them they are suffering from a serious condition. Therefore, we should end with, 'So in my opinion . . .' Of course, they are free to reject the suggested course of action.

Relatives

These deserve the same consideration that we give to patients. We hope that they will give encouragement, support and help to the patient throughout the management of the condition requiring treatment.

Occasionally there is conflict between the demands of the patient and those of the relatives. What do you say if a patient demands that you do not disclose what is happening, while the relatives press you for information? Your contract is with the patient and you must honour that relationship. The relatives may ask you not to give certain information to the patient. Again, judge for yourself the best course, on the patient's behalf.

COLLEAGUES

A vital professional duty is to inform colleagues about matters of patient care. Always write up notes, avoiding abbreviations, jargon and opinionated remarks that might be misinterpreted. Sign and date them. When you hand over before you go off duty, inform the on-call doctor personally of any outstanding problems.

If you have had a discussion with a patient about the future, or about treatment, ensure that you tell the nurses and your seniors. There is nothing that under-

mines the confidence of patients more than being given different information from different people.

Included in this category are all those with whom you come into professional contact – doctors of all grades, students, nurses, physiotherapists, technicians, managers, clerical staff, porters, cleaners and tradesmen. Do not draw a line of 'importance', below which you do not acknowledge people, or bolster your dignity by trying to diminish others. Each of us counts as just one.

One of the most important qualities we have is our self-esteem. When we fail to carry out a task conscientiously we expect to be reprimanded. When we perform well, we rightly hope to be congratulated. If you expect to be acknowledged, remember there are others that hope you will acknowledge and encourage them.

IMPARTING BAD NEWS

Communicating with ill or distressed people requires great sensitivity. Your behaviour should be influenced by your feelings of sympathy and compassion. Our reactions may be modified if we are able to enter our patient's personality in our imagination and think how we would feel if we were in a similar situation; this is termed empathy (Greek *em* = in + *pathos* = feeling, suffering). Obviously we cannot always achieve this but in making the effort we can identify the likely reactions and apprehension of the patient and respond sensitively.

We have the duty to keep our patients and any close relatives informed of what is happening, and what it means. This often entails telling them that recovery is failing, the patient has developed a complication, or our investigations reveal severe and perhaps terminal disease. You may be the only doctor present and are therefore responsible for dealing with the problem.

Try to do so in a calm and private area. Ask someone to take over your 'bleep', so you cannot be interrupted. It is usually valuable to have a nurse with you so that she can tell her colleagues what has been said.

Do not necessarily state the information in an initial outburst but first determine how much knowledge the patient already has.

Some doctors avoid this difficult subject by ignoring it. In the past, many patients did not wish to know, and again, some still resist being told bad news. In recent years patients have become more knowledgeable, ask direct questions, and may demand to be told everything that is known about the situation and the consequences.

As often happens when there is change, there may be an over-swing. It is sometimes stated that the information belongs to the patient and the doctor has no right to withhold it. Do not dismiss the minority who do not wish to be told the whole truth, by forcing information on them immediately.

In human relations we must retain a sense of balance and sensitivity. Rigid blanket rules are inappropriate. Just as in our personal life we try to avoid pouring out sensitive bad news, so we need to be as considerate to our patients and allow them to dictate the way in which we inform them. To suddenly force 'the truth' on another human being is as cruel as a physical assault.

The founder of the hospice movement in Britain, Cecily Saunders, stated: 'The patient, not the doctor, or the nurse, or the relative, must retain control of information to suit his needs.' Our duty is to interpret the patient's often unspoken signals and be governed by them.

Look at the patient's expression as you approach. You are also being carefully studied in return, for hints of what you are about to say. If possible, start with some positive information or ask how the patient feels. Now the patient has the opportunity to channel the discussion.

In response to your first greeting, the patient may steadfastly not ask any questions. You must judge from your previous conversations whether to make any tentative statement or whether to defer it until later. Occasionally a very anxious patient blurts out the words, 'I want to know everything,' but their eyes are begging for reassurance that all is well. Do not immediately pour out the whole potentially devastating news; such a patient may become deeply and even hysterically depressed.

As far as possible allow the patient to ask the questions so that you can answer and explain their implications at a rate that the patient can cope with them. Be ready to defer answering questions that are not asked.

Provided you are sympathetic and sensitive, you are unlikely to make gross mistakes. Those who are told very serious news and later asked what was said, often give a different and more optimistic version, if they are unable to cope with the full truth. There are some patients who indicate that they fully understand the circumstances but do not wish to have them spelled out in concrete terms. Respect their wishes.

Never leave a patient without hope or support. If treatment such as operation cannot be employed it is possible to say, 'Operation is not appropriate but I shall continue to care for you.'

Remember that the news may be more distressing for the relatives and friends than for the patient, because they are not only sad for the patient but they are desolate at the prospect of being left alone. However, the information belongs to the patient, not the relatives. Ensure that you do not disclose anything to them against the patient's wishes.

Now write in the notes exactly what has passed between you and inform your colleagues including the family doctor and the nurses.

Summary

1. There are no rigid or absolute rules; be sensitive to the patient's signals.
2. Communication is more than mere words.
3. Give patients time to absorb your remarks, and time to respond in their own way.
4. As you prepare to give patients information, enquire how much they already know.
5. Recognize and honour the (often non-verbal) signs that patients do not wish to have more information forced on them at this time.
6. Keep your colleagues informed about the information passed between you and the patients.

 ### Further reading

Buckman R 1992 How to break bad news. Papermac, London

Lloyd M, Bor R 1996 Communication skills for medicine. Churchill Livingstone, Edinburgh

Myerscough P R 1992 Talking with patients. Oxford University Press, Oxford

47

The surgical logbook

D. Baker

Objectives

- **Understand the importance of maintaining a logbook.**
- **Understand how and what information to collect in your logbook.**
- **Know how to analyse the collected data.**
- **Recognize the difficulties in keeping a logbook.**

INTRODUCTION

A surgical logbook is a record of the activity you have undertaken. Although important during training it remains a central part of the routine throughout your career. Of the different parts of a surgeon's job, the most easy to record are:

- Operations performed
- Patients seen in clinic
- Patients admitted and seen while in hospital.

This chapter will concentrate on logging actual operations undertaken. Although this is the most commonly kept record, the other two records are important, as surgeons see and treat many more patients than they actually operate on. The outcome of patients who have surgical problems and are not operated on is as important as the outcome of those operated on.

WHY KEEP A LOGBOOK?

1. Like airline pilots it is every surgeon's duty to have the self-discipline to keep a record of the procedures they have performed. Although not yet a legal requirement, it is a requirement of the Surgical Colleges to keep a logbook during training. This is because it is necessary to demonstrate that there has

been adequate training in an operation or procedure before a surgeon can be considered fit to undertake it independently. Likewise it will soon be necessary to demonstrate that a surgeon, once a consultant, has continued to undertake this procedure adequately if they are to be allowed to continue to perform it.

2. The logbook provides a source of self-auditing surgical practice. For example, if there has been a series of wound infections when performing a particular procedure, it is the surgeon who needs to identify and rectify this.

3. For the trainee, a logbook identifies strengths and weaknesses in individual training. For example, if it can be demonstrated that significant numbers of one procedure have been undertaken successfully, but that there are deficiencies in another procedure, this gives quantitative data during the regular formal appraisal for further training in the latter rather than the former.

4. For the trainer, the logbook helps assess training standards within the specific posts of a surgical training rotation. For example, if an early trainee shows from his log that he has been undertaking major procedures at night on his own without supervision this should be investigated. Perhaps the trainee is very able, or perhaps the trainer requires further tuition on the training of surgeons!

HOW TO COLLECT THE INFORMATION

Information for the logbook is collected as a spreadsheet or grid of data divided into rows and columns. Each operative case occupies a row with all the information about the case occupying separate columns. There are several logbooks of different complexity. At its most simple the logbook can be a lined school exercise book with vertical lines drawn in, dividing the pages into rows and columns. The Royal Surgical Colleges have logbooks and there are several computer packages covering a wide range of prices that can be purchased that are suitable for both personal computers

(PC) and palm top computers. The computerized log-book offers the considerable advantage of being able to analyse the data quickly and present it in clear neat tables.

 Key point

It is not the logbook's complexity, type or cost that makes it a good logbook, but what information is collected and the accuracy and completeness of that collection.

WHAT INFORMATION TO COLLECT

The operative information collected varies with your expertise and interest. This will change and develop throughout your career. However, some core information is always necessary. This includes:

Patients details

The patients' name, age or date of birth, sex and hospital number need to be recorded. It is important to collect this information as without it your log can never be externally audited (see quality assurance below) and it would be impossible to trace a patient's notes or occasionally the patient themselves if, for example, you are subsequently following-up your results. Nevertheless, you must not infringe the patient's personal rights and let this information become publicly available, as the same ethical and legal restrictions on ensuring patient confidentiality apply here as elsewhere in surgery.

Demographic details

A column for the hospital and operation date and time are needed. Morbidity and mortality outcomes are affected by whether the case was planned or an emergency. Recording this can be difficult, as the definitions are not always clear, and cases which need to be done quickly may be done on an 'emergency' list or on the next routine list.

Staff involvement

The different role you and members of the team play in the operation can be recorded. This includes who performed the operation and your level of involvement. Who was the most senior person involved in the surgery? Some people record who was involved in the anaesthetic, but few surgeons record the scrub nurse details, although hospital records nearly always contain this information.

Operation details

Level of anaesthesia

The detail recorded depends on you, but whether the case was under general or local anaesthesia is a minimum.

The type of operation

Use at least three columns, each getting subsequently more specialized and specific. For example, if the training programme involves rotating though several different surgical specialities, the first column could indicate this by recording the speciality such as orthopaedics, neurosurgery, plastic surgery. The second column could identify sub-specialities; for example, within general surgery there are several sub-specialities including breast surgery, colorectal surgery, biliary surgery, vascular surgery, endocrine surgery. The third column could be the actual operation performed. There are specific codes (OPCS codes) for each operation; these have been developed by the Office for Population Censuses and Surveys and, if recorded, they ensure uniformity between cases and thus accurate subsequent analysis. Most consultant surgeons have copies of the OPCS codes.

Remember it is your logbook and you can collect whatever information you want. No procedure is too minor; for example, you may wish to keep a record of all the rigid sigmoidoscopies you perform or central lines you insert.

The outcome of surgery

It is important and necessary to record all complications that occur. A perioperative death is one that occurs within 30 days of surgery and needs to be recorded. Deaths early in the postoperative period are usually remembered and recorded, but deaths 3 weeks after surgery are not always related to the operations and the temptation not to record them must be resisted. With complications that can be related directly to the surgery, such as wound dehiscence, postoperative haemorrhaging, wound infections and anastomotic leaks there is also a strong temptation not to record them as there is a feeling of admitting to a weakness in your surgical ability. With more general complications, such as urinary tract infections and deep vein thrombosis, there is a temptation to consider these as not being related to the surgery. They are! Your logbook is your confidential record of events and it is up to you who you allow to see it.

 Key point

The only way to avoid complications is not to operate. Be honest with yourself and record all complications.

ANALYSING THE DATA

The logbook contains a vast wealth of information from which many facts about training and, subsequently, surgical practice can be drawn. Analysing what you have done can be an exceptionally informative and often enjoyable reflection on your progress. Before starting to analyse your data, clearly determine what information is needed. For example, while in training it is important to know the number of operations you have done, their size, the degree of urgency and the level of supervision received. Using the above layout, this information can be extracted either manually or with the aid of a personal computer.

PROBLEMS WITH KEEPING A LOGBOOK

Accuracy and completeness of data collection

Inaccurate and incompletely kept logbooks are a waste of time. In order to avoid this an enthusiasm to keep an accurate record of operative activities is vital. Several thing help ensure this:

1. Get into a routine. Discipline yourself to fill your logbook in every time, say when you leave theatre or every night just before going to bed. It is very easy to get behind and give up.
2. Collect the data soon after the event while it is still fresh in the mind. Collect the data little by little as operations are done. If you only do it once a month, cases may be missed and the data will not be accurate.
3. Collect the data from its original source, i.e. from what you know happened in theatre and not from the operating room logbook or the hospital computer record of admissions and discharges as this information will not be as accurate nor provide the exact details required.
4. Include all operations. As training progresses there is a tendency to exclude minor procedures such as sebaceous cyst excisions, which have been undertaken several times before. Avoid this temptation and continue to record all operations you do, however big or small. Failure to do so results in an inaccurate and incomplete logbook.
5. Record all complications. The psychological difficulty in admitting *all* your surgical complications in your logbook has already been discussed.
6. Analyse the data regularly. One reason why logbooks are not kept up to date centres around a failure to regularly analyse the contained data. All surgeons are keen to assess their progress to identify strengths as well as weaknesses. Regular analysis of the data is therefore important and gratifying. It shows the true worth of keeping the logbook and stimulates accuracy and completeness in data collection.
7. Quality assurance. Checking the accuracy and completeness of your data collection requires dedication but is well worthwhile. Every 3 months or so obtain a list of operations you have been involved in from another source such as the operating room logbook and check this against your record. Your record should be more accurate and complete than any other list. If not, data collection is inadequate.

Problems with data analysis

Analysis takes too long

If the logbook data is stored in a paper book, analysis is done manually by counting through each case. This will take time once there are several years of cases. If the log is stored on a computerized spreadsheet, analysis time is considerably shortened. However, a limited basic knowledge of computers and computer spreadsheet analysis is necessary first. This should never be considered a hurdle and all surgeons in training should be prepared to sacrifice the single afternoon required to obtain these skills.

Analysis appears incomplete

Assuming complete data collection, a lack of uniformity between cases in recording similar data may result in a failure to detect all cases. For example, if abdominal aortic aneurysm repairs are sometimes recorded as 'aneurysm', and at other times as 'AAA' and other times under the OPCS code L1940, computer analysis looking only for 'aneurysm' will miss cases coded with either 'AAA' or L1940.

The logbook is lost

Always keep at least one recently updated copy of your logbook separate from the original.

CONCLUSIONS

Keeping a record of your surgical activities is a central part of the discipline of being a surgeon. It requires dedication to ensure its accuracy and completeness, but if well done you have a valuable record of your activities as a surgeon.

Summary

1. Keeping a record of all surgical activity is an integral part of a surgeon's job, both while in training and later in professional life.
2. On every procedure, keep information relating to the patients details, the site and time of the operation, the procedure undertaken and by whom and, importantly, record all complications.
3. Ensure that the data is collected quickly, accurately and completely.
4. Analyse and review your progress regularly.

48

The MRCS examination

R. C. G. Russell

Objectives

- **Understand the philosophy of the MRCS.**
- **Understand the nature of the examination.**
- **Know how to pass the examination.**

INTRODUCTION

This examination is designed to assess the knowledge gained during basic surgical training; it is but part of a programmed learning course which is organized by the Royal College of Surgeons to assist basic surgical trainees cover the syllabus which is designed to contain appropriate knowledge for those of you beginning surgical training. The course covers essential surgical knowledge, including the basic science knowledge necessary to gain an understanding of surgical disease. Thus the examination is not divided according to traditional boundaries of anatomy, physiology and pathology separate from clinical surgery, but strives to integrate these subjects as a coherent whole. Although the viva is called 'applied surgical anatomy and operative surgery', the topics discussed may legitimately stray from these confines to illustrate a particular point. It is important that you understand a subject and you avoid rote learning with minimal understanding.

We prefer that you work continuously during your training and elect to take the examination in parts such as the MCQ at one year and the clinical and vivas at the end of the second year. The content of the examination does not vary so that the core knowledge you learn for the MCQ is tested again in the viva, with the opportunity to establish that you understand the subject which will have become part of your working day experience.

Ideally, examinations in surgery should objectively test whether you have all the aptitudes required of a surgeon; unfortunately, the qualities required of you as a surgeon have not been defined, and attempts to do so have not proven successful because the role of a surgeon is markedly varied and hence attractive. The unifying requirement of these roles is, however, that of knowledge. Without knowledge, appropriate decisions cannot be made and the technical skills of the surgeons are put to waste. Tests of cognition and factual knowledge can be assessed with fair objectivity. The reproducibility of these new tests is carefully monitored to ensure that the standard remains stable between examinations and care is taken to ensure you are exposed to most parts of the syllabus. How you use that knowledge to make accurate diagnoses and sensible decisions, and to plan effective management is more difficult to determine. Deductive ability is not learned except through experience, and is an important part of clinical practice; this knowledge is tested in the clinical examination and in the viva. In the examination, the initial response to a prime question invariably requires factual knowledge, while the supplementary questions require the application of clinical experience and deductive reasoning. For this reason the examiner may stray away from what is strictly within the required body of knowledge, as your patients do not always present according to the textbook, and that application of knowledge is frequently required in the clinical setting.

All those of you who have reached this stage in your medical career have sufficient mental ability to pass this examination but many of you fail to apply yourselves to the task of preparation appropriately. Too great an emphasis on facts learned slavishly and without understanding leads to disappointment. The knowledge you require is acquired in clinical practice by reading around the clinical situations you encounter, together with studious attention to the content (especially the breadth) of the syllabus. The examination is designed to test the whole syllabus; deliberate avoidance of part of that requirement will reap just rewards. Particular attention to clinical examination is essential for a good performance in the clinical part of the examination. It is not difficult to guess the type of case that will be encountered – time spent thinking how you will examine each of these clinical scenarios will ensure a confident performance. Similarly, practice at answering questions in a viva is essential preparation, and time spent thinking about approach is time well spent. The approach to this examination is that of developing a strategy of defining what you are going to learn, marshalling your knowledge, and then practising the presentation of that knowledge in a manner which will score the maximum points.

Passing the examination

- **Define your learning targets**
- **Marshall your knowledge**
- **Practice presentation**
- **Cover the whole syllabus**
- **Prepare your clinical examination**
- **Practice your viva technique**

THE FORMAT

The examination is held twice yearly, and is subdivided into three parts: the *MCQ examination* which takes place in April and October, the *clinical examination* which is held in three or four centres around the country during May and November, and the *viva voce examination* which takes place at the Royal College of Surgeons in June and December. The exact dates of the examinations are published in the examination calendar which can be obtained from the Examinations Department in the various Colleges. The first MCQ examination of the London College was held in April 1997 and the second in October 1997. The first clinical examination was held in May 1998 and the first viva in June 1998. It is no longer possible to take the old FRCS examination as the last examination in applied basic sciences was held in January 1998 and new candidates can no longer register for that examination. The second part of the CSIG examination will continue until the year 2000 to ensure that all those who are eligible will have the opportunity to complete the examination.

THE EXAMINATION (Table 48.1)

You may sit the MCQ examination of the MRCS during the first year of your senior house officer appointment, but the clinical examination cannot be sat until you have completed 20 months of clinical training in recognized appointments, and the viva examination after 22 months of training. Once you have sat the clinical examination you must complete the examination within 2 years – thus you may have up to four attempts. To take the examination without adequate preparation is therefore unwise. The exact details of eligibility will vary from time to time, hence *you are strongly advised to check these rules at an early stage* of your preparation for the examination.

THE MULTIPLE CHOICE PAPERS

Multiple choice questions are well known. What is not always appreciated is that there are variations in the format and marking system. The simplest form is a 'stem' or statement inviting you to select the most appropriate answer to a proposal or question from five possibilities. One or more of the proffered answers may be 'distracters' so that a decision has to be made whether each statement is right or wrong.

The marking system may vary from College to College. Marks are gained for correct answers. In the old Applied Basic Sciences MCQ, marks were deducted for the wrong answer, but in line with most modern examinations this process of so-called negative marking has been withdrawn so that now marks will not be deducted for an incorrect answer. *It behoves you to answer all questions as this will maximize the chance of scoring a pass mark.*

Multiple choice questions have the merit that knowledge over a wide area can be tested, and indeed each of the two papers has been designed to cover the whole field of their respective syllabus – the morning paper the 'core modules' of the curriculum and the afternoon paper the 'systems modules'. Many questions will be

Table 48.1	The examination		
Part	Sitting	Timing	Location
MCQ I and II	April, October	Any time	Multiple centres
Clinical	May, November	20 months	Multiple centres
Viva voce	June, December	22 months	Royal College, London

asked from each module according to a previously designed protocol. In order to avoid the MCQ containing rare or obscure parts to a question, each stem may have a variable number of parts; it is hoped that this will improve the quality of the question and should not confuse the candidate. A long question has no implication regarding importance or otherwise of the topic. In order that the meaning of certain words may not prove confusing, a glossary of terms is given to you when you apply to sit the examination, and is incorporated in the question sheet at the time of the examination. Thus, terms such as *common* have a specific meaning which should be adhered to when answering the question.

A new departure for this examination is the use of *extended matching questions*. Their objective is to test a degree of clinical judgement: a theme is stated, such as 'abdominal pain', followed by a list of options. Under the list of options there is a guiding statement such as, 'For each of the following vignettes select the most likely option. Each option may be used once, more than once, or not at all.' There follows several case descriptions – these descriptions require careful reading as the options are similar, and the immediate option that comes to mind may not fit all the facts. An example is given below.

Key points

- **Read the questions carefully**
- **Answer all the questions**
- **Leave adequate time to mark the answer card accurately**

THE CLINICAL EXAMINATION

As the examination is held in several centres simultaneously, it is necessary to have a more structured format than previously in order to ensure that the examination is not only similar between centres but is reproducible and of the same standard over a series of examinations. The examination consists of five separate bays or sections. Two examiners are associated with each bay; one asks the questions whilst the other observes your performance and makes notes about the conduct of the interview. You spend 10 minutes in each of the four bays dealing with clinical topics, and 15 minutes in the communications bay. You will be in a group of eight candidates and no one will leave until the whole group has completed the examination. Communication between groups of candidates is discouraged so that information cannot be passed between those taking the examination.

> **Box 48.1 Example of extended matching question**
>
> **Theme: postoperative complications**
> *Options:*
> a. Tension pneumothorax
> b. Unstable angina
> c. Septicaemia
> d. Acute massive pulmonary embolism
> e. Myocardial infarction
>
> *For each of the clinical vignettes described below, select the single most likely postoperative complication from the options listed above. Each option may be used once, more than once or not at all.*
>
> 1. A man of 75 had emergency surgery for a perforated diverticulum of the sigmoid colon. Twenty-four hours after operation he was peripherally warm, hypotensive (95/40 mmHg), and oliguric. The ECG was within normal limits.
> 2. A man of 75 had a hip fracture treated by hemiarthroplasty. In the history it was apparent that he had fallen a couple of days before he presented. He received subcutaneous heparin from the time of admission. Six days after operation he became hypotensive (95/75 mmHg) and was blue, cold and clammy, with a high central venous pressure. He had inverted T waves in lead III.
> 3. A man of 75 had a laparoscopic cholecystectomy. The following day he was noted to be peripherally cold with a tachycardia. He had crackles at the lung bases. The ECG showed Q waves and ST segment elevation in the chest leads.
>
> *Answers: 1 – c, 2 – d, 3 – e*

Bay 1 The aim of this bay is to determine the ability of the candidate to identify palpable or superficial lumps, including skin lesions. The candidate is expected to be able to describe the morphology and anatomy of the lesion with accuracy, and to describe its layer of origin when appropriate. For example, you will be asked to demonstrate why a lesion is arising from the skin or the subcutaneous tissues or an underlying structure such as the thyroid. The examiner explores the differential diagnosis as is done on a ward round or in outpatients. The use of simple investigations is considered as is the part played by such tests in clarification of the diagnosis. It is expected that you will see between three and five patients within the 10 minute period, thus the time you have to examine the patient is limited and direct answers to questions are required. The

> **Box 48.2   Format of the clinical examination**
>
> *Bay 1* Short cases
> *Bay 2* Orthopaedics
> *Bay 3* Vascular
> *Bay 4* Abdomen and chest
> *Bay 5* Communication

method of the examination is important, and an efficient and professional approach scores well. The observing examiner is able to quickly pick up the clinical competence of the candidate by their clinical behaviour. At the end of the 10 minutes the examiners have 2 minutes to agree a mark for the candidate.

Bay 2. This bay tests your ability to take a history in the musculoskeletal system and undertake an examination of any part of the musculoskeletal system. Your findings should be interpreted to reach a possible diagnosis. Investigation results and X-rays may be shown to corroborate the diagnosis. One examiner is an orthopaedic surgeon and the other a non-orthopaedic surgeon. Two or three patients will be seen in this bay in the 10 minute period.

Bay 3. This bay deals with the circulatory system. A detailed knowledge of the surgical treatment is not required but an indication that you understand the principles of the treatment of vascular disease will be assessed. One of the examiners is a vascular surgeon while the other is from another speciality. Again, two or three patients will be seen in this bay in the 10 minute period.

Bay 4. The aim of this bay is to determine your ability to examine the chest and abdomen, describe the physical findings, and demonstrate a sound knowledge of the process of investigation which is likely to produce a differential diagnosis. Results of relevant investigations are shown and discussed. One examiner will be a general surgeon and the other may be from any speciality. The examiners will aim to show the candidate three or four conditions during this 10 minute period.

Bay 5. This part of the examination is an entirely new part of the clinical assessment, the aim of which is to assess communications skills. A vignette or clinical scenario will be given to you. You will then approach the relative or patient (played by an actor trained in this type of role-play) who will either ask questions about a relative, or enquire about their own disease ('Have I got cancer?'), or you may be required to gain consent from the 'patient' for a particular procedure to be done. The two examiners observe and determine according to

predetermined guidelines (which will vary according to the scenario) how you perform. Not only will your approach to the patient be marked but also the level of knowledge required of the vignette will be assessed; thus, incorrect information given to the patient will be scored adversely. The scenario is designed to mimic the real clinical situation.

 Key point

> **A professional and competent approach to the patient with clear specific answers scores.** *Practice is required.*

Marking

Each examiner awards marks on a 0–5 points basis with the pair of examiners agreeing on the final mark for each bay. The communication bay is given equal weighting to the clinical examination bays. Three is the pass mark for each bay and therefore 15 is the pass mark for the whole examination. Candidates with a marginal fail may be discussed by the examiners when they meet at the end of the day to collate the marks. You are marked and assessed individually by the five pairs of examiners without reference to other candidates. No account is taken of performance in the MCQ examination so that there is no compensation between parts of the examination; indeed, the examiners have no knowledge of these results.

 Key points

* **Be polite to the patient**
* **Examine professionally**
* **Present with thoughtfulness**

THE VIVA VOCE EXAMINATION

> The viva covers the whole syllabus and it covers the basic sciences.

The examination consists of three separate viva examinations each of which has two parts. The first part of the viva commences with a basic scientist whose questioning begins with a basic science topic and moves towards a clinical subject, while the second part is conducted by a clinician who emphasizes clinical topics but may well extend his question towards the underlying principles. Just as the clinical examination is structured, so also is the viva examination, with set questions and approved answers. The questions have largely been preset with suggestions for supplementary topics to delve more deeply into a particular subject. The emphasis is to cover as much as possible of the syllabus during the course of the examination. To achieve this you are given a subject sheet on which are marked the areas covered in each viva so that the topics discussed in the three vivas do not overlap. In turn, the examiners are given sufficient questions to ensure that there are a wide selection of topics available for consideration.

(a) Applied surgical anatomy and operative surgery viva

You will face three examiners. One is the anatomist who starts the questions, and two are surgeons – one will be chairman and observer, and the other will scrutinize the logbook, taking the second part of the viva on topics drawn from your personal experience recorded in the logbook. It is a prerequisite for entry into the examination that you maintain a record of the procedures which you have assisted or have been helped to do. Any procedure recorded in the book can be the basis for questions along the lines of principles rather than precise operative technique. The viva will last 20 minutes; 10 minutes on anatomy and 10 minutes on operative surgery.

Key point

Logbooks must be contemporary records; their importance will increase as part of continuous assessment.

As prompts, the examiners will have bones, live models, prosections, instruments, and pictures depicting X-rays, MRI scans, CT scans, and operating theatre environments and equipment. There are no histology slides, but pictures of histology slides are available.

A mark is given for each part of the viva; the chairman and individual examiners of parts one and two agree the final mark.

(b) Applied physiology and critical care viva

The candidate faces two pairs of examiners – one a physiologist, the other a surgeon. The viva consists of two 10-minute parts; the first part starts with the physiologist who will cover three core subjects, often aided by the use of simple charts or diagrams based on clinical conditions. The candidate then changes tables for

the second part and faces a new pair of examiners who are unaware of their performance in the first part of this viva. The surgeon examiner covers questions based on critical care and applied physiology. Prompts for these examiners include charts (vital signs, fluid balance, etc.), laboratory results, ECG traces and radiographs.

Each part of this viva is given a separate mark which is agreed between the acting and observing examiners at each table.

(c) Clinical pathology and principles of surgery viva

This viva relates to the pathology and principles of surgery; it should be noted that the order of the vivas is variable due to the logistics of the examination. You will be asked to take a topic sheet from table to table to ensure coverage of the whole syllabus. As for the applied physiology and critical care viva you are examined by two pairs of examiners, one of each being a pathologist and the other a surgeon. The first part is started by the pathologist who will cover at least three subjects within the fields of histology, haematology, microbiology and biochemistry, with questions migrating from basic to clinical pathology. After 10 minutes you move to a second table for examination on the principles of surgery. There is a strong basic science input into this viva, with emphasis on principles.

Again, each part of the viva is given a separate mark agreed by each pair, with the second pair of examiners being unaware of the mark awarded by the first.

Marking

At the end of each session the marks will be collated – six separate marks each in the range of 1–5, from the 11 examiners. A pass mark of 18 is required for the successful completion of the examination, although a candidate with 17 marks who has failed only one part may be raised to a pass mark at the discretion of the examiners. Performance in other parts of the examination will not be taken into account; emphasis is laid on the large number of examiners who are in contact with you during the course of the day as a counterbalance to individual bias. A review group of examiners with the examinations secretariat carefully monitors the examination and the examiners to ensure that the quality of the examination is such that it is a fair test of the candidates' performance.

Examiners' performance is monitored by a review group.

Key points

- **Learn the whole syllabus**
- **Learn basic sciences**
- **Think before speaking**

YOU – THE CANDIDATE

It is a truism that the outcome of an examination depends on you and your knowledge. Alas, many candidates do not do their knowledge or themselves justice because their behaviour on the day portrays either an uncertainty or a brash overconfidence which worry the examiner. After all, the examiner is responsible for ensuring that only those of professional competence are passed and therefore able to practice at an increasingly independent level. The public demand is for higher rather than lower standards and this will inevitably be reflected in the standards demanded of the candidate. The excuse that the candidate is nervous is no longer an acceptable plea and allowance cannot be made for such by the examiners, for stress of the emergency in theatre or in the accident room may be every bit as great. Preparation is the key to overcome this problem and a disciplined approach to the clinical examination and questioning in the viva pays great dividends.

> The public demands on professional competence are ever greater and this must be reflected in examination standards.

HOW TO PASS

The clinical examination

The first principle in the clinical and viva examinations is to conduct yourself as a professional, and to treat the examiner with respect but as an equal. If you do not understand what is required of you in the clinical examination, or if the question in the viva is imprecise, ask for clarification.

In the clinical examination, start by introducing yourself to the patient and ask their permission to examine the part of the patient requested by the examiner. Unless you are forbidden to do so, ask about the history of any lesion and any other relevant history.

Next, carry out a systematic examination of the part which you have been asked to examine. This examination should be carried out according to the protocol that you have worked out – during your preparation for

the clinical examination you should have worked out how you will examine each part of the body for the common conditions and indeed practised this on numerous occasions during the performance of your routine ward work. Ensure that you did not cause pain during the examination and watch the patient's face for any grimace. If you do accidentally cause pain, apologies to the patient and gain their confidence. Beware of 'spot diagnoses', and even if you are confident that you have made an accurate immediate diagnosis, examine the lesion carefully so that you can justify your confidence. When you have finished your examination, think … marshall your findings and give a clear account of them. Unless asked, do not blurt out the 'spot diagnosis' as you just might be wrong! Even though you may be asked to concentrate on a single area do not fail to take in the general appearance of the patient. Their age, gender and general condition will influence treatment decisions. Consider whether a more extended examination is requisite; for example, if you find an enlarged lymph node you should examine the whole reticulo-endothelial system, or, if you find vascular disease you should examine the whole cardiovascular system, but before doing so explain to the examiner what you are about to do and why, as time may not allow such a complete approach.

Before speaking to the examiner ... think

- **Completeness of the examination**
- **Adequacy of history**
- **Diagnosis – differential**
  – verification
- **Treatment strategy**
- **What to say – to patient**
  – to examiner

When you are sure that you have answers to the questions, *thank the patient* and turn to the examiner indicating that you are ready. The above process may sound detailed, but it should be performed simultaneously with your examination. You are then able to tell the examiner your findings and the diagnosis with the evidence for your conclusion. This process cannot be learnt without practice – *the amount of practice you have undertaken is obvious to the examiner.*

If you are unsure of the diagnosis state in order the relevant findings. For example, state both in area and in depth where a lump is, its attachments, size, shape, surface consistency, fluctuations, tenderness, and any other features. Never try to re-examine the patient unless asked to do so by the examiner. If there is anything you have omitted, state this and admit the error.

It is essential to practice for the communication bay. The bay tries to imitate typical clinical situations: it is not intended to be a harrowing emotional experience unless you turn it into such. So much about examinations concerns thinking under pressure, a feature which is easier if there is a good basis of knowledge and practice. The vignettes will outline common clinical situations such as breaking bad news, informing patients of their situation, getting consent for procedures, and speaking with relatives. A structured approach conveying fact with empathy is required; this bay is about clinical knowledge.

The viva examination

You will meet no less than seven examiners during the course of the day, with a further five who will assess your progress; it is unlikely you will be able to fool all these examiners with superficial or inadequate knowledge, and it is equally unlikely that you will be able to charm them all by your personality, however effervescent! Thus you are back to a strict professional format based on a sound knowledge of your subject. The examiner starts with a straightforward question. Your response to that question sets the tone of the viva so a careful measured reply is required. The examiner does not know you so that each interview starts from the baseline; the variable will be you and it is your performance that determines the mark. Some candidates consider that minimal knowledge will suffice; this is a dangerous strategy as it behoves you to gain points so that if there is a genuine gap in knowledge in one area, good marks elsewhere compensate. The examiners are trained to use the whole range of the marking system to genuinely reflect the candidates' performance, so that deficiency in the answers to basic questions will be marked down while good answers will be marked up – examiners will tend to give a mark for each question, and hence the final mark will reflect the sum of those marks; it is hoped that this will make the examination more reproducible and encourage you to concentrate on answering concisely and accurately. A very slow response in which little ground is covered will inevitably mean you fail to score. The examiner is encouraged to cover three topics as a minimum during the 10 minutes and hence sudden changes in a subject which is going well or badly have no meaning except that the examiner is doing his job and covering as much of the subject as possible to give you a fair test of your knowledge of the subject as a whole.

If you do not know the answer to an important question do not bluff as you can waste important time. It is better to admit you do not know but, if pressed, try to work out an answer on a logical basis. An examiner will not expect you to know everything but occasionally high marks can be scored for logical thought in the elucidation of a problem – this is particularly true in physiology and critical care. If you make a mistake, admit it and start again. Do not let your confidence be shaken as you can always make up on another viva.

The logbook is required for the operative surgery viva. To come to the examination with an untidy book and incomplete summary sheets tempts the examiner's patience. It is a simple part of preparation and portrays clearly your attitude as a professional person. Your logbook repays study. It will be the basis of your operative surgery viva so familiarity with the procedures that you have described is important, especially understanding the principles of any operation with which you have been involved. There are certain important surgical procedures which you are expected to know; for instance, life saving operations such as the management of traumatically sustained wounds or the competent accomplishment of small intestinal anastomoses. An important part of your preparation is to see for yourself these procedures in your hospital. If there are difficulties in arranging this confer with your surgical tutor.

Summary

Multiple choice questions test only your cognitive (factual) capabilities. Clinical examinations test your psychomotor and interpersonal skills. Viva voce examinations display your affective skills to the examiners as well as your cognitive skills. In the clinical and viva voce examinations the good examiner will test your decision-making skills. The only objective test is that of your factual knowledge. Most of the qualities that are amenable to objective testing are but a part of the professional surgeon's duties, yet without that factual knowledge a professional is but a charlatan; it is this knowledge which will guide the surgeon to make the right decisions to treat the patient appropriately. It is fashionable to decry examinations and emphasize continuous assessment. Alas, the ability of surgeons continuously to assess their trainees has been poor and not reproducible – often to the detriment of the trainee. The MRCS examination has been designed to test the knowledge that is required, or thought to be required, of the basic surgical trainee. To be effective it

Summary (contd.)

must change with the requirements of the trainee, and indeed, the examination has a review group to monitor the examination and its content. The examination candidate is a vital part of this review, and any candidate with concerns about the examination should discuss these with the Examination Department with a view to improving the procedure. After all, when you have passed the examination, you are a member of the Royal College of Surgeons and concerned that the standards of surgery are maintained as a protection for the patient and the reputation of your College.

To pass the examination
- Assess what you have to learn
- Gain that knowledge with understanding
- Practice again and again
- Present yourself professionally
- Propound your knowledge

Intercollegiate speciality examinations

A. O. Mansfield

INTRODUCTION

The Senate of Surgery is composed of four surgical Royal Colleges of the British Isles and representatives of all the SAC speciality associations, of which there are ten (including accident and emergency).

One intercollegiate activity which stems from senate is the Joint Committee for Intercollegiate Examinations (JCIE) and there is an examination in each of the ten specialities.

These examinations are taken after completion of at least 4 years of higher surgical training in that speciality with the exception of urology which is 3 years, and there must be documented evidence of a satisfactory 4 year assessment (3rd year in urology).

Candidates must all have completed basic surgical training and acquired the associated diploma, e.g. MRCS/AFRCS, and so this examination concentrates on the speciality. It is designed to test theoretical knowledge in that speciality and clinical experience and understanding. Operative skills are assessed by the trainer and knowledge of the operations in that speciality will be tested in the examination.

Success in the examination is signalled by a suffix to the FRCS in that speciality and is an essential prerequisite for the acquisition of the certificate of completion of specialist training and for entry onto the specialist register.

Details of requirements and the examination vary between specialities and the regulations can be obtained from Intercollegiate Speciality Boards, Central Administration Office, 3 Hill Square, Edinburgh, EH8 9DR, Tel: 0131-662 9333, Fax: 0131-662 9444. As regulations may change, it is wise to ensure that you consult the up-to-date documents. This chapter is a broad guide and not a substitute for the regulations. At present the examinations are conducted two or three times a year and the location will vary.

THE COMPONENTS OF THE EXAMINATION

Clinical

Most of the examinations include a clinical examination. This can include both the long case and short case type of clinical test.

MCQ

Three speciality examinations currently have an MCQ section and other specialities are considering the addition of this type of examination.

Spot test

An objective spot test is part of some of the examinations. This type of test may consist of clinical slides, X-rays, other test results, charts, etc. and the candidate may be asked about the diagnosis, investigations, management, treatment options, prognosis, etc.

Vivas (orals)

The area likely to be included in each viva is laid down in the regulations for that speciality and may include:

- Subspeciality interests
- Basic science
- Operative surgery

- Academic vivas
  (These four areas are an opportunity to assess your critical appraisal of published papers and in some to give the opportunity to present your own contribution)
- Practical test (at present only one board provides this).

PREPARATION

Basic science

All the examinations will expect a high level of knowledge of the basic sciences, anatomy, physiology, pathology etc, which are relevant to practice in that speciality.

Anatomy

Anatomical knowledge is a prerequisite for every surgical procedure and should be refreshed at every opportunity from anatomical texts, computer programmes, cadaver dissections and operative textbooks. Operative experience will be sought at every opportunity.

Physiology

Physiology relevant to pre- and postoperative care essentially means a broad understanding with supplementary in-depth knowledge of that which is specially applicable to your speciality. Those with whom you come in to day-to-day contact (e.g., anaesthetists, diabetic specialists, radiologists, etc.) will have specialist physiological knowledge and the physiological basis on which investigations and managements are based is important in selecting appropriate tests, e.g. the physiological changes in the kidney brought about by intravenous contrast agents.

Pathology

Similarly, all aspects of pathology need to be pursued and this extends well beyond histopathology to include cell biology, haematology, biochemistry and so on. Genetics, embryology, metabolism are specifically mentioned in some of the regulations.

Clinical preparation

Your patients

They are and will continue to be the source of your continuing and life-long learning.

Miss no opportunity to see, talk to and examine patients. There is no substitute.

Persuade senior colleagues to discuss, demonstrate and explain aspects of signs, symptoms, pathology, investigations and management. These contacts will stimulate the pursuit of such problems in the medical literature.

 Key points

Practise, practise, practise examining patients, presenting and interpreting your findings, and justifying your intended management to senior colleagues, for assessment.

Textbooks on your specialty
Surgical literature

Knowledge of the recent surgical literature in closely related aspects of care and in associated concerns such as the results of trials, the effectiveness of treatments, and the appropriateness of investigations.

Evidence has always been the basis on which we practise and there is now increased pressure to ensure that our practice is evidence-based and there is an unprecedented opportunity to access that information.

Your own records

Keeping and reviewing records: logbooks are required for all the examinations but should be seen as a valuable learning opportunity. They should allow critical appraisal of your practice and may identify areas of need both in your training and in your studying. Where gaps are evident or deficiencies noted these can often be addressed. Get a colleague to look at and criticize your logbook and to identify the gaps which you need to fill. A candidate with a subspeciality interest in coloproctology had never done a colonoscopy. Although such an omission may be a criticism of the training programme it was an easily identifiable defect that might well have been overcome by arranging to spend a week or two with an expert. It is your career and this shortened training period is the basis on which your future depends.

Meetings

Presenting cases and literature reviews and critically analysing management.

Operative experience

Take every opportunity to assist the good operative surgical teachers. The grapevine will tell you who they are and they may well be glad of an extra assistant and perhaps flattered to have been sought out.

Feedback

Look for feedback at every opportunity.

THE EXAMINATION

If you have been in a recognized training programme and have taken every opportunity to obtain extra experience and knowledge then the examination will not be a major hurdle.

The clinical cases will usually be problems with which you are familiar or which will provide a stimulating discussion. If you approach them in the way you would if asked to give an opinion about a patient under another team in your own hospital you will strike the right level.

Concentrate the opinion, advice, management which you advocate on that particular patient so that the examiner can assess your ability to select what is appropriate in a particular set of circumstances rather than the textbook answer.

In everyday clinical practice co-morbidity is the deciding factor in many cases – so too in examinations.

Be prepared to demonstrate your communication skills if asked to explain an investigation or operation to a patient.

Informed consent is such a crucial factor of surgical practice that you may reasonably be asked to discuss the topics you would need to explain to a patient.

Postoperative problems or complications may well form part of the clinical as well as the oral examination as current patients with on-going problems will usually feature in the examination.

Summary

1. Obtain the up-to-date regulations.
2. Ensure you have a good foundation of basic sciences.
3. Prepare and practise the skills required for each section of the examination.
4. Read widely around the subject and know the evidence.
5. Critically assess your experience.
6. Obtain feedback on your performance from colleagues.
7. Remember that this is a speciality and not a subspeciality examination.

Index